PRETERM BIRTH - MOTHER AND CHILD

Edited by **John C. Morrison**

Preterm Birth - Mother and Child
Edited by John C. Morrison

Published by InTech
Janeza Trdine 9, 51000 Rijeka, Croatia

Publishing Process Manager Anja Filipovic

Technical Editor Teodora Smiljanic

Cover Designer InTech Design Team

Additional hard copies can be obtained from orders@intechopen.com

Preterm Birth - Mother and Child, Edited by John C. Morrison
p. cm.
ISBN 978-953-307-828-1

For EU product safety concerns:
IN TECH d.o.o., Prolaz Marije Krucifikse Kozulić 3, 51000 Rijeka, Croatia,
info@intechopen.com or visit our website at intechopen.com.

Meet the editor

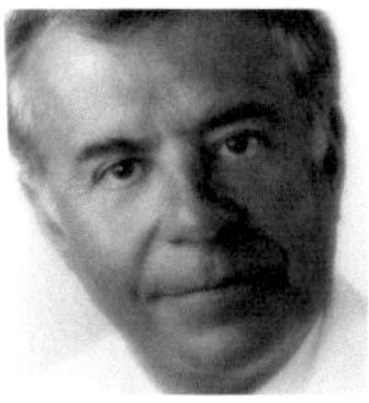

Dr Morrison is Professor Emeritus of Obstetrics, Gynecology and Pediatrics at the University of Mississippi Medical Center in Jackson, Mississippi. Over the past 30 years, he has served as Chairman of Obstetrics and Gynecology and Chief of Maternal-Fetal Medicine. He specializes in Obstetrics and Gynecology, Maternal-Fetal Medicine and is the former president of the Society of Maternal-Fetal Medicine, The Central Association of Obstetrics and Gynecology, The Southern Perinatal Association, and the South Central Obstetrics/Gynecology Society. He has published over 500 peer-reviewed journal articles, 100 book chapters, and 3 textbooks concerning Obstetrics and Gynecology and Maternal-Fetal Medicine. He has received over sixty research grants as principal investigator or co-investigator, and holds six patents in these areas. He has also served on the editorial board of the Journal of Perinatology, the Journal of Maternal-Fetal Investigation, Southern Medical Journal, American Journal of Obstetrics and Gynecology, Obstetrics and Gynecology International.

Contents

Preface

"...the black of the zebra fish, my past struggles
the white, my strengths
the blue of my zebra fish, my hope."

Hollidae Robinson, 2011

Clinicians have struggled with the ravages of preterm birth for decades, even centuries, but we have solved many issues through our scientific strengths and there remains considerable hope of reducing the number of preterm births in the future. While there are a multitude studies and books regarding preterm birth, both in the obstetric and the neonatal/pediatric literature, what is missing is the integration of data, from obstetrics through neonatal course, into pediatrics as the neonate transverses childhood. Certainly, pediatricians might wonder why obstetricians cannot keep the baby in utero longer, while obstetricians are rarely apprised of the continued progress of the baby once it is delivered.

Obstetricians do not actually know what goes on after the delivery any more than many pediatricians know about what happened during pregnancy, as well as labor, and delivery. This dialogue between specialties is crucial in the battle against preterm birth. While obstetrician looks for causes of preterm birth and strategies for preventing it, the neonatologist searches for treatments for the complications of preterm birth while the pediatrician seeks therapy for long-term morbidity of preterm birth on each organ system of the child. Clearly there needs to be more linkages between the specialties that are divided by birth.

This is especially true when confronted with preterm birth because it is certainly problematic for the obstetrician, the neonatologist, and the pediatrician in addition to the hospital, family and society in general.

The ultimate goal of this needed dialogue between specialties is to offset the effects or after-effects of preterm birth. In spite of medical advances, preterm birth is still all too common, and it's ramifications are staggering. Babies that are born preterm, especially before 32 weeks gestation, are associated with the majority of neonatal morbidity and mortality. Preterm delivery before 37 weeks is all too common (i.e., 8-10% of births in the United States). The reasons for early delivery are varied. For example, fetal disease, such as severe growth restriction, oligohydramnios, or abnormal fetal health assessment tests, may dictate that the infant should be delivered even when it is extremely preterm. Also, maternal factors such as diabetes, preeclampsia, cardiopulmonary disorders, trauma and others may also require early delivery. Similarly, obstetric complications such as preterm labor, preterm premature rupture of the membranes (usually with preterm labor), as well as cervical insufficiency among others, all may lead to birth before 37 weeks. Finally, preterm births may result from iatrogenic causes. Many times, late preterm births (34-37 weeks), occur when the physician deems the baby is near enough to term that attempting preventive treatment should not be undertaken or when the patient refuses treatment (i.e., tocolytics).

If the linkages of all these causes of preterm birth are heterogeneous, certainly the etiology of preterm labor also comes in many forms. Preterm labor may occur because of the inflammation, infection, uterine overdistention, cervical insufficiency, illicit drug use, uterine malformations, etc. Complicating matters further; treatment of many causes is usually empiric; since no common etiologic thread is known. Therefore, in women contracting with idiopathic preterm labor, tocolytics are used to stop the contractions rather than using idiologic medications (although none are available) to directly treat the disorder itself, instead of merely treating uterine activity. Lastly, it is difficult to study the treatment modalities, as they last for months. For example, if a patient is treated for acute preterm labor at 26 weeks with intravenous tocolytics, and the contractions are successfully stopped, the effect of that treatment is over within a few hours as the medicine exits the maternal circulation quickly. Continuous tocolytic medications given orally have the problems of patient compliance, and if no treatment is given the risk of recurrent preterm labor and early delivery is high. Unfortunately, the highly successful treatment for prolonging pregnancy with low dose terbutaline administered by continuous infusion pump is no longer available in the U.S.

Another problem with preterm birth is the data itself. Some material in articles and practically all the data in books offer information that, while new when written, becomes old in the 1-2 years it takes to publish the results of the latest findings and getting it in the hands of the reader. This is where electronic publishing can be so helpful, as a bridge between researchers and practitioners. The goals for this book on preterm birth are several. First, the subject of preterm birth should be covered from the obstetric, neonatal, and pediatric perspective. Second, the data should be cutting edge, well referenced, and always related to clinical circumstances for the practitioner. Thirdly, via electronic publishing, the data on this subject should be online within a few months of acceptance of each chapter rather than a year or more it takes with traditional publishing. Fourthly, this methodology also should enable the authors to continually update the chapters electronically as new findings become available. Instead of sending off for reprints, obtaining interlibrary loans for references, buying a new textbook, or subscribing to new journals, the data on preterm birth is here reading all at the right price – and it is free.

I wish to thank Ms. Rosemarie McMillon for her tireless work in compiling and assisting in editing each and every chapter. Without her contribution, this book could not have become a reality.

Finally, I dedicate this book to Rita D. Morrison. What I am and have accomplished, what our children and grandchildren are and will become, what our life is and will be, is because of you; the strongest of the steel magnolias: my wife.

John C. Morrison
University of Mississippi Medical Center,
Jackson, MS,
USA

1

Assisted Reproduction and Preterm Birth

Offer Erez[1], Ruth Beer-Weisel[1], Tal Rafaeli-Yehudai[1],
Idit Erez-Weiss[2] and Moshe Mazor[1]
[1]*Department of Obstetrics and Gynecology "B" Soroka University Medical Center, School of Medicine, Faculty of Health Sciences, Ben Gurion University of the Negev, Beer Sheva,*
[2]*Department of Family Medicine, School of Medicine, Faculty of Health Sciences, Ben Gurion University of the Negev, Beer Sheva, Israel*

1. Introduction

Preterm parturition is a syndrome (Romero, Gomez *et al.*, 1997; Romero R, Espinoza J *et al.*, 2004) that is one of the leading causes for perinatal morbidity and mortality. Moreover, prematurity is a leading cause for neonatal mortality, as well as short and long term morbidity. The incidence of preterm delivery is constantly increasing, crossing the 12% in the USA, and it's annual cost reached 26.2 billion US dollars in 2005, posing a huge burden on public health (Institute of Medicine (US) Committee on Understanding Premature Birth and Assuring Healthy Outcomes, 2007).

Prematurity can be either spontaneous due to preterm labor with intact membranes (PTL) or preterm prelabor rupture of the chorioamniotic membranes (preterm PROM); or indicated, meaning induced preterm delivery by the medical team due to maternal (i.e. preeclampsia) or fetal (growth restriction, non-reassuring fetal heart rate tracing) indication (Goldenberg, Culhane *et al.*, 2008). The incidence of the latter group, especially after 34 weeks of gestation, is constantly rising (Ananth, Joseph *et al.*, 2005; Ananth and Vintzileos, 2006a; Ananth, Getahun *et al.*, 2006).

Emerging contributors for the increasing rate of preterm birth are assisted reproduction technologies (Institute of Medicine (US) Committee on Understanding Premature Birth and Assuring Healthy Outcomes, 2007). The use of infertility treatments has risen dramatically in the past 20 years; between 1996 and 2003, the number of cycles of Assisted reproductive technologies (ART) nearly doubled from 64,681 to 122,872. The number of live births resulting from conceptions achieved by the use of ARTs more than doubled from 14,507 to 35,785 (Institute of Medicine (US) Committee on Understanding Premature Birth and Assuring Healthy Outcomes, 1980). This has been associated with the trend to delay childbearing, indeed, more than 50 percent of these women were 35 years of age or older. In recent years, an unintended consequence of the use of these technologies, multiple gestations and the increased risk for preterm delivery, has become a focus of attention, and the institute of Medicine in the USA has concluded that "Fertility treatments are a significant contributor to preterm birth among both multiple and singleton pregnancies." (Institute of

Medicine (US) Committee on Understanding Premature Birth and Assuring Healthy Outcomes, 2007).

The mechanisms in which assisted reproduction technologies increases the risk for preterm birth are still under investigation. Aside the contribution of ART to the increase number of multiple gestations (especially twins) that increases the risk for preterm delivery; The mechanisms leading to preterm delivery in singleton gestations conceived through ART have not been thoroughly investigated. Preliminary evidence suggests that some of the underlying maternal conditions that lead to infertility (i.e. inflammation and insulin resistance) may contribute to this observation.

The current chapter will explore the epidemiology, underlying mechanisms, and possible tools for the prevention of preterm delivery in pregnancies conceived by assisted reproduction.

2. Infertility: Treatments, epidemiology and trends

2.1 Definitions

The most commonly used definition of infertility is a failure to conceive after 12 months of regular, unprotected intercourse. However, existing definitions of infertility lack uniformity, rendering comparisons of prevalence between countries or over time problematic. The absence of an agreed definition also compromises clinical management and undermines the impact of research findings. Gurunath at al suggested that the definition will be based on the duration of trying for pregnancy coupled with female age. (Gurunath, Pandian *et al.*, 2011) According to the report of The Centers for Disease Control and Prevention (CDC), in 2002, 7% of married couples in which the woman was of reproductive age (2.1 million couples) reported that they had not used contraception for 12 months and the woman had not become pregnant. Many of these patients are treated by ARTs. These technologies are defined by the CDC as procedures in which the ovum and the sperm are handled in the laboratory. During the past few decades several options of ART have developed including: 1) in vitro fertilization (IVF); 2) intra-cytoplasmic sperm injection (ICSI); 3) gamete intra-fallopian transfer (GIFT) and 4) zygote intra-fallopian transfer (ZIFT) (Centers for Disease Control and Prevention 2008).

2.2 What is the magnitude of ART utilization in developed countries?

The use of infertility treatments has risen dramatically in the past 10 years and has been associated with the trend to delay childbearing. Today, over 1% of all infants born in the United States every year are conceived using ART; and the number of ART cycles performed has nearly doubled, from 87,636 cycles in 1999 to 148,055 in 2008. Similarly, the number of live-birth in 2008 (46,326) was more than twice the number recorded 1999 (21,746). Because in many of the ART pregnancies more than one infant is born alive (e.g., twins, triplets), the total number of infants born is greater than the number of live-birth. The trend in the number of infants delivered after ART cycles was in accord to the trends observed in the number of pregnancies and live-births. Thus, the number of infants born in 2008, (61,426) was more than twice than the 30,629 that were delivered in 1999 (Figure 1).

Outside the USA, The Canadian Assisted Reproductive Technologies Register (CARTR), in its 2007 annual publication, reported a 12% increase in the total number of ART cycles, and an increase in the rate of clinical pregnancies and live-birth, along with a decrease in high-order multiple births in comparison to these parameters in 2006 (Gunby, Bissonnette *et al.*,

2011). While in Europe, according to the 10th annual European Society of Human Reproduction and Embryology (ESHRE) publication the reported number of ART cycles has increased, with a marginal increase in pregnancy rates, even though fewer embryos were transferred and the multiple delivery rates have declined (1994). This report includes 20 countries, where all clinics report their activity to the IVF register. Altogether, a total of 359,110 cycles were performed in a population of 422.5 million, corresponding to 850 cycles per million inhabitants. The IVF cycles rates of clinical pregnancy per ovum aspiration and per embryo transfer were 29.0 and 32.4%, respectively; while the corresponding ICSI cycles rates were 29.9 and 33.0%, respectively (1994). In spite of the new guidelines, transferring of 2 embryos is still the most prevalent choice in the European Union.

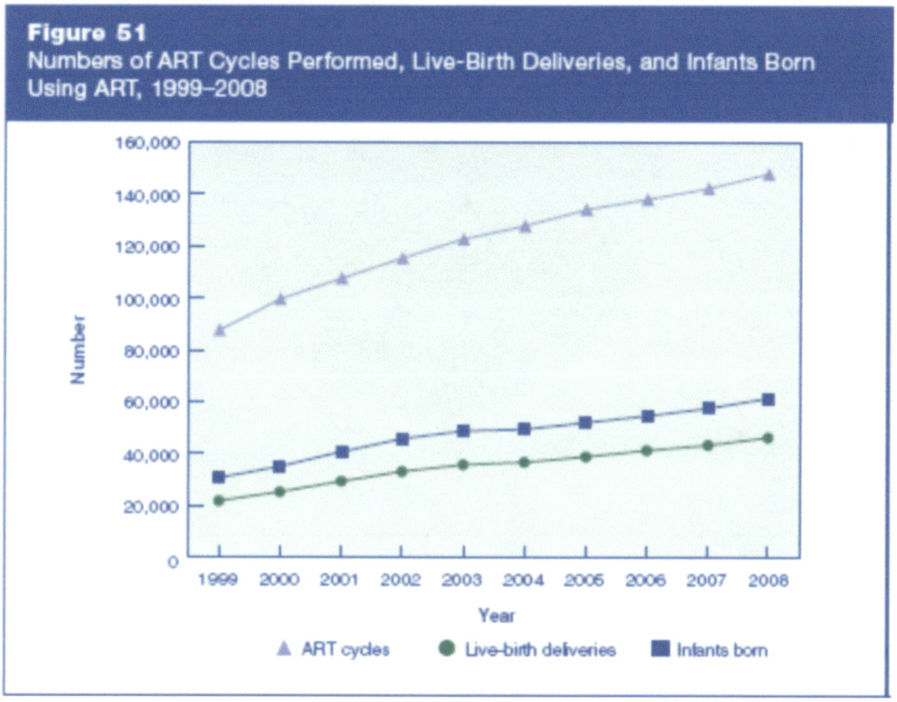

Fig. 1. Number of ART cycles performed, live-birth delivery, and infants born used ART, 1999-2008 From Centers for Disease Control and Prevention, American Society for Reproductive Medicine, Society for Assisted Reproductive Technology. 2006 Assisted Reproductive Technology Success Rates: National summary and fertilityNclinic reports. Atlanta: Centers for Disease Control and Prevention,2008.

ART often is categorized according to whether the procedure used a woman's own eggs (self) or eggs from another woman (donor) and according to whether the embryos used were newly fertilized (fresh) or previously fertilized, frozen, and then thawed (frozen). For approximately 71% of ART cycles performed in USA in 2008, self-fresh eggs or embryos were used. ART cycles that used self-frozen embryos were the next most common type, accounting for approximately 17% of the total. In about 12% of cycles, eggs or embryos were donated by another woman (Figure 2).

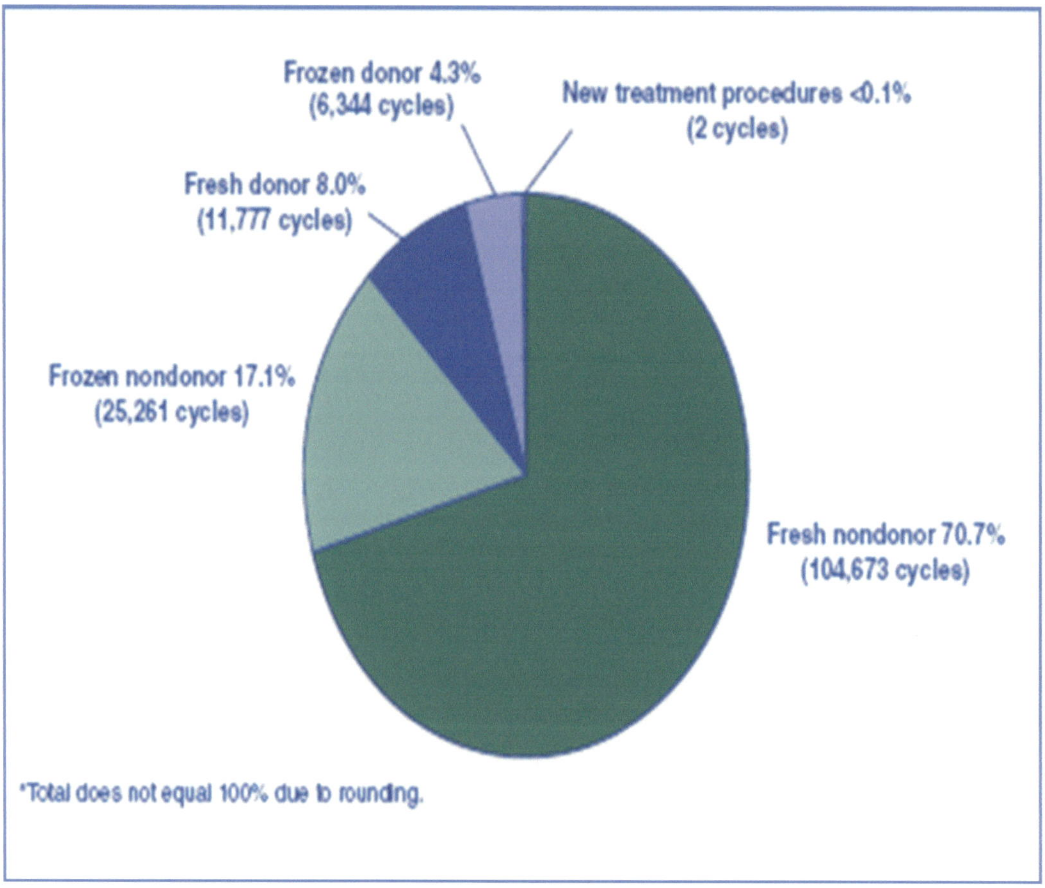

Fig. 2. Distribution of ART cycles according to the source of the ovum and whether the cycle was fresh or frozen. (CDC 2008, USA).

The average age of women using ART services in the USA in 2008 was 36. However, the largest group of women using ART services were women younger than 35, representing approximately 39% of all ART cycles performed in 2008. Approximately 21% of ART cycles were performed in women aged 35–37, 20% in women aged 38–40, 10% in women aged 41–42, 6% in women aged 43–44, and 5% among women older than 44 (Figure 4). In Europe, the age distribution of women treated with IVF varied across the continent. In some countries, more than 20% of women were aged 40 years or older (Greece, Ireland, Italy, Macedonia, Montenegro, Serbia and Switzerland), whereas in Bulgaria, Czech Republic, Lithuania, Norway, Poland, Portugal, and Ukraine <10% were 40 years or older. (ESHRE,2006)

The success rate of ART decreases with age, indeed, pregnancy rates decreased from 28.2% in women aged ≤34, to 9.6% at the age ≥40 years. A similar trend was seen for the delivery rates (26.6%, and 8.6%). In egg donation cycles, the recipients were aged 40 years or more in 50.0% of cases, in almost all countries. Pregnancy and delivery rates in oocyte recipients were comparable across different age groups. (ESHRE,2006)

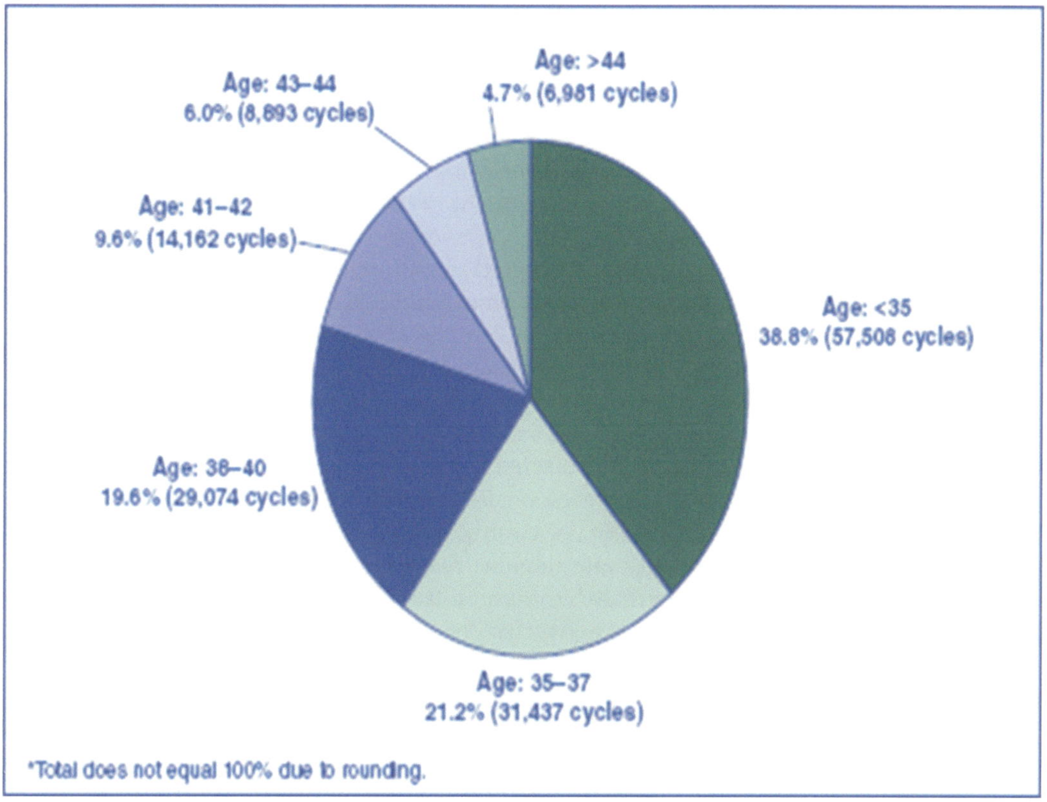

Fig. 3. Maternal age distribution among patients undergoing ART cycles. CDC 2008 USA.

3. The effect of maternal age on reproduction and pregnancy outcome

The average fertility rate (live births per 1,000 women of childbearing age 15-44 years) in USA from 1991-2008 is about 66.5, with mild fluctuations over the years. When it is divided in subgroups by maternal age, the birth rate has declined for women under 30-s on the other hand among women in their 30's- 40's the fertility rate had steadily increased from 1978 onward. In the last three decades a new group of women aged 50 and over has increased more than 10 percent annually since 1997 (Martin, Hamilton *et al.*, 2010). The trend in the fertility rate among European women is somewhat different. From the 1960s up to the beginning of the 21st century, the number of live births in the Europe declined sharply. However, from 2002 onward there has been a modest rebound in the number of live births born in this continent. As with the American women, the late increase during the last years may be, in part, attributed to a catching-up process following a general pattern of postponing the child bearing age. When women give birth later in life, the total fertility rate first indicates a decrease in fertility, followed later by a recovery (Atkinson and Marlier, 2010). For example, in Finland the rate of women giving birth after the age of 35 increased from 16.7%in 1997 to 19.2% in 2007 (Lampinen, Vehvilainen-Julkunen *et al.*, 2009). The corresponding mean maternal age in Japan between 1970 and 2000 increased from 25.6 to 28.0 years (Mathews and Hamilton, 2002).

Delaying childbearing may be attributed to several reasons, beginning with the longer life span, greater accessibility to education and career opportunities for women, and the existence of effective means of birth control (Stein, 1985; Berkowitz, Skovron *et al.*, 1990). Men and women recognized the direct relationship between older maternal age and the declined in fertility (Tough, Benzies *et al.*, 2006; Tough, Benzies *et al.*, 2007), however, there is a popular concept that IVF treatment can reverse the effects of age (Maheshwari, Porter *et al.*, 2008). Interestingly, along with acknowledgment in the success of ART there is a lack of awareness regarding the effect of maternal age over perinatal complications during pregnancy. Women are not aware of the increased risk of preeclampsia, stillbirth, caesarean delivery, multiple births and preterm delivery associated with delayed childbirth to elderly stages of life (Tough, Benzies *et al.*, 2006; Tough, Benzies *et al.*, 2007).

Postponement of motherhood beyond 35 years of age influences many aspects of reproduction from conceiving through embryonic implantation all the way until delivery. The effect of maternal age on her ability to conceive is well documented. Populations that do not use contraceptives and practice unprotected intercourse give the best estimation of the ability of normal women to conceive. Based on 10 different populations living between the 17th and the 20th Centuries that did not use contraceptives, Menken et al (Menken, Trussell *et al.*, 1986) reported that the fertility rate remains relatively stable until a woman is in her late 30s and then decreases substantially from more than 400 pregnancies per 1000 women per year at the age of 30, to only 100 pregnancies per 1000 women per year by the age of 45. The decline in fertility as a function of women's age was also demonstrated in a donor insemination programmed in which the cause of infertility was related to male factors alone and the women were assumed to be normal. Pregnancy rates at 1 year declined from 74% among women below the age of 30 years to 61.5% among women aged 31–35 years and 55.8% among women aged 36–41 years (Schwartz and Mayaux, 1982).

After conceiving, the risk of spontaneous miscarriage increases as a function of maternal age. In a prospective population-based register linkage study, involving 12,221,546 pregnancies of 634,272 Danish women from 1978 to 1992, older maternal age was a significant risk factor for spontaneous pregnancy loss irrespective of the number of previous miscarriages and parity. The risk of a spontaneous abortion in women aged 20–24 years was 8.9% and it climbed up to 74.7% in those aged 45 years or older (Nybo Andersen, Wohlfahrt *et al.*, 2000). Ben Kroon et all performed a cytogenetic evaluation for the products of conception obtained from patients with first trimester abortion who had a dilatation and curettage (D&C). The rate of embryos with aneuploidy in women aged ≥35 years was significantly higher than that of those younger than 35 years (45.7%, vs. 34.8%, respectively; P=.018) (Kroon, Harrison *et al.*, 2011). The derived rates apply to women whose only risk factor is advanced maternal age. The categories analyzed were trisomy 21 (Down's syndrome), Trisomy 18 (Edwards' syndrome), trisomy 13 (Patau's syndrome), 47XXY (Klinefelter's syndrome), 47,XXX, and a group of other clinically significant abnormalities that were considered collectively. The rate of all these chromosomal abnormalities in this study was about five per 1,000 at age 35 years, 15 per 1,000 at age 40 years, and 50 per 1,000 at age 45 years (Hook, Cross *et al.*, 1983). Savva et al (Savva, Walker *et al.*, 2010) reviewed the records of prenatal and postnatal diagnoses from seven UK regional congenital anomaly registers and two Australian registers from 1997 to 2004. These dataset included 4.5 million deliveries, of which 975 diagnosed as having trisomy 13 and 2254 had trisomy 18. In addition, the authors reported that since 1989 until 1996 there was an increase, by 13% in the rate of trisomy 13 and by 25% in the rate of trisomy 18. These findings are consistent with those predicted to be associated with the increases in maternal age (Savva, Walker *et al.*, 2010).

The link between Down syndrome and advanced maternal age deserves special attention. This association was already reported by Penrose in the mid 1930's (Penrose, 1933; Penrose, 1934). Lately, Graves Allen et al (Allen, Freeman *et al.*, 2009) examined the origin of the meiotic error leading to the association between maternal age and chromosome 21 non-disjunction. They emphasis that the a significant association between advanced maternal age and chromosome 21 non-disjunction was restricted to meiotic errors in the egg and was not observed in sperm or in post-zygotic mitotic errors. The authors reported that the advanced maternal age was significantly associated with a higher rate of non-disjunction in both meiosis I (MI) and meiosis II (MII). Indeed, compared to mothers of euploid neonates, mothers of infants with trisomy 21 due to MI non-disjunction were 8.5 times more likely to be ≥40 years old than 20–24 years old at the birth of the index case (95% CI = 5.6–12.9). Where non-disjunction occurred in MII, mothers were 15.1 times more likely to be ≥40 years (95% CI = 8.4–27.3) (Allen, Freeman *et al.*, 2009).

Women's age has a major impact on the rate of chronic maternal diseases and pregnancy outcome. Indeed, the rate of diabetes increases with maternal age. The 2010 National Vital Statistics Reports reported that in 2007 the rate of diabetes among USA mothers under the age of 20 was 14.0 per 1,000, and it increases almost 7 times higher to 100.5 per 1,000 in women over the age of 40 (Table 1). Similar trends were reported regarding the rate of chronic hypertension. The prevalence of this disease increases from 3.9 per 1000 in women younger than 20 years old to 32.2 per 1000 in women older than 40. In contrast to the linear association between diabetes, as well as chronic hypertension and maternal age, the incidence of gestational hypertension as a function of maternal age has a U shape curve with a prevalence of 41.8 per 1000 among patients under 20 years and 50.1 per 1000 for women over 40, and the lowest incidence is between 20-35 years old. Similarly to the National Vital Statistics Reports, a different population based cohort involving 1,160,000 women delivered during a 2-year period found increased rate of preeclampsia and gestational diabetes among women aged 40 years or older in comparison to those aged 20-29 (Gilbert, Nesbitt *et al.*, 1999). Yogev et al (Yogev, Melamed *et al.*, 2010) stratified the rate of pregnancy complication according to maternal age with a special attention to women aged ≥45 years (n = 177) with an additional subgroup analysis of women aged 45-49 years with those women aged ≥50 years. Similar to previous studies the authors reported that the rates of gestational diabetes mellitus and hypertensive complications of pregnancy were increased among women aged 45 years and older.

Maternal age also influences perinatal outcome, small-for-gestational age births (SGA) are common and can have serious immediate consequences for the infant (Das and Sysyn, 2004; Salem, Levy *et al.*, 2011). They have also been associated with the development of a range of chronic diseases in subsequent adult life (Nepomnyaschy and Reichman, 2006; Barker, 2004). There is an association between maternal age and the delivery of an SGA neonate. In the FASTER trial, patients aged 35-39 years were at increased risk to a deliver low birthweight neonate (adjusted OR 1.6) (Cleary-Goldman, Malone *et al.*, 2005). In addition, Salem- Yaniv et al, in a retrospective population based study found a significant increase in low birth weight among older women (35–40 and above 40 years of age) in comparison to women younger than 35 years old (Salem, Levy *et al.*, 2011).

Maternal age	Diabetes per 1,000 live births in specified group	Chronic Hypertension per 1,000 live births in specified group
All ages	44.8	11.0
Under 20 years	14.0	3.9
20–24 years	25.9	6.4
25–29 years	42.4	9.9
30–34 years	59.5	13.6
35–39 years	78.6	20.4
40–54 years	100.5	32.2

Table 1. Number and rate of live births to mothers with selected risk factors during pregnancy, obstetric procedures, characteristics of labor and delivery, and congenital anomalies, by age and race and Hispanic origin of mother: United States, 2007. (National Vital Statistics Reports, Volume 58, Number 24, August 9, 2010)

The Human Fertilization and Embryology Authority database was examined in order to ascertain the predictors of live birth in all IVF cycles undertaken in the UK between 2003 and 2007 (n = 144,018). This study has found that the odds of low birth weight were reduced with increasing maternal age and with a history of a previous pregnancy (either spontaneous or following IVF) (Nelson and Lawlor, 2011). Similarly to these findings, Erez et al reported that among patients with twin gestation who conceived through ART the rate of preeclampsia was higher in women younger than 35 years old than in older parturient (Erez, Vardi *et al.*, 2006). These reports suggest that among patients who suffers from infertility the background maternal illness may be more severe and with clinical implication that is additive to the effect of maternal age.

Advanced maternal age also influences the rate of preterm delivery. Jacobsson et al examined the Swedish Medical Birth Register, managed by the National Board of Health and Welfare, contains data on 1,566,313 deliveries that are more than 99% of all births in Sweden during the last 15-years. The rate of preterm delivery before 37 and 34 weeks among women 20-29 were compared to those of women age 40-44 years and above 45 years (Jacobsson, Ladfors *et al.*, 2004). The authors reported that the rate of preterm birth increases with maternal age. Indeed, after adjustment to confounding factors women aged 40-44 years old had an odds ratio of 1.54 (95% CI 1.47-1.60), while those who were ≥ 45 years had an odds of 1.63 (95% CI 1.32-2.00) to deliver before 37 weeks of gestation (Jacobsson, Ladfors *et al.*, 2004). Similar data where published also by others (Cleary-Goldman, Malone *et al.*, 2005; Salem, Levy *et al.*, 2011).

Women ≥ 35 years have a significantly higher rate of fetal death than their younger counterparts. Fretts and colleagues documented that the fetal death rate decreased by more than 70 percent over the past 30 years among white Canadian women. Although the absolute stillbirth rate declined significantly for women of all ages and parity groups, older women remained at higher risk for fetal death, even after controlling for diabetes, hypertension, and placental abruption (Fretts, Schmittdiel *et al.*, 1995). This report was in accord with other publications regarding the increased rate of fetal demise among older women (Jacobsson, Ladfors *et al.*, 2004; Cleary-Goldman, Malone *et al.*, 2005). In contrast, among nulliparous patients advanced maternal age was not an independent risk factor for perinatal mortality (Salem, Levy *et al.*, 2011).

The increasing numbers of pregnancies at advanced maternal age influences the rising rate of cesarean birth. Among 57,426 primiparous women who gave birth in Victoria, Australia, in 2005 and 2006, older patients were more likely to give birth by cesarean section in comparison to younger primiparous women (Carolan, Davey *et al.*, 2011). Salem-Yaniv at al reported that in comparison to women younger than 35 years old, those aged 35–40 have an almost a threefold increase in the rate of cesarean deliveries among nulliparous patients (38.2%) and close to a fivefold increase among women over 40 years (63.3%) (Salem, Levy *et al.*, 2011). Similar results were published by the National Vital Statistics Reports UA. Among 4,316,233 women that delivered during the year 2007, older maternal age was associated to delivery through cesarean section (under 20 22.7% 35-39 41.8%: 40-54 47.7%) (Martin, Hamilton *et al.*, 2010). This increasing risk of cesarean birth associated with advancing maternal age is of importance, because the proportion of women who are delaying childbearing is growing, and in addition, the cesarean delivery rate is increasing (Martin, Hamilton *et al.*, 2010).

4. Pregnancy outcome in patients conceived through assisted reproduction

IVF pregnancies are associated with an increased risk for obstetrics complication including gestational diabetes, preeclampsia, placenta previa and neonatal intensive care admission (Shevell, Malone *et al.*, 2005; Chen, Wen *et al.*, 2009; Nelson and Lawlor, 2011). A prospective database from a large multicenter investigation of singleton pregnancies demonstrated that the use of IVF was associated with a significant increase in the risk to develop preeclampsia (OR 2.7; 95% CI 1.7–4.4), placental abruption (OR 2.4; 95% CI 1.1–5.2), placenta previa (OR 6.0; 95% CI 3.4–10.7), and risk of cesarean delivery (OR 2.3; 95% CI 1.8–2.9) (Shevell, Malone *et al.*, 2005). A different prospective cohort study that included singleton IVF/ICSI pregnancies had more than 4-fold increased risk of stillbirth compared with spontaneously conceived singleton pregnancies (Wisborg, Ingerslev *et al.*, 2010a). There is a strong evidence to support the association between IVF treatments and preterm birth. Indeed, ART are independently associated with preterm birth in singleton as well as in twin gestation.

5. The association between preterm birth and assisted reproduction

Preterm delivery is the leading cause for perinatal morbidity and mortality worldwide (Goldenberg, Culhane *et al.*, 2008). The annual societal economic burden associated with preterm birth in the United States exceeded $26.2 billion in 2005 (Institute of Medicine (US) Committee on Understanding Premature Birth and Assuring Healthy Outcomes, 2007). Preterm birth is associated with short and long term maternal and fetal sequel. The mothers are at risk of recurrent preterm birth and cardiovascular disease later in life. (Nardi, Zureik *et al.*, 2006; Smith, Pell *et al.*, 2001) The premature newborn is at risk for acute (i.e. respiratory distress syndrome, necrotizing enterocolitis, and intraventricular hemorrhage) and chronic (i.e. retinopathy of prematurity, cerebral palsy, broncho pulmonary dysplasia) illness, as well as social and behavioral maladjustment later in life. (Moster, Lie *et al.*, 2008) The prevalence of preterm birth varies from 6% to 15% of all deliveries depending on the geographical and demographical characteristics of the population tested. (Romero, Mazor *et al.*, 1994; Martin, Hamilton *et al.*, 2009; Slattery and Morrison, 2002).

In Europe the rate of preterm deliveries varies from 5% to 9% (Slattery and Morrison, 2002), while the rate of preterm birth in the United States reached 12.8% by 2006 (Martin, Hamilton *et al.*, 2009), 20% higher than in 1990. Of interest, while the rate of early (<34 weeks) preterm birth remained relatively constant (2.9% among singleton and 3.3% to 3.6% among multiple gestations) the rate of late preterm birth (34-37 weeks) increased among singleton by 19.1% (from 6.1% to 8.1%) and by 24.7% among all pluralities from 1990 to 2005 (Martin, Hamilton *et al.*, 2007) (Figure 4).

Preterm delivery can be either spontaneous or medically induced (indicated) regardless of the gestational age at delivery. Spontaneous preterm birth account for 75% of all preterm deliveries (Meis, Ernest *et al.*, 1987; Meis, Goldenberg *et al.*, 1998; Meis, Michielutte *et al.*, 1995) and can be the end result of three main clinical presentations: 1) preterm labor with intact membranes; 2) preterm prelabor rupture of membranes (preterm PROM); and 3) cervical insufficiency. (McElrath, Hecht *et al.*, 2008) Indicated preterm birth results from medical intervention due to maternal or fetal complications that necessitate medical intervention. (Ananth and Vintzileos, 2006b; Mazaki-Tovi, Romero *et al.*, 2007; Meis, Michielutte *et al.*, 1995; Ananth and Vintzileos, 2006a; Ananth, Getahun *et al.*, 2006) Although many studies have focused on the rate of preterm birth, (1999; Joseph, Kramer *et al.*, 1998; Vintzileos, Ananth *et al.*, 2002) an important consideration is whether these deliveries are the result of spontaneous labor or "indicated" preterm deliveries. The need for this distinction is based on the premise that the risk factors for recurrent preterm PROM, preterm labor with intact membranes, preeclampsia, and/or SGA are different. However, recent observations suggest that there may be overlap among these conditions, (Ananth and Vintzileos, 2006a; Ananth, Getahun *et al.*, 2006) so that a patient with an "indicated" preterm birth may also be at risk for spontaneous preterm birth (Ananth and Vintzileos, 2006a; Ananth, Getahun *et al.*, 2006). The converse may also be true (i.e. that a patient with a spontaneous preterm birth is at risk for an "indicated" preterm birth in a subsequent pregnancy).

Assisted reproduction technologies are emerging contributors for the increasing rate of preterm birth. The use of infertility treatments has risen dramatically in the past 20 years; between 1996 and 2003, the number of cycles of ART nearly doubled from 64,681 to 122,872 (Institute of Medicine (US) Committee on Understanding Premature Birth and Assuring Healthy Outcomes, 2007). The number of live births resulting from conceptions achieved by the use of ARTs more than doubled from 14,507 to 35,785. This has been associated with the trend to delay childbearing, indeed, more than 50 percent of these women were 35 years of age or older. In recent years, an unintended consequence of the use of these technologies, multiple gestations and the increased risk for preterm delivery, has become a focus of attention. Indeed, the institute of Medicine in the USA has concluded that "Fertility treatments are a significant contributor to preterm birth among both multiple and singleton pregnancies." (Institute of Medicine (US) Committee on Understanding Premature Birth and Assuring Healthy Outcomes, 2007).

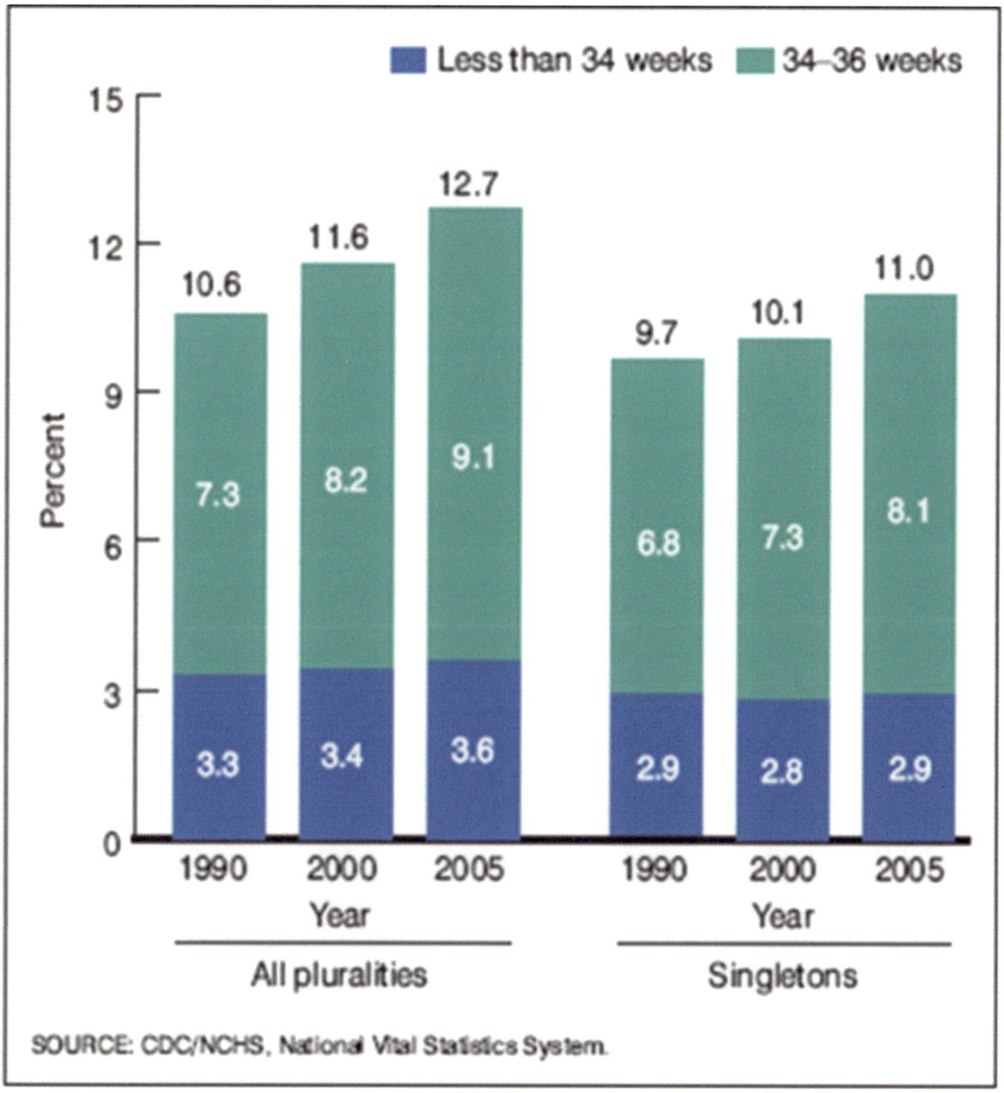

Fig. 4. Chances over time in the rate of preterm birth according to gestational age at delivery and the number of fetuses.

ART are associated with increased rate of pregnancy complication. Several questions are being raised in regard with this topic:1) what are the causes or mechanisms leading for such complications? Is it the treatment or the underlying maternal condition that leads to infertility? 2) Are these complications due to multiple gestation or they affect also singleton gestations? 3) Is there an association with between the ART protocol and adverse pregnancy outcome?

5.1 The association between ART and multiple gestations

There is a direct relationship between the rise in the use of assisted reproduction and the increasing rate of multiple gestations. This trend is mostly due to the transfer of multiple embryos. In spite of the new regulation regarding the maximal embryos transferred during IVF cycle. In 2008, among the ART cycles that used fresh non-donor eggs or frozen-thawed embryos and progressed to the embryo transfer stage, approximately 38% involved the transfer of three or more embryos, about 13% of cycles involved the transfer of four or more embryos, and approximately 4% of cycles involved the transfer of five or more embryos. In addition, ART conceived pregnancies have a higher rate of zygotic splitting in cycles were a single embryo was transferred resulting in increased rate of monochorionic twins than spontaneously conceived pregnancies (Blickstein, Jones *et al.*, 2003; Blickstein, Verhoeven *et al.*, 1999). Among the 38,631 pregnancies that resulted from ART cycles using fresh non-donor eggs or embryos, approximately 61% were singleton, 29% were twins, and about 4% were triplets or more. Approximately 32% of the pregnancies ending in live births produced more than one infant (30% twins and approximately 2% triplets or more). This compares with a multiple-infant birth rate of slightly more than 3% in the general U.S. population Figure 5.

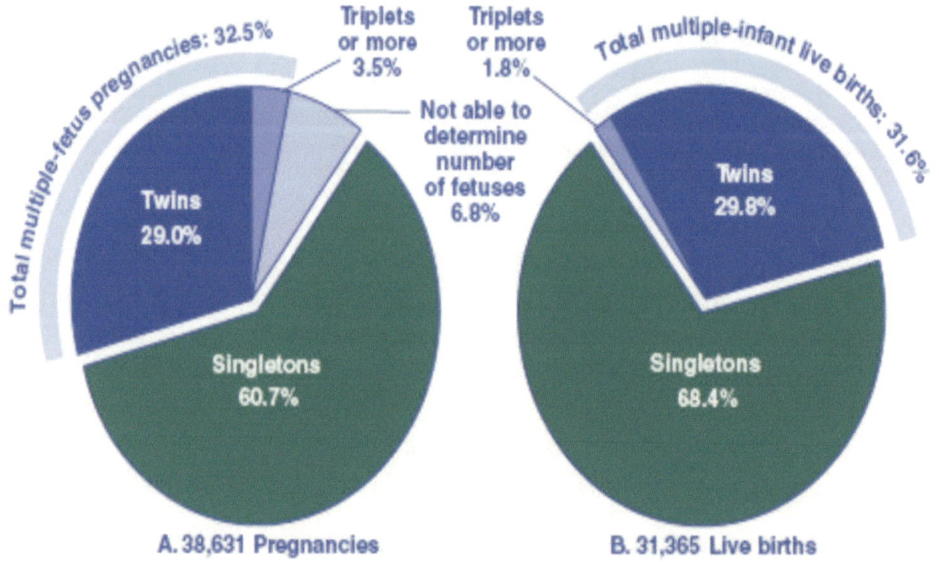

Fig. 5. Risk of having multi-frtus pregnancies and multiple infant live birth from ART cycles using fresh non-donor eggs or embryos-US CDC 2008.

The proportions of multiple birth in Europe is lower than in the USA, and is declining in the recent years. Indeed, the proportion of singleton, twin and triplet deliveries after IVF and ICSI combined was 79.2, 19.9 and 0.9%, respectively. This gives a total multiple delivery rates of 20.8% compared with 21.8% in 2005 and 22.7% in 2004 (ESHRE, 2006). In an effort to reduce the number of higher-order multiple pregnancies, the American society for reproductive medicine (ASRM) and the Society for Assisted Reproductive Technology Data (SART) have developed guidelines for the number of embryos to be transferred in IVF cycle.

5.1.1 What is the effect of the mode of conception on the risk for preterm birth in twin gestations?

Twin and higher order of multiple gestation are at increased risk to deliver preterm. Nevertheless, the effect of mode of conception on the prematurity rate in twin pregnancies is under continues debate. Several studies have stated that twin pregnancies conceived through ART have similar perinatal complication rate (Zaib-un-Nisa, Ghazal-Aswad *et al.*, 2003; Boulet, Schieve *et al.*, 2008). In contrast, other studies and number of meta-analysis demonstrated no difference between spontaneously and ART conceived twin (Daniel, Ochshorn *et al.*, 2000; Wright, Schieve *et al.*, 2003; Wright, Schieve *et al.*, 2004; Wang, Sullivan *et al.*, 2005; Pinborg, 2005; Allen, Wilson *et al.*, 2006; Reddy, Wapner *et al.*, 2007; Chan, Mannino *et al.*, 2007; A B and M K, 2008; Shebl, Ebner *et al.*, 2009; Hansen, Colvin *et al.*, 2009; Weghofer, Klein *et al.*, 2009; Rossi and D'Addario, 2011; Morcel, Lavoue *et al.*, 2010). Verstraelen et al reported in a population based cohort study, that pregnancies conceived by ART have a persistent increased risk for preterm delivery (Figure 6), even after correction for birth year, maternal age, parity, and for infant sex, caesarean delivery, zygosity, and chorionicity (Verstraelen, Goetgeluk *et al.*, 2005).

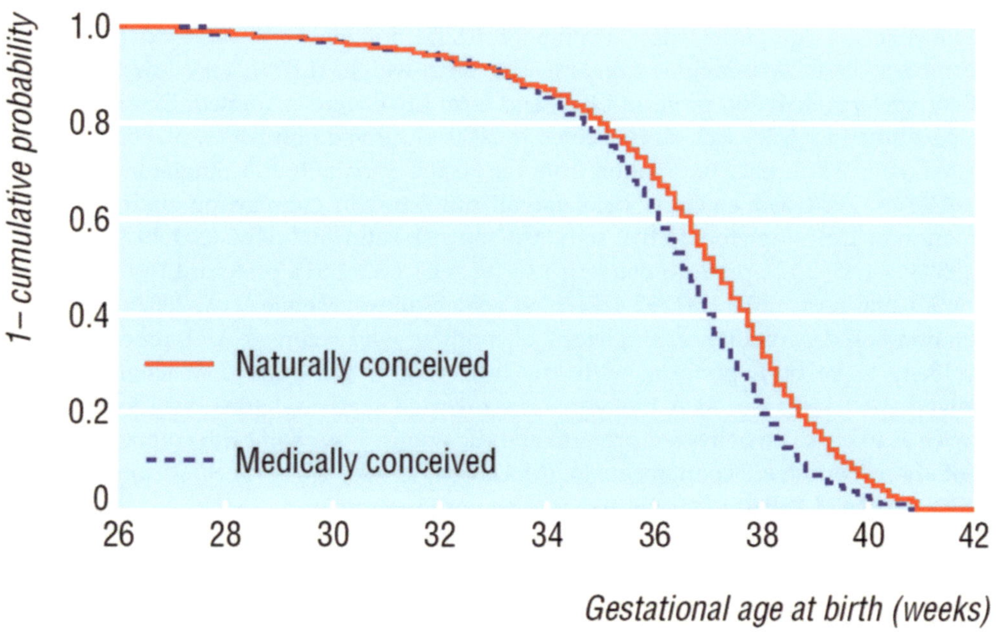

Fig. 6. Kaplan-Meier plot of gestational length in naturally conceived (n=2915) and medically conceived (n=1453) twins. Adopted from Verstraelen H et al. BMJ, 2005; 331: 1173.with permeation.

In addition, Erez et al in a population based cohort study reported that ARTs are an independent risk factor for preterm birth after adjustment to parity, rupture of membranes, severe preeclampsia (Erez, Mayer *et al.*, 2008). In a systematic review and meta-analysis including eleven case-control studies that involved 2303 IVF twins and 2326 spontaneously conceived twins, as well as, three cohort studies that involved at least 1509 IVF twins IVF twins have an increase risk for PTB from 32 to 36 weeks of gestation compared with spontaneously conceived twins who were matched for maternal age (OR, 1.48; 95% CI, 1.05-2.10). The OR for PTB at< 37 weeks of gestation in studies that also matched for parity was similar and approached statistical significance at a 5% level of significance (OR, 1.47; 95% CI, 1.01-2.44). The origin of the increase in PTB has yet to be determined (McDonald, Han *et al.*, 2010). Collectively these studies suggest that in comparison to spontaneously conceived twin gestations, twin pregnancies that result from ART are at increased for preterm birth especially between 32-36 weeks of gestation.

5.2 Are singleton ART pregnancies at increased risk for preterm birth?

One of the major questions regarding the association between ART and preterm birth was whether this effect is mainly due to the increase in the rate of multiple pregnancies or is it relevant also for singleton gestations (Jackson, Gibson *et al.*, 2004; McGovern, Llorens *et al.*, 2004; Schieve, Meikle *et al.*, 2002). Mounting evidence suggest that singleton pregnancies conceived following ART are at increased risk for preterm birth. Indeed: 1) In a Prospective follow-up study done in Denmark, including a total of 20,080 liveborn singletons, in comparison to fertile women, those who conceived following IVF/ICSI had a significant increase in the risk of preterm and very preterm delivery (Wisborg, Ingerslev *et al.*, 2010b). 2) Schieve et al compared the outcome of 62,551 infants born after ART treatments performed in 1996-2000. Secular trends in low birth weight (LBW), very low birth weight (VLBW), preterm delivery, preterm LBW, and term LBW were examined. Detailed analyses were performed for 6,377 infants conceived in 2000. Observed numbers were compared with expected using a reference population from the 2000 U.S. natality file. Singleton infants born after ART in 2000 had elevated risks for all outcomes in comparison with the general population of U.S. singletons: LBW standardized risk ratio 1.62 (95% CI 1.49, 1.75), VLBW 1.79 (95% CI 1.45, 2.12), preterm delivery 1.41 (95% CI 1.32, 1.51), preterm LBW 1.74 (95% CI 1.57, 1.90), and term LBW 1.39 (95% CI 1.19, 1.59) (Schieve, Meikle *et al.*, 2002). 3) In a USA population based surveillance, singletons of mothers who received ART procedures were more likely to be born preterm, with low birthweight, and SGA than singleton infants conceived spontaneously. 4) A meta-analysis revealed that singletons born following IVF are twice as likely to be delivered preterm and die within 1 week of birth compared with the risk of those conceived spontaneously (McGovern et al., 2004). 5) Singletons conceived through the use of IVF are twice as likely to be born preterm and die within 1 week of birth as those not conceived through IVF and 2.7 times more likely to have a low birth weight (Hampton, 2004). 6) A meta-analysis that compiled information from 12,283 singleton births resulting from IVF pregnancies and 1.9 million spontaneously conceived singleton births noted a twofold increase in the risk of preterm delivery (Jackson et al., 2004). 7) According to the CDC report among the infants conceived through the use of ART, singletons that resulted from fetal reduction (either spontaneous or medically) had a higher rate of preterm birth (19%) than those who started as a singleton gestation (12%) (Figure 7).

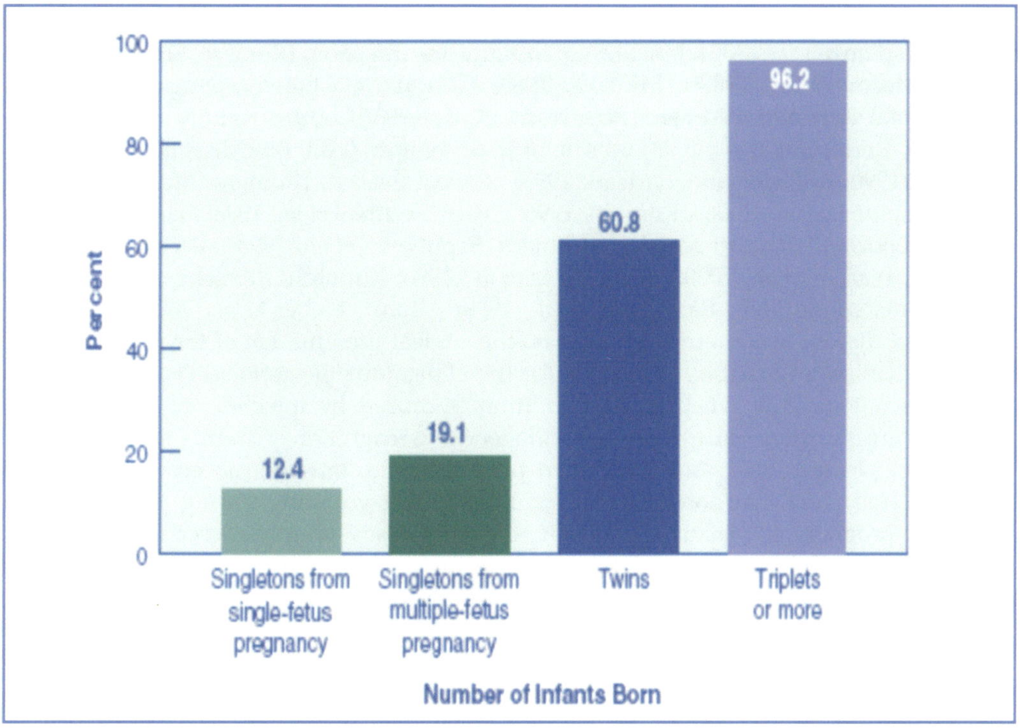

Fig. 7. Proportion of preterm birth resulting from ART cycles using fresh non-donor eggs or embryos, by number of infants born-USA, CDC 2008.

5.3 What are the possible mechanisms associated with the increased risk for preterm birth in ART pregnancies?

The mechanisms in which assisted reproduction technologies increases the risk for preterm birth are still under investigation. Aside the contribution of ART to the increase number of multiple gestations (especially twins) that increases the risk for preterm delivery; the mechanisms leading to preterm delivery in singleton gestation conceived by ART have not been thoroughly investigated yet. Preliminary evidence suggests that underlying maternal conditions that may lead to infertility including insulin resistance and inflammation may contribute to this observation.

5.3.1 Preterm parturition as a syndrome

The implicit paradigm that has governed much of the study of preterm parturition is that term and preterm labor are fundamentally the same process except for the gestational age at which they occur (Romero, Espinoza *et al.*, 2004a; Romero, Espinoza *et al.*, 2006b) and share a 'common pathway'. The common pathway of human parturition is defined as the anatomical, physiological, biochemical, endocrinological, immunological, and clinical events that occur in the mother and/or fetus in both term and preterm labor. The fundamental difference between term and preterm parturition is that the former results from physiological activation of the common pathway, while preterm labor arises from pathological processes that extemporaneously activate one or more of the components of the common pathway of parturition.

Preterm labor (PTL) is the clinical presentation of different underlying mechanisms, (Romero, Espinoza *et al.*, 2004c) including: intrauterine infection, (Romero, Sirtori *et al.*, 1989; Romero, Mazor *et al.*, 1988b; Minkoff, 1983; Goncalves, Chaiworapongsa *et al.*, 2002) uteroplacental ischemia, (Romero, Sepulveda *et al.*, 1993; Combs, Katz *et al.*, 1993; Arias, 1990; Arias, Rodriquez *et al.*, 1993) uterine over-distention, (Hill, Breckle *et al.*, 1987; Phelan, Park *et al.*, 1990; Besinger and Carlson, 1995) cervical disease, (Romero, Mazor *et al.*, 1993; Romero, Espinoza *et al.*, 2006a; Romero, 1996; Heath, Southall *et al.*, 1998; Hassan, Romero *et al.*, 2000) abnormal allograft reaction, (Romero, Sepulveda *et al.*, 1993) allergic phenomena, (Holloway, Warner *et al.*, 2000; Jones, Miles *et al.*, 1996; Rudolph, Reinicke *et al.*, 1993) and endocrine disorders. (Belt, Baldassare *et al.*, 1999; Allport, Pieber *et al.*, 2001) The current taxonomy of disease in obstetrics is based on the clinical presentation of the mother and not on the mechanism of disease responsible for the clinical manifestations. The term 'preterm labor' does not indicate whether the condition is caused by infection, a vascular insult, uterine overdistension, an abnormal allogeneic recognition, stress, or some other pathological process. The same applies to pre-eclampsia, intrauterine growth restriction, fetal death, recurrent abortions, as well as, nausea and vomiting during pregnancy, and failure to progress in labor, in which the diagnoses simply describe the clinical manifestations without consideration of the specific etiology. The lack of recognition that these conditions simply represent a collection of signs and symptoms with little reference to the underlying mechanisms of disease may be responsible for the expectation that one diagnostic test and treatment will detect and cure each of these conditions. This has implications for the fundamental understanding of the biology of preterm parturition and the clinical strategies to diagnose, treat, and prevent spontaneous preterm labour (Romero, Espinoza *et al.*, 2004a; Romero, Espinoza *et al.*, 2006b).

5.3.2 Intrauterine Infection and/or inflammation

Systemic and subclinical infections are a leading cause of preterm birth. Indeed, pyelonephritis and pneumonia are frequently associated with the onset of premature labor and delivery. (Benedetti, Valle *et al.*, 1982; Cunningham, Morris *et al.*, 1973; Fan, Pastorek *et al.*, 1987; Finland and Dublin T.D., 1939; Gilles, Lawson *et al.*, 1969; Herd and Jordan, 1981; Hibbard, Thrupp *et al.*, 1967; Kass, 1962; Madinger, Greenspoon *et al.*, 1989; McLane, 1939; Oxhorn, 1955; Stevenson, Glasko A.J. *et al.*, 1951; Wing and Troppoli D.V., 1930) Similarly, subclinical intrauterine infection is a frequent and important mechanism of disease leading to premature contraction, preterm labor and preterm birth. (Minkoff, 1983; Romero, Mazor *et al.*, 1988a; Bang, 1987; Fidel, Jr., Romero *et al.*, 1994; Kullander, 1977; McDuffie, Jr., Sherman *et al.*, 1992; McKay and Wong, 1963; Rieder and Thomas, 1960; Romero, Munoz *et al.*, 1994; Skarnes and Harper, 1972; Takeda and Tsuchiya I., 1953; Zahl and Bjerknes, 1943; Gomez, Ghezzi *et al.*, 1995; Romero, Sirtori *et al.*, 1989; Goncalves, Chaiworapongsa *et al.*, 2002) Microbiological and histo-pathological studies suggest that infection-related inflammation may account for 25 to 40% of cases of preterm deliveries.

Goncalves et al (Goncalves, Chaiworapongsa *et al.*, 2002) studied the rate of positive amniotic fluid cultures for microorganisms in women with preterm labor and intact membranes. The authors reviewed the results of amniotic fluid cultures from 33 studies and the prevalence of microbial invasion of amniotic fluid among patients with preterm labor was 12.8% (Goncalves, Chaiworapongsa *et al.*, 2002; Romero, Espinoza *et al.*, 2002), and about 50% of them were polymicrobial. The rate of microbial invasion of the amniotic cavity in patients with preterm labor and intact membrane is gestational age dependant. It is as high as 45% at 23-26 weeks and decreases to 11.5% at 31-34 weeks of gestation (Watts, Krohn *et al.*, 1992). Thus, the earlier the gestational age at preterm birth, the more likely that microbial invasion of the amniotic cavity is present (Watts, Krohn *et al.*, 1992). In preterm PROM, the prevalence of a positive amniotic fluid culture for microorganisms is approximately 32.4%. (Goncalves, Chaiworapongsa *et al.*, 2002; Romero, Espinoza *et al.*, 2002) However, when amniocenteses were performed at the time of the onset of labor, 75% of patients had microbial invasion of the amniotic cavity (Romero, Quintero *et al.*, 1988), suggesting that some patients are already infected prior to the clinical rupture of membranes, while others are infected after the membrane have ruptured. The rate of microbial invasion of amniotic cavity among women presenting with a cervical insufficiency in the mid-trimester is around 33% (range 13%-52%) (Romero, Gonzalez *et al.*, 1992; Bujold, Morency *et al.*, 2008) and 45% to 51% in the early third trimester (Bujold, Morency *et al.*, 2008). In addition, a recent study has demonstrated that while only 8% of patients with cervical insufficiency had a positive amniotic fluid culture, 80% have intra-amniotic inflammation determined by a positive rapid MMP-8 kit (Lee, Romero *et al.*, 2008). Patients with intra-amniotic inflammation and negative amniotic fluid culture had a shorter amniocentesis-to-delivery interval and a lower gestational age at delivery than patients without intra-amniotic infection/inflammation. In twin gestations, microbial invasion of the amniotic cavity occurs in 11.9% of patients presenting with preterm labor and deliver preterm (Romero, Manogue *et al.*, 1989; Romero, Mazor *et al.*, 1988b). The most common microbial organisms isolated from the amniotic fluid of patients with preterm parturition were genital mycoplasmas , *Fusobacterium* species *Streptococcus agalactiae, Petostreptococcus spp., Fusobacterium spp., Staphylococcus aureus, Gardenerella vaginalis, Streptococcus viridans,* and *Bacterioides spp.* (Alanen, 1998; Hitti, Riley *et al.*, 1997; Averbuch, Mazor *et al.*, 1995; Carroll, Papaioannou *et al.*, 1996; Cotton, Hill *et al.*, 1984; Coultrip and Grossman, 1992; Garite, Freeman *et al.*, 1979; Zlatnik, Cruikshank *et al.*, 1984; Romero, Quintero *et al.*, 1988; Romero, Gonzalez *et al.*, 1992)

The association between infection and/or inflammation and preterm birth in ART pregnancies is implied from recently published data. A prospective cohort study that included 144,018 treatment cycles reported that tubal causes of infertility were associated with increased odds of preterm birth (Nelson and Lawlor, 2011). Kamiyama et al (Kamiyama, Teruya *et al.*, 2004) reported that among women undergoing IVF-ET, those who had endotoxin concentrations > 200 pg/mL in menstrual effluent did not conceive, while 30% of those with lower endotoxin concentrations got pregnant. Thus, preexisting endometrial microbial invasion with Gram negative bacteria is associated with failure of IVF-ET, either because of failure of implantation or the induction of sub clinical spontaneous abortion (Romero, Espinoza *et al.*, 2004b). Endotoxin is a component of the cell wall of Gram negative bacteria and its detection in biological fluid is evidence of microbial invasion of a sterile compartment such as the amniotic cavity. An increased concentration in non-sterile body fluids such as cervical mucus or vaginal fluid is an indication of enlarged Gran-negative microbial population and has been reported in women with bacterial vaginosis (Romero, Espinoza *et al.*, 2004b).

5.3.2.1 Bacterial vaginosis and preterm birth

Bacterial vaginosis is a risk factor for spontaneous preterm birth with intact or ruptures membranes (Leitich, Bodner-Adler *et al.*, 2003). The rate of bacterial vaginosis during pregnancy is 15-20%; however, 50% of these patients are asymptomatic. A meta-analysis

(Leitich, Bodner-Adler *et al.*, 2003) of 18 studies (20,232 patients) concluded that bacterial vaginosis was associated with an increased risk for preterm delivery < 37 weeks of gestation (OR 2.19, 95%CI 1.54-3.12), and this effect was significant among singleton gestations, as well as among low and high risk pregnancies for preterm delivery. Detection of bacterial vaginosis <16 weeks of pregnancy was associated with an increased risk for preterm birth (OR 7.55, 95%CI 1.8-31.65) (Leitich, Bodner-Adler *et al.*, 2003). Bacterial vaginosis was also found to be associated with intra-amniotic infection, histologic chorioamnionitis, preterm PROM, first trimester losses in women who conceived after in vitro fertilization, and second trimesters abortions, as well as post cesarean section endometritis and wound infection (Vidaeff and Ramin, 2006; Newton, Piper *et al.*, 1997; Ralph, Rutherford *et al.*, 1999; Llahi-Camp, Rai *et al.*, 1996; Watts, Krohn *et al.*, 1990; Watts, Eschenbach *et al.*, 1989; Chaim, Mazor *et al.*, 1997).

Patients who undergo IVF treatments have a rate of bacterial vaginosis of about 25% (Liversedge, Turner *et al.*, 1999; Wilson, Ralph *et al.*, 2002) which is higher than that observed in other groups of patients (11-15%) (Eschenbach, Gravett *et al.*, 1984; Pavletic, Wolner-Hanssen *et al.*, 1999; Eschenbach, 1993; McGregor, Allen *et al.*, 2001; McGregor and French, 2000; Sobel, 2000; Ugwumadu, 2002). Moreover, bacterial vaginosis was more common among infertile patients with tubal occlusion (Wilson, Ralph *et al.*, 2002), which is independently associated with an increased risk for preterm birth (Nelson and Lawlor, 2011). Bacterial vaginosis was also more common in unovulatory women and those with unexplained infertility than in infertile couples due to male factor or endometriosis (Wilson, Ralph *et al.*, 2002).

Randomized clinical trials for the prevention of preterm birth by antibiotic treatment of patients with bacterial vaginosis have yielded contradictory results (McDonald, O'Loughlin *et al.*, 1997; Kekki, Kurki *et al.*, 2001; Ugwumadu, Manyonda *et al.*, 2003; Guaschino, Ricci *et al.*, 2003; Okun, Gronau *et al.*, 2005; Shennan, Crawshaw *et al.*, 2006; McDonald, Brocklehurst et al., 2005; Carey, Klebanoff *et al.*, 2000). The randomized placebo control trial of the NICHD MFMU network included 1953 women with bacterial vaginosis who were assigned to treatment with oral metronidazol or placebo (Carey, Klebanoff *et al.*, 2000). Treatment with metronidazol was not associated with a significant reduction in the rate of preterm birth. Moreover, a sub-analysis of high risk patients for preterm delivery demonstrated a higher rate of preterm delivery and preterm PROM in the treatment group (Carey, Klebanoff *et al.*, 2000). A Cochrane review concluded that, overall, antibiotic treatment of bacterial vaginosis did not reduce the risk for preterm birth; however, treatment before 20 weeks of gestation may reduce the risk for preterm delivery < 37 weeks (OR 0.72 95%CI 0.55-0.95) (McDonald, Brocklehurst *et al.*, 2007). In conclusion, treatment of bacterial vaginosis before 20 weeks of gestation in patients with a history of previous preterm birth, may reduce the risk for preterm PROM and low birthweight.

5.3.3 Utero-placenta ischemia

Abnormal placentation and vascular lesions in the fetal and maternal sides of the placenta are the second most prevalent lesions observed in patients who deliver preterm (Arias, Rodriquez *et al.*, 1993). Several possible mechanisms can lead to such findings including vaginal and decidual bleeding, spontaneous or iatrogenic death of intrauterine sibling, and uterine vascular changes such as atherosclerosis that are more prevalent in older parturient.

First trimester bleeding among patients with singleton gestation who conceived by ART was associated with an increased risk for: 1) recurrent second-trimester (OR 4.56, 95% CI = 2.76–7.56) and third-trimester bleeding (OR 2.85, 95% CI = 1.42– 5.73); 2) preterm PROM (OR 2.44, 95% CI 1.38–4.31); 3) preterm contractions (OR 2.27, 95% CI 1.48–3.47) as well as increased the risk for preterm birth (OR 1.64, 95%CI = 1.05–2.55) and extreme preterm birth (OR 3.05, 95%CI 1.12–8.31); and 4) NICU admissions (OR 1.75, 95% CI 1.21–2.54) (De Sutter, Bontinck *et al.*, 2006). The origin of vaginal bleeding associated with preterm birth can be either decidual or placental.

Vascular pathology is one of the mechanisms leading to decidual hemorrhage and subsequent preterm birth. Arias et al (Arias, Rodriquez *et al.*, 1993) reported the rate of vascular lesions in placentae of patients with preterm labor was 34% and 35% of those with PROM, in comparison to only in 12% in those of women who delivered at term. The rate of failure of transformation of spiral arteries is higher among patients and preterm labor with intact membranes as well as those with preterm PROM than in patients who delivered at term (Kim, Bujold *et al.*, 2003; Kim, Chaiworapongsa *et al.*, 2002; Romero, Kusanovic *et al.*, 2011; Lockwood, Krikun *et al.*, 2007). Moreover, the changes in the uterine vasculature associated with maternal age contribute as well for the vascular pathology. Indeed, Crawford et al (Crawford, Davis *et al.*, 1997) studied whether uterine artery atherosclerosis is associated with known cardiovascular risk factors in women undergoing hysterectomy. Among the 59 premenopausal women, 55.9% had intimal thickening, 40.7% had simple plaques and 3.7% had complex lesions in the uterine artery samples. Among postmenopausal women, 40% had intimal fibrosis, 20% had simple plaques, and 40% had complex lesions. Postmenopausal status was correlated strongly with the presence of advanced atherosclerotic disease ($P < 0.001$). Postmenopausal women had significantly greater intimal area ($P = 0.01$), intimal area/medial area ($P = 0.002$), intimal area/vessel area ($P = 0.002$), maximal intimal thickness/medial thickness ($P = 0.01$), and significantly less medial thickness ($P < 0.001$). A significant linear correlation existed between age and the intimal/medial ratio among premenopausal women ($P = 0.04$) and postmenopausal women ($P = 0.01$). Patients with electrocardiogram (ECG) abnormalities had significantly greater intimal/medial area as well ($P = 0.02$). Hypertension was associated with complex lesions among the postmenopausal patients ($P = 0.01$). Preoperative cholesterol levels greater than 200 mg/dL were associated with greater intimal thickness ($P = 0.05$) and intimal thickness/medial thickness ($P = 0.03$) (Crawford, Davis *et al.*, 1997). Moreover, Naeye et al (Naeye, 1983) reported that sclerotic lesions in the myometrial arteries are a possible cause of underperfusion because the proportion of arteries with these lesions increased from 11% at age 17 to 19 years to 83% after the age of 36. This finding is in accord with the report that uterine artery PI during pregnancy increases with maternal age (Pirhonen, Bergersen *et al.*, 2005). These observations are supported also by the clinical findings including an increased rate of SGA neonates among patients with preterm labor and intact membranes as well as those with preterm PROM, and the higher prevalence of low birthweight in ART pregnancies.

Decidual bleeding is thought to play a role in the pathogenesis of preterm labor and preterm PROM leading to preterm birth. Indeed, hemosiderin deposition, that are regarded as a marker for bleeding are found in the decidua and retro-chorionic hematoma formation is present in 37.5% of patients who deliver preterm after PROM between 22 and 32 weeks of gestation, and 36% of patients with preterm delivery and intact membranes (Salafia, Lopez-Zeno *et al.*, 1995). In contrast these lesions are found only in 0.8% of placentas of those who deliver at term.

The effect of decidual bleeding on the activation of premature uterine contractions and/or rupture of membranes is thought to be mediated by thrombin (Lockwood, Krikun et al., 2007; Lockwood, Paidas *et al.*, 2009). The decidua is reach with tissue factor the most potent activator of the coagulation cascade. Thus, any minor decidual bleeding activates the coagulation cascade leading to the generation of thrombin thrombin (Stephenson, Lockwood et al.,2005; Lockwood, Toti *et al.*, 2005; Sarno, Schatz *et al.*, 2006; Lockwood, Krikun et al., 2007). Evidence in support of the increase activation of the coagulation cascade among patients with preterm labor and intact membranes as well as women with preterm PROM include: 1) women with spontaneous preterm labor without intra-amniotic infection or inflammation and women with vaginal bleeding who delivered preterm, have a lower median maternal plasma protein Z (a co factor of protein Z dependent protease inhibitor that inhibits the activity of factor X) than that of normal pregnant women (Kusanovic, Espinoza *et al.*, 2007); 2) regardless to the presence of intra-amniotic infection/inflammation, women with preterm labor and intact membranes have a higher median tissue factor activity and a lower median tissue factor pathway inhibitor than those with a normal pregnancy 3) patients with preterm PROM have a higher median maternal plasma tissue factor concentration and a lower median TFPI concentrations than normal pregnant women (Erez, Espinoza *et al.*, 2008); 4) patients with PTL as well as those with preterm PROM have a higher median maternal plasma thrombin-antithrombin III concentration than that of women with a normal pregnancy (Chaiworapongsa, Espinoza *et al.*, 2002; Elovitz, Baron *et al.*, 2001; Rosen, Kuczynski *et al.*, 2001); and 5) maternal plasma thrombin-antithrombin III complex concentration in the mid trimester were lower in patients about to deliver preterm than in those who subsequently delivered at term (Hackney, Catov *et al.*, 2010).

Moreover, increased thrombin generation was detected not only in the maternal circulation but also in the amniotic fluid (Erez,Romero,et al.,2009). Women with preterm labor who delivered preterm had a higher median thrombin anti-thrombin III concentration than those who delivered at term (Erez, Romer *et al.*, 2009). This was particularly evident among those without intra-amniotic infection/inflammation, in which elevated amniotic fluid of thrombin anti-thrombin complex concentrations were associated with a shorter amniocentesis to delivery interval and a lower gestational age at delivery than those with normal or low concentrations of this complex (Erez,Romero,et al.,2009). A vanishing twin can be an additional possible source for increase intrauterine thrombin generation that may lead to preterm birth. Indeed, vanishing twins among women who conceived by IVF/ICSI was associated with a higher rate of preterm birth <37 and <32 weeks of gestation, especially in the vanishing of the twin occur in later stages of gestation (Pinborg, Lidegaard *et al.*, 2005). A possible explanation for this observation is the report that intrauterine fetal demise is associated with an increased intra-amniotic thrombin generation (Erez, Gotsch *et al.*, 2009). This may be the case also in patients with a vanishing twin, meaning, the increased thrombin generation associated with the dissolving of the dead twin increases the risk for preterm delivery of the surviving fetus.

Thrombin can activate preterm parturition through several mechanisms: 1) it has a uterotonic activity, indeed, the administration of a whole blood into a non-pregnant uterus generated uterine contractions that were not evident when saline or heparinzed blood were introduced into the uterine cavity (Elovitz, Saunders *et al.*, 2000; Elovitz, Baron *et al.*, 2001); 2) thrombin and activated coagulation factor X can induce pro inflammatory cytokines production (IL-6 and IL-1) that may leads to prostaglandins generation and premature myometrial activation and contractions (Lockwood, Toti *et al.*, 2005); and 3) thrombin activates matrix degrading enzymes such as matrix metalloproteneinases (MMPs) 1, 3 and 9 that can degrade the chorioamniotic membranes leading to rupture of membranes (Rosen, Schatz *et al.*, 2002; Stephenson, Lockwood et al., 2005).

5.3.4 Uterine over-distention

Women with a multiple pregnancy are at increased risk for spontaneous preterm labor and preterm birth. Intra-amniotic pressure remains relatively constant throughout gestation despite the growth of the fetus and placenta. This has been attributed to progressive myometrial relaxation due to the effects of progesterone and endogenous myometrial relaxants such as nitric oxide (Sladek, Westerhausen-Larson *et al.*, 1999). Stretching can, however, induce increased myometrial contractility (Laudanski and Rocki, 1975), prostaglandin release (Kloeck and Jung, 1973), expression of gap junction protein or connexin-43 (Ou, Orsino *et al.*, 1997), and increased oxytocin receptor in pregnant and non-pregnant myometrium (Ou, Chen *et al.*, 1998). The stretch-induced contraction- associated protein gene expression during pregnancy is inhibited by progesterone (Ou, Orsino *et al.*, 1997). The effect of stretch increases in late gestation and is maximal during labor as a consequence of the relative reduction in uterine growth compared with fetal growth and of the declining circulating and/or local concentrations of progesterone (Ticconi and Lye, 2002; Chow and Lye, 1994; Ou, Orsino *et al.*, 1997).

Mechanical stress induces activation of integrin receptors (Tzima, del Pozo *et al.*, 2001), stretch-activated calcium channels (Holm, Rich *et al.*, 2000; Farrugia, Holm *et al.*, 1999), phosphorylation of platelet-derived growth factor receptor (Hu, Bock *et al.*, 1998) and activation of G proteins (Li and Xu, 2000; Hu, Bock *et al.*, 1998). Once mechanical force is sensed, it leads to activation of protein kinase C and mitogen- activated protein kinases, increased gene expression of c-fos and c-jun, and enhanced binding activity of transcription factor activator protein-1 (Shynlova, Oldenhof *et al.*, 2002; Oldenhof, Shynlova *et al.*, 2002; Mitchell and Lye, 2002; Mitchell and Lye, 2001; Piersanti and Lye, 1995; Lefebvre, Piersanti *et al.*, 1995). Other effects of physical forces relevant to myometrium include increased expression of prostaglandin H synthase 2 (Wu, Ma *et al.*, 1999), superoxide dismutase, and nitric oxide synthase. The nature of force/pressure-sensing mechanisms of the myometrium has yet to be determined. A role for integrins and their ligands has been proposed for other organs (Shyy and Chien, 2002; Lee, Millward-Sadler *et al.*, 2002). Stretch may not only induce increased myometrial contractility but may also modify the contractile response through 'mechanoelectrical feedback' similar to the one reported in the heart. The chorioamniotic membranes are distended by 40% at 25–29 weeks of gestation, 60% at 30–34 weeks of gestation, and 70% at term (Millar, Stollberg *et al.*, 2000). Stretching of the membranes in vitro induces histological changes characterized by elongation of the amnion cells and increased production of collagenase activity and IL-8 (Maradny, Kanayama *et al.*, 1996; Maehara, Kanayama *et al.*, 1996), while stretching of amnion cells in culture results in increased production of prostaglandin E2 (Kanayama and Fukamizu, 1989). Recent studies using an in vitro cell culture model for fetal membrane distension revealed upregulation of IL-8 and pre-B-cell colony-enhancing factor (Nemeth, Tashima *et al.*, 2000). When fetal membrane explants were distended in an in vitro distension device to mimic the situation in vivo, and the gene expressions of distended explants were compared with that of nondistended explants, three genes, namely IL enhancer binding factor 2, huntingtin-interacting protein 2, and interferon-stimulated gene encoding a 54 kDa protein, were found to be upregulated (Nemeth, Millar *et al.*, 2000). Collectively, these observations suggest that mechanical forces associated with uterine overdistension may result in activation of mechanisms leading to membrane rupture.

5.3.5 Insulin resistance

The association between infertility and maternal insulin resistance is well documented and polycystic ovary disease is its classical feature (Lobo, 1995; Barbieri, 1992; Ruutiainen and Seppala, 1991; Franks, Robinson *et al.*, 1996; Davison, 1998; Taylor, 1998; Sills, Perloe *et al.*, 2000; Scarpitta and Sinagra, 2000; Gutmann and Corson, 2001; Nestler, Stovall *et al.*, 2002; Moran and Norman, 2002; Ben-Shlomo, 2003). Indeed, these patients have a higher rate of infertility or sub fertility. The rate of pregnancy complications among patients with polycystic ovary disease is increased and women with PCOS demonstrated a significantly higher risk of developing gestational diabetes [odds ratio (OR) 2.94; 95% CI: 1.70–5.08], gestational hypertension (OR 3.67; 95% CI: 1.98–6.81), pre-eclampsia (OR 3.47; 95% CI: 1.95–6.17) and preterm birth (OR 1.75; 95% CI: 1.16–2.62). Their babies had a significantly higher risk of admission to a neonatal intensive care unit (OR 2.31; 95% CI: 1.25–4.26) and a higher perinatal mortality (OR 3.07; 95% CI: 1.03–9.21), unrelated to multiple births (Boomsma, Eijkemans *et al.*, 2006). Thus these findings suggest that insulin resistance may contribute to preterm birth in twin gestations especially among patients with PCOS. The exact mechanisms leading to preterm birth due to maternal insulin resistance are not clear, recent reports suggest that alteration in adipocytokines may be involved in this process (Mazaki-Tovi, Romero *et al.*, 2008; Mazaki-Tovi, Romero *et al.*, 2009a; Mazaki-Tovi, Romero *et al.*, 2009b; Mazaki-Tovi, Romero *et al.*, 2010; Mittal, Romero *et al.*, 2009).

5.3.6 Endocrine effect of ART

The controlled ovarian hyperstimulation during ART cycles has endocrine implication that may contribute to the increasing rate of preterm birth in these patients. Human Chorionic Gonadotropin (hCG) induces the secretion of relaxin by the corpus luteum (Kristiansson, Svardsudd *et al.*, 1996; Weiss, Goldsmith *et al.*, 1993). Due to the ovarian hyperstimulation during ART cycle the maternal luteal mass is more prominent than that observed during spontaneously conceived pregnancies resulting in the significant increase in relaxin secretion in response to hCG, and indeed, pregnancies following ART were associated with hyper relaxinemia (Kristiansson, Svardsudd *et al.*, 1996; Weiss, Goldsmith *et al.*, 1993). Higher maternal relaxin concentrations were found to be significantly associated with preterm birth (Iams, Goldsmith *et al.*, 2001; Vogel, Salvig *et al.*, 2001; Vogel, Glavind-Kristensen *et al.*, 2002). Relaxin acts by promoting collagenolysis through inducing the activity of matrixmetaloproteinase (MMP) 1-3 and inhibiting tissue inhibitor of metalloprotease-1 (TIMP-1) (Palejwala, Stein *et al.*, 2001); the net effect is remodeling and ripening of the uterine cervix and increased uterotonic activity. Progesterone can counter act relaxin activity by inducing an anti-inflammatory response and decrease the MMP concentrations and uterine contractility (Palejwala, Stein *et al.*, 2001).

6. Prevention of preterm birth

The prevention of preterm birth is one of the major objectives of modern obstetrics. In the US there is an initiative to reduce the rate of preterm birth to 6.1% by 2010, and the March of Dimes has made this topic its main field of interest. In spite of all efforts, at present there is

no specific treatment for spontaneous preterm birth and this is attributed to the syndromic nature of preterm delivery that cannot be resolved by a single medication or intervention.
Currently there is wide agreement regarding the beneficial effect of two treatments: (1) the administration of corticosteroids for patients at risk for preterm birth to reduced acute neonatal morbidity; and (2) prophylactic antibiotic treatment for patients with preterm PROM that has occurred from 24 to 32 weeks of gestation (Mercer, Miodovnik *et al.*, 1997; Kenyon, Taylor *et al.*, 2001) but not for preterm labor with intact membranes (Kenyon, Brocklehurst *et al.*, 2008). This treatment has been proven to prolong pregnancy and reduce the rate of acute neonatal morbidity in patients with preterm PROM (Kenyon, Brocklehurst *et al.*, 2008). However, the results of the follow up of children after 7 years were as follows: (1) In children who were born after preterm PROM, neither antibiotic regime was associated with a significant effect on the overall level of behavioral, medical status and academics achievements (Kenyon, Pike *et al.*, 2008). (2) In contrast, prophylactic antibiotic treatment of patients with preterm labor had a negative effect on the children's outcome at the age of 7. Treatment with erythromycin was associated with increased functional impairment of children of mother with preterm labor and intact membranes (Kenyon, Pike *et al.*, 2008). The more worrisome outcome was the higher rate of cerebral palsy among children whose mothers were treated with erythromycin (OR 1.93, 95% CI 1.21–3.09) as well as in those treated with co-amoxicalve (OR 1.69, 95% CI 1.07–2.67) (Kenyon, Pike *et al.*, 2008). Thus, prophylactic antibiotic treatment should not be administrated to patients and preterm labor with intact membranes.
Yet, these treatments are targeted to reduce the rate of complications rather than to prevent the "disease". In the recent years, attempts to prevent spontaneous preterm birth are mainly by two approaches: (1) the administration of progesterone to patients with a history of preterm birth or with a short sonographic cervix; and (2) placement of a cerclage for cervical os insufficiency.

6.1 Progesterone for the prevention of preterm birth

Progestogens administration for the prevention of recurrent abortion or preterm birth has been a subject of investigation (Papiernik-Berkhauer, 1970; LEVINE, 1964; BISHOP, RICHARDS *et al.*, 1950; BISHOP and RICHARDS, 1952; Check, Chase *et al.*, 1987; Tognoni, Ferrario *et al.*, 1980; Gerhard, Gwinner *et al.*, 1987; Johnson, Austin *et al.*, 1975; Hauth, Gilstrap, III *et al.*, 1983; Yemini, Borenstein *et al.*, 1985; Hartikainen-Sorri, Kauppila *et al.*, 1980; Breart, Lanfranchi *et al.*, 1979) and meta-analyses (Daya, 1989; Goldstein, Berrier *et al.*, 1989; Keirse, 1990) or several decades. However, progesterone gained a wide acceptance as a valid treatment for the prevention of preterm birth (2003) only after the publication of the studies by da Fonseca (da Fonseca, Bittar *et al.*, 2003) and the NICHD MFMU (Meis, Klebanoff *et al.*, 2003) who investigated its efficacy in the prevention of preterm birth in women with a history of preterm delivery.
Da Fonseca et al. (da Fonseca, Bittar *et al.*, 2003) reported the results of a randomized, double-blinded, placebo-controlled study including 142 high-risk singleton pregnancies including patients with: (1) at least one previous spontaneous preterm birth; (2) prophylactic cervical cerclage; or (3) a uterine malformation. The patients were randomized to receive either daily vaginal suppository of micronized progesterone (100 mg) or placebo, from 24 to 34 weeks of gestation. The rate of preterm delivery <37 weeks and <34 weeks was lower in the progesterone group than in the placebo group (<37 weeks, progesterone: 13.8% vs.

placebo: 28.5%, *p*=0.03; and < 34 weeks, progesterone: 2.8% vs. 18.6%, *p*=0.002) (da Fonseca, Bittar *et al.*, 2003). The authors concluded that prophylactic vaginal progesterone appeared to reduce the rate of preterm delivery in women at high risk for preterm birth (da Fonseca, Bittar *et al.*, 2003).

The NICHD-MFMU network (Meis, Klebanoff *et al.*, 2003) reported the results of a multicenter double-blind, placebo-controlled clinical trial testing whether 17-hydroxy progesterone caproate (OHPC) administration can reduce the rate of preterm delivery in patients with a history of spontaneous preterm birth. The patients were enrolled at 16 to 20 weeks of gestation and randomly assigned in a 2:1 ratio to receive either a weekly injection of 250 mg of 17-OHPC or a weekly injection of placebo until delivery or 36 weeks of gestation. Treatment with 17-OHPC significantly reduced the rate of preterm delivery at less than 37 weeks, less than 35 weeks, and less than 32 weeks of gestation (<37 weeks, RR 0.66; 95% CI 0.54–0.81; <35 weeks, RR 0.67; 95% CI 0.48–0.93; and <32 weeks, RR 0.58; 95% CI 0.37–0.91]. Moreover, neonates born to women treated with 17-OHPC had significantly lower rates of NEC, IVH and need for supplemental oxygen (Meis, Klebanoff *et al.*, 2003). Thus, among women at high risk for preterm delivery, a weekly injection of 17-OHPC resulted in a reduction in the rate of recurrent preterm birth and several neonatal complications (Meis, Klebanoff *et al.*, 2003). The beneficial effect of 17-OHPC and vaginal progesterone in the reduction of preterm birth and of 17-OHPC in the reduction of the rate of neonates with low birth weight were further supported by systematic reviews meta-analyses and a Cochrane review (Sanchez-Ramos, Kaunitz *et al.*, 2005; Dodd, Crowther *et al.*, 2005; Coomarasamy, Thangaratinam *et al.*, 2006; Mackenzie, Walker *et al.*, 2006; Dodd, Flenady *et al.*, 2006).

In 2007, three new randomized clinical trials on the efficacy of progestogens in preventing preterm birth were reported (Rouse, Caritis *et al.*, 2007; O'Brien, Adair *et al.*, 2007; Fonseca, Celik *et al.*, 2007). The recent randomized clinical trials yielded conflicting results. O'Brien et al (O'Brien, Adair *et al.*, 2007) reported the results of a multinational, randomized, double-blind, placebo-controlled trial of progesterone vaginal gel administration to patients with a history of spontaneous preterm birth between 20 to 35 weeks of gestation. Women were randomized, between 18 to 22 completed weeks of gestation, to receive daily treatment of progesterone vaginal polycarbophil-based gel (Crinone®, 8%, 90 mg) or placebo (Replens®) that were self-administered either until delivery, 37 weeks of gestation, or the occurrence of PROM. Vaginal progesterone did not reduce the rate of preterm birth at ≤32, ≤35, or ≤37 weeks of gestation. Moreover, there were no differences in the neonatal and maternal outcomes (O'Brien, Adair *et al.*, 2007).

The beneficial effect of progesterone in patients with a sonographic short cervix has been recently reported (Facchinetti, Paganelli *et al.*, 2007). A randomized prospective clinical trial (Facchinetti, Paganelli *et al.*, 2007) in which women with preterm labor and intact membranes (25 to 33 6/7 weeks) were allocated to either observation or IM administration of 341 mg of 17-OHPC twice a week until 36 weeks of gestation or delivery was performed. Patients allocated to receive 17-OHPC had a longer sonographic cervical length than those in the observation group (Facchinetti, Paganelli *et al.*, 2007); suggesting that progesterone may have major effects on the uterine cervix.

Fonseca et al. (Fonseca, Celik *et al.*, 2007) reported the results of a randomized clinical trial evaluating the efficacy of vaginal progesterone in reducing the rate of preterm birth in women with a sonographic short cervix (≤15 mm by transvaginal ultrasound between 20 to 25 weeks of gestation). Women were allocated to daily vaginal administration of 200 mg of micronized progesterone or placebo (safflower oil) from 24 to 34 weeks. The frequency of spontaneous preterm delivery <34 weeks was significantly lower in the progesterone group than that in patients allocated to placebo (19.2% vs. 34.4%; p=0.007) (Fonseca, Celik *et al.*, 2007). A secondary analysis of this trial indicated that among women without a history of delivery <34 weeks, the incidence of preterm birth was significantly lower in women receiving progesterone than in those allocated to placebo (RR 0.57, 95% CI 0.35-0.93) suggesting that progesterone may be beneficial to patients with a sonographic short cervix even without a history of preterm birth (Fonseca, Celik *et al.*, 2007).

The secondary retrospective analysis (Defranco, O'Brien *et al.*, 2007) of the study by O'Brien et al (O'Brien, Adair *et al.*, 2007). supports the findings of Fonseca et al (Fonseca, Celik *et al.*, 2007) that patients with a short cervix may benefit from vaginal progesterone administration. However, the authors (Defranco, O'Brien *et al.*, 2007) reported that vaginal progesterone gel may have a beneficial effect in reducing preterm delivery <32 weeks of gestation at a sonographic cervical length of <28 mm (Defranco, O'Brien *et al.*, 2007). These findings imply that the cutoff of 15 mm may be too stringent and progesterone may also work in women with a longer cervix. As the frequency of a cervix of ≤15 mm is 1.7% but that of <28 mm is about 10% (Iams, Goldenberg *et al.*, 1996; Iams, Goldenberg *et al.*, 2001; Iams, Johnson *et al.*, 1995), this could expand the therapeutic range of progesterone.

The study of De Franco et al (Defranco, O'Brien *et al.*, 2007) provides the first hint that vaginal progesterone administration may improve infant outcome in properly selected patients. The frequency of NICU admission was lower in women with a cervical length of ≤30 mm and <28 mm and who had received progesterone treatment than in those allocated to placebo. The same was the case for the duration of NICU length of stay (Defranco, O'Brien *et al.*, 2007). However, these conclusions must be considered tentative because they derive from a secondary analysis which is intended to be hypothesis-generating.

In contrast to the results in singleton gestations, the administration of progesterone for the prevention of preterm birth in twin gestation had no beneficial effect. Hartikainen-Sorri et al (Hartikainen-Sorri, Kauppila *et al.*, 1980) more than twenty-five years ago, and recently Rouse et al (Rouse, Caritis *et al.*, 2007) reported the results of a multicenter, placebo-controlled, double-blind, randomized clinical trials of 17-OHPC for prevention of preterm birth in twin pregnancies. Both studies concluded that there was no beneficial effect of 17-OHPC administration for the prevention of preterm birth in twin gestation.

6.2 The role of cervical cerclage in the prevention of preterm birth

Keeping with the view that cervical insufficiency is a mechanical disorder of the cervix, placement of a cervical stitch (cerclage) has been proposed as a treatment for this disorder. The clinical value of cervical cerclage has been subject of many observational and randomized clinical trials (To, Palaniappan *et al.*, 2002; 1993; Althuisius, Dekker *et al.*, 2002; Althuisius, Dekker *et al.*, 2000; Althuisius, Dekker *et al.*, 2001; Althuisius, Dekker *et al.*, 2003; Lazar, Gueguen *et al.*, 1984; To, Alfirevic *et al.*, 2004) and systematic reviews (Belej-Rak, Okun *et al.*, 2003; Drakeley, Roberts *et al.*, 2003a; Drakeley, Roberts *et al.*, 2003b). Yet controversies still exist regarding the subset of patients who will benefit from cerclage.

The current evidence suggests the following: (1) Women who are at low risk for preterm delivery (by history) and have a sonographic short cervix (≤15 mm) will not benefit from cerclage (To, Alfirevic *et al.*, 2004). (2) The benefit of cerclage in women who have a high risk for preterm birth, both by history and a sonographic short cervix observed during the current pregnancy, is controversial (Berghella, Odibo *et al.*, 2004; Rust, Atlas *et al.*, 2000;

Rust, Atlas *et al.*, 2001; Althuisius, Dekker *et al.*, 2000; Althuisius, Dekker *et al.*, 2001). However, a recent randomize clinical trial conducted by the NICHD MFM network among patients with a prior preterm birth <34 weeks of gestation. Patients with a cervical length <25 mm randomly assigned to cerclage reported a beneficial effect of cerclage (Owen, Hankins *et al.*, 2009). This benefit was highly concentrated in women with very short cervical length (<15 mm) (Owen, Hankins *et al.*, 2009). (3) Among patients at risk for preterm delivery, serial sonographic examinations of the cervix followed by cerclage in those who shortened the cervix is a reasonable alternative to prophylactic placement of cerclage based upon uncontrolled studies (Guzman, Forster *et al.*, 1998; To, Alfirevic *et al.*, 2004; Higgins, Kornman *et al.*, 2004). (4) The role of prophylactic cerclage in high-risk patients without a sonographic short cervix for the prevention of preterm delivery/midtrimester abortion (by history) is unclear (1993; Althuisius, Dekker *et al.*, 2001; Lazar, Gueguen *et al.*, 1984; Odibo, Elkousy *et al.*, 2003; Rush, Isaacs *et al.*, 1984). (5) In one trial, emergency cerclage combined with indomethacin administration appeared to reduce the rate of preterm delivery in patients with the clinical presentation of "cervical insufficiency" (Althuisius, Dekker *et al.*, 2003). This evidence indicates that only patients with the clinical presentation of "acute cervical insufficiency" and those with a previous history consistent with "cervical insufficiency" or spontaneous preterm birth and a progressive shortening of the cervix demonstrated by ultrasound may benefit from cerclage placement (Althuisius, Dekker *et al.*, 2001; Althuisius, Dekker *et al.*, 2003; Berghella, Rafael *et al.*, 2011; Berghella, Keeler *et al.*, 2010; Owen, Hankins *et al.*, 2009). The inflammatory status of the endocervix may be an additional criterion to identify those patients that could benefit from cerclage placement and those for whom this intervention may be harmful. (Sakai, Shiozaki *et al.*, 2006)

6.3 The role of progesterone in primary prevention of preterm birth

A recent study by Hassan et al (Hassan, Romero *et al.*, 2011)raised for the first time the possibility of primary prevention of preterm delivery. The study included patients with a short cervix (cervical length between 10-20 mm) who were randomized at 19-24 weeks to the administration of daily vaginal progesterone gel vs. placebo, regardless to their obstetrical history. 32,091 were screened, of them 733 had a short cervix, and 465 were randomized. Women at the progesterone group had a significant reduction in the rate of preterm birth before 33 weeks of gestation and a significant lower rate of neonatal complications in comparison to those in the placebo group (Hassan, Romero *et al.*, 2011). Thus, cervical length is an effective risk assessment tool for the identification of patients at risk for preterm birth and vaginal progesterone gel can prevent preterm delivery in a significant portion of patients with a short cervix.

7. Summary

Assisted reproduction aids a substantial proportion of women to conceive and deliver, however, these pregnancies are at increased risk for preterm birth. Some of the mechanisms leading to preterm parturition in these patients are inherited from the nature of conception like multiple gestations along with their complications. In addition, especially among singleton gestations, ART are an independent risk factor for preterm delivery and this may result from the underlying mechanisms leading to maternal infertility like infection/inflammation of the genital tract as well as other mechanisms. Thus, women who conceived following ART cycles should be followed and treated as a patient at risk for preterm birth.

8. References

[1] (1993) Final report of the Medical Research Council/Royal College of Obstetricians and Gynaecologists multicentre randomised trial of cervical cerclage. MRC/RCOG Working Party on Cervical Cerclage. Br J Obstet Gynaecol, 100, 516-523.

[2] (1999) Preterm singleton births--United States, 1989-1996. MMWR Morb Mortal Wkly Rep, 48, 185-189.

[3] (1994b) Abstracts of the 10th annual meeting of the European Society of Human Reproduction and Embryology. Brussels, Belgium, 27-29 June 1994. Hum Reprod, 9 Suppl 4:1-227., 1-227.

[4] (2003) ACOG Committee Opinion. Use of progesterone to reduce preterm birth. Obstet Gynecol, 102, 1115-1116.

[5] (1994a) Abstracts of the 10th annual meeting of the European Society of Human Reproduction and Embryology. Brussels, Belgium, 27-29 June 1994. Hum Reprod, 9 Suppl 4:1-227., 1-227.

[6] (2008) Centers for Disease Control and Prevention, American Society for Reproductive Medicine, Society for Assisted Reproductive Technology. 2006 Assisted Reproductive Technology Success Rates: National summary and fertility clinic reports. In Centers for Disease Control and Prevention, pp. 1-584.

[7] Baxi A and Kaushal M (2008) Outcome of twin pregnancies conceived after assisted reproductive techniques. J Hum Reprod Sci, 1, 25-28.

[8] Alanen A (1998) Polymerase chain reaction in the detection of microbes in amniotic fluid. Ann Med, 30, 288-295.

[9] Allen EG, Freeman SB, Druschel C, Hobbs CA, O'Leary LA, Romitti PA, Royle MH, Torfs CP, and Sherman SL (2009) Maternal age and risk for trisomy 21 assessed by the origin of chromosome nondisjunction: a report from the Atlanta and National Down Syndrome Projects. Hum Genet, 125, 41-52.

[10] Allen VM, Wilson RD, and Cheung A (2006) Pregnancy outcomes after assisted reproductive technology. J Obstet Gynaecol Can, 28, 220-250.

[11] Allport VC, Pieber D, Slater DM, Newton R, White JO, and Bennett PR (2001) Human labour is associated with nuclear factor-kappaB activity which mediates cyclo-oxygenase-2 expression and is involved with the 'functional progesterone withdrawal'. Mol Hum Reprod, 7, 581-586.

[12] Althuisius S, Dekker G, Hummel P, Bekedam D, Kuik D, and van GH (2002) Cervical Incompetence Prevention Randomized Cerclage Trial (CIPRACT): effect of therapeutic cerclage with bed rest vs. bed rest only on cervical length. Ultrasound Obstet Gynecol, 20, 163-167.

[13] Althuisius SM, Dekker GA, Hummel P, Bekedam DJ, and van Geijn HP (2001) Final results of the Cervical Incompetence Prevention Randomized Cerclage Trial (CIPRACT): therapeutic cerclage with bed rest versus bed rest alone. Am J Obstet Gynecol, 185, 1106-1112.

[14] Althuisius SM, Dekker GA, Hummel P, and van Geijn HP (2003) Cervical incompetence prevention randomized cerclage trial: emergency cerclage with bed rest versus bed rest alone. Am J Obstet Gynecol, 189, 907-910.

[15] Althuisius SM, Dekker GA, van Geijn HP, Bekedam DJ, and Hummel P (2000) Cervical incompetence prevention randomized cerclage trial (CIPRACT): study design and preliminary results. Am J Obstet Gynecol, 183, 823-829.

[16] Ananth CV, Getahun D, Peltier MR, Salihu HM, and Vintzileos AM (2006) Recurrence of spontaneous versus medically indicated preterm birth. Am J Obstet Gynecol, 195, 643-650.
[17] Ananth CV, Joseph KS, Oyelese Y, Demissie K, and Vintzileos AM (2005) Trends in preterm birth and perinatal mortality among singletons: United States, 1989 through 2000. Obstet Gynecol, 105, 1084-1091.
[18] Ananth CV and Vintzileos AM (2006a) Epidemiology of preterm birth and its clinical subtypes. J Matern Fetal Neonatal Med, 19, 773-782.
[19] Ananth CV and Vintzileos AM (2006b) Maternal-fetal conditions necessitating a medical intervention resulting in preterm birth. Am J Obstet Gynecol, 195, 1557-1563.
[20] Arias F (1990) Placental insufficiency: an important cause of preterm labor and preterm premature ruptured membranes. Presented at the 10th Annual Meeting of the Society of Perinatal Obstetricians, 23–27 January 1990, Houston, TX, USA.
[21] Arias F, Rodriquez L, Rayne SC, and Kraus FT (1993) Maternal placental vasculopathy and infection: two distinct subgroups among patients with preterm labor and preterm ruptured membranes. Am J Obstet Gynecol, 168, 585-591.
[22] Atkinson AB and Marlier E (2010) Income and living conditions in Europe., European Union, 2010.
[23] Averbuch B, Mazor M, Shoham-Vardi I, Chaim W, Vardi H, Horowitz S, and Shuster M (1995) Intra-uterine infection in women with preterm premature rupture of membranes: maternal and neonatal characteristics. Eur J Obstet Gynecol Reprod Biol, 62, 25-29.
[24] Bang B (1987) The etiology of epizootic abortion. J Comp Anthol Ther, 10, 125.
[25] Barbieri RL (1992) Hyperandrogenism: new insights into etiology, diagnosis, and therapy. Curr Opin Obstet Gynecol, 4, 372-379.
[26] Barker DJ (2004) The developmental origins of adult disease. J Am Coll Nutr, 23, 588S-595S.
[27] Belej-Rak T, Okun N, Windrim R, Ross S, and Hannah ME (2003) Effectiveness of cervical cerclage for a sonographically shortened cervix: a systematic review and meta-analysis. Am J Obstet Gynecol, 189, 1679-1687.
[28] Belt AR, Baldassare JJ, Molnar M, Romero R, and Hertelendy F (1999) The nuclear transcription factor NF-kappaB mediates interleukin-1beta-induced expression of cyclooxygenase-2 in human myometrial cells. Am J Obstet Gynecol, 181, 359-366.
[29] Ben-Shlomo I (2003) The polycystic ovary syndrome: what does insulin resistance have to do with it? Reprod Biomed Online, 6, 36-42.
[30] Benedetti TJ, Valle R, and Ledger WJ (1982) Antepartum pneumonia in pregnancy. Am J Obstet Gynecol, 144, 413-417.
[31] Berghella V, Keeler SM, To MS, Althuisius SM, and Rust OA (2010) Effectiveness of cerclage according to severity of cervical length shortening: a meta-analysis. Ultrasound Obstet Gynecol, 35, 468-473.
[32] Berghella V, Odibo AO, and Tolosa JE (2004) Cerclage for prevention of preterm birth in women with a short cervix found on transvaginal ultrasound examination: a randomized trial. Am J Obstet Gynecol, 191, 1311-1317.

[33] Berghella V, Rafael TJ, Szychowski JM, Rust OA, and Owen J (2011) Cerclage for short cervix on ultrasonography in women with singleton gestations and previous preterm birth: a meta-analysis. Obstet Gynecol, 117, 663-671.
[34] Berkowitz GS, Skovron ML, Lapinski RH, and Berkowitz RL (1990) Delayed childbearing and the outcome of pregnancy. N Engl J Med, 322, 659-664.
[35] Besinger R and Carlson N (1995) The physiology of preterm labor. In Keith L, Papiernik E, Keith D, and Luke B (eds) Multiple Pregnancy: Epidemiology, Gestation and Perinatal Outcome. Parthenon Publishing, London, p. 415.
[36] BISHOP PM and RICHARDS NA (1952) Habitual abortion; further observations on the prophylactic value of progesterone pellet implantation. Br Med J, 1, 244-246.
[37] BISHOP PM, RICHARDS NA, and DOLL R (1950) Habitual abortion; prophylactic value of progesterone pellet implantation. Br Med J, 2, 130-133.
[38] Blickstein I, Jones C, and Keith LG (2003) Zygotic-splitting rates after single-embryo transfers in in vitro fertilization. N Engl J Med, 348, 2366-2367.
[39] Blickstein I, Verhoeven HC, and Keith LG (1999) Zygotic splitting after assisted reproduction. N Engl J Med, 340, 738-739.
[40] Boomsma CM, Eijkemans MJ, Hughes EG, Visser GH, Fauser BC, and Macklon NS (2006) A meta-analysis of pregnancy outcomes in women with polycystic ovary syndrome. Hum Reprod Update, 12, 673-683.
[41] Boulet SL, Schieve LA, Nannini A, Ferre C, Devine O, Cohen B, Zhang Z, Wright V, and Macaluso M (2008) Perinatal outcomes of twin births conceived using assisted reproduction technology: a population-based study. Hum Reprod, 23, 1941-1948.
[42] Breart G, Lanfranchi M, Chavigny C, Rumeau-Rouquette C, and Sureau C (1979) A comparative study of the efficiency of hydroxyprogesterone caproate and of chlormadinone acetate in the prevention of premature labor. Int J Gynaecol Obstet, 16, 381-384.
[43] Bujold E, Morency AM, Rallu F, Ferland S, Tetu A, Duperron L, Audibert F, and Laferriere C (2008) Bacteriology of amniotic fluid in women with suspected cervical insufficiency. J Obstet Gynaecol Can, 30, 882-887.
[44] Carey JC, Klebanoff MA, Hauth JC, Hillier SL, Thom EA, Ernest JM, Heine RP, Nugent RP, Fischer ML, Leveno KJ et al (2000) Metronidazole to prevent preterm delivery in pregnant women with asymptomatic bacterial vaginosis. National Institute of Child Health and Human Development Network of Maternal-Fetal Medicine Units. N Engl J Med, 342, 534-540.
[45] Carolan M, Davey MA, Biro MA, and Kealy M (2011) Older maternal age and intervention in labor: a population-based study comparing older and younger first-time mothers in Victoria, Australia. Birth, 38, 24-29.
[46] Carroll SG, Papaioannou S, Ntumazah IL, Philpott-Howard J, and Nicolaides KH (1996) Lower genital tract swabs in the prediction of intrauterine infection in preterm prelabour rupture of the membranes. Br J Obstet Gynaecol, 103, 54-59.
[47] Chaim W, Mazor M, and Leiberman JR (1997) The relationship between bacterial vaginosis and preterm birth. A review. Arch Gynecol Obstet, 259, 51-58.
[48] Chaiworapongsa T, Espinoza J, Yoshimatsu J, Kim YM, Bujold E, Edwin S, Yoon BH, and Romero R (2002) Activation of coagulation system in preterm labor and preterm premature rupture of membranes. J Matern Fetal Neonatal Med, 11, 368-373.

[49] Chan OT, Mannino FL, and Benirschke K (2007) A retrospective analysis of placentas from twin pregnancies derived from assisted reproductive technology. Twin Res Hum Genet, 10, 385-393.

[50] Check JH, Chase JS, Nowroozi K, Wu CH, and Adelson HG (1987) Progesterone therapy to decrease first-trimester spontaneous abortions in previous aborters. Int J Fertil, 32, 192-193.

[51] Chen XK, Wen SW, Bottomley J, Smith GN, Leader A, and Walker MC (2009) In vitro fertilization is associated with an increased risk for preeclampsia. Hypertens Pregnancy, 28, 1-12.

[52] Chow L and Lye SJ (1994) Expression of the gap junction protein connexin-43 is increased in the human myometrium toward term and with the onset of labor. Am J Obstet Gynecol, 170, 788-795.

[53] Cleary-Goldman J, Malone FD, Vidaver J, Ball RH, Nyberg DA, Comstock CH, Saade GR, Eddleman KA, Klugman S, Dugoff L et al (2005) Impact of maternal age on obstetric outcome. Obstet Gynecol, 105, 983-990.

[54] Combs CA, Katz MA, Kitzmiller JL, and Brescia RJ (1993) Experimental preeclampsia produced by chronic constriction of the lower aorta: validation with longitudinal blood pressure measurements in conscious rhesus monkeys. Am J Obstet Gynecol, 169, 215-223.

[55] Coomarasamy A, Thangaratinam S, Gee H, and Khan KS (2006) Progesterone for the prevention of preterm birth: a critical evaluation of evidence. Eur J Obstet Gynecol Reprod Biol, 129, 111-118.

[56] Cotton DB, Hill LM, Strassner HT, Platt LD, and Ledger WJ (1984) Use of amniocentesis in preterm gestation with ruptured membranes. Obstet Gynecol, 63, 38-43.

[57] Coultrip LL and Grossman JH (1992) Evaluation of rapid diagnostic tests in the detection of microbial invasion of the amniotic cavity. Am J Obstet Gynecol, 167, 1231-1242.

[58] Crawford BS, Davis J, and Harrigill K (1997) Uterine artery atherosclerotic disease: histologic features and clinical correlation. Obstet Gynecol, 90, 210-215.

[59] Cunningham FG, Morris GB, and Mickal A (1973) Acute pyelonephritis of pregnancy: A clinical review. Obstet Gynecol, 42, 112-117.

[60] da Fonseca EB, Bittar RE, Carvalho MH, and Zugaib M (2003) Prophylactic administration of progesterone by vaginal suppository to reduce the incidence of spontaneous preterm birth in women at increased risk: a randomized placebo-controlled double-blind study. Am J Obstet Gynecol, 188, 419-424.

[61] Daniel Y, Ochshorn Y, Fait G, Geva E, Bar-Am A, and Lessing JB (2000) Analysis of 104 twin pregnancies conceived with assisted reproductive technologies and 193 spontaneously conceived twin pregnancies. Fertil Steril, 74, 683-689.

[62] Das UG and Sysyn GD (2004) Abnormal fetal growth: intrauterine growth retardation, small for gestational age, large for gestational age. Pediatr Clin North Am, 51, 639-54, viii.

[63] Davison RM (1998) New approaches to insulin resistance in polycystic ovarian syndrome. Curr Opin Obstet Gynecol, 10, 193-198.

[64] Daya S (1989) Efficacy of progesterone support for pregnancy in women with recurrent miscarriage. A meta-analysis of controlled trials. Br J Obstet Gynaecol, 96, 275-280.

[65] De Sutter P, Bontinck J, Schutysers V, Van der EJ, Gerris J, and Dhont M (2006) First-trimester bleeding and pregnancy outcome in singletons after assisted reproduction. Hum Reprod, 21, 1907-1911.

[66] Defranco EA, O'Brien JM, Adair CD, Lewis DF, Hall DR, Fusey S, Soma-Pillay P, Porter K, How H, Schakis R et al (2007) Vaginal progesterone is associated with a decrease in risk for early preterm birth and improved neonatal outcome in women with a short cervix: a secondary analysis from a randomized, double-blind, placebo-controlled trial. Ultrasound Obstet Gynecol, 30, 697-705.

[67] Dodd JM, Crowther CA, Cincotta R, Flenady V, and Robinson JS (2005) Progesterone supplementation for preventing preterm birth: a systematic review and meta-analysis. Acta Obstet Gynecol Scand, 84, 526-533.

[68] Dodd JM, Flenady V, Cincotta R, and Crowther CA (2006) Prenatal administration of progesterone for preventing preterm birth. Cochrane Database Syst Rev, CD004947.

[69] Drakeley AJ, Roberts D, and Alfirevic Z (2003b) Cervical stitch (cerclage) for preventing pregnancy loss in women. Cochrane Database Syst Rev, CD003253.

[70] Drakeley AJ, Roberts D, and Alfirevic Z (2003a) Cervical cerclage for prevention of preterm delivery: meta-analysis of randomized trials. Obstet Gynecol, 102, 621-627.

[71] Elovitz MA, Baron J, and Phillippe M (2001) The role of thrombin in preterm parturition. Am J Obstet Gynecol, 185, 1059-1063.

[72] Elovitz MA, Saunders T, scher-Landsberg J, and Phillippe M (2000) Effects of thrombin on myometrial contractions in vitro and in vivo. Am J Obstet Gynecol, 183, 799-804.

[73] Erez O, Espinoza J, Chaiworapongsa T, Gotsch F, Kusanovic JP, Than NG, Mazaki-Tovi S, Vaisbuch E, Papp Z, Yoon BH et al (2008) A link between a hemostatic disorder and preterm PROM: a role for tissue factor and tissue factor pathway inhibitor. J Matern Fetal Neonatal Med, 21, 732-744.

[74] Erez O, Gotsch F, Mazaki-Tovi S, Vaisbuch E, Kusanovic JP, Kim CJ, Chaiworapongsa T, Hoppensteadt D, Fareed J, Than NG et al (2009) Evidence of maternal platelet activation, excessive thrombin generation, and high amniotic fluid tissue factor immunoreactivity and functional activity in patients with fetal death. J Matern Fetal Neonatal Med, 22, 672-687.

[75] Erez O, Mayer A, Shoham-Vardi I, Dukler D, and Mazor M (2008) Primiparity, assisted reproduction, and preterm birth in twin pregnancies: a population based study. Arch Gynecol Obstet, 277, 311-317.

[76] Erez O, Romer R, Vaisbuch E, Chaiworapongsa T, Kusanovic JP, Mazaki-Tovi S, Gotsch F, Gomez R, Maymon E, Pacora P et al (2009) Changes in amniotic fluid concentration of thrombin-antithrombin III complexes in patients with preterm labor: evidence of an increased thrombin generation. J Matern Fetal Neonatal Med, 22, 971-982.

[77] Erez O, Vardi IS, Hallak M, Hershkovitz R, Dukler D, and Mazor M (2006) Preeclampsia in twin gestations: association with IVF treatments, parity and maternal age. J Matern Fetal Neonatal Med, 19, 141-146.

[78] Eschenbach DA (1993) Bacterial vaginosis and anaerobes in obstetric-gynecologic infection. Clin Infect Dis, 16 Suppl 4:S282-7., S282-S287.

[79] Eschenbach DA, Gravett MG, Chen KC, Hoyme UB, and Holmes KK (1984) Bacterial vaginosis during pregnancy. An association with prematurity and postpartum complications. Scand J Urol Nephrol Suppl, 86:213-22., 213-222.

[80] Facchinetti F, Paganelli S, Comitini G, Dante G, and Volpe A (2007) Cervical length changes during preterm cervical ripening: effects of 17-alpha-hydroxyprogesterone caproate. Am J Obstet Gynecol, 196, 453-454.
[81] Fan YD, Pastorek JG, Miller JM, Jr., and Mulvey J (1987) Acute pyelonephritis in pregnancy. Am J Perinatol, 4, 324-326.
[82] Farrugia G, Holm AN, Rich A, Sarr MG, Szurszewski JH, and Rae JL (1999) A mechanosensitive calcium channel in human intestinal smooth muscle cells. Gastroenterology, 117, 900-905.
[83] Fidel PL, Jr., Romero R, Wolf N, Cutright J, Ramirez M, Araneda H, and Cotton DB (1994) Systemic and local cytokine profiles in endotoxin-induced preterm parturition in mice. Am J Obstet Gynecol, 170, 1467-1475.
[84] Finland M and Dublin T.D. (1939) Pneumococcic pneumonia complicating pregnancy and the puerperium. JAMA, 112, 1027-1032.
[85] Fonseca EB, Celik E, Parra M, Singh M, and Nicolaides KH (2007) Progesterone and the risk of preterm birth among women with a short cervix. N Engl J Med, 357, 462-469.
[86] Franks S, Robinson S, and Willis DS (1996) Nutrition, insulin and polycystic ovary syndrome. Rev Reprod, 1, 47-53.
[87] Fretts RC, Schmittdiel J, McLean FH, Usher RH, and Goldman MB (1995) Increased maternal age and the risk of fetal death. N Engl J Med, 333, 953-957.
[88] Garite TJ, Freeman RK, Linzey EM, and Braly P (1979) The use of amniocentesis in patients with premature rupture of membranes. Obstet Gynecol, 54, 226-230.
[89] Gerhard I, Gwinner B, Eggert-Kruse W, and Runnebaum B (1987) Double-blind controlled trial of progesterone substitution in threatened abortion. Biol Res Pregnancy Perinatol, 8, 26-34.
[90] Gilbert WM, Nesbitt TS, and Danielsen B (1999) Childbearing beyond age 40: pregnancy outcome in 24,032 cases. Obstet Gynecol, 93, 9-14.
[91] Gilles HM, Lawson JB, Sibelas M, Voller A, and Allan N (1969) Malaria, anaemia and pregnancy. Ann Trop Med Parasitol, 63, 245-263.
[92] Goldenberg RL, Culhane JF, Iams JD, and Romero R (2008) Epidemiology and causes of preterm birth. Lancet, 371, 75-84.
[93] Goldstein P, Berrier J, Rosen S, Sacks HS, and Chalmers TC (1989) A meta-analysis of randomized control trials of progestational agents in pregnancy. Br J Obstet Gynaecol, 96, 265-274.
[94] Gomez R, Ghezzi F, Romero R, Munoz H, Tolosa JE, and Rojas I (1995) Premature labor and intra-amniotic infection. Clinical aspects and role of the cytokines in diagnosis and pathophysiology. Clin Perinatol, 22, 281-342.
[95] Goncalves LF, Chaiworapongsa T, and Romero R (2002a) Intrauterine infection and prematurity. Ment Retard Dev Disabil Res Rev, 8, 3-13.
[96] Guaschino S, Ricci E, Franchi M, Frate GD, Tibaldi C, Santo DD, Ghezzi F, Benedetto C, Seta FD, and Parazzini F (2003) Treatment of asymptomatic bacterial vaginosis to prevent pre-term delivery: a randomised trial. Eur J Obstet Gynecol Reprod Biol, 110, 149-152.
[97] Gunby J, Bissonnette F, Librach C, and Cowan L (2011) Assisted reproductive technologies (ART) in Canada: 2007 results from the Canadian ART Register. Fertil Steril, 95, 542-547.

[98] Gurunath S, Pandian Z, Anderson RA, and Bhattacharya S (2011) Defining infertility--a systematic review of prevalence studies. Hum Reprod Update.
[99] Gutmann JN and Corson SL (2001) Female reproductive endocrinology at the turn of the millennium. Int J Fertil Womens Med, 46, 101-115.
[100] Guzman ER, Forster JK, Vintzileos AM, Ananth CV, Walters C, and Gipson K (1998) Pregnancy outcomes in women treated with elective versus ultrasound-indicated cervical cerclage. Ultrasound Obstet Gynecol, 12, 323-327.
[101] Hackney DN, Catov JM, and Simhan HN (2010) Low concentrations of thrombin-inhibitor complexes and the risk of preterm delivery. Am J Obstet Gynecol, 203, 184-186.
[102] Hansen M, Colvin L, Petterson B, Kurinczuk JJ, de KN, and Bower C (2009) Twins born following assisted reproductive technology: perinatal outcome and admission to hospital. Hum Reprod, 24, 2321-2331.
[103] Hartikainen-Sorri AL, Kauppila A, and Tuimala R (1980) Inefficacy of 17 alpha-hydroxyprogesterone caproate in the prevention of prematurity in twin pregnancy. Obstet Gynecol, 56, 692-695.
[104] Hassan SS, Romero R, Berry SM, Dang K, Blackwell SC, Treadwell MC, and Wolfe HM (2000) Patients with an ultrasonographic cervical length < or =15 mm have nearly a 50% risk of early spontaneous preterm delivery. Am J Obstet Gynecol, 182, 1458-1467.
[105] Hassan SS, Romero R, Vidyadhari D, Fusey S, Baxter JK, Khandelwal M, Vijayaraghavan J, Trivedi Y, Soma-Pillay P, Sambarey P et al (2011) Vaginal progesterone reduces the rate of preterm birth in women with a sonographic short cervix: a multicenter, randomized, double-blind, placebo-controlled trial. Ultrasound Obstet Gynecol, 38, 18-31.
[106] Hauth JC, Gilstrap LC, III, Brekken AL, and Hauth JM (1983) The effect of 17 alpha-hydroxyprogesterone caproate on pregnancy outcome in an active-duty military population. Am J Obstet Gynecol, 146, 187-190.
[107] Heath VC, Southall TR, Souka AP, Elisseou A, and Nicolaides KH (1998) Cervical length at 23 weeks of gestation: prediction of spontaneous preterm delivery. Ultrasound Obstet Gynecol, 12, 312-317.
[108] Herd N and Jordan T (1981) An investigtion of malaria during pregnancy in Zimbabwe. Afr J Med, 27, 62.
[109] Hibbard L, Thrupp L, Summeril S, Smale M, and Adams R (1967) Treatment of pyelonephritis in pregnancy. Am J Obstet Gynecol, 98, 609-615.
[110] Higgins SP, Kornman LH, Bell RJ, and Brennecke SP (2004) Cervical surveillance as an alternative to elective cervical cerclage for pregnancy management of suspected cervical incompetence. Aust N Z J Obstet Gynaecol, 44, 228-232.
[111] Hill LM, Breckle R, Thomas ML, and Fries JK (1987) Polyhydramnios: ultrasonically detected prevalence and neonatal outcome. Obstet Gynecol, 69, 21-25.
[112] Hitti J, Riley DE, Krohn MA, Hillier SL, Agnew KJ, Krieger JN, and Eschenbach DA (1997) Broad-spectrum bacterial rDNA polymerase chain reaction assay for detecting amniotic fluid infection among women in premature labor. Clin Infect Dis, 24, 1228-1232.

[113] Holloway JA, Warner JO, Vance GH, Diaper ND, Warner JA, and Jones CA (2000) Detection of house-dust-mite allergen in amniotic fluid and umbilical-cord blood. Lancet, 356, 1900-1902.

[114] Holm AN, Rich A, Sarr MG, and Farrugia G (2000) Whole cell current and membrane potential regulation by a human smooth muscle mechanosensitive calcium channel. Am J Physiol Gastrointest Liver Physiol, 279, G1155-G1161.

[115] Hook EB, Cross PK, and Schreinemachers DM (1983) Chromosomal abnormality rates at amniocentesis and in live-born infants. JAMA, 249, 2034-2038.

[116] Hu Y, Bock G, Wick G, and Xu Q (1998) Activation of PDGF receptor alpha in vascular smooth muscle cells by mechanical stress. FASEB J, 12, 1135-1142.

[117] Iams JD, Goldenberg RL, Meis PJ, Mercer BM, Moawad A, Das A, Thom E, McNellis D, Copper RL, Johnson F et al (1996) The length of the cervix and the risk of spontaneous premature delivery. National Institute of Child Health and Human Development Maternal Fetal Medicine Unit Network. N Engl J Med, 334, 567-572.

[118] Iams JD, Goldenberg RL, Mercer BM, Moawad AH, Meis PJ, Das AF, Caritis SN, Miodovnik M, Menard MK, Thurnau GR et al (2001) The preterm prediction study: can low-risk women destined for spontaneous preterm birth be identified? Am J Obstet Gynecol, 184, 652-655.

[119] Iams JD, Goldsmith LT, and Weiss G (2001) The preterm prediction study: maternal serum relaxin, sonographic cervical length, and spontaneous preterm birth in twins. J Soc Gynecol Investig, 8, 39-42.

[120] Iams JD, Johnson FF, Sonek J, Sachs L, Gebauer C, and Samuels P (1995) Cervical competence as a continuum: a study of ultrasonographic cervical length and obstetric performance. Am J Obstet Gynecol, 172, 1097-1103.

[121] Institute of Medicine (US) Committee on Understanding Premature Birth and Assuring Healthy Outcomes; Behrman RE, Butler AS, editors. Preterm Birth: Causes, Consequences, and Prevention. Washington (DC): National Academies Press (US); 2007.

[122] Jackson RA, Gibson KA, Wu YW, and Croughan MS (2004) Perinatal outcomes in singletons following in vitro fertilization: a meta-analysis. Obstet Gynecol, 103, 551-563.

[123] Jacobsson B, Ladfors L, and Milsom I (2004a) Advanced maternal age and adverse perinatal outcome. Obstet Gynecol, 104, 727-733.

[124] Johnson JW, Austin KL, Jones GS, Davis GH, and King TM (1975) Efficacy of 17alpha-hydroxyprogesterone caproate in the prevention of premature labor. N Engl J Med, 293, 675-680.

[125] Jones AC, Miles EA, Warner JO, Colwell BM, Bryant TN, and Warner JA (1996) Fetal peripheral blood mononuclear cell proliferative responses to mitogenic and allergenic stimuli during gestation. Pediatr Allergy Immunol, 7, 109-116.

[126] Joseph KS, Kramer MS, Marcoux S, Ohlsson A, Wen SW, Allen A, and Platt R (1998) Determinants of preterm birth rates in Canada from 1981 through 1983 and from 1992 through 1994. N Engl J Med, 339, 1434-1439.

[127] Kamiyama S, Teruya Y, Nohara M, and Kanazawa K (2004) Impact of detection of bacterial endotoxin in menstrual effluent on the pregnancy rate in in vitro fertilization and embryo transfer. Fertil Steril, 82, 788-792.

[128] Kanayama N and Fukamizu H (1989) Mechanical stretching increases prostaglandin E2 in cultured human amnion cells. Gynecol Obstet Invest, 28, 123-126.
[129] Kass E (1962) Maternal urinary tract infection. NY State J Med, 1, 2822-2826.
[130] Keirse MJ (1990) Progestogen administration in pregnancy may prevent preterm delivery. Br J Obstet Gynaecol, 97, 149-154.
[131] Kekki M, Kurki T, Pelkonen J, Kurkinen-Raty M, Cacciatore B, and Paavonen J (2001) Vaginal clindamycin in preventing preterm birth and peripartal infections in asymptomatic women with bacterial vaginosis: a randomized, controlled trial. Obstet Gynecol, 97, 643-648.
[132] Kenyon S, Brocklehurst P, Jones D, Marlow N, Salt A, and Taylor D (2008) MRC ORACLE Children Study. Long term outcomes following prescription of antibiotics to pregnant women with either spontaneous preterm labour or preterm rupture of the membranes. BMC Pregnancy Childbirth, 8:14., 14.
[133] Kenyon S, Pike K, Jones DR, Brocklehurst P, Marlow N, Salt A, and Taylor DJ (2008) Childhood outcomes after prescription of antibiotics to pregnant women with spontaneous preterm labour: 7-year follow-up of the ORACLE II trial. Lancet, 372, 1319-1327.
[134] Kenyon SL, Taylor DJ, and Tarnow-Mordi W (2001) Broad-spectrum antibiotics for preterm, prelabour rupture of fetal membranes: the ORACLE I randomised trial. ORACLE Collaborative Group. Lancet, 357, 979-988.
[135] Kim YM, Bujold E, Chaiworapongsa T, Gomez R, Yoon BH, Thaler HT, Rotmensch S, and Romero R (2003) Failure of physiologic transformation of the spiral arteries in patients with preterm labor and intact membranes. Am J Obstet Gynecol, 189, 1063-1069.
[136] Kim YM, Chaiworapongsa T, Gomez R, Bujold E, Yoon BH, Rotmensch S, Thaler HT, and Romero R (2002) Failure of physiologic transformation of the spiral arteries in the placental bed in preterm premature rupture of membranes. Am J Obstet Gynecol, 187, 1137-1142.
[137] Kloeck FK and Jung H (1973) In vitro release of prostaglandins from the human myometrium under the influence of stretching. Am J Obstet Gynecol, 115, 1066-1069.
[138] Kristiansson P, Svardsudd K, von SB, and Wramsby H (1996) Supraphysiological serum relaxin concentration during pregnancy achieved by in-vitro fertilization is strongly correlated to the number of growing follicles in the treatment cycle. Hum Reprod, 11, 2036-2040.
[139] Kroon B, Harrison K, Martin N, Wong B, and Yazdani A (2011) Miscarriage karyotype and its relationship with maternal body mass index, age, and mode of conception. Fertil Steril, 95, 1827-1829.
[140] Kullander S (1977) Fever and parturition. An experimental study in rabbits. Acta Obstet Gynecol Scand Suppl, 77-85.
[141] Kusanovic JP, Espinoza J, Romero R, Hoppensteadt D, Nien JK, Kim CJ, Erez O, Soto E, Fareed J, Edwin S et al (2007) Plasma protein Z concentrations in pregnant women with idiopathic intrauterine bleeding and in women with spontaneous preterm labor. J Matern Fetal Neonatal Med, 20, 453-463.
[142] Lampinen R, Vehvilainen-Julkunen K, and Kankkunen P (2009) A review of pregnancy in women over 35 years of age. Open Nurs J, 3:33-8., 33-38.

[143] Laudanski T and Rocki W (1975) The effects on stretching and prostaglandin F2alpha on the contractile and bioelectric activity of the uterus in rat. Acta Physiol Pol, 26, 385-393.

[144] Lazar P, Gueguen S, Dreyfus J, Renaud R, Pontonnier G, and Papiernik E (1984) Multicentred controlled trial of cervical cerclage in women at moderate risk of preterm delivery. Br J Obstet Gynaecol, 91, 731-735.

[145] Lee HS, Millward-Sadler SJ, Wright MO, Nuki G, Al-Jamal R, and Salter DM (2002) Activation of Integrin-RACK1/PKCalpha signalling in human articular chondrocyte mechanotransduction. Osteoarthritis Cartilage, 10, 890-897.

[146] Lee SE, Romero R, Park CW, Jun JK, and Yoon BH (2008) The frequency and significance of intraamniotic inflammation in patients with cervical insufficiency. Am J Obstet Gynecol, 198, 633-638.

[147] Lefebvre DL, Piersanti M, Bai XH, Chen ZQ, and Lye SJ (1995) Myometrial transcriptional regulation of the gap junction gene, connexin-43. Reprod Fertil Dev, 7, 603-611.

[148] Leitich H, Bodner-Adler B, Brunbauer M, Kaider A, Egarter C, and Husslein P (2003) Bacterial vaginosis as a risk factor for preterm delivery: a meta-analysis. Am J Obstet Gynecol, 189, 139-147.

[149] LEVINE L (1964) HABITUAL ABORTION. A CONTROLLED STUDY OF PROGESTATIONAL THERAPY. West J Surg Obstet Gynecol, 72:30-6., 30-36.

[150] Li C and Xu Q (2000) Mechanical stress-initiated signal transductions in vascular smooth muscle cells. Cell Signal, 12, 435-445.

[151] Liversedge NH, Turner A, Horner PJ, Keay SD, Jenkins JM, and Hull MG (1999) The influence of bacterial vaginosis on in-vitro fertilization and embryo implantation during assisted reproduction treatment. Hum Reprod, 14, 2411-2415.

[152] Llahi-Camp JM, Rai R, Ison C, Regan L, and Taylor-Robinson D (1996) Association of bacterial vaginosis with a history of second trimester miscarriage. Hum Reprod, 11, 1575-1578.

[153] Lobo RA (1995) Polycystic ovary syndrome/hyperandrogenic chronic anovulation. Adv Endocrinol Metab, 6:167-91., 167-191.

[154] Lockwood CJ, Krikun G, Rahman M, Caze R, Buchwalder L, and Schatz F (2007a) The role of decidualization in regulating endometrial hemostasis during the menstrual cycle, gestation, and in pathological states. Semin Thromb Hemost, 33, 111-117.

[155] Lockwood CJ, Paidas M, Murk WK, Kayisli UA, Gopinath A, Huang SJ, Krikun G, and Schatz F (2009) Involvement of human decidual cell-expressed tissue factor in uterine hemostasis and abruption. Thromb Res, 124, 516-520.

[156] Lockwood CJ, Toti P, Arcuri F, Paidas M, Buchwalder L, Krikun G, and Schatz F (2005) Mechanisms of abruption-induced premature rupture of the fetal membranes: thrombin-enhanced interleukin-8 expression in term decidua. Am J Pathol, 167, 1443-1449.

[157] Mackenzie R, Walker M, Armson A, and Hannah ME (2006) Progesterone for the prevention of preterm birth among women at increased risk: a systematic review and meta-analysis of randomized controlled trials. Am J Obstet Gynecol, 194, 1234-1242.

[158] Madinger NE, Greenspoon JS, and Ellrodt AG (1989) Pneumonia during pregnancy: has modern technology improved maternal and fetal outcome? Am J Obstet Gynecol, 161, 657-662.
[159] Maehara K, Kanayama N, Maradny EE, Uezato T, Fujita M, and Terao T (1996) Mechanical stretching induces interleukin-8 gene expression in fetal membranes: a possible role for the initiation of human parturition. Eur J Obstet Gynecol Reprod Biol, 70, 191-196.
[160] Maheshwari A, Porter M, Shetty A, and Bhattacharya S (2008) Women's awareness and perceptions of delay in childbearing. Fertil Steril, 90, 1036-1042.
[161] Maradny EE, Kanayama N, Halim A, Maehara K, and Terao T (1996) Stretching of fetal membranes increases the concentration of interleukin-8 and collagenase activity. Am J Obstet Gynecol, 174, 843-849.
[162] Martin JA, Hamilton BE, Sutton PD, Ventura SJ, Menacker F, Kirmeyer S, and Munson ML (2007) Births: Final Data for 2005. Natl Vital Stat Rep, 56, 1-104.
[163] Martin JA, Hamilton BE, Sutton PD, Ventura SJ, Mathews TJ, and Osterman MJ (2010) Births: Final Data for 2008. Natl Vital Stat Rep, 59, 1-72.
[164] Martin JA, Hamilton BE, Sutton PD, Ventura SJ, Menacker F, Kirmeyer S, and Mathews TJ (2009) Births: Final Data for 2006. Natl Vital Stat Rep, 57, 1-121.
[165] Mathews TJ and Hamilton BE (2002) Mean age of mother, 1970-2000. Natl Vital Stat Rep, 51, 1-13.
[166] Mazaki-Tovi S, Romero R, Kusanovic JP, Erez O, Gotsch F, Mittal P, Than NG, Nhan-Chang CL, Hamill N, Vaisbuch E et al (2008) Visfatin/Pre-B cell colony-enhancing factor in amniotic fluid in normal pregnancy, spontaneous labor at term, preterm labor and prelabor rupture of membranes: an association with subclinical intrauterine infection in preterm parturition. J Perinat Med, 36, 485-496.
[167] Mazaki-Tovi S, Romero R, Kusanovic JP, Erez O, Pineles BL, Gotsch F, Mittal P, Gabor TN, Espinoza J, and Hassan SS (2007) Recurrent preterm birth. Semin Perinatol, 31, 142-158.
[168] Mazaki-Tovi S, Romero R, Vaisbuch E, Erez O, Chaiworapongsa T, Mittal P, Kim SK, Pacora P, Gotsch F, Dong Z et al (2009a) Maternal plasma visfatin in preterm labor. J Matern Fetal Neonatal Med, 22, 693-704.
[169] Mazaki-Tovi S, Romero R, Vaisbuch E, Erez O, Mittal P, Chaiworapongsa T, Kim SK, Pacora P, Yeo L, Gotsch F et al (2009b) Dysregulation of maternal serum adiponectin in preterm labor. J Matern Fetal Neonatal Med, 22, 887-904.
[170] Mazaki-Tovi S, Romero R, Vaisbuch E, Kusanovic JP, Erez O, Mittal P, Gotsch F, Chaiworapongsa T, Than NG, Kim SK et al (2010) Adiponectin in amniotic fluid in normal pregnancy, spontaneous labor at term, and preterm labor: a novel association with intra-amniotic infection/inflammation. J Matern Fetal Neonatal Med, 23, 120-130.
[171] McDonald H, Brocklehurst P, and Parsons J (2005b) Antibiotics for treating bacterial vaginosis in pregnancy. Cochrane Database Syst Rev, CD000262.
[172] McDonald HM, Brocklehurst P, and Gordon A (2007) Antibiotics for treating bacterial vaginosis in pregnancy. Cochrane Database Syst Rev, CD000262.
[173] McDonald HM, O'Loughlin JA, Vigneswaran R, Jolley PT, Harvey JA, Bof A, and McDonald PJ (1997) Impact of metronidazole therapy on preterm birth in women with bacterial vaginosis flora (Gardnerella vaginalis): a randomised, placebo controlled trial. Br J Obstet Gynaecol, 104, 1391-1397.

[174] McDonald SD, Han Z, Mulla S, Ohlsson A, Beyene J, and Murphy KE (2010) Preterm birth and low birth weight among in vitro fertilization twins: a systematic review and meta-analyses. Eur J Obstet Gynecol Reprod Biol, 148, 105-113.
[175] McDuffie RS, Jr., Sherman MP, and Gibbs RS (1992) Amniotic fluid tumor necrosis factor-alpha and interleukin-1 in a rabbit model of bacterially induced preterm pregnancy loss. Am J Obstet Gynecol, 167, 1583-1588.
[176] McElrath TF, Hecht JL, Dammann O, Boggess K, Onderdonk A, Markenson G, Harper M, Delpapa E, Allred EN, and Leviton A (2008) Pregnancy disorders that lead to delivery before the 28th week of gestation: an epidemiologic approach to classification. Am J Epidemiol, 168, 980-989.
[177] McGovern PG, Llorens AJ, Skurnick JH, Weiss G, and Goldsmith LT (2004) Increased risk of preterm birth in singleton pregnancies resulting from in vitro fertilization-embryo transfer or gamete intrafallopian transfer: a meta-analysis. Fertil Steril, 82, 1514-1520.
[178] McGregor JA, Allen KG, Harris MA, Reece M, Wheeler M, French JI, and Morrison J (2001) The omega-3 story: nutritional prevention of preterm birth and other adverse pregnancy outcomes. Obstet Gynecol Surv, 56, S1-13.
[179] McGregor JA and French JI (2000) Bacterial vaginosis in pregnancy. Obstet Gynecol Surv, 55, S1-19.
[180] McKay DG and Wong TC (1963) The effect of bacterial endotoxin on the placenta of the rat. Am J Pathol, 42, 357-377.
[181] McLane CM (1939) Pyelitis of pregnancy: a five-year study. Am J Obstet Gynecol, 38, 117.
[182] Meis PJ, Goldenberg RL, Mercer BM, Iams JD, Moawad AH, Miodovnik M, Menard MK, Caritis SN, Thurnau GR, Bottoms SF et al (1998) The preterm prediction study: risk factors for indicated preterm births. Maternal-Fetal Medicine Units Network of the National Institute of Child Health and Human Development. Am J Obstet Gynecol, 178, 562-567.
[183] Meis PJ, Klebanoff M, Thom E, Dombrowski MP, Sibai B, Moawad AH, Spong CY, Hauth JC, Miodovnik M, Varner MW et al (2003) Prevention of recurrent preterm delivery by 17 alpha-hydroxyprogesterone caproate. N Engl J Med, 348, 2379-2385.
[184] Meis PJ, Michielutte R, Peters TJ, Wells HB, Sands RE, Coles EC, and Johns KA (1995) Factors associated with preterm birth in Cardiff, Wales. II. Indicated and spontaneous preterm birth. Am J Obstet Gynecol, 173, 597-602.
[185] Meis P, Ernest J, Moore M, Michielutte R, Sharp P, and Buescher PA (1987) Regional program for prevention of premature birth in northwestern North Carolina. American Journal of Obstetrics & Gynecology, 157, 550-556.
[186] Menken J, Trussell J, and Larsen U (1986) Age and infertility. Science, 233, 1389-1394.
[187] Mercer BM, Miodovnik M, Thurnau GR, Goldenberg RL, Das AF, Ramsey RD, Rabello YA, Meis PJ, Moawad AH, Iams JD et al (1997) Antibiotic therapy for reduction of infant morbidity after preterm premature rupture of the membranes. A randomized controlled trial. National Institute of Child Health and Human Development Maternal-Fetal Medicine Units Network. JAMA, 278, 989-995.
[188] Millar LK, Stollberg J, DeBuque L, and Bryant-Greenwood G (2000) Fetal membrane distention: determination of the intrauterine surface area and distention of the fetal membranes preterm and at term. Am J Obstet Gynecol, 182, 128-134.

[189] Minkoff H (1983) Prematurity: infection as an etiologic factor. Obstet Gynecol, 62, 137-144.
[190] Mitchell JA and Lye SJ (2002) Differential expression of activator protein-1 transcription factors in pregnant rat myometrium. Biol Reprod, 67, 240-246.
[191] Mitchell JA and Lye SJ (2001) Regulation of connexin43 expression by c-fos and c-jun in myometrial cells. Cell Commun Adhes, 8, 299-302.
[192] Mittal P, Romero R, Mazaki-Tovi S, Tromp G, Tarca AL, Kim YM, Chaiworapongsa T, Kusanovic JP, Erez O, Than NG et al (2009) Fetal membranes as an interface between inflammation and metabolism: increased aquaporin 9 expression in the presence of spontaneous labor at term and chorioamnionitis. J Matern Fetal Neonatal Med, 22, 1167-1175.
[193] Moran LJ and Norman RJ (2002) The obese patient with infertility: a practical approach to diagnosis and treatment. Nutr Clin Care, 5, 290-297.
[194] Morcel K, Lavoue V, Beuchee A, Le LD, Poulain P, and Pladys P (2010) Perinatal morbidity and mortality in twin pregnancies with dichorionic placentas following assisted reproductive techniques or ovarian induction alone: a comparative study. Eur J Obstet Gynecol Reprod Biol, 153, 138-142.
[195] Moster D, Lie RT, and Markestad T (2008) Long-term medical and social consequences of preterm birth. N Engl J Med, 359, 262-273.
[196] Naeye RL (1983) Maternal age, obstetric complications, and the outcome of pregnancy. Obstet Gynecol, 61, 210-216.
[197] Nardi O, Zureik M, Courbon D, Ducimetiere P, and Clavel-Chapelon F (2006) Preterm delivery of a first child and subsequent mothers' risk of ischaemic heart disease: a nested case-control study. Eur J Cardiovasc Prev Rehabil, 13, 281-283.
[198] Nelson SM and Lawlor DA (2011) Predicting live birth, preterm delivery, and low birth weight in infants born from in vitro fertilisation: a prospective study of 144,018 treatment cycles. PLoS Med, 8, e1000386.
[199] Nemeth E, Millar LK, and Bryant-Greenwood G (2000) Fetal membrane distention: II. Differentially expressed genes regulated by acute distention in vitro. Am J Obstet Gynecol, 182, 60-67.
[200] Nemeth E, Tashima LS, Yu Z, and Bryant-Greenwood GD (2000) Fetal membrane distention: I. Differentially expressed genes regulated by acute distention in amniotic epithelial (WISH) cells. Am J Obstet Gynecol, 182, 50-59.
[201] Nepomnyaschy L and Reichman NE (2006) Low birthweight and asthma among young urban children. Am J Public Health, 96, 1604-1610.
[202] Nestler JE, Stovall D, Akhter N, Iuorno MJ, and Jakubowicz DJ (2002) Strategies for the use of insulin-sensitizing drugs to treat infertility in women with polycystic ovary syndrome. Fertil Steril, 77, 209-215.
[203] Newton ER, Piper J, and Peairs W (1997) Bacterial vaginosis and intraamniotic infection. Am J Obstet Gynecol, 176, 672-677.
[204] Nybo Andersen AM, Wohlfahrt J, Christens P, Olsen J, and Melbye M (2000) Maternal age and fetal loss: population based register linkage study. BMJ, 320, 1708-1712.
[205] O'Brien JM, Adair CD, Lewis DF, Hall DR, Defranco EA, Fusey S, Soma-Pillay P, Porter K, How H, Schackis R et al (2007) Progesterone vaginal gel for the reduction of recurrent preterm birth: primary results from a randomized, double-blind, placebo-controlled trial. Ultrasound Obstet Gynecol, 30, 687-696.

[206] Odibo AO, Elkousy M, Ural SH, and Macones GA (2003) Prevention of preterm birth by cervical cerclage compared with expectant management: a systematic review. Obstet Gynecol Surv, 58, 130-136.

[207] Okun N, Gronau KA, and Hannah ME (2005) Antibiotics for bacterial vaginosis or Trichomonas vaginalis in pregnancy: a systematic review. Obstet Gynecol, 105, 857-868.

[208] Oldenhof AD, Shynlova OP, Liu M, Langille BL, and Lye SJ (2002) Mitogen-activated protein kinases mediate stretch-induced c-fos mRNA expression in myometrial smooth muscle cells. Am J Physiol Cell Physiol, 283, C1530-C1539.

[209] Ou CW, Chen ZQ, Qi S, and Lye SJ (1998) Increased expression of the rat myometrial oxytocin receptor messenger ribonucleic acid during labor requires both mechanical and hormonal signals. Biol Reprod, 59, 1055-1061.

[210] Ou CW, Orsino A, and Lye SJ (1997) Expression of connexin-43 and connexin-26 in the rat myometrium during pregnancy and labor is differentially regulated by mechanical and hormonal signals. Endocrinology, 138, 5398-5407.

[211] Owen J, Hankins G, Iams JD, Berghella V, Sheffield JS, Perez-Delboy A, Egerman RS, Wing DA, Tomlinson M, Silver R et al (2009) Multicenter randomized trial of cerclage for preterm birth prevention in high-risk women with shortened midtrimester cervical length. Am J Obstet Gynecol, 201, 375-378.

[212] Oxhorn H (1955) The changing aspects of pneumonia complicating pregnancy. Am J Obstet Gynecol, 70, 1057.

[213] Palejwala S, Stein DE, Weiss G, Monia BP, Tortoriello D, and Goldsmith LT (2001) Relaxin positively regulates matrix metalloproteinase expression in human lower uterine segment fibroblasts using a tyrosine kinase signaling pathway. Endocrinology, 142, 3405-3413.

[214] Papiernik-Berkhauer E (1970) Etude en double aveugle d'un medicament prevenant la survenue prematurée de l'accouchement chez des femmes 'a risque eleve' d'accouchement premature. In Edition Schering, Serie IV, fiche 3.pp. 65-68.

[215] Pavletic AJ, Wolner-Hanssen P, Paavonen J, Hawes SE, and Eschenbach DA (1999) Infertility following pelvic inflammatory disease. Infect Dis Obstet Gynecol, 7, 145-152.

[216] Penrose LS (1933) The relative effects of paternal and maternal age in Mongolism. J Genet, 27, 219-224.

[217] Penrose LS (1934) The relative aetiological importance of birth order and maternal age in Mongolism. Proc R Soc B Biol Sci, 115, 431-450.

[218] Phelan JP, Park YW, Ahn MO, and Rutherford SE (1990) Polyhydramnios and perinatal outcome. J Perinatol, 10, 347-350.

[219] Piersanti M and Lye SJ (1995) Increase in messenger ribonucleic acid encoding the myometrial gap junction protein, connexin-43, requires protein synthesis and is associated with increased expression of the activator protein-1, c-fos. Endocrinology, 136, 3571-3578.

[220] Pinborg A (2005) IVF/ICSI twin pregnancies: risks and prevention. Hum Reprod Update, 11, 575-593.

[221] Pinborg A, Lidegaard O, la Cour FN, and Andersen AN (2005) Consequences of vanishing twins in IVF/ICSI pregnancies. Hum Reprod, 20, 2821-2829.

[222] Pirhonen J, Bergersen TK, Abdlenoor M, Dubiel M, and Gudmundsson S (2005) Effect of maternal age on uterine flow impedance. J Clin Ultrasound, 33, 14-17.
[223] Ralph SG, Rutherford AJ, and Wilson JD (1999) Influence of bacterial vaginosis on conception and miscarriage in the first trimester: cohort study. BMJ, 319, 220-223.
[224] Reddy UM, Wapner RJ, Rebar RW, and Tasca RJ (2007) Infertility, assisted reproductive technology, and adverse pregnancy outcomes: executive summary of a National Institute of Child Health and Human Development workshop. Obstet Gynecol, 109, 967-977.
[225] Rieder RF and Thomas L (1960) Studies on the mechanisms involved in the production of abortion by endotoxin. J Immunol, 84, 189-193.
[226] Romero R, Espinoza J, Mazor M, and Chaiworapongsa T (2004) The preterm parturition syndrome. In Critchely H, Bennett P, and Thornton S (eds) Preterm Birth. RCOG Press, London, pp. 28-60.
[227] Romero R, Gomez R, Mazor M, Ghezzi F, and Yoon BH (1997) The preterm labor syndrome. In Elder MG, Romero R, and Lamont RF (eds) Preterm labor. Churchill Livingstone, New York, NY, pp. 29-49.
[228] Romero R, Mazor M, Wu Y, Sirtori M, Oyarzun E, Mitchell M, and Hobbins J (1988a) Infection in the pathogenesis of preterm labor. Seminars in Perinatology, 12, 262-279.
[229] Romero R (1996) The child is the father of the man. Prenat Neonat Med, 1, 8-11.
[230] Romero R, Espinoza J, Mazor M, and Chaiworapongsa T (2004a) The preterm parturition syndrome. In Critchley C, Bennet P, and Thornton S (eds) Preterm Birth. RCOG Press, London, pp. 28-60.
[231] Romero R, Espinoza J, Chaiworapongsa T, and Kalache K (2002) Infection and prematurity and the role of preventive strategies. Semin Neonatol, 7, 259-274.
[232] Romero R, Espinoza J, Erez O, and Hassan S (2006a) The role of cervical cerclage in obstetric practice: can the patient who could benefit from this procedure be identified? Am J Obstet Gynecol, 194, 1-9.
[233] Romero R, Espinoza J, Kusanovic J, Gotsch F, Hassan S, Erez O, Chaiworapongsa T, and Mazor M (2006b) The preterm parturition syndrome. BJOG, 113 Suppl 3, 17-42.
[234] Romero R, Espinoza J, and Mazor M (2004b) Can endometrial infection/inflammation explain implantation failure, spontaneous abortion, and preterm birth after in vitro fertilization? Fertil Steril, 82, 799-804.
[235] Romero R, Espinoza J, Mazor M, and Chaiworapongsa T (2004c) The preterm parturition syndrome. In Critchley H, Bennett P, and Thornton S (eds) Preterm Birth. RCOG Press, London, pp. 28-60.
[236] Romero R, Gonzalez R, Sepulveda W, Brandt F, Ramirez M, Sorokin Y, Mazor M, Treadwell MC, and Cotton DB (1992) Infection and labor. VIII. Microbial invasion of the amniotic cavity in patients with suspected cervical incompetence: prevalence and clinical significance. Am J Obstet Gynecol, 167, 1086-1091.
[237] Romero R, Kusanovic JP, Chaiworapongsa T, and Hassan SS (2011) Placental bed disorders in preterm labor, preterm PROM, spontaneous abortion and abruptio placentae. Best Pract Res Clin Obstet Gynaecol, 25, 313-327.
[238] Romero R, Manogue KR, Mitchell MD, Wu YK, Oyarzun E, Hobbins JC, and Cerami A (1989) Infection and labor. IV. Cachectin-tumor necrosis factor in the amniotic fluid of women with intraamniotic infection and preterm labor. Am J Obstet Gynecol, 161, 336-341.

[239] Romero R, Mazor M, and Gomez R (1993) Cervix, incompetence and premature labor. Fetus, 3, 1.
[240] Romero R, Mazor M, Munoz H, Gomez R, Galasso M, and Sherer DM (1994) The preterm labor syndrome. Ann N Y Acad Sci, 734, 414-429.
[241] Romero R, Mazor M, Wu YK, Sirtori M, Oyarzun E, Mitchell MD, and Hobbins JC (1988b) Infection in the pathogenesis of preterm labor. Semin Perinatol, 12, 262-279.
[242] Romero R, Munoz H, Gomez R, Ramirez M, Araneda H, Cutright J, Wolf N, Cotton D, and Fidel PL (1994) Antibiotic therapy reduces the rate of infection-induced preterm delivery and perinatal mortality. In p. 390.
[243] Romero R, Quintero R, Oyarzun E, Wu YK, Sabo V, Mazor M, and Hobbins JC (1988) Intraamniotic infection and the onset of labor in preterm premature rupture of the membranes. Am J Obstet Gynecol, 159, 661-666.
[244] Romero R, Sepulveda W, Baumann P, Yoon BH, Brandt F, Gomez R, Mazor M, Sorokin Y, and Cotton D (1993) The preterm labor syndrome: Biochemical, cytologic, immunologic, pathologic, microbiologic, and clinical evidence that preterm labor is a heterogeneous disease. In p. 288.
[245] Romero R, Sirtori M, Oyarzun E, Avila C, Mazor M, Callahan R, Sabo V, Athanassiadis AP, and Hobbins JC (1989) Infection and labor. V. Prevalence, microbiology, and clinical significance of intraamniotic infection in women with preterm labor and intact membranes. Am J Obstet Gynecol, 161, 817-824.
[246] Rosen T, Kuczynski E, O'Neill LM, Funai EF, and Lockwood CJ (2001) Plasma levels of thrombin-antithrombin complexes predict preterm premature rupture of the fetal membranes. J Matern Fetal Med, 10, 297-300.
[247] Rosen T, Schatz F, Kuczynski E, Lam H, Koo AB, and Lockwood CJ (2002) Thrombin-enhanced matrix metalloproteinase-1 expression: a mechanism linking placental abruption with premature rupture of the membranes. J Matern Fetal Neonatal Med, 11, 11-17.
[248] Rossi AC and D'Addario V (2011) Neonatal outcomes of assisted and naturally conceived twins: systematic review and meta-analysis. J Perinat Med.
[249] Rouse DJ, Caritis SN, Peaceman AM, Sciscione A, Thom EA, Spong CY, Varner M, Malone F, Iams JD, Mercer BM et al (2007) A trial of 17 alpha-hydroxyprogesterone caproate to prevent prematurity in twins. N Engl J Med, 357, 454-461.
[250] Rudolph MI, Reinicke K, Cruz MA, Gallardo V, Gonzalez C, and Bardisa L (1993) Distribution of mast cells and the effect of their mediators on contractility in human myometrium. Br J Obstet Gynaecol, 100, 1125-1130.
[251] Rush RW, Isaacs S, McPherson K, Jones L, Chalmers I, and Grant A (1984) A randomized controlled trial of cervical cerclage in women at high risk of spontaneous preterm delivery. Br J Obstet Gynaecol, 91, 724-730.
[252] Rust OA, Atlas RO, Jones KJ, Benham BN, and Balducci J (2000) A randomized trial of cerclage versus no cerclage among patients with ultrasonographically detected second-trimester preterm dilatation of the internal os. Am J Obstet Gynecol, 183, 830-835.
[253] Rust OA, Atlas RO, Reed J, van GJ, and Balducci J (2001) Revisiting the short cervix detected by transvaginal ultrasound in the second trimester: why cerclage therapy may not help. Am J Obstet Gynecol, 185, 1098-1105.

[254] Ruutiainen K and Seppala M (1991) Polycystic ovary syndrome: evolution of a concept. Curr Opin Obstet Gynecol, 3, 326-335.
[255] Sakai M, Shiozaki A, Tabata M, Sasaki Y, Yoneda S, Arai T, Kato K, Yamakawa Y, and Saito S (2006) Evaluation of effectiveness of prophylactic cerclage of a short cervix according to interleukin-8 in cervical mucus. Am J Obstet Gynecol, 194, 14-19.
[256] Salafia CM, Lopez-Zeno JA, Sherer DM, Whittington SS, Minior VK, and Vintzileos AM (1995) Histologic evidence of old intrauterine bleeding is more frequent in prematurity. Am J Obstet Gynecol, 173, 1065-1070.
[257] Salem YS, Levy A, Wiznitzer A, Holcberg G, Mazor M, and Sheiner E (2011) A significant linear association exists between advanced maternal age and adverse perinatal outcome. Arch Gynecol Obstet, 283, 755-759.
[258] Sanchez-Ramos L, Kaunitz AM, and Delke I (2005) Progestational agents to prevent preterm birth: a meta-analysis of randomized controlled trials. Obstet Gynecol, 105, 273-279.
[259] Sarno JL, Schatz F, Lockwood CJ, Huang ST, and Taylor HS (2006) Thrombin and interleukin-1beta regulate HOXA10 expression in human term decidual cells: implications for preterm labor. J Clin Endocrinol Metab, 91, 2366-2372.
[260] Savva GM, Walker K, and Morris JK (2010) The maternal age-specific live birth prevalence of trisomies 13 and 18 compared to trisomy 21 (Down syndrome). Prenat Diagn, 30, 57-64.
[261] Scarpitta AM and Sinagra D (2000) Polycystic ovary syndrome: an endocrine and metabolic disease. Gynecol Endocrinol, 14, 392-395.
[262] Schieve LA, Meikle SF, Ferre C, Peterson HB, Jeng G, and Wilcox LS (2002) Low and very low birth weight in infants conceived with use of assisted reproductive technology. N Engl J Med, 346, 731-737.
[263] Schwartz D and Mayaux MJ (1982) Female fecundity as a function of age: results of artificial insemination in 2193 nulliparous women with azoospermic husbands. Federation CECOS. N Engl J Med, 306, 404-406.
[264] Shebl O, Ebner T, Sir A, Sommergruber M, and Tews G (2009) The role of mode of conception in the outcome of twin pregnancies. Minerva Ginecol, 61, 141-152.
[265] Shennan A, Crawshaw S, Briley A, Hawken J, Seed P, Jones G, and Poston L (2006) A randomised controlled trial of metronidazole for the prevention of preterm birth in women positive for cervicovaginal fetal fibronectin: the PREMET Study. BJOG, 113, 65-74.
[266] Shevell T, Malone FD, Vidaver J, Porter TF, Luthy DA, Comstock CH, Hankins GD, Eddleman K, Dolan S, Dugoff L et al (2005) Assisted reproductive technology and pregnancy outcome. Obstet Gynecol, 106, 1039-1045.
[267] Shynlova OP, Oldenhof AD, Liu M, Langille L, and Lye SJ (2002) Regulation of c-fos expression by static stretch in rat myometrial smooth muscle cells. Am J Obstet Gynecol, 186, 1358-1365.
[268] Shyy JY and Chien S (2002) Role of integrins in endothelial mechanosensing of shear stress. Circ Res, 91, 769-775.
[269] Sills ES, Perloe M, and Palermo GD (2000) Correction of hyperinsulinemia in oligoovulatory women with clomiphene-resistant polycystic ovary syndrome: a review of therapeutic rationale and reproductive outcomes. Eur J Obstet Gynecol Reprod Biol, 91, 135-141.

[270] Skarnes RC and Harper MJ (1972) Relationship between endotoxin-induced abortion and the synthesis of prostaglandin F. Prostaglandins, 1, 191-203.
[271] Sladek SM, Westerhausen-Larson A, and Roberts JM (1999) Endogenous nitric oxide suppresses rat myometrial connexin 43 gap junction protein expression during pregnancy. Biol Reprod, 61, 8-13.
[272] Slattery MM and Morrison JJ (2002) Preterm delivery. Lancet, 360, 1489-1497.
[273] Smith GC, Pell JP, and Walsh D (2001) Pregnancy complications and maternal risk of ischaemic heart disease: a retrospective cohort study of 129,290 births. Lancet, 357, 2002-2006.
[274] Sobel JD (2000) Bacterial vaginosis. Annu Rev Med, 51:349-56., 349-356.
[275] Stein ZA (1985) A woman's age: childbearing and child rearing. Am J Epidemiol, 121, 327-342.
[276] Stephenson CD, Lockwood CJ, Ma Y, and Guller S (2005a) Thrombin-dependent regulation of matrix metalloproteinase (MMP)-9 levels in human fetal membranes. J Matern Fetal Neonatal Med, 18, 17-22.
[277] Stevenson CS, Glasko A.J., and Gillespie EC (1951) Treatment of typhoid in pregnancy with chloramphenicol (chloromycetin). JAMA, 146, 1190.
[278] Takeda Y and Tsuchiya I. (1953) Studies on the pathological changes caused by the injection of the Shwartzman filtrate and the endotoxin into pregnant rabbits. Jap J Exper Med, 21, 9-16.
[279] Taylor AE (1998) Polycystic ovary syndrome. Endocrinol Metab Clin North Am, 27, 877-902, ix.
[280] Ticconi C and Lye SJ (2002) Placenta and fetal membranes in human parturition and preterm delivery--a workshop report. Placenta, 23 Suppl A:S149-52., S149-S152.
[281] To MS, Alfirevic Z, Heath VC, Cicero S, Cacho AM, Williamson PR, and Nicolaides KH (2004) Cervical cerclage for prevention of preterm delivery in women with short cervix: randomised controlled trial. Lancet, 363, 1849-1853.
[282] To MS, Palaniappan V, Skentou C, Gibb D, and Nicolaides KH (2002) Elective cerclage vs. ultrasound-indicated cerclage in high-risk pregnancies. Ultrasound Obstet Gynecol, 19, 475-477.
[283] Tognoni G, Ferrario L, Inzalaco M, and Crosignani PG (1980) Progestagens in threatened abortion. Lancet, 2, 1242-1243.
[284] Tough S, Benzies K, Fraser-Lee N, and Newburn-Cook C (2007) Factors influencing childbearing decisions and knowledge of perinatal risks among Canadian men and women. Matern Child Health J, 11, 189-198.
[285] Tough S, Benzies K, Newburn-Cook C, Tofflemire K, Fraser-Lee N, Faber A, and Sauve R (2006) What do women know about the risks of delayed childbearing? Can J Public Health, 97, 330-334.
[286] Tzima E, del Pozo MA, Shattil SJ, Chien S, and Schwartz MA (2001) Activation of integrins in endothelial cells by fluid shear stress mediates Rho-dependent cytoskeletal alignment. EMBO J, 20, 4639-4647.
[287] Ugwumadu A, Manyonda I, Reid F, and Hay P (2003) Effect of early oral clindamycin on late miscarriage and preterm delivery in asymptomatic women with abnormal vaginal flora and bacterial vaginosis: a randomised controlled trial. Lancet, 361, 983-988.

[288] Ugwumadu AH (2002) Bacterial vaginosis in pregnancy. Curr Opin Obstet Gynecol, 14, 115-118.
[289] Verstraelen H, Goetgeluk S, Derom C, Vansteelandt S, Derom R, Goetghebeur E, and Temmerman M (2005) Preterm birth in twins after subfertility treatment: population based cohort study. BMJ, 331, 1173.
[290] Vidaeff AC and Ramin SM (2006) From concept to practice: the recent history of preterm delivery prevention. Part II: Subclinical infection and hormonal effects. Am J Perinatol, 23, 75-84.
[291] Vintzileos AM, Ananth CV, Smulian JC, Scorza WE, and Knuppel RA (2002) The impact of prenatal care in the United States on preterm births in the presence and absence of antenatal high-risk conditions. Am J Obstet Gynecol, 187, 1254-1257.
[292] Vogel I, Glavind-Kristensen M, Thorsen P, Armbruster FP, and Uldbjerg N (2002) S-relaxin as a predictor of preterm delivery in women with symptoms of preterm labour. BJOG, 109, 977-982.
[293] Vogel I, Salvig JD, Secher NJ, and Uldbjerg N (2001) Association between raised serum relaxin levels during the eighteenth gestational week and very preterm delivery. Am J Obstet Gynecol, 184, 390-393.
[294] Wang YA, Sullivan EA, Black D, Dean J, Bryant J, and Chapman M (2005) Preterm birth and low birth weight after assisted reproductive technology-related pregnancy in Australia between 1996 and 2000. Fertil Steril, 83, 1650-1658.
[295] Watts DH, Eschenbach DA, and Kenny GE (1989) Early postpartum endometritis: the role of bacteria, genital mycoplasmas, and Chlamydia trachomatis. Obstet Gynecol, 73, 52-60.
[296] Watts DH, Krohn MA, Hillier SL, and Eschenbach DA (1990) Bacterial vaginosis as a risk factor for post-cesarean endometritis. Obstet Gynecol, 75, 52-58.
[297] Watts DH, Krohn MA, Hillier SL, and Eschenbach DA (1992) The association of occult amniotic fluid infection with gestational age and neonatal outcome among women in preterm labor. Obstet Gynecol, 79, 351-357.
[298] Weghofer A, Klein K, Stammler-Safar M, Barad DH, Worda C, Husslein P, and Gleicher N (2009) Severity of prematurity risk in spontaneous and in vitro fertilization twins: does conception mode serve as a risk factor? Fertil Steril, 92, 2116-2118.
[299] Weiss G, Goldsmith LT, Sachdev R, Von HS, and Lederer K (1993) Elevated first-trimester serum relaxin concentrations in pregnant women following ovarian stimulation predict prematurity risk and preterm delivery. Obstet Gynecol, 82, 821-828.
[300] Wilson JD, Ralph SG, and Rutherford AJ (2002) Rates of bacterial vaginosis in women undergoing in vitro fertilisation for different types of infertility. BJOG, 109, 714-717.
[301] Wing ES and Troppoli D.V. (1930) The intrauterine transmission of typhoid. JAMA, 95, 405.
[302] Wisborg K, Ingerslev HJ, and Henriksen TB (2010b) In vitro fertilization and preterm delivery, low birth weight, and admission to the neonatal intensive care unit: a prospective follow-up study. Fertil Steril, 94, 2102-2106.
[303] Wisborg K, Ingerslev HJ, and Henriksen TB (2010a) IVF and stillbirth: a prospective follow-up study. Hum Reprod, 25, 1312-1316.

[304] Wright VC, Schieve LA, Reynolds MA, and Jeng G (2003) Assisted reproductive technology surveillance--United States, 2000. MMWR Surveill Summ, 52, 1-16.
[305] Wright VC, Schieve LA, Reynolds MA, Jeng G, and Kissin D (2004) Assisted reproductive technology surveillance--United States, 2001. MMWR Surveill Summ, 53, 1-20.
[306] Wu WX, Ma XH, Yoshizato T, Shinozuka N, and Nathanielsz PW (1999) Differential expression of myometrial oxytocin receptor and prostaglandin H synthase 2, but not estrogen receptor alpha and heat shock protein 90 messenger ribonucleic acid in the gravid horn and nongravid horn in sheep during betamethasone-induced labor. Endocrinology, 140, 5712-5718.
[307] Yemini M, Borenstein R, Dreazen E, Apelman Z, Mogilner BM, Kessler I, and Lancet M (1985) Prevention of premature labor by 17 alpha-hydroxyprogesterone caproate. Am J Obstet Gynecol, 151, 574-577.
[308] Yogev Y, Melamed N, Bardin R, Tenenbaum-Gavish K, Ben-Shitrit G, and Ben-Haroush A (2010) Pregnancy outcome at extremely advanced maternal age. Am J Obstet Gynecol, 203, 558-7.
[309] Zahl PA and Bjerknes C (1943) Induction of decidua-placental hemorrhage in mice by the endotoxins of certain gram-negative bacteria. Proc Soc Exper Biol Med, 54, 329-332.
[310] Zaib-un-Nisa S, Ghazal-Aswad S, and Badrinath P (2003) Outcome of twin pregnancies after assisted reproductive techniques--a comparative study. Eur J Obstet Gynecol Reprod Biol, 109, 51-54.
[311] Zlatnik FJ, Cruikshank DP, Petzold CR, and Galask RP (1984) Amniocentesis in the identification of inapparent infection in preterm patients with premature rupture of the membranes. J Reprod Med, 29, 656-660.

2

Environmental Exposures, Genetic Susceptibility and Preterm Birth

Regina Grazuleviciene, Jone Vencloviene, Asta Danileviciute, Audrius Dedele and Gediminas Balcius
Vytautas Magnus University
Lithuania

1. Introduction

Preterm births cause a large public-health burden because of its high prevalence, leading cause of neonatal morbidity and mortality, and environmental hazards is considered to be a potential risk factors (Adams et al., 2000; Bloom et al., 2001; Tucker & McGuire, 2004; Colvin et al. 2004; Fraser et al. 2004; Murphy et al. 2004). The frequency of preterm births is about 12–13% in the USA and 5–9% in many other developed countries; however, the rate of preterm birth has increased in many locations (Goldenberg et al., 2008). Thus, to elicit of risk factors that could predict high risk of preterm birth represents a challenge to practitioners and researchers. The increasing rate of preterm birth in recent decades, despite improvements in health care, creates an impetus to better understand and prevent this disorder. The identification of women at increased risk of preterm delivery is an important challenge. Preterm birth likely depends on a number of interacting factors, including genetic, epigenetic, and environmental risk factors (Windham et al., 2000; Plunkett & Muglia, 2008). The epidemiological data suggested that both genetic factors and socioenvironmental factors may influence preterm birth (Wang et al., 2000; Nukui et al., 2004; Lewis et al., 2006; Suh et al., 2008).

Genetic studies may identify stable over time markers, which can predict preterm birth in genetically susceptible subjects and the gene-environment studies may explain how the variations in the human genome (polymorphisms) can modify the effects of exposures to environmental health hazards (Kelada et al., 2003). Given individual genetic variations of pregnant women and different environmental exposures, the study may reveal women group susceptible to environmental hazards and may explain the differences in risk of preterm birth among individuals exposed to a particular environmental toxicant (Rothman et al., 2001). Furthermore, enhanced understanding of pathologic mechanisms may allow the development of interventions that can be used to prevent or treat preterm birth.

To date, however, only a relatively few studies on the association of gene-environment interactions with preterm birth have been published (Wang et al., 2002; Genc et al., 2004; Macones et al., 2004).

Experimental and epidemiologic studies provide evidence that a number of drinking water disinfection by-products (DBPs), including trihalomethanes (THM), may be associated with adverse pregnancy outcomes. Epidemiological studies suggested that pregnant women exposed to water containing elevated THM concentrations may be at greater risk for adverse pregnancy outcomes, including fetal growth, but findings of the studies to date have been inconsistent (Nieuwenhuijsen et al., 2000; Graves et al., 2001; Bove et al., 2002). The relationship between DBPs exposure and reproductive health outcomes remains unclear, mainly owing to limitations in the crude exposure assessment in most studies (Tardiff et al., 2006; Yang et al., 2007; Nieuwenhuijsen et al., 2009).

A recent meta-analysis of epidemiologic studies data on the association of THMs concentration in water and birth outcome, without taking into account exposure routes, concluded that there was little or no evidence for associations between THM concentration and prematurity and fetal growth, and that the uncertainties-relating particularly to exposure that may have affected them (Grellier et al., 2010). In addition, some epidemiological studies show little evidence for an association between THM and preterm birth, term low birth weight and other adverse birth outcomes (Bove et al., 2002; Hinckley et al., 2005; Nieuwenhuijsen et al., 2009). These epidemiological studies of reproductive outcomes had relied on different methods of assessing exposure, which presents difficulties in making comparisons between investigations and in generalizing results. The inconsistency of the association between exposure to THM and birth outcomes also could be related to both - qualitative and quantitative differences in exposure between the compared studies (Jaakkola et al., 2001). So, a major challenge in studies that examine the association between DBPs in drinking water and pregnancy outcomes is the accurate representation of a subject's exposure (King et al., 2004).

Seeking to improve the exposure assessment, studies have begun to incorporate behavioural determinants of different routes of exposure to DBPs such as dermal absorption and inhalation during bathing and showering, and ingestion of drinking water (Savitz et al. 2006; Hoffman et al., 2008; MacLehose et al., 2008). In our previous prospective Kaunas cohort study, which incorporated of different routes of exposure to THMs, we found dose–response relationships for entire pregnancy and trimester-specific gestational THMs and chloroform internal dose for low birth weight and reduction in birth weight (Grazuleviciene et al., 2011).

The epidemiological studies concluded that, while there appears to be suggestive evidence associating elevated total THM levels with some adverse reproductive outcomes, evidence for relationships with preterm birth and fetal growth is inconclusive and inconsistent (Richardson et al., 2003; Lewis et al., 2006; Grellier et al., 2010).

Most of the previous investigations have evaluated crude THM exposure; these studies differed on control of maternal characteristics that could also to be associated with adverse pregnancy outcomes; these studies did not evaluated genetic susceptibility to individual THM in relation to adverse pregnancy outcomes. Polymorphic variation in metabolic genes involved in detoxification of xenobiotics may explain some of the variation in individual susceptibility to the adverse effects of pollutants on preterm birth.

There is now some evidence concerning adverse effects of traffic-related air pollution on pregnancy outcomes and infant health. The evidence is suggestive of causality for the association of birth weight with air pollution, although for preterm birth and fetal growth, the current evidence is insufficient to infer a causal relationship and effects were not always consistent between studies Maisonet et al., 2001; Maroziene & Grazuleviciene, 2002; Sram et al., 2005; Dugandzic et al., 2006). Nitrogen dioxide (NO_2) is considered as a marker for air pollution from traffic associated with health effects (Belander et al., 2001; Rijnders et al.,

2001). In addition, a number of epidemiological studies have found various level relationships between exposures to traffic-related air pollution and birth outcomes, particularly for NO_2 and particulate matter, suggesting that exposure to these air pollutants may increase a woman's risk for preterm birth (Bobak, 2000; Maroziene & Grazuleviciene, 2002; Leem et al., 2006; Llop et al., 2010; Gehring et al., 2011).

The biological mechanisms by which air pollutants may interfere with the processes of prenatal development are still not clear. Several potential mechanisms have been hypothesised, including increased maternal susceptibility to inflammation, oxidative stress (Mohorovic, 2004; Becker et al., 2005; Risom et al., 2005), haematological factors (e.g., blood viscosity) (Pekkanen et al., 2000; Liao et al., 2005;) and the direct effect of specific pollutants on foetal development or on DNA and its transcription (Perera et al., 1999; Sram et al., 1999). Nitrogen dioxide is capable of oxidising tissue components (e.g., proteins, lipids) and of suppressing the antioxidant protective systems of organism (Sagai & Ichinose, 1991). Increased lipid peroxidation in the maternal and/or foetal compartment has been found in preterm birth (Moison et al., 1993). It was suggested that maternal exposure to NO_2 can increase the risk of pregnancy complications through stimulation of the formation of cell damaging lipid peroxides and from decrease in maternal antioxidant reserves (Tabacova et al., 1998). Recently a few potential biological mechanisms have been described through which air pollution could influence pregnancy outcomes, such as the induction inflammation of placenta, respiratory system and cardiovascular mechanisms of oxidative stress, coagulation, endothelial function, and hemodynamic responses (Kannan et al., 2006).

A crucial aspect of the study of prenatal exposure to air pollutants is the identification of vulnerable periods to the detrimental effects of the exposure during pregnancy and sensitive subjects (Hackley et al., 2007; Woodruff et al., 2009). Molecular epidemiological studies suggest possible biological mechanisms for the effect on preterm birth and intrauterine growth retardation (Shin, 2008). Population-based study data showed that 25% of the variation in preterm birth was explained by maternal genetic factors, fetal genetic factors only marginally influenced the variation in liability, while 70% of the variation in preterm birth was explained by the environmental effects (Svensson et al., 2009). More research is needed to clarify the role of traffic-related hazards on preterm birth, as well as their interactions with other environmental hazards and with specific genetic factors affecting maternal susceptibility.

In the present study, using individual cohort study data and adjusting for many important risk factors for preterm birth, we evaluated the effect of trimester-specific gestational THM internal dose and residential NO_2 exposure for preterm birth among genetically susceptible women. In our study individual exposure to THM was estimated as total internal dose based on monitoring of tap water THM levels and detailed water use behaviours. Controlling for influence of potential confounding variables, we seek to investigate whether the polymorphisms of metabolic genes GSTT1 and GSTM1 affect the association of maternal exposures to THMs and NO_2 with preterm birth risk.

2. Methods

We conducted a prospective cohort study of 4,161 pregnant women in Kaunas (Lithuania). We used tap water THM concentrations, geocoded maternal address at birth, individual information on drinking water ingestion, showering and bathing, and uptake factors of THMs in blood, to estimate an internal dose of THM. We estimated maternal residential exposure to NO2 by Airviro dispersion models during entire pregnancy, and three pregnancy trimesters and used logistic regression to evaluate the relationship between internal THM dose and NO2 exposure and preterm birth controlling for potential confounding variables. To investigate whether the polymorphisms of metabolic genes GSTT1 and GSTM1 affect the association of maternal exposure to THMs and NO2 with preterm birth risk, a nested case-control study on preterm birth occurrence among 682 women with genotyping of GSTT1 and GSTM1 polymorphisms was conducted.

2.1 Participant recruitment and outcome assessment

We conducted a prospective cohort study of pregnant women in Kaunas city, Lithuania. On their first visit to a general practitioner, all pregnant women living in Kaunas city between 2007 and 2009 were invited to join the cohort. The women were enrolled in the study only if they consented to participate in the cohort. The study ethics complied with the Declaration of Helsinki (1996). The research protocol was approved by the Lithuanian Bioethics Committee and an oral informed consent was obtained from all subjects. In total 5,405 women were approached; 79% of them agreed to participate in the study.

The first interview was completed during the first pregnancy trimester. The median gestational age at interview was 8 weeks. The interview queried women regarding demographics, residence and job characteristics, chronic diseases (cardiovascular, hypertension, diabetes, renal), reproductive history, including date of last menstrual period, previous preterm delivery. We also asked the women to report their age (less than 20 years, 20–29 years, 30 years, and more), educational level (primary, secondary, university), marital status (married not married), smoking (non-smoker, smoker at least one cigarette per day), alcohol consumption (0 drinks per week, at least one drink per week), blood pressure (<140/80 mm/Hg, ≥140 or ≥ 90 mm/Hg), body mass index (<25 kg/m2, 25–30 kg/m2, >30 kg/m2), and other potential risk factors for preterm birth. Adjustment for these variables was made for studies of various subgroups. The women also were examined by ultrasound to determine the gestational age of the foetus.

A special water consumption and water use habits questionnaire was used to interview the 4,260 women who agreed to participate in the study; 76.4% of them were interviewed during the third pregnancy trimester before delivery at the hospital and 23.6% by telephone within the first month after delivery. Consumption was ascertained for three types of water: cold tape water or dinks made from cold tap water; boiled tap water (tea, coffee, and other); and bottled water, used at home, at work, other. In addition, number of showers, baths, swimming pools weekly, and their average length was asked of all subjects. The interviews were conducted by trained nurses who did not know the THM exposure status and birth outcome.

Pregnancy outcomes were abstracted from the medical records. Preterm birth was defined as infant's whose gestational age was less than 37 weeks. Gestational age of the foetus was estimated as the difference between the delivery date and the date of the last menstruation as reported by the women at the beginning of their pregnancies, and of an ultrasound examination. The reference group was defined as all term births (born at >37 weeks of gestation).

Women with multiple pregnancies (150), having inconsistent or invalid data for dating the pregnancy (5) or estimating THM exposure (mostly students moved out of the city during pregnancy, 839) or with newborn birth weight above 4,500 g (75) were excluded. We restricted our analyses to infants born with a birth weight below 4,500 g, leaving data for 3,341 women in the final analysis.

2.2 THM exposure assessment

The Kaunas city municipal drinking water is supplied by four water treatment plants system. The each treatment plant water supplied system is constituted of only one subsystem (i.e., one chlorination, and branchy water supplied to the users). Groundwater sources are used for the whole water supply system.

However, the four water treatment plants, which disinfected ground water with sodium hypochlorite (chlorine dose 0.26–0.91 mg/L, residual chlorine 0–0.22 mg/L), produced different concentrations of THMs in finished water. One treatment plant (Petrasiunai) supplied finished water with higher levels of THMs ("high level THM site," 54.9% subjects), and the three other plants supplied finished water with lower levels of all THMs ("low level THM site"). Water samples were collected four times per year over a 3-year study period (2007–2009) in the morning in three locations: close to the treatment plant, at 5 km, and at 10 km or more from every treatment plant. A total of 85 water samples were collected from 12 monitoring sites in four water supply zones for THM analysis.

Samples were analysed at the University of the Aegean, Greece, by using gas chromatography with electron captures detection (Nikolaou et al., 2005). Measurements included specific values for the four regulated THMs (chloroform, bromoform, bromodichloromethane, and dibromochloromethane). We calculated the mean quarterly THM constituent concentrations for water zones and subsequently, depending on the TTHM levels within each zone, assigned "low level" and "high level" sites. We used tap water THM concentration, derived as the average of quarterly sample values over the time that the pregnancy occurred from all sampling sites located in the each distribution system, and geocoded maternal address at birth to assign the individual women residential exposure index. Estimates of exposure index to total and specific THMs from drinking water were tabulated first as an average level at the tap over the pregnancy period; this measure was then categorized at the tertiles of the distribution for birth outcomes. In addition, trimester-specific analyses were conducted. We combined every subject's residential exposure index and water-use questionnaire data to assess individual exposure through ingestion of THMs. Women were asked to indicate the cup or glass size and number of cups or glasses of tap water consumed per day, including hot and cold beverages made from tap water. With this information, we calculated daily amounts of hot and cold tap water ingested. Integration of the information on residential THM levels (μg/L), ingested amounts (L/day), and modifications by heating using an estimated uptake factor of 0.00490 to derive an integrated index of blood concentration, expressed in micrograms per day (μg/d) (Savitz et al., 2006; Whitaker et al., 2003).

The actual algorithms of internal dose from ingestion were:

chloroform level (μg/l) × water consumption (l/day) × 0.00490196 μg/μg/l;

brominated THM level (μg/l) × water consumption (l/day) × 0.00111848 μg/μg/l.

We assumed a null THM level for any bottled water consumption since in local bottled water production chlorination and ozonation is not used.

Finally, we addressed dermal absorption and inhalation by considering showering and bathing alone and combined with ingestion. We multiplied residential THM levels (μg/L) by frequency and average duration of bathing or showering per day (min/day) and calculated each mother's trimester-specific and entire pregnancy average daily uptake of THM internal dose (μg/d). We derived indices of daily uptake by integrating THM concentrations, duration of bathing and showering reported in a questionnaire administered

to study participants, and estimated uptake factors of 0.001536 and 0.001321 of THMs in blood per minute per microgram from showering and bathing, respectively (Backer et al., 2000; Lynberg et al., 2001). The uptake factors of THMs individual constituents were assessed on the relative changes in blood levels after 10 minutes exposure (after versus before ingestion 1 L of tap water, 10 minutes showering, and 10 minutes bathing). The actual algorithms of internal dose from showering and bathing were:
min/day showering × μg/l chloroform in water × 0.001536261 μg/min/μg/l,
min/day showering × μg/l brominated THM in water × 0.001352065 μg/min/μg/l,
min/day bathing × μg/l chloroform in water × 0.001320755 μg/min/μg/l,
min/day bathing × μg/l brominated THM in water × 0.00129571 μg/min/μg/l
We then used average daily total uptakes in our analysis as continuous and categorized variables. We calculated tertiles of THM internal dose. This gave first (0.0025–0.0386 μg/d), second (0.0386–0.3496 μg/d), and third (0.3496–2.4040 μg/d) tertiles for average TTHM uptake. To reduce exposure misclassification errors in the subsequent analysis, we used a subset of women who through the entire pregnancy did not change their address.

2.3 NO_2 exposure assessment

In this study exposure to ambient NO_2 pollution estimates at each cohort number home address was assigned using GIS and AIRVIRO dispersion model, developed by the Swedish Meteorological and Hydrological (Airviro User Documentation 1997). The model integrates emissions inventories, meteorological data (wind direction and speed, temperature), background pollution measurements as input parameters and land use. Kaunas streets NO_2 emission data were used to create emission database within AIRVIRO Air Quality Management System. Gaussian plume dispersion simulations were run for a model domain encompassing the entire city area on a course grid resolution.

Geographic data for the Kaunas city streets, its type were measured by combination GIS and manual measurements. Total traffic counts and its composition (calculated as cars/day time's km street length) were measured based on the 2008 Municipal traffic-count data for Kaunas. If no counts were available for specific street, the numbers were estimated by a person with local information about the traffic conditions based on comparison with roads on which data were available. Traffic count data were available for 80% of the streets nearest to cohort addresses.

To attribute the NO_2 exposure to every study subject, the health data base and the environmental NO_2 pollution data base were joined. Every subject's full street address and residential NO_2 pollution level measurement data, and the current residence history data were combined to assess the individual NO_2 pollution exposure. A GIS assigning NO_2 pollution level was used for every woman by applying different GIS functions and possibilities. First, the study subjects data were converted to a database file structure for use in GIS software (ArcInfo version 9.3, ESRI). Geocoding was performed to obtain latitude and longitude coordinates for each patient's home address. Initially, 63 % records were matched and 37 % were left unmatched. All unmatched records were reviewed and corrected, leading to another 37 % matched addresses (total of 3287). Then, a spatial join was perform that allows the GIS user to append the attributes of one data layer (patient address points) to the attributes of another layer (nitrogen dioxide) assessed with AIRVIRO. We established the individual outdoor NO_2 exposure during three trimesters and entire pregnancy for every subject at the geocoded residential address.

2.4 Genotyping

Within the prospective cohort study, a nested case-control study on preterm birth occurrence among 682 women with genotyping of GSTT1 and GSTM1 polymorphisms was conducted. This study was assumed to identify gene–environment interaction that increases the risk of preterm delivery. We investigated the association between the risk of preterm delivery and each metabolic gene of glutathione *S*-transferases mu 1 (GSTM1) and theta 1 (GSTT1) along with exposure to THM and NO_2. The GSTM1-null and GSTT1-null genotypes were identified by the multiplex polymerase chain reaction (PCR) in peripheral blood DNA samples.

For genetic analysis maternal blood samples were collected in vials containing EDTA and stored at a temperature of −20 °C. DNA was purified from the peripheral blood using DNA purification kits (SORPOclean Genomic DNA Extraction Kit, Vilnius, Lithuania). DNA concentrations were quantified with a spectrophotometer (Eppendorrf BioPhotometer, 61310488, Hamburg, Germany). The GSTM1- and GSTT1-null genotypes were identified by the multiplex polymerase chain reaction (PCR) in peripheral blood DNA samples. Multiplex PCR was performed as described by Arand et al. (1998) to determine the present (at least 1 allele present: AA or Aa) or absent (complete deletion of both alleles: aa) of GSTM1 and GSTT1 genes. PCR condition could be found elsewhere (Grazuleviciene et al., 2009).

2.5 Statistical analysis

The data analysis compared the preterm birth of low, medium and high exposed women to THMs. We used logistic regression to estimate adjusted odds ratios (ORs) and 95-percent confidence intervals (CIs) for preterm birth and the various exposure indices. We categorized TTHM internal dose in tertiles and evaluated the possible relationship between increases in preterm birth risk for an increase in estimated TTHM internal dose. We ran multivariate logistic regression models for the TTHMs, chloroform, dibromochloromethane, and bromodichloromethane for the total pregnancy and trimester specific periods. We also used multiple linear regressions for TTHM internal dose analysis as continuous variable to evaluate the relationship, if any between preterm birth and every 1 µg/d increase in TTHM internal dose.

In the logistic regression models for preterm birth outcome, using personal data of the cohort sample, we assessed a variety of potential confounders identified by univariate analysis. Further, we examined the association of THM exposure and preterm birth with a multivariable analysis controlling for effect of major covariates that changed the adjusted ORs for THM by 10% or more. The adjusted preterm birth outcome analyses included maternal smoking, education, family status, chronic diseases, previous preterm birth, stress and infant birth year.

The effect of ambient NO_2 exposure on preterm birth was estimated by logistic regression. We grouped the NO_2 concentrations into three categories (tertiles) and applied the exposure variable as both categorical and continuous parameters. We used exposure levels in the 1st tertile as the reference category (low exposure) and then also conducted an analysis of continuous exposure parameters on the basis of an increase of 10 $\mu g/m^3$ in NO_2 concentrations. We calculated crude and adjusted odds ratios (OR) and their 95 % confidence intervals (CIs) of preterm birth exposure categories. Statistical analyses were performed with SPSS software for Windows version 13.

To investigate whether the polymorphisms of metabolic genes GSTT1 and GSTM1 affect the association of maternal exposure to THMs and NO_2 with preterm birth risk, a nested case-control study data on preterm birth occurrence among 682 women with genotyping of

GSTT1 and GSTM1 polymorphisms was analysed. Logistic regression analyses were performed to explore the impact of each gene, THM and NO_2 exposure and their effect on the risk of preterm birth. The subgroups were defined by maternal genotype for GSTT1 (present, absent) and GSTM1 (present, absent) and maternal exposure to THM status during pregnancy (above median/below median). We run multivariate logistic regression models for the TTHMs, chloroform, dibromochloromethane, and bromodichloromethane for total gestational and trimester-specific periods, while adjusting for potential confounders. Similarly we run analysis for the NO_2. We used logistic regression to estimate adjusted odds ratios (ORs) and 95-percent confidence intervals (CIs) for preterm birth, and the various exposure indices.

We estimated the exposure effect for GSTT1 (present, absent) and GSTM1 (present, absent) genotypes by a multivariable analysis controlling for influence of major covariates that changed the adjusted ORs for NO_2 by 10% or more. Two-tailed statistical significance was evaluated by using a p value of 0.05. All statistical analyses were carried out using the SPSS software for Windows version 12.0.1.

3. Results

3.1 Daily THM uptake

The mean tap water THM level in the low level site from three water treatment plants was 1.3 μg/L, and in the high level site (Petrasiunai) 21.9 μg/L (Table 1). The estimated individual total uptake of THMs ranged between 0.0025 and 2.40 μg/d. The total chloroform uptake ranged between 0.0013 and 2.13 μg/d. Mothers supplied with water who had a higher chloroform concentration generally also had a higher total internal dose. Daily uptake of bromodichloromethane ranged between 0.0001 and 0.34 μg/d and dibromochloromethane ranged between 0 and 0.064 μg/d. Bromoform was below the limit of detection.

Tap water sampling sites	TTHMs[c] Mean (SD[d])	$CHCl_3$ Mean (SD)	$CHBr_2Cl$ Mean (SD)	$CHBrCl_2$ Mean (SD)
All sites	9.8 (12.4)	7.8 (10.2)	0.3 (0.5)	1.7 (2.2)
Low THM level[a]	1.3 (1.2)	0.9 (1.0)	0.1 (0.2)	0.3 (0.5)
High THM level[b]	21.9 (10.9)	17.7 (9.0)	0.5 (0.6)	3.6 (2.1)

[a]Viciunai, Eiguliai, Kleboniskis. [b]Petrasiunai.
[c]TTHMs = total trihalomethanes: the sum of $CHCl_3$ (chloroform), $CHBr_2Cl$ dibromochloromethane), and $CHBrCl_2$ (bromodichloromethane).
[d]SD = standard deviation.

Table 1. Mean THM levels (μg/L) by sampling site and water supply zone

3.2 Preterm birth risk factors

The women recruited were predominantly Lithuanian in ethnic origin (97.4%) and did not smoke (93.1%) (Table 2). The mean age was 28.4 years, and the women tended to be highly educated (54.3% with a university degree). In general, mothers who were single, less educated, had previous preterm delivery, or reported a chronic stress delivered a higher proportion of preterm birth infants. We did not find a difference in preterm birth between water filter users and non-users.

Risk factors	Characteristics	All participants N(%)	Preterm birth N(%)
Maternal age	< 20 years	95 (2.8)	4 (2.1)
	20–29 years	1961 (58.7)	107 (55.7)
	≥ 30 years	1285 (38.5)	81 (42.2)
Marital status*	Married	2744 (82.1)	147 (76.6)
	Not married	597 (17.9)	45 (23.4)
Maternal education*	Primary school	166 (5.0)	16 (8.4)
	Secondary school	1361 (40.7)	88 (45.8)
	University degree	1814 (54.3)	88 (45.8)
Maternal smoking	Non-smoker	3110 (93.1)	176 (91.7)
	Smoker	231 (6.9)	16 (8.3)
Paternal smoking	Non-smoker	1748 (52.9)	88 (46.1)
	Smoker	1558 (47.1)	103 (53.9)
Alcohol consumption	No	3142 (94.0)	182 (94.8)
	Yes	199 (6.0)	10 (5.2)
Blood pressure (mm/Hg)	<140/80	2882 (86.3)	163 (84.9)
	≥140 or ≥ 90	459 (13.7)	29 (15.1)
Ethnic group	Lithuanian	3254 (97.4)	191 (99.5)
	Other	87 (2.6)	1 (0.5)
Parity	No child	1507 (45.1)	85 (44.3)
	≥ 1 child	1834 (54.9)	107 (55.7)
Infant gender	Male	1714 (51.3)	92 (47.9)
	Female	1627 (48.7)	100 (52.1)
Current residence	1–4 years	1401 (41.9)	84 (43.7)
	5–9 years	841 (25.2)	46 (24.0)
	≥ 10 years	1099 (32.9)	62 (32.3)
Work exposure	No	3048 (91.2)	177 (92.2)
	Yes	293 (8.8)	15 (7.8)
Chronic disease	No	2527 (75.6)	136 (70.8)
	Yes	814 (24.4)	56 (29.2)
Previous preterm delivery*	No	3279 (98.1)	180 (93.7)
	Yes	62 (1.9)	12 (6.3)
Socio economic status	Low income	1010 (30.2)	68 (35.4)
	Medium income	1824 (54.6)	95 (49.5)
	High income	507 (15.2)	29 (15.1)
Body mass index (kg/m^2)	<25 Normal	1974 (59.1)	118 (61.5)
	25–30 Overweight	947 (28.3)	49 (25.5)
	30 Obesity	420 (12.6)	25 (13.0)
Water filter	Yes	1015 (30.4)	64 (33.3)
	No	2326 (69.6)	128 (66.7)
Water supply area	Petrasiunai	1835 (54.9)	114 (59.3)
	Other	1506 (45.1	78 (40.7)
Birth year*	2007	681 (20.4)	48 (25.0)
	2008	1711 (51.2)	78 (40.6)
	2009	949 (28.4)	66 (34.4)
Maternal stress*	No	2432 (72.8)	128 (66,7)
	Yes	909 (27.2)	64 (33.3)

*$p<0.05$.

Table 2. Distribution of Kaunas cohort study subjects for various characteristic

The analysis by TTHM internal dose tertiles showed, that most characteristics of the exposure groups were similar (Table 3). There were no differences in social and demographic characteristics, health behaviour, pregnancy history, and maternal diseases. However, paternal smoking and alcohol consumption differed between exposure groups. All subjects of high THM exposure group were served by Petrasiunai water treatment plant while 99.8% subjects of low exposure group were served by other water treatment plants. Among 3,341 singleton infant, 192 (5.7%) were classified as preterm birth. The proportion of premature birth cases tended to be higher among women of medium and high THM exposure to compare to low THM exposure.

3.3 Association between THM internal dose and preterm birth risk

Using total gestational and trimester-specific daily uptakes tertiles of TTHM and individual THMs continuous variables, we examined the association between internal dose and preterm birth risk (Table 4). In THMs analysis by tertile, preterm birth risk tended to increase by increasing internal dose, however, data for TTHM and chloroform were not consistent. TTHM and chloroform analysed as continuous variables (increase of 0.1 μg/d) showed slightly elevated, but statistically non-significant increase in risk of preterm birth in all pregnancy trimesters. However, we found dose-response relationships for the first and second trimester's bromodichloromethane and dibromochloromethane internal dose and risk for preterm birth. The adjusted odds ratio for third tertile vs. first tertile dibromochloromethane internal dose of first trimester was 2.06, 95% CI 1.28–3.31; of second trimester the OR was 1.84, 95% CI 1.04–3.26; the OR per every 0.01 μg/d increase in dibromochloromethane internal dose was 1.28, 95% CI 1.04–1.57 and 1.21, 95% CI 1.01–1.45,respectively, for first and second trimester. The trend was not statistically significant when dibromochloromethane exposure were examined. The analyses were adjusted for the variables that have had effect on preterm birth risk: family status, maternal education, smoking, alcohol consumption, stress, previous preterm delivery, and infant birth year.

We used THM internal dose median level as a cut off (above median vs. below median) in a genetic polymorphism analyses. When GSTM1 genotype was considered, the association between exposure to THM and preterm birth differed by genotype: OR for preterm birth among women exposed to TTHM above median during the second trimester pregnancy was 1.03 (95% CI 0.52–2.06) and 2.07 (95% CI 1.00–4.35) for the present and absent genotype, respectively. The findings were similar for chloroform and bromodichloromethane: in carriers of GSTM1-0 genotype exposure was associated with higher OR than in carriers of GSTM1-1 genotype for all three trimesters. However, these findings were not evident when the dibromochloromethane exposures were analyzed. The OR for preterm birth among women exposed to dibromochloromethane during the second trimester was 4.33 (95% CI 1.69–11.10) and 1.69 (95% CI 0.0.78–3.64) for the present and absent genotypes, respectively.

The findings suggest that carriers of the GSTT1-0 genotype and exposed to TTHM, chloroform and bromodichloromethane had an increased risk for preterm birth compared to carriers of the GSTT1-1 genotype: the ORs during the second trimester among woman GSTT1-1 genotype carriers were 1.03–1.17, while among GSTT1-0 genotype carriers ORs were 2.46–3.08. Exposure to dibromochloromethane during the second trimester among carriers of the GSTT1-1 genotype was associated with an OR of 2.89, 95% CI 1.46–5.69, and among carriers of the GSTT1-0 genotype produced an OR of 1.42, 95% CI 0.43–4.64.

Risk factors	Characteristics	Low THM N (%)	Medium THM N (%)	High THM N (%)
Maternal age	< 20 years	19 (1.8)	17 (1.5)	23 (2.1)
	20–29 years	652 (60.1)	688 (59.7)	658 (59.6)
	≥ 30 years	414 (39.2)	447 (38.8)	423 (38.3)
Marital status	Married	876 (80.7)	958 (83.2)	910 (82.4)
	Not married	209 (19.3)	194 (16.8)	194 (17.6)
Maternal education	Primary school	59 (5.4)	50 (4.3)	57 (5.2)
	Secondary school	454 (41.8)	465 (40.4)	442 (40.0)
	University degree	572 (52.7)	637 (55.3)	605 (54.8)
Maternal smoking	Non-smoker	1003 (92.4)	1076 (93.4)	1031 (93.4)
	Smoker	82 (7.6)	76 (6.6)	73 (6.6)
Paternal smoking*	Non-smoker	574 (53.4)	629 (55.4)	545 (49.8)
	Smoker	501 (46.6)	507 (44.6)	550 (50.2)
Alcohol consumption*	No	1000 (92.2)	1094 (95.0)	1048 (94.9)
	Yes	85 (7.8)	58 (5.0)	56 (5.1)
Blood pressure (mm/Hg)	<140/80	969 (89.3)	1020 (88.5)	977 (88.5)
	≥140 or ≥ 90	116 (10.7)	132 (11.5)	127 (11.5)
Ethnic group	Lithuanian	1054 (97.1)	1117 (97.0)	1082 (98.1)
	Other	31 (2.9)	35 (3.0)	21 (1.9)
Parity	No child	492 (45.3)	499 (43.3)	516 (46.7)
	≥ 1 child	593 (54.7)	653 (56.7)	588 (53.3)
Infant gender	Male	559 (51.5)	611 (53.0)	544 (49.3)
	Female	526 (48.5)	541 (47.0)	560 (50.7)
Current residence	1–4 years	437 (40.3)	492 (42.7)	472 (42.8)
	5–9 years	257 (23.7)	288 (25.0)	296 (26.8)
	≥ 10 years	391 (36.0)	372(32.3)	336 (30.4)
Work exposure	No	996 (91.8)	1053 (91.4)	999 (90.5)
	Yes	89 (8.2)	99 (8.6)	105 (9.5)
Chronic disease	No	825 (76.0)	858 (74.5)	844 (76.4)
	Yes	260 (24.0)	294 (25.5)	260 (23.6)
Previous preterm	No	1069 (98.5)	1123 (97.5)	1087 (98.5)
	Yes	16 (1.5)	29 (2.5)	17 (1.5)
Socio economic status	Low income	335 (30.9)	337 (29.3)	338 (30.6)
	Medium income	582 (53.6)	642 (55.7)	600 (54.3)
	High income	168 (15.5)	173 (15.0)	166 (15.0)
Body mass index (kg/m^2)	<25 Normal	618 (57.0)	677 (58.8)	679 (61.5)
	25–30 Overweight	329 (30.3)	334 (29.0)	284 (25.7)
	30 Obesity	138 (12.7)	141 (12.2)	141 (12.8)
Water filter	Yes	341 (31.4)	336 (29.2)	338 (30.6)
	No	744 (68.6)	816 (70.8)	766 (69.4)
Water supply area*	Petrasiunai	2 (0.2)	728 (63.3)	1105 (100.0)
	Other	1084 (99.8)	422 (36.7)	0 (0.0)
Birth year*	2007	266 (24.5)	91 (7.9)	324 (29.3)
	2008	524 (48.3)	680 (59.1)	507 (45.9)
	2009	296 (27.3)	379 (33.0)	274 (24.8)
Maternal stress	No	794 (73.1)	848 (73.7)	790 (71.5)
	Yes	292 (26.9)	302 (26.3)	315 (28.5)
Preterm birth	No	1032 (95.0)	1079 (93.8)	1038 (93.9)
	Yes	54 (5.0)	71 (6.2)	67 (6.1)

*p<0.05.

Table 3. Distribution of Kaunas cohort study subjects for various characteristic by THM exposure

THM dose tertile limits (μg/d)	Cases	Controls	Entire pregnancy OR (95% CI)	I trimester OR (95% CI)	II trimester OR (95% CI)	III trimester OR (95% CI)
THM						
0.0025-0.0386	54	1032	1	1	1	1
0.0386-0.3496	71	1079	1.35 (0.93-1.96)	1.51 (1.04-2.18)	1.34 (0.92-1.95)	1.47 (1.01-2.14)
0.3496-2.4040	67	1038	1.24 (0.85-1.80)	1.09 (0.74-1.61)	1.18 (0.81-1.72)	1.10 (0.76-1.59)
Continuous (0.1μg/d)			1.02 (0.98-1.07)	1.01 (0.97-1.06)	1.03 (0.98-1.07)	1.02 (0.98-1.07)
Chloroform						
0.0013-0.0249	55	1035	1	1	1	1
0.0249-0.2868	73	1072	1.38 (0.95-2.02)	1.65 (1.13-2.42)	1.38 (0.94-2.02)	1.67 (1.13-2.47)
0.2868-2.1328	64	1042	1.14 (0.78-1.66)	1.15 (0.78-1.69)	1.16 (0.79-1.68)	1.20 (0.82-1.76)
Continuous (0.1μg/d)			1.03 (0.97-1.08)	1.01 (0.96-1.07)	1.03 (0.98-1.08)	1.03 (0.98-1.08)
BDCM						
0.0001-0.0124	62	1029	1	1	1	1
0.0124-0.0501	61	1085	1.02 (0.70-1.49)	1.26 (0.87-1.83)	1.21 (0.83-1.76)	1.02 (0.70-1.50)
0.0501-0.3359	69	1035	1.17 (0.82-1.68)	1.27 (0.88-1.85)	1.32 (0.91-1.90)	1.11 (0.78-1.60)
Continuous (0.01μg/d)			1.02 (0.99-1.05)	1.02 (0.98-1.06)	1.02 (0.98-1.06)	1.02 (0.99-1.05)
DBCM						
0.0000-0.0000	64	1051	1	1	1	1
0.0000-0.0039	59	1065	1.40 (0.82-2.39)	1.51 (0.91-2.51)	1.79 (1.03-3.13)	0.83 (0.51-1.36)
0.0039-0.0644	69	1033	1.67 (0.97-2.85)	2.06 (1.28-3.31)	1.84 (1.04-3.26)	1.11 (0.70-1.77)
Continuous (0.01μg/d)			1.20 (0.99-1.46)	1.28 (1.04-1.57)	1.21 (1.01-1.45)	1.12 (0.94-1.32)

Adjusted for: family status, smoking, education, alcohol consumption, stress, previous preterm birth, and infant bPirth year.

Table 4. Preterm birth adjusted OR and 95% confidence intervals for entire pregnancy and trimester-specific internal THM dose

THM exposure*	GSTM1-1 GS (95% PI)	GSTM1-0 GS (95% CI)	GSTT1-1 GS (95% CI)	GSTT1-0 GS (95% CI)
TTHM				
Entire pregnancy	1.00 (0.50–1.99)	1.86 (0.89–3.88)	1.06 (0.61–1.83)	2.55 (0.82–7.97)
First trimester	1.05 (0.53–2.10)	1.91 (0.91–4.01)	1.13 (0.65–1.96)	2.46 (0.79–7.67)
Second trimester	1.03 (0.52–2.06)	2.07 (1.00–4.35)	1.17 (0.67–2.03)	2.46 (0.80–7.68)
Third trimester	1.00 (0.50–2.00)	1.59 (0.77–3.28)	0.99 (0.87–1.72)	2.30 (0.76–6.99)
Chloroform				
Entire pregnancy	1.00 (0.50–1.99)	1.83 (0.88–3.81)	1.05 (0.61–1.83)	2.46 (0.79–7.67)
First trimester	1.04 (0.52–2.07)	1.86 (0.88–3.91)	1.11 (0.64–1.92)	2.46 (0.79–7.67)
Second trimester	1.03 (0.52–2.06)	1.97 (0.94–4.15)	1.14 (0.65–1.97)	2.66 (0.85–8.29)
Third trimester	1.00 (0.50–2.01)	1.69 (0.82–3.49)	1.03 (0.59–1.78)	2.49 (0.82–7.60)
BDCM**				
Entire pregnancy	1.06 (0.53–2.13)	1.66 (0.80–3.45)	1.03 (0.59–1.79)	2.63 (0.85–8.09)
First trimester	1.01 (0.51–2.01)	1.56 (0.76–3.22)	0.98 (0.56–1.69)	2.52 (0.83–7.65)
Second trimester	1.11 (0.55–2.21)	1.66 (0.80–3.45)	1.03 (0.59–1.79)	3.08 (0.97–9.75)
Third trimester	1.06 (0.53–2.13)	1.69 (0.81–3.51)	1.04 (0.60–1.80)	2.63 (0.85–8.09)
DBCM**				
Entire pregnancy	2.02 (0.85–4.79)	1.61 (0.76–3.42)	1.76 (0.93–3.34)	1.37 (0.43–4.38)
First trimester	7.35 (2.62–20.6)	2.81 (1.21–6.52)	4.29 (2.06–8.93)	2.47 (0.68–8.95)
Second trimester	4.33 (1.69–11.1)	1.69 (0.78–3.64)	2.89 (1.46–5.69)	1.42 (0.43–4.64)
Third trimester	2.51 (0.99–6.39)	1.34 (0.62–2.89)	1.88 (0.97–3.66)	0.96 (0.29–3.11)

*Referent group bellow median.
Adjusted for: family status, smoking, education, stress, previous preterm birth, and infant birth year.

Table 5. Preterm birth adjusted OR and 95% confidence intervals for trimester-specific and entire pregnancy internal THM dose according to maternal polymorphisms in the GST gene

3.4 Distribution preterm birth risk factors by NO_2 exposure levels

Distribution of pregnancy outcomes and NO_2 pollution levels are presented in Figure 1. The mean levels of NO_2 to which the women were exposed outside their homes throughout their pregnancies ranged from 5.3 to 36.0 μg/m³. Table 6 shows the prevalence of distribution of Kaunas cohort study subjects for various characteristic by nitrogen dioxide exposure. There were no differences in social and demographic characteristics, health behaviour, pregnancy history, maternal diseases and health behaviour between the three NO_2 exposure groups.

Risk factors	All participants N(%)	Low NO_2 N (%)	Medium NO_2 N (%)	High NO_2 N (%)
Maternal age				
< 20 years	95 (2.8)	34 (3.0)	31 (2.9)	28 (2.6)
20–29 years	1935 (58.8)	655 (58.3)	663 (61.2)	617 (56.8)
≥ 30 years	1264 (38.4)	434 (38.6)	389 (35.9)	441 (40.6)
Marital status				
Married	2707 (82.2)	920 (81.9)	888 (82.0)	899 (82.8)
Not married	585 (17.8)	203 (18.1)	195 (18.0)	187 (17.2)
Maternal education				
Primary school	162 (4.9)	52 (4.6)	55 (5.1)	55 (5.1)
Secondary school	1340 (40.7)	483 (43.0)	412 (38.0)	445 (41.0)
University degree	1790 (54.4)	588 (52.4)	616 (56.9)	586 (54.0)
Maternal smoking				
Non-smoker	3066 (93.1)	1049 (93.4)	1009 (93.2)	1008 (92.8)
Smoker	226 (6.9)	74 (6.6)	74 (6.8)	78 (7.2)
Paternal smoking				
Non-smoker	1721 (52.8)	589 (52.6)	593 (55.4)	539 (50.5)
Smoker	1536 (47.2)	530 (47.4)	477 (44.6)	529 (49.5)
Alcohol consumption				
No	3095 (94.0)	1054 (93.9)	1016 (93.8)	1025 (94.4)
Yes	197 (6.0)	69 (6.1)	67 (6.2)	61 (5.6)
Blood pressure				
<140/80 mm/Hg	2841 (86.3)	989 (88.1)	925 (85.4)	927 (85.4)
≥140 or ≥ 90 mm/Hg	451 (13.7)	134 (11.9)	158 (14.6)	159 (14.6)
Ethnic group				
Lithuanian	3205 (97.4)	1094 (97.4)	1054 (97.3)	1057 (97.3)
Other	87 (2.6)	29 (2.6)	29 (2.7)	29 (2.7)
Parity				
No child	1487 (45.2)	493 (43.9)	500 (46.2)	494 (45.5)
≥ 1 child	1805 (54.8)	630 (56.1)	583 (53.8)	592 (54.5)
Infant gender *				
Male	1690 (51.3)	615 (54.8)	543 (50.1)	532 (49.0)
Female	1602 (48.7)	508 (45.2)	540 (49.9)	554 (51.0)
Current residence				
1–4 years	1381 (42.0)	480 (42.7)	468 (43.2)	433 (39.9)
5–9 years	831 (25.2)	266 (23.7)	256 (23.6)	309 (28.5)
≥ 10 years	1080 (32.8)	377 (33.6)	359 (33.1)	344 (31.7)

Work h/week during 1st trimester				
Nonemployed				
<10 h.	537 (16.0)	172 (15.3)	161 (14.9)	194 (17.9)
10-20 h.	305 (9.3)	102 (9.1)	104 (9.6)	99 (9.1)
20-40 h.	138 (4.2)	45 (4.0)	40 (3.7)	53 (4.9)
> 40 h.	1785 (54.2)	597 (53.2)	612 (56.5)	576 (53.0)
	537 (16.3)	207 (18.4)	166 (15.3)	164 (15.1)
Chronicle disease				
No	2487 (75.5)	847 (75.4)	839 (77.5)	801 (73.8)
Yes	805 (24.5)	276 (24.6)	244 (22.5)	285 (26.2)
Previous preterm				
No	3231 (98.1)	1102 (98.1)	1061 (98.0)	1068 (98.3)
Yes	61 (1.9)	21 (1.9)	22 (2.0)	18 (1.7)
Socio economic status				
Low income	994 (30.2)	344 (30.6)	300 (27.7)	350 (32.2)
Medium income	1799 (54.6)	605 (53.9)	623 (57.5)	571 (52.6)
High income	499 (15.2)	174 (15.5)	160 (14.8)	165 (15.2)
Body mass index				
<25 Normal	1951 (59.3)	663 (59.0)	642 (59.3)	646 (59.5)
25–30 Overweight	926 (28.1)	320 (28.5)	309 (28.5)	297 (27.3)
30 Obesity	415 (12.6)	140 (12.5)	132 (12.2)	143 (13.2)
Birth year*				
2007	671 (20.4)	205 (18.3)	209 (19.3)	257 (23.7)
2008	1688 (51.3)	572 (50.9)	551 (50.9)	565 (52.0)
2009	933 (28.3)	346 (30.8)	323 (29.8)	264 (24.3)
Maternal stress				
No	2397 (72.8)	830 (73.9)	782 (72.2)	785 (72.3)
Yes	891 (27.2)	293 (26.1)	301 (27.8)	301 (27.7)
Preterm birth				
No	3105 (94.3)	1061 (94.5)	1026 (94.7)	1018 (93.7)
Yes	187 (5.7)	62 (5.5)	57 (5.3)	68 (6.3)

*$p<0.05$

Table 6. Distribution of Kaunas cohort study subjects for various characteristic by nitrogen dioxide exposure

3.5 Association between NO_2 exposure and preterm birth risk

In crude analyses, we found consistently higher, statistically non-significant, ORs for preterm birth before 37 weeks associated with higher NO_2 levels during the entire pregnancy and during the three trimesters of pregnancy (Table 7). Fully adjusted models by trimesters revealed exposure–response relationships for the entire pregnancy and trimester-specific NO_2 tertile and risk for preterm birth, however, none of these associations reached statistical significance. After adjustment for confounding variables, strongest relation between preterm birth and NO_2 levels was in the first and in the second trimesters of pregnancy. The OR for preterm birth among women exposed to third tertile NO_2 during the first trimester was 1.28 (95% CI 0.87–1.90) and 1.42 (95% CI 0.96–2.11) for the second trimester, respectively, to compare to the first NO_2 exposure tertile. During the third pregnancy trimester third NO_2 exposure tertile was associated with OR 1.12 (95% CI 0.76–1.67), compared with the lowest NO_2 exposure. Using a continuous measure, we found that the risk of preterm birth for entire pregnancy tended to increase by 22 % (adjusted OR = 1.22, 95% CI 0.94–1.56) per every 10 $\mu g/m^3$ increase in NO_2 concentrations. There was no statistically significant association between preterm birth and NO_2 exposure.

NO_2 exposure tertiles	Preterm birth (<37 weeks)		Control (>37 weeks)		Crude odds ratio	Adjusted* odds ratio
	N	%	N	%	OR (95% CI)	OR (95% CI)
Entire pregnancy						
1st tertile (6.4-18.7 μg/m³)	50	5.0	958	95.0	1	1
2nd tertile (18.7-23.7 μg/m³)	50	4.9	966	95.1	0.99 (0.66-1.48)	0.99 (0.66-1.49)
3rd tertile (23.7-44.3 μg/m³)	67	6.8	922	93.2	1.39 (0.96-2.03)	1.44 (0.98-2.11)
Continuous variable (per 10 μg/m³ increase in concentration)					1.19 (0.93-1.53)	1.22 (0.94-1.56)
First trimester						
1st tertile (5.3-16.7 μg/m³)	55	5.2	994	94.8	1	1
2nd tertile (16.7-24.0 μg/m³)	51	5.2	921	94.8	1.00 (0.68-1.48)	1.04 (0.70-1.55)
3rd tertile (24.0-53.2 μg/m³)	61	6.1	931	93.9	1.18 (0.81-1.72)	1.28 (0.87-1.90)
Continuous variable (per 10 μg/m³ increase in concentration)					1.07 (0.88-1.28)	1.11 (0.91-1.35)
Second trimester						
1st tertile (5.3-16.7 μg/m³)	47	4.8	936	95.2	1	1
2nd tertile (16.7-24.5 μg/m³)	56	5.4	989	94.6	1.13 (0.76-1.68)	1.15 (0.77-1.73)
3rd tertile (24.5-53.2 μg/m³)	64	6.5	921	93.5	1.38 (0.94-2.04)	1.42 (0.96-2.11)
Continuous variable (per 10 μg/m³ increase in concentration)					1.14 (0.95-1.37)	1.15 (0.96-1.39)
Third trimester						
1st tertile (5.3-16.7 μg/m³)	53	5.1	977	94.2	1	1
2nd tertile (16.7-24.2 μg/m³)	58	5.7	958	94.2	1.12 (0.76-1.64)	1.12 (0.76-1.66)
3rd tertile (24.2-51.9 μg/m³)	56	5.8	911	94.6	1.13 (0.77-1.67)	1.12 (0.76-1.67)
Continuous variable (per 10 μg/m³ increase in concentration)					1.10 (0.92-1.32)	1.09 (0.90-1.31)

Adjusted for: maternal smoking, education, family status, chronic diseases, previous preterm birth, stress, gender, and birth year. Parity below 4 children.

Table 7. Crude and adjusted odds ratios (OR) and their 95% confidence intervals (CI) for preterm birth by trimester-specific and entire pregnancy NO_2 exposure

Genotype	NO2 tertiles limits (μg/m³)	Total N	Preterm birth (%)	Crude OR 95% CI	Adjusted* OR 95% CI
GSTT1-1	I tertile (5.3-16.7)	171	16 (9.4)	1	1
	II tertile (16.7-24.5)	146	14 (9.6)	1.03 (0.48-2.18)	1.05 (0.47-2.36)
	III tertile (24.5-53,2)	187	25 (13.4)	1.50 (0.77-2.90)	1.64 (0.80-3.38)
GSTT1-0	I tertile (5.3-16.7)	46	6 (13.0)	1	1
	II tertile (16.7-24.5)	30	5 (16.7)	1.33 (0.37-4.83)	1.21 (0.27-5.44)
	III tertile (24.5-53,2)	26	9 (34.6)	3.53 (1.09-11.5)	5.44 (1.29-22.9)
GSTM1-1	I tertile (5.3-16.7)	107	12 (11.2)	1	1
	II tertile (16.7-24.5)	96	6 (6.3)	0.53 (0.19-1.47)	0.50 (0.17-1.44)
	III tertile (24.5-53,2)	111	17 (15.3)	1.43 (0.65-3.16)	1.42 (0.62-3.26)
GSTM1-0	I tertile (5.3-16.7)	110	10 (9.1)	1	1
	II tertile (16.7-24.5)	80	13 (16.3)	1.94 (0.80-4.68)	1.90 (0.68-5.25)
	III tertile (24.5-53,2)	102	17 (16.7)	2.00 (0.87-4.60)	2.65 (1.03-6.83)

* Adjusted for: maternal smoking, education, family status, chronic diseases, previous preterm birth, stress, and birth year.

Table 8. Crude and adjusted associations as odds ratios (OR) of NO_2 exposure during entire pregnancy with preterm birth by maternal genotypes

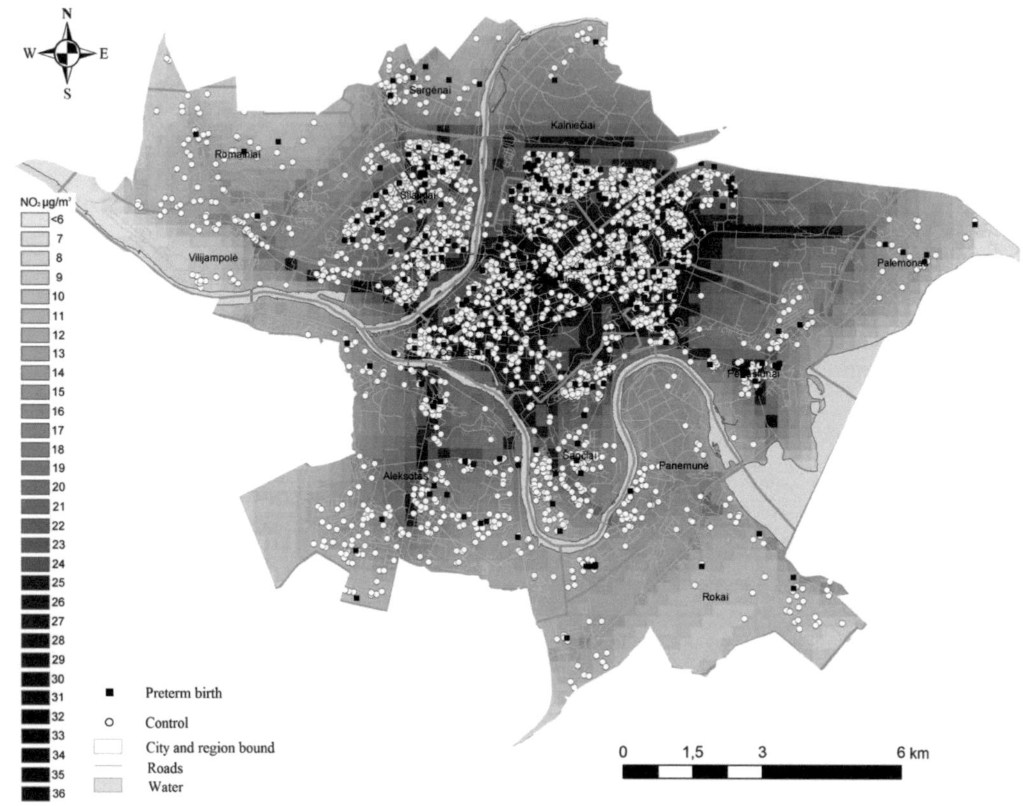

Fig. 1. Modelled NO_2 concentration and geocoded study subjects addresses

4. Discussion

4.1 Trihalomethanes effects

We conducted a prospective cohort study to examine the effects of internal dose of THM during the entire pregnancy and during three trimesters on preterm births before 37 weeks. TTHM and chloroform analysed as continuous variables (increase of 0.1 µg/d) showed slightly elevated, but statistically non-significant increase in risk of preterm birth in all pregnancy trimesters. However, we found dose-response relationships for the first and second trimester's bromodichloromethane and dibromochloromethane internal dose and risk for preterm birth. The adjusted ORs for third tertile vs. first tertile dibromochloromethane internal dose of first trimester was 2.06, 95% CI 1.28–3.31; of second trimester the OR was 1.84, 95% CI 1.04–3.26. The probability of delivering a preterm birth infant was elevated by 28% per every 0.01 µg/d increase in dibromochloromethane internal dose (OR 1.28, 95% CI 1.04-1.57) and by 21% (OR 1.21, 95% CI 1.01-1.45), respectively, for first and second trimester. The lack of statistically significant effects for other TTHM constituents may be due to low exposure because of low levels, and lack of power in our study sample.

Consistent with other recent studies (Källén & Robert; 2000; Lewis et al., 2007; Nieuwenhuijsen et al., 2009) our findings suggest that THM exposures might increase the risk of preterm birth. The epidemiological evidence for an association between exposure to THM and preterm birth is relatively inconsistent. A number of prior investigations have evaluated crude exposure during the pregnancy. An epidemiological study reported a statistically significant increased risk of delivering a preterm birth infant among women users of chlorinated with sodium hypochlorite water vs. no chlorinated water, with OR of 1.09 (CI 1.01-1.17) (Källén and Robert; 2000). Some authors found no association between preterm birth and THM (Aggazzotti et al., 2004; Hinckley et al., 2005). Some authors find small increases in gestation age with increased TTHM exposure and with both chloroform and BDCM (Wright et al., 2003; 2004). A negative association during the second trimester were reported, however, women who depended on a governmental source of payment for prenatal care were at increased risk when exposed at high levels TTHM late in gestation (OR 1.39; 95% CI, 1.06-1.81) (Lewis et al., 2007).

Lack of a consistent effect of the epidemiologic studies may be result of a study design, be a result of exposure misclassification or inadequate control for confounding variables, or a lack of power in studies sample, or actual lack of an effect of DBP on reproductive effects. This study offered advancement in individual internal dose assessment based on residential THM levels, detailed water use behaviours and exposure during pregnancy. Every subject's exposure indices were estimated as daily internal dose of the THM constituents (mg/d) and birth outcome effects were assessed by using indices categorical variable and also as a continuous variable. An additional strength of our study is that pregnant women were prospectively followed, and did not move during pregnancy. This allowed collection of self reported data on potential confounding covariates and decreased of exposure misclassification errors. However, there is a possibility of confounding in our study, because of lack information on maternal nutrition, infection diseases, and occupational physical exposures (Magann et al., 2005). Furthermore, lack of information regarding the validity of the internal dose assessment models that we used is one of the limitations of this study, but again validity studies are difficult to conduct and are expensive.

4.2 Maternal GSTT and GSTM genotypes effects

Our study adds to the findings of researchers who studied genetic polymorphism along with to environmental toxicants (Nukui et al., 2004; Suh et al., 2008) in showing effect modification between mothers with and without GSTT1- and GSTM1- genotype variant and response to the environmental hazards. Adjusted ORs for preterm birth among women exposed to TTHM above median internal dose during the second trimester pregnancy was 1.03 (95% CI 0.52-2.06) and 2.07 (95% CI 1.00-4.35) for the present and absent GSTM1 genotype, respectively. The findings suggest that carriers of the GSTT1-0 genotype and exposed to TTHM, chloroform and bromodichloromethane had an increased risk for preterm birth compared to carriers of the GSTT1-1 genotype: the ORs during the second trimester among woman GSTT1-1 genotype carriers were 1.03-1.17, while among GSTT1-0 genotype carriers ORs were 2.46-3.08. Our data indicated that individuals with GSTT1 and GSTM1 null genotypes tended to be more susceptible to THM exposure.

Our findings raises the possibility that the effect of TTHM exposure on preterm birth may be associated with one or two variant alleles for the GSTT and GSTM genes involved in the metabolism of low doses of THMs. Further tests with larger sample sizes are needed to verify these observations.

Although the effects of unmeasured risk factors could not be excluded with certainty, our findings suggest that genetically determined differences in maternal detoxification may contribute to the risk of preterm birth. In particular, women carriers of GSTT1 or GSTM1 null genotypes and exposed to high levels of NO_2 during the pregnancy were at a higher risk for preterm birth to compare to the GSTT1-1 and GSTM1-1 genotypes carriers. We observed a statistically significant association between maternal GSTT1 null genotype (OR 5.44, 95% CI 1.29–22.9) and GSTM1 null genotype (OR 2.65, 95% CI 1.03–6.83) and the risk for preterm birth infants in the presence of maternal NO_2 exposure of third tertile during pregnancy. This result provided evidence for a gene–environment interaction regarding a risk for preterm birth.

To the best of our knowledge, this is the first study to explore the synergistic effect of the GSTT1 and GSTM1 polymorphism and exposure to NO_2 on preterm birth. Limitations in interpreting these results include: there are other external exposures which we did not measure; the presence of internal uncontrolled exposures; GSTT1 and GSTM1 genes are linked to other genes responsible for preterm birth.

4.3 NO_2 exposure effects

Our findings provide little support to the hypothesis of an adverse effect of maternal exposure to NO_2 during pregnancy on preterm birth. NO_2 exposure during entire pregnancy and during the three trimesters of pregnancy tended to be associated with increase in risk of preterm birth after adjustment for the main possible confounders: maternal smoking, education, family status, chronic diseases, previous preterm birth, stress, infant gender, and birth year. In this study we also were able to estimate residential NO_2 exposure to every cohort study subject during pregnancy trimesters and to control for effect of change residence during pregnancy. Adjusted odds ratios for preterm birth for entire pregnancy exposed to third tertile NO_2 was found to be 1.44, 95% CI 0.98–2.11. The risk of preterm birth tended to increase by 22% (adjusted OR = 1.22, 95% CI 0.94–1.56) per 10 $\mu g/m^3$ increase in NO_2 concentrations. A limited statistical power of the study may be associated with a low prevalence of preterm birth in our cohort (5.7 %) and also be a consequence of low NO_2 exposure level, since only a low percentage of pregnant women were exposed to the levels exceeding established limit value of the annual mean NO_2 concentration (40 $\mu g/m^3$).

The results of the study confirm to a data of epidemiological studies performed in other countries. The reported NO_2 effect on preterm birth was small with odds ratios in the range 1.1–1.2 per 10 $\mu g/m^3$ increase in NO_2 levels or effect was not found (Gehring et al. 2011; Liu et al. 2003; Hansen et al. 2006; Ritz et al. 2007). Association of NO_2 exposure and increased risk of preterm birth was reported during different trimesters (Bobak 2000; Lee et al. 2003). A study in Valencia, Spain, find that highest association between NO_2 levels during pregnancy and preterm birth was found in second trimester (1.11, 95 % CI 1.03- 1.21) (Llop et al. 2010). Consistent with the findings of a cohort study in Vancouver, Canada where association between preterm birth and NO_2 concentrations was found during different periods of pregnancy (Liu et al. 2003), our findings suggest that NO_2 exposure might increase the risk of preterm birth.

In our previous study we found a moderately increased preterm birth risk for NO_2 exposures estimated at the entire residential district level (Maroziene and Grazuleviciene 2002). Adjusted ORs of preterm birth for the medium and high NO_2 tertile exposures were OR = 1.14 (95% CI 0.77–1.68) and OR = 1.68 (95% CI 1.15–2.46), respectively. Using a continuous measure, the risk of preterm birth increased by 25% (adjusted OR = 1.25, 95% CI 1.07–1.46) per 10 $\mu g/m^3$ increase in NO_2 concentrations.

Potential mechanisms by which air pollution might increase preterm birth include inflammation, endotelian dysfunction, endocrine disruption and genetic polymorphisms (Slama et al., 2010; Suh et al., 2008; Yorifuji et al., 2011).

Consistent with our finding, some previous studies found that exposure to maternal smoking or high levels of particulate matter in the presence of the GSTM1 null genotype is associated with the adverse birth outcomes (Sram et al., 2006; Suh et al., 2008; Grazuleviciene et al., 2009).

To make progress, this research field needs input from molecular epidemiology, toxicology, exposure assessment, and epidemiology, especially to aid in the identification and exposure assessment of reproductive-toxic agents in water and ambient air, and in the development of early markers of adverse reproductive outcomes. Additional research that clearly defines the mechanisms by which risk factors are related to preterm birth is crucial. Improved understanding of these mechanisms should allow clinicians to design appropriate interventions so that the incidence of preterm birth and related fetal and neonatal morbidity and mortality will be reduced. Improved methods of characterizing patients based on etiology that allow for the evaluation of multiple candidate genes simultaneously are most likely to be successful in identifying genetic susceptibility that increase the risk for preterm birth. Futher research should focus on the use of individual environmental exposures and genetic susceptibility in the studies of environmental toxicants effects on birth outcomes.

5. Conclusion

This study presented epidemiological evidence for a dose-response relationship between dibromochloromethane internal dose and the risk for preterm birth. The analyses were adjusted for the confounding variables that have had effect on preterm birth risk: single women, low maternal education, smoking, alcohol consumption, stress, previous preterm delivery, and infant birth year. In addition, increased THM internal dose tended to increase preterm birth risk and maternal GSTM1 and GSTT1 genotypes modified the THM exposure effects on preterm birth. Furthermore, we found an association between exposure to high levels of NO_2 during pregnancy and the presence of the GSTM1 null and GSTT1 null genotypes for the risk of preterm birth, providing evidence that both genetic and environmental factors determine complex traits such as preterm delivery. Genes involved in metabolic detoxification processes such as GSTM1 and GSTT1 may be treated as candidate risk factors for preterm birth.

6. Acknowledgment

We appreciate the contributions of the staff at Department of Obstetric and Gynaecology, Kaunas University of Medicine for providing health data. We also thank Maria Kostopoulou-Karadanelli and Stuart W Krasner for THM analyses and consultations.

7. References

Adams, MM., Elam-Evans, LD., Wilson, HG. & Gilbertz, DA. (2000). Rates of and factors associated with recurrence of preterm delivery. *The Journal of the American Medical Association,* Vol. 283, No. 12, pp. 1629-1630.

Aggazzotti, G., Righi, E., Fantuzzi, G., Biasotti, B., Ravera, G., Kanitz, S., Barbone, F., Sansebastiano, G., Battaglia, MA., Leoni, V., Fabiani, L., Triassi, M. & Sciacca, S. (2004). Chlorination by-products (CBPs) in drinking water and adverse pregnancy outcomes in Italy. *Journal of Water Health,* Vol 2, No 4, pp. 233–247.

Airviro Users Documentation. (1997). Swedish Meteorological and Hydrological Institute, Sweden.

Arand, M., Mühlbauer, R., Hengstler, J., Jäger, E., Fuchs, J., Winkler, L. & Oesch F. (1996). A multiplex polymerase chain reaction protocol for the simultaneous analysis of the glutathione S-transferase GSTM1 and GSTT1 polymorphisms. *Analytical Biochemistry,* Vol. 236, No 1, pp. 184–186.

Backer, LC., Ashley, DL., Bonin, MA., Cardinali, FL., Kieszak, SM. & Wooten, JV. (2000). Household exposures to drinking water disinfection by-products: whole blood trihalomethane levels. *Journal of Exposure Analysis and Environmental Epidemiology,* Vol. 10, No. 4, pp. 321–326.

Becker, S., Dailey, LA., Soukup, JM., Grambow, SC., Devlin, RB. & Huang, YCT. (2005). Seasonal variations in air pollution particle-induced inflammatory mediator release and oxidative stress. *Environmental Health Perspectives,* Vol. 113, No. 8, pp. 1032-1038.

Bellander, T., Berglind, N., Gustavsson, P., Jonson, T., Nyberg, F., Pershagen, G. & Järup, L. (2001). Using geographic information system to assess individual historical exposure to air pollution from traffic and house heating in Stockholm. *Environmental Health Perspectives,* Vol. 109. No. 6, pp. 633–639.

Bloom, SL., Yost, NP., McIntire ,DD. & Leveno, KJ. (2001). Recurrence of preterm birth in singleton and twin pregnancies. *Obstetrics and Gynecology,* Vol. 98, No. 3, pp. 379–385.

Bobak, M. (2000). Outdoor air pollution, low birth weight, and prematurity. *Environmental Health Perspectives,* Vol. 108, No. 2, pp. 173-176.

Bove, F., Shim, Y. & Zeitz, P. (2002). Drinking water contaminants and adverse pregnancy outcomes: a review. *Environmental Health Perspective,* Vol. 110, No. S11, pp. 61–74.

Colvin, M., Mcguire, W. & Fowlie, PW. (2004). Neurodevelopmental outcomes after preterm birth. *British Medical Journal,* Vol. 329, No. 7479, pp. 1390-1393.

Declaration of Helsinki. (1996). Recommendations guiding physicians in biomedical research involving human subjects. *British Medical Journal,* Vol. 313, No. 7070, pp. 1448-1449.

Dugandzic, R., Dodds, L., Stieb, D. & Smith-Doiron, M. (2006). The association between low level exposures to ambient air pollution and term low birth weight: a retrospective cohort study. *Environmental Health: A Global Access Science Source, Vol.* 5, No. 3, pp. 1-8. Published online 2006 February 17. doi: 10.1186/1476-069X-5-3.

Fraser, J., Walls, M. & Mcguire, W. (2004). Respiratory complications of preterm birth. *British Medical Journal,* Vol. 329, No. 7472, pp. 962-965.

Gehring, U., Wijga, AH., Fischer, P., de Jongste, JC., Kerkhof, M., Koppelman ,GH., Smit, HA. & Brunekreef, B. (2011). Traffic-related air pollution, preterm birth and term birth weight in the PIAMA birth cohort study. *Environmental Research,* Vol. 111, No. 1, pp. 125–135.

Genc, MR., Onderdonk, AB., Vardhana, S., Delaney, ML., Norwitz, ER., Tuomala, RE., Paraskevas, L-R. & Witkin, SS. (2004). Polymorphism in intron 2 of the interleukin-1 receptor antagonist gene, local midtrimester cytokine response to vaginal flora, and subsequent preterm birth. *American Journal of Obstetrics and Gynecology,* Vol. 191, No. 4, pp. 1324-1330.

Goldenberg, RL., Culhane, JF., Iams, JD. & Romero, R. (2008). Epidemiology and causes of preterm birth. *The Lancet,* Vol. 371, No. 9606, pp. 75-84.

Graves, CG., Matanoski, GM. & Tardiff, RG. (2001). Weight of evidence for an association between adverse reproductive and developmental effects and exposure to disinfection by-products: a critical review. *Regulatory Toxicology and Pharmacology,* Vol. 34, No. 2, pp. 103–124.

Grazuleviciene, R., Danileviciute, A., Nadisauskiene, R. & Vencloviene, J. (2009). Maternal smoking, GSTM1 and GSTT1 polymorphism and susceptibility to adverse pregnancy outcomes. *International Journal of Environmental Research and Public Health.* Vol. 6, No. 3, pp. 1282-1297.

Grazuleviciene, R., Nieuwenhuijsen, MJ., Vencloviene, J., Kostopoulou-Karadanelli, M., Krasner, SW., Danileviciute, A., Balcius, G. & Kapustinskiene, V. (2011). Individual exposures to drinking water trihalomethanes, low birth weight and small for gestational age risk: a prospective Kaunas cohort study. *Environmental Health,* Vol. 10, pp. 1-32. doi:10.1186/1476-069X-10-32.

Grellier, J., Bennett, J., Patelarou, E., Smith, RB., Toledano, MB., Rushton, L., Briggs, DJ. & Nieuwenhuijsen, MJ. (2010). Exposure to disinfection by-products, fetal growth, and prematurity: a systematic review and meta-analysis. *Epidemiology,* Vol. 21, No. 3, pp. 300-313.

Hackley, B., Feinstein, A. & Dixon, J. (2007). Air pollution: impact on maternal and perinatal health. *Journal of Midwifery and Women's Health,* Vol. 52, No. 5, pp. 435–443.

Hansen, C., Neller, A,. Williams, G. & Simpson, R. (2006). Maternal exposure to low levels of ambient air pollution and preterm birth in Brisbane, Australia. *An International Journal of Obstetrics and Gynaecology,* Vol. 113, No.8, pp. 935-941.

Hinckley, AF., Bachand, AM. & Reif, JS. (2005). Late pregnancy exposures to disinfection by-products and growth-related birth outcomes. *Environmental Health Perspective, Vol.* 113, No. 12, pp. 1808–1813.

Hoffman, CS., Mendola, P., Savitz, DA., Herring, AH., Loomis. D., Hartmann, KE., Singer, PC., Weinberg, HS. & Olshan, AF. (2008). Drinking water disinfection by-product exposure and fetal growth. *Epidemiology,* Vol.19, No.5, pp. 729–737.

Jaakkola, JJ., Magnus, P., Skrondal, A., Hwang, BF., Becher, G. & Dybing, E. (2001). Foetal growth and duration of gestation relative to water chlorination. *Occupational and Environmental Medicine,* Vol. 58, No. 7, pp. 437-442.

Kallen, BA. & Robert, E. (2000). Drinking water chlorination and delivery outcome-a registry-based study in Sweden. *Reproductive Toxicology,* Vol. 14, No. 4, pp. 303-309.

Kannan, S., Misra, DP., Dvonch, JT. & Krishnakumar, A. (2006). Exposures to airborne particulate matter and adverse perinatal outcomes: a biologically plausible mechanistic framework for exploring potential effect modification by nutrition. Environmental Health Perspectives, Vol. 114, No. 11, pp. 1636-1642.

Kelada, SN., Eaton, DL., Wang, SS., Rothman, NR. & Khoury, MJ. (2003). The role of genetic polymorphism in environmental health. *Environ Health Perspect,* Vol. 111, No. 8, pp. 1055–1064.

King, WD., Dodds, L., Armson, BA., Allen, AC., Fell, DB. & Nimrod, C. (2004). Exposure assessment in epidemiologic studies of adverse pregnancy outcomes and disinfection byproducts. *Journal of Exposure Analysis and Environmental Epidemiology,* Vol. 14, No. 6, pp. 466-472.

Lee, BE., Ha, EH., Park, HS., Kim, YJ., Hong, YC., Kim, H. & Lee, JT. (2003). Exposure to air pollution during different gestational phases contributes to risk of low birth weight risk. *Human Reproduction,* Vol. 18, No. 3, pp. 638–643.

Leem, JH., Kaplan, BM., Shim, YK., Pohl, HR., Gotway, CA., Bullard, SM., Rogers, JF., Smith, MM. & Tylenda, CA. (2006). Exposures to air pollutants during pregnancy and preterm delivery. *Environmental Health Perspectives,* Vol. 114, No. 6, pp. 905-910.

Lewis, C., Suffet, IH., Hoggatt, K. & Ritz, B. (2007). Estimated effects of disinfection by-products on preterm birth in a population served by a single water utility. *Environmental Health Perspective,* Vol. 115, No. 2, pp. 290-295.

Lewis, C., Suffet, IH. & Ritz, B. (2006). Estimated effects of disinfection by-products on birth weight in a population served by a single water utility. *American Journal of Epidemiology,* Vol. 163, Vo. 1, pp. 38–47.

Liu, S., Krewski, D., Shi, Y., Chen, Y. & Burnett, RT. (2003). Association between gaseous ambient air pollutants and adverse pregnancy outcomes in Vancouver, Canada. *Environmental Health perspectives,* Vol. 111, No. 14, pp. 1773-1778.

Llop, S., Ballester, F., Estarlich, M., Esplugues, A., Rebagliato, M. & Iñiguez, C. (2010). Preterm birth and exposure to air pollutants during pregnancy. *Environmental Research,* Vol. 110, No. 8, pp. 778–785.

Lynberg, M., Nuckols, JR., Langlois, P., Ashley, D., Singer, P., Mendola, P., Wilkes, C., Krapfl, H., Miles, E., Speight, V., Lin, B., Small, L., Miles, A., Bonin, M., Zeitz, P., Tadkod, A., Henry, J. & Forrester, MB. (2001). Assessing exposure to disinfection by-products in women of reproductive age living in Corpus Christi, Texas, and Cobb County, Georgia: descriptive results and methods. *Environmental Health Perspectives,* Vol. 109, No. 6, pp. 597–604.

MacLehose, RF., Savitz, DA., Herring, AH., Hartmann, KE., Singer, PC. & Weinberg, HS. (2008). Drinking water disinfection by-products and time to pregnancy. *Epidemiology*, Vol. 19, No. 3, pp. 451–458.

Macones, GA., Parry, S., Elkousy, M., Clothier, B., Ural, SH. & Strauss, JF. (2004). A polymorphism in the promoter region of TNF and bacterial vaginosis: Preliminary evidence of gene environment interaction in the etiology of spontaneous preterm birth. *American Journal of Obstetrics and Gynecology,* Vol. 190, No. 6, pp. 1504-1508.

Magann, EF., Evans, SF., Chauhan, SP., Nolan, TE., Henderson, J., Klausen, JH., Newnham, JP. & Morrison, JC. (2005). The effects of standing, lifting and noise exposure on preterm birth, growth restriction, and perinatal death in healthy low-risk working military women. *Journal of Maternal- Fetal and Neonatal Medicine,* Vol. 18, No. 3, pp. 155-162.

Maisonet, M., Bush, TJ., Correa, A. & Jaakkola, JJ. (2001). Relation between ambient air pollution and low birth weight in the northeastern United States. *Environmental Health Perspectives,* Vol. 109, No. S3, pp. 351-356.

Maroziene, L., & Grazuleviciene, R. (2002). Maternal exposure to low-level air pollution and pregnancy outcomes: a population-based study. *Environmental Health,* Vol. 1. No. 6, pp. 1–13.

Mohorovic, L. (2004). First two months of pregnancy—critical time for preterm delivery and low birth weight caused by adverse effects of coal combustion toxics. *Early Human Development,* Vol. 80, No. 2, pp. 115-123.

Moison, RM., Palinckx, JJ., Roest, M., Houdkamp, E. & Berger, HM. (1993). Induction of lipid peroxidation of pulmonary surfactant by plasma of preterm babies. *The Lancet*, Vol. 341, No. 8837, pp. 79-82.

Murphy, DJ., Fowlie, PW. & Mcguire, W. (2004). Obstetric issues in preterm birth. *British Medical Journal,* Vol. 329, No. 7469, pp. 783-786.

Nieuwenhuijsen, MJ., Grellier, J., Smith, R., Iszatt, N., Bennett, J., Best, N. & Toledano, M. (2009). The epidemiology and possible mechanisms of disinfection by-products in drinking water. *Philosophical Transaction. Series A, Mathemathical, Physical and Enginieric Science,* Vol. 367, No. 1904, pp. 4043–4076.

Nieuwenhuijsen, MJ., Toledano, MB., Eaton, NE., Fawell, J. & Elliott, P. (2000). Chlorination disinfection by-products in water and their association with adverse reproductive outcomes, a review. *Occupational and Environmental Medicine*, Vol. 57, No. 2, pp. 73–85.

Nikolaou, A., Golfinopoulos, S., Rizzo, L., Lofrano, G., Lekkas, T. & Belgiorno, V. (2005). Optimisation of analytical methods for the determination of DBPs: Application to drinking waters from Greece and Italy. *Desalination,* Vol. 176, No. 1-3, pp. 25–36.

Nukui, T., Day, RD., Sims, CS., Ness, RB. & Romkes, M. (2004). Maternal/newborn GSTT1 null genotype contributes to risk of preterm, low birth weight infants. *Pharmacogenetics,* Vol. 14, No. 9, pp. 569–576.

Pekkanen, J., Brunner, EJ., Anderson, HR., Tiittanen, P. & Atkinson, RW. (2000). Daily concentrations of air pollution and plasma fibrinogen in London. *Occupational and Environmental Medicine,* Vol. 57, No. 12, pp. 818-822.

Perera, FP., Jedrychowski, W., Rauh, V. & Whyatt, RM. (1999). Molecular epidemiologic research on the effects of environmental pollutants on the fetus. *Environmental Health Perspective,* Vol. 107, No. S3, pp. 451-460.

Plunkett, J. & Muglia, LJ. (2008). Genetic contributions to preterm birth: Implications from epidemiological and genetic association studies. *Annals of Medicine,* Vol. 40, No. 3, pp. 167–195.

Richardson, SD. (2003). Disinfection by-products and other emerging contaminants in drinking water. *Trends in Analytic Chemistry,* Vol. 22, No. 10, pp. 666-684.

Rijnders, E., Janssen, NA., van Vliet, PH. & Brunekreef, B. (2001). Personal and outdoor nitrogen dioxide concentrations in relation to degree of urbanization and traffic density. *Environmental Health Perspective,* Vol. 109, No. S3, pp. 411–417.

Ritz, B., Wilhelm, M., Hoggatt, KJ. & Ghosh, JKC. (2007). Ambient Air Pollution and Preterm Birth in the Environment and Pregnancy Outcomes Study at the University of California, Los Angeles. *American Journal of Epidemiology,* Vol. 166, No. 9, pp. 1045-1052.

Rothman, N., Wacholder, S., Caporaso, NE., Garcia-Closas, M., Buetow, K. & Fraumeni, JF. Jr. (2001). The use of common genetic polymorphisms to enhance the epidemiologic study of environmental carcinogens. *Acta Biochimica et Biophysica,* Vol. 147, No. 2, pp. C1–C10.

Sagai, M., & Ichinose, T. (1991). Experimental study on lipid peroxide formation and tumor-promoting effects of nitrogen dioxide and ozone. *In: Oxidative Damage and Repair (Edited by: Davies KTA) Oxford, UK: Pergamon* 1991, 511-516.

Savitz, DA., Singer, PC., Herring, AH., Hartmann, KE., Howard, S., Weinberg, HS. & Makarushka, C. (2006). Exposure to drinking water disinfection by-products and pregnancy loss. *American Journal of Epidemiology,* Vol. 164, No. 11, pp. 1043–1051.

Shin, JC. (2008). Genetics of preterm birth. *Journal of Women's Medicine,* Vol. 1, No. 2, pp. 61-70.

Slama, R., Gräbsch, C., Lepeule, J., Siroux, V., Cyrys, J., Sausenthaler, S., Herbarth, O., Bauer, M., Borte, M., Wichmann, HE. & Heinrich, J. (2006). Maternal fine particulate matter exposure, polymorphism in xenobiotic-metabolizing genes and offspring birth weight. *Reproductive Toxicology,* Vol. 30, No. 4, pp. 600-12.

Sram, RJ., Binkova, B., Dejmek, J. & Bobak, M. (2005). Ambient air pollution and pregnancy outcomes: a review of the literature. *Environmental Health Perspectives,* Vol. 113, No. 4, pp. 375–382.

Sram, RJ., Binkova, B., Dejmek, J., Chvatalova, I., Solansky, I. & Topinka, J. (2006). Association of DNA adducts and genotypes with birth weight. *Mutatation Research,* Vol. 608, No. 2, pp. 121–128.

Sram, RJ., Binkova, B., Rossner, P., Rubes, J., Topinka, J. & Dejmek, J. (1999). Adverse reproductive outcomes from exposure to environmental mutagens. *Mutatation Research,* Vol. 428, No. 1-2, pp. 203-215.

Suh, YJ., Ha, EH., Park, H., Kim, YJ., Kime, H. & Hong, YC. (2008). GSTM1 polymorphism along with PM10 exposure contributes to the risk of preterm delivery. *Mutation Research,* Vol. 656, No. 1-2, pp. 62–67.

Svensson, AC., Sandin, S., Cnattingius, S., Reilly, M., Pawitan, Y., Hultman, CM. & Lichtenstein, P. (2009). Maternal Effects for Preterm Birth: A Genetic Epidemiologic Study of 630,000 Families. *American Journal of Epidemiology,* Vol. 170, No. 11, pp. 1365–1372.

Tabacova, S., Baird, DD. & Balabaeva, L. (1998). Exposure to oxidized nitrogen: lipid peroxidation and neonatal health risk. *Archives of Environmental Health,* Vol. 53, No.3, pp. 214-221.

Tardiff, RG., Carson, ML. & Ginevan, ME. (2006). Updated weight of evidence for an association between adverse reproductive and developmental effects and exposure to disinfection by-products. *Regulatory Toxicology and Pharmacology,* Vol. 45, No. 2, pp. 185–205.

Tucker, J. & Mcguire, W. (2004). Epidemiology of preterm birth. *British Medical Journal,* Vol. 329, No. 7467, pp. 675-678.

Wang, X., Chen, D., Niu, T., Wang, Z., Wang, L., Ryan, L., Smith, T., Christiani, DC., Zuckerman, B. & Xu, X. (2000). Genetic susceptibility to benzene and shortened gestation: evidence of gene–environment interaction. *American Journal of Epidemiology,* Vol. 152, No. 8, pp. 693–700.

Wang, X., Zuckerman, B., Pearson, C., Kaufman, G., Chen, C., Wang, G., Niu, T., Wise, PH., Bauchner, H. & Xu, X. (2002). Maternal cigarette smoking, metabolic gene polymorphism, and infant birth weight. *The Journal of American Medical Association,* Vol. 287, No. 2, pp. 195–202.

Whitaker, HJ., Nieuwenhuijsen, MJ., Best, NG. (2003). The relationship between water concentrations and individual uptake of chloroform: a simulation study. *Environmental Health Perspective,* Vol. 111, No. 5, pp. 688–694.

Windham, GC., Hopkins, B., Fenster, L. & Swan, SH. (2000). Prenatal active or passive tobacco smoke exposure and the risk of preterm delivery or low birth weight. *Epidemiology,* Vol. 11, No.4, pp. 427–433.

Woodruff, TJ., Parker, JD., Darrow, LA., Slama, R., Bell, ML., Choi, H., Glinianaia, S., Hoggatt, KJ., Karr, CJ., Lobdell, DT. & Wilhelm, M. (2009). Methodological issues in studies of air pollution and reproductive health. *Environmental Research,* Vol. 109, No. 3, pp. 311–320.

Wright, JM., Schwartz, J. & Dockery, DW. (2002). Effect of trihalomethane exposure on fetal development. *Occupational and Environmental Medicine,* Vol. 60, No. 3, pp. 173–180.

Wright, JM., Schwartz, J. & Dockery, DW. (2004). The effect of disinfection by-products and mutagenic activity on birth weight and gestational duration. *Environmental Health Perspectives,* Vol. 112, No. 8, pp. 920–925.

Yang, CY., Xiao, ZP., Ho, SC., Wu, TN. & Tsai, SS. (2007). Association between trihalomethane concentrations in drinking water and adverse pregnancy outcome in Taiwan. *Environmental Research,* Vol. 104, No. 3, pp. 390–395.

Yorifuji, T., Naruse, H., Kashima, S., Ohki, S., Murakoshi, T., Takao, S., Tsuda, T. & Doi, H. (2011). Residential proximity to major roads and preterm births. *Epidemiology,* Vol. 22, No. 1, pp. 74-80.

3

Clinical Risk Factors for Preterm Birth

Ifeoma Offiah, Keelin O'Donoghue and Louise Kenny
Anu Research Centre, Cork University Maternity Hospital
Ireland

1. Introduction

1.1 Definitions

Preterm birth (PTB) refers to the birth of a baby that occurs before 37 completed weeks of gestation. PTB can be further sub-categorized as late preterm delivery- 34 to 36 completed weeks gestation, moderately preterm- 32 to 34 completed weeks, very preterm- less than 32 weeks, and extremely preterm- less than 28 weeks gestation (Lockwood, et al., 2011). Preterm birth can also be defined by birth weight: low birth weight- less than 2500g, very low birth weight- 1500g, and extremely low birth weight- less than 1000g (Lockwood, et al., 2011).

1.2 Significance

Preterm birth is an increasingly common complex condition with multiple risk factors (Allen, 2008) and has substantial medical, psychological, economic and social impacts. It is the leading cause of infant mortality in the United States. Compared with term neonates, mortality rates for preterm (less than 37 weeks) and very preterm infants (less than 32 weeks) are 15-fold and 75-fold higher respectively (Mathews, et al., 2004). The organs most commonly affected by preterm delivery are the lungs, as the lungs are one of the last organs to develop in utero. Preterm birth is also the most important determinant of short and long term morbidity in infants and children, and can have serious long term health consequences, such as cerebral palsy, blindness, developmental difficulties, including cognitive, sensory, learning and language deficits (Allen, 2008). The younger the gestation, the greater the risk of severe morbidity. The EPIPAGE study group reported a twofold increased prevalence of hyperactivity, inattention and peer problems in very preterm birth children at school ages when compared to children born at term (Delobel-Ayoub, et al., 2009). Additionally, preterm birth and low birth weight is associated with cardiovascular disease in adult life (Barker, et al., 1993).

1.3 Incidence

Significant progress has been made in the care of premature infants, but not in reducing the prevalence of preterm birth (Goldenberg, et al., 2008). In the United States, there has been a 21% rise in the rate of preterm births since 1990, which peaked in 2006 with 12.8% of all 4 million annual live births born at less than 37 weeks of gestation (Russell, et al., 2007). The incidence in Europe and other developed countries lies between 5-9% (Goldenberg, et al., 2008). East Asian and Hispanic women typically have a low pre-term birth rate. However, the incidence of preterm birth continues to rise. Part of this escalation is due to the increased

indicated preterm delivery of artificially conceived multiple pregnancies, which account for 15-20% of all pre-term births (Goldenburg, et al., 2008).
Preterm birth is the principal cause of infant mortality in developed countries. One in 8 births in the United States in 2005 were preterm, compared to 1 in 18 births in Ireland and Finland. The infant mortality rate in Ireland in 2010 was 3.89 per 1000 live births and in the United States 6.8 per 1000 live births. The main cause of the United States' high infant mortality rate when compared with Europe is the very high percentage of preterm births in the United States, the period when infant mortality is greatest (Mac Dorman & Mathews, 2010).

1.4 Economic implications

The cost associated with providing care for preterm infants, who may spend numerous months in hospital, has significant implications for the economy. In the UK, 75% of neonatal deaths, and the majority of neonatal intensive care admissions, are due to preterm infants.
A nationwide survey carried out by Russell and colleagues in 2001, regarding the hospital cost of preterm infants showed that in the United States, in 2001, 4.6 million infants were hospitalized, costing $12.4 billion. Of these, 8% of hospitalizations were for preterm or low birth weight infants, the hospital care cost of which totaled $5.8 billion. This represents 47% of the costs for all infant hopitalizations. This cost is partly explained by the increased cost of caring for a preterm infants in hospital, $15,100, and an extremely preterm infant, $65,600, versus $600 for an uncomplicated newborn. Additionally, preterm infants and extremely preterm infant have, on average, an increased length of stay in hospital than uncomplicated newborns: 12.9 days and 42.2 days versus 1.9 days respectively (Russell, et al., 2007). This data suggests that major infant and paediatric cost savings can be achieved by the identification and prevention of preterm birth.

2. Risk factors

Several factors have been identified that are associated with preterm birth. These include intrauterine inflammation/ infection, uterine overdistension, uteroplacental ischaemia / haemorrhage, and stress. However, an association does not establish causality.
Mothers exposed to high levels of psychological or social stresses are at increased risk of pre-term birth. Additionally, exposure to severe life events, has also been linked to very and extremely pre-term births. Clinical depression, possibly due to its associated increase in smoking, alcohol and drug use also plays a role in increasing pre-term birth as mediated by these behaviours. Tobacco use alone increases the pre-term birth rate by almost 2 fold, due to the associated increased risk of small for gestational age and placental abruption. There are also marked ethnic differences in the incidence and aetiology of preterm birth, with African American women being consistently at increased risk of preterm birth compared to native white women.
As the cause of labour still remains elusive, the exact cause of preterm birth is also uncertain.
Approximately 30–35% of preterm births are indicated or iatrogenic due to medical or obstetric complications, 40–45% are related to spontaneous preterm labour, and 25–30% to preterm prelabour rupture of membranes (PPROM). Spontaneous pre-term birth is most

commonly caused by pre-term labour in Caucasians, and PPROM in black women indicating the existence of potentially different causative mechanisms. This chapter will review the current literature on established and putative risk factors for spontaneous preterm labour and PPROM.

2.1 Previous preterm birth

The risk of preterm birth is increased among women who have had a previous preterm birth (Iams et al., 1998). Previous preterm birth is the strongest risk factor for repeated preterm delivery and recurrences often occur at a similar gestational age, with around 70% delivering within 2 weeks of the gestational age of their first preterm delivery (Bloom, et al., 2001). Yet, the majority of mothers who have had a preterm delivery will go on to have a subsequent term delivery. Term births decrease the risk of PTB in subsequent pregnancies. Some risk factors of preterm delivery, if not adequately treated or permanent, persist in subsequent pregnancies.

Given the strong risk of recurrence, the genetic aspects of preterm delivery have become a matter of keen interest. Several studies suggest that a new partner between pregnancies reduces the risk of preterm delivery. A study carried out by Li suggested that among women with a preterm delivery at gestational age less than 34 weeks, changing partners resulted in a 33% reduction in the risk of preterm delivery in the subsequent pregnancy, compared to those who did not change partners (Li, 1999). However, a change in partners may reflect an association with long inter-pregnancy intervals rather than the influence of the partner's genetics *per se.* A more recent and extensive study of this hypothesis suggested that fathers contributed little to the preterm delivery risk (Wilcox, et al., 2008).

Genetic researchers have instead concentrated on both maternal and fetal genes, as poor perinatal outcomes can, in principle, be affected by both the maternal genotype and the fetal genotype (Wilcox, et al., 2008). It is obvious that fetal genes can affect fetal wellbeing. However, the role of maternal genetics in fetal health and pregnancy outcome is more subtle.

Wilcox et al, 2008, carried out a study to investigate familial recurrence of preterm birth, and analyze the relative contributions of maternal and fetal genotypes to the risk of preterm delivery. They concluded that the recurrence risk of preterm birth was transmitted through the mother, with a higher risk if the mother was born preterm herself. There was no increased risk with the father's previous history or genetic input (Wilcox, et al., 2008). Other studies implicate a significant increase in risk to children, whose older siblings were affected by preterm birth, due to maternal and /or fetal genetic influences (Plunkett, et al., 2008). This increased risk still persists even after adjustment for common non-genetic environmental risk factors in families.

2.2 Iatrogenic preterm delivery

Iatrogenic preterm delivery accounts for more than 30% of all preterm deliveries. The preterm birth rate continues to escalate in many countries worldwide because of an increase in the indicated preterm births rate (Goldenberget al., 2008). Pre-eclampsia and placental abruption affects approximately 7% and 1% of all pregnancies, respectively. Along with intrauterine growth restriction and premature rupture of the membranes, they represent the most common reasons for indicated preterm delivery (Goldenberg, 2008, Plunket, 2008). Multiple gestations make up 10% of all preterm births, the majority of which, (50%), are delivered preterm due to medical indications (Moutquin, 2003). The Obstetrician has to weigh up the benefits of allowing the pregnancy to continue in order to achieve improved perinatal outcome for the preterm infant, against delivering the fetus early for the health of the mother and infant. In 1995, The American College of Obstetricians and Gynecologists reported a survival rate for newborns at 34 weeks gestation as being within 1% of those born at or beyond 37 weeks (Hauth, 2006).

2.3 Preterm prelabour rupture of membranes

Preterm Prelabour Rupture of Membranes (PPROM) complicates only 2% of pregnancies but is associated with 40-45% of preterm deliveries. It can occur spontaneously or can be iatrogenic following invasive procedures such as diagnostic amniocentesis or cervical surgery. PPROM together with spontaneous preterm labour accounts for almost 75% of all cases of preterm birth. At less than 37 weeks' gestation rupture of the membranes places the mother and the fetus at increased risk of short-term and long-term morbidity and mortality.
The three causes of neonatal death associated with PPROM are prematurity, sepsis and pulmonary hypoplasia. Women with intrauterine infection deliver earlier than non-infected women and infants born with sepsis have a mortality rate four times higher than those without sepsis (RCOG, Green-top Guideline No. 44, 2010).
The decision to deliver the fetus prematurely or to manage the pregnancy expectantly following a diagnosis of PPROM requires careful assessment of the dangers related to prematurity in pregnancies delivered earlier compared with the development of intrauterine infection in those pregnancies managed expectantly. Since the 1970s expectant management has been the standard treatment for PPROM (Alexander & Cox, 1996). Controversy exists over the gestational age at which expectant management should be abandoned and active interventions to effect delivery pursued. The Royal College of Obstetricians and Gynaecologists, Green-top Guideline, No. 44, recommend delivery at 34 weeks' gestation due to the increased risk of chorioamnionitis thereafter (RCOG, Green-top Guideline No. 44, 2010).

2.4 Antepartum haemorhage

Vaginal bleeding in early pregnancy has been consistently shown to be an independent risk factor for preterm delivery. One study quotes a two-fold increase in the risk of preterm birth in mothers who had bleeding in the first trimester of pregnancy compared to mothers with no vaginal bleeding (Williams, et al., 1991). Even women with only light vaginal bleeding were also at a significantly increased risk of preterm birth (Berkowitz, et al., 1983).
Antepartum haemorrhage in the second or third trimester of pregnancy is an important risk factor for preterm birth. A bloody show is benign and does not contribute to preterm birth. Other causes of antepartum haemorrhage, including placental abruption and placenta praevia, although they represent a minority of cases of antepartum haemorrhage (Chan & To, 1999), are more ominous and if left untreated could potentially lead to the death of the fetus and mother. Other non-obstetric causes of antepartum haemorrhage, such as bleeding from the lower genital tract or rectal bleeding need to be carefully excluded. Antepartum haemorrhage of unknown origin remains the most common cause of bleeding in pregnancy, accounting for more than 50% of all cause of antepartum haemorrhage (Chan & To, 1999).
A retrospective analysis into the timing of preterm birth and antepartum haemorrhage showed that the risk of preterm delivery, although higher with associated uterine contractions, was still significant even without contractions: 62.5% versus 13.6% (Leung, et al., 2001).

2.4.1 Abruption

Evidence exists that correlates decidual bleeding with chronic uteroplacental vascular pathologic processes (Salafia, et al., 1995). Implantation of the human blastocyst involves trophoblastic invasion deep into the decidual cells of the uterus. Shallow invasion leads to inadequate decidual vascular formation and subsequent poor uteroplacental blood flow (Lockwood, et al., 2009). Placental ischaemia occurs and is implicated in the pathogenesis of placental abruption and of preterm birth (Vintzileos, 2008, Ananth, et al., 2007). Decidual bleeding at the time of formation of the placenta is associated with preterm birth through an increased risk of PPROM (Harger, 1990).

2.5 Excessive uterine distention

Polyhydramnios, multiple gestations, and other reasons of excessive uterine distention are well studied risk factors for PTB. Over stretching of the uterine muscle induces the formation of gap junctions, upregulation of oxytocin receptors, and production of prostaglandin E2 and F2 and myosin light chain kinase, which are critical events preceding uterine contractions and cervical dilation (Ou, CW., & Orsino A. 1997).

2.5.1 Abnormal amniotic fluid volumes

Abnormal amniotic fluid volumes is associated with poor perinatal outcome. The incidence of polyhydramnios, an excess amount of amniotic fluid, ranges from 1- 2% of all pregnancies depending on the diagnostic criteria used (Hill, et al., 1987, Bundgaard, et al., 2007). It is caused by fetal malformation, such as gastrointestinal obstruction, in the majority of cases, followed closely by maternal diabetes mellitus. Other causes such as fetal anaemia and congenital infection play a less significant role (Beloosesky & Ross, 2010). Polyhydramnios causes uterine overdistension and thus predisposes pregnancies to preterm delivery. Complications associated with oligohydramnios include skeletal deformations, contractures and pulmonary hypoplasia. Preterm delivery in fetuses with no congenital anomalies, either spontaneous preterm birth or medically indicated due to maternal or fetal complications, occurs in more than 62% of cases of oligohydramnios, compared to 8% in pregnancies with normal liquor volumes (Petrozella, et al, 2011).

2.5.2 Multiple gestations

Multiple gestations are high-risk pregnancies, which are often complicated by preterm birth, low birth weight, neonatal morbidity and perinatal, neonatal and infant mortality. Twins and higher order multiple pregnancies account for only 2 to 3% of all births, but make up more than 17% of late preterm births, and 23% of very preterm births (Blickstein, 2006). The average birth age of most multiple gestations occurs in the late preterm period due to the occurrence of spontaneous onset of labour and iatrogenic preterm birth. 50% of all twins and more than 90% of triplets are born premature. 36% of triplets are delivered before 32 weeks gestation (Blickstein, 2006). Of the preterm pregnancies, twins are also at increased risk of being born at an earlier gestation than singleton pregnancies (Gardner, et al., 1995). Determination of chorionicity is important as the risk of preterm birth in dichorionic twins before 32 weeks is 5.5% and in monochorionic twins, 9% (Krampl & Klein, 2007). Iatrogenic preterm birth in monochorionic twins significantly increases the number of preterm deliveries in this type of twinning as obstetric and maternal complications are particularly high (Lee, et al., 2006). The most concerning complication associated with monochorionicity

is twin to twin transfusion syndrome (TTTS). The management of these pregnancies is controversial especially regarding the optimal timing of delivery. Some recommend preterm delivery of monochorionic diamniotic twins, even without TTTS or other anomalies, due to the high incidence (ranging from 3.6% to 4.6%) of unexpected intrauterine fetal death despite intensive fetal monitoring after 32 weeks of gestation (Lee, et al., 2008, Barigye, et al., 2005).
The endocrine environment produced by multiple gestations may also be a contributing factor. Multiple gestations produce a higher amount of estrogen, progesterone, and sex steroids compared to singleton pregnancies (Robinson, 2011). Increased steroid production in multiple pregnancies may play a role in initiation of preterm labor. In particular, higher peripheral levels of relaxin, associated with multiple gestations, may cause cervical insufficiency, with subsequent PTB (Weiss, et al., 1993).
The emergence of assisted reproduction technologies has increased the rate of multiple gestations.
The pathophysiology for preterm birth in multiple gestations, particularly higher order multiple gestations, may be related to uterine over-distension and increased intrauterine volume, or related complications such as cervical incompetence. Healthcare professionals should endeavor to reduce the risk of multiple gestation and pre-term labour through appropriate monitoring of patients treated with fertility drugs and limiting the number of embryos transferred. Reduction of multiple gestations, particularly high order multi-fetal pregnancies, may improve neonatal outcome.

2.6 Uterine trauma/anomalies

Uterine abnormalities predispose to preterm birth, due to the inability of uterus to hold the pregnancy until term. Uterine leiomyomas are the most common abnormalities observed. Pregnancies with uterine duplication anomalies, such as bicornuate uteri are more likely to be complicated by preterm birth at less than 34 weeks gestation, 29% versus a preterm birth rate of 3% at 34 weeks, with normal uteri (Cooney, et al., 1998). Unicornuate uteri, although rare, (1: 4020) carries with it the poorest overall obstetric outcome with a preterm birth rate of 20.1% (Reichman, et al., 2009).

2.6.1 Uterine leiomyoma

Leiomyoma, better known as uterine fibroids, are benign smooth muscle neoplasms of the uterus. They arise in women of reproductive age, and in most cases are asymptomatic. Reports of an increase in the size of uterine fibroids during pregnancy have been inconsistent throughout the literature (Aharoni, 1988, Lev-Toaff, 1987, Strobel 1994). Those that do increase in pregnancy do so in the first trimester (Ouyang, 2006). The most common recognized complication of uterine fibroids in pregnancy is pain, affecting approximately 10% of women with fibroids (Rasmussen & Knudsen, 1994).
There appears to be a small increase in the rate of preterm birth in pregnant women with uterine fibroids. This risk is further increased if there are multiple fibroids present in the uterus or if placentation has occurred next to or overlying a submucosal fibroid (Lev-Toaff). Various theories have been proposed regarding the relationship between preterm birth and fibroids. These include a localized increase in oxytocin levels and premature contractility when a gravid fibroid uterus reaches a certain size, as fibroid uteri are assumed to be less distensible than non-fibroid uteri (Ouyang, 2011). Myomectomy should be considered on an individual basis in women with a pregnancy complication or an adverse pregnancy outcome presumed due to fibroids prior to future pregnancies.

2.6.2 Diethylstilbestrol

Diethylstilbestrol is a synthetic non-steroidal estrogen, initially produced for the treatment of postmenopausal symptoms and endometriosis. Historically, it was used in pregnant women with the incorrect assumption that it would reduce the rate of miscarriage and preterm birth.

In 1971 a case series, published by the *New England Journal of Medicine* emerged linking Diethylstilbestrol (DES) to female offspring genital tract neoplasia via transplacental carcinogenesis 15 to 22 years later (Herbst, et al., 1971). Subsequent studies into its use confirmed a predisposition to clear cell adenocarcinoma of the vagina and cervical intraepithelial neoplasia in female offspring (Hatch, et al., 2001, Troisi, et al., 2007). Women exposed to DES in-utero were also found to be at higher risk of infertility, preterm birth and adverse pregnancy outcomes. This has been attributed to the increased risk of abnormalities of the uterus, such as t-shaped uterus and uterine fibroids seen in DES daughters (Kaufman, et al., 2000). Its use in pregnant women was subsequently discontinued.

2.6.3 Previous cervical surgery

Cervical incompetence is dilatation and effacement of the cervix prior to term, which contributes to the loss of an otherwise healthy pregnancy. It is relatively rare accounting for 1-2% of all pregnancies in the United States, but up to 25% of all mid trimester losses. Risk factors for cervical incompetence include previous cervical surgery, and history of second trimester pregnancy loss.

The risk of preterm birth is significantly increased in women who have had cervical surgery, most notably with cone biopsies (conization) or Large Loop Excision of the Transformation Zone (LLETZ) (Kristensen, et al., 1994). In a retrospective study carried out on 624 women, who delivered post loop electrosurgical excision procedure, Jakobsson et al, found that the risk of preterm birth was higher following larger biopsies or repeated procedures, with a two and five-fold increase respectively (Jakobsson, et al., 2009). A subsequent study on the subject found that it was the presence of cervical intra-epithelial neoplasia 3 (CIN3) as opposed to cervical surgery *per se* that contributes to the increased the risk of preterm birth: women with CIN3 were significantly more likely to have spontaneous preterm birth compared with those without CIN, 11% versus 6% respectively (Shanbhag, et al., 2009). It is therefore important to consider that the social risk factors that predispose to CIN rather than cervical surgery alone may increase preterm birth rates in women undergoing LLETZ procedures.

2.6.4 History of second trimester termination of pregnancy

Speculation exists regarding the effects of termination of pregnancy as an independent risk factor for adverse obstetric outcomes. First and indeed second trimester termination of pregnancies have historically been considered minor procedures, with little thought paid to future pregnancies or fertility. Termination of pregnancies is a very common event, occurring in 21.3 out of every 1000 women per year in the United States in 2000 (Finer & Henshaw 2003). Suspected mechanisms that predispose to preterm birth associated with termination of pregnancies include introduction of infection, with formation of uterine adhesions, and secondly, damage to the cervix leading to cervical incompetence. A systematic review of research into birth outcomes for women with a history of termination of pregnancy found that the procedure was associated with a small but statistically significant risk of preterm birth, in comparison to mothers who had never had a termination (8.7% versus 6.8% respectively). Additionally, the risk of both preterm birth and low birth weight was increased with an increasing number of pregnancy terminations (Shah & Zao, 2009). When considering these results, it is important to note that many of the other risk factors, such as smoking and low maternal body mass index, related to adverse pregnancy outcomes in this group of women undergoing termination of pregnancy.

2.7 Psychological stressors

The mechanisms involved in the psychosocial associations of preterm birth are not well understood. Research on psychosocial factors and preterm birth has accumulated rapidly in recent years. Some psychosocial factors implicated in the aetiology of preterm birth include major life events, chronic stress, maternal anxiety, personal racism, and lack of support (Behrman & Butler, 2007).

2.7.1 Major life event

Exposure to severe life events has been linked to very and extremely pre-term births. Khashan and colleagues carried out a study evaluating the influence of exposure to severe life events and preterm, very preterm and extremely preterm birth. Exposures were defined as death or serious illness in close relatives 6 months prior to conception or in the first or second trimester of pregnancy. In their cohort of 1.35 million singleton live births, they found that maternal exposure to severe life events contributed significantly to the risk of preterm birth; severe life events in close relatives increased the preterm birth rate by 16%, while if the severe life event involved an older child, the risk of preterm and very preterm birth was increased by 23% and 59% respectively (Khashan et al, 2009).

2.7.2 Work related stressors

With the increasing number of mothers who continue to work late into their pregnancy, occupational stress is hypothesized to be an important contributor to adverse reproductive outcomes, both for mother and baby (Mutambudzi et al., 2011). Physical stressors such as shift work, long hours standing, and heavy lifting have been consistently associated with increased risk of preterm birth (Gold et al 1994). Theoretically, having and being able to maintain a job, is an indicator in itself of a higher socioeconomic status, which has an inverse effect on preterm birth rates. Recent studies have found no increase in the rate of preterm birth and employment, but these are mainly studies carried out in developed countries, where physical strain and hazardous working conditions are not the norm.

2.7.3 Behavioral stressors

Behavioral stressors such as smoking, alcohol and illicit drug use, poor eating habits, sexual and physical activity, are of great importance as modifiable risk factors, as their elimination can lead to an effective reduction in the preterm birth rate. These behaviors pose specific challenges in establishing a cause and effect relationship because of their inherent complexity (Behrman & Butler, 2007). In addition, unfavorable health activities tend to cluster: for example women with poor diets often have other potentially detrimental behaviors, such as a lack of physical activity, and vice versa (Behrman & Butler, 2007).

In the UK in 2004, 25% of all adults were smokers (NHS). 17% of mothers continued to smoke throughout pregnancy, whilst 49% of smoking mothers gave up before or during pregnancy (NHS). Studies have shown that lower or stressful socioeconomic status contributes significantly to persisting to smoke during pregnancy (Weaver, 2007). Smoking is strongly related to placental abruption, reduced birth weight and infant mortality, however, the relationship of cigarette smoking to preterm birth is somewhat modest and not completely replicable (Behrman & Butler, 2007). Its influence on pregnancy outcomes, like preterm birth, is most notable in the third trimester and there is no increased risk detected in mothers who smoke prior to the onset, or in the early stages of pregnancy (Behrman & Butler, 2007).

High levels of alcohol use during pregnancy have detrimental effects on fetal development and subsequent neonatal survival. Women who have more than one drink a day are at an increased risk of preterm labour. According to a study carried out by Albertsen et al., 2004, the relative risk of preterm delivery and very preterm birth, <32 completed weeks, among women who had seven or more drinks a week during pregnancy was 1.77 and 3.26 respectively, compared to non-drinkers. If less than 4 units a week of alcohol was consumed, then there was no increased risk of preterm birth (Albertsen et al., 2004). Due the differing effects of alcohol on the fetus depending on the amount consumed and the limitations associated with self-reporting, the relationship between alcohol and preterm birth remains unclear.

Illicit drug use, especially cocaine, has been widely implicated as an important cause of preterm birth. Cocaine use in the United States rose from 3.2% in 1972 to 12.5% in 1985, and continues to rise (Rouse, 1991). Antenatal cocaine users experience significantly increased risk of preterm birth compared with that for non-users, with an odds ratio of 3.38 (Gouin, 2011). Marijuana smoking does not appear to significantly increase the risk of preterm labour. Its adverse effects come mainly from the inhalation of combustion material (Behrman & Butler, 2007).

Repeatedly, evidence shows that mothers who live a favorable lifestyle are at a reduced risk of adverse pregnancy outcome, including a reduction in the risk of preterm labour (Behrman & Butler, 2007). Continued efforts are required to better understand and therefore define the aspects of a positive lifestyle that are associated with a reduced risk of preterm birth.

2.8 Ethnicity

Preterm birth, the primary predictor of prenatal morbidity and mortality can result from diverse biologic and sociodemographic variables (Al-Eissa, & Ba'Aqeel, 1994). The infant mortality rate for non-Hispanic Black mothers in 2002 was 13.9 per 1000 live births. This is a huge difference from the rate for non-Hispanic White mothers: 5.8 per 1000 live births (Mathews, et al., 2004). Chronic stress is a more prominent feature in the daily lives of Black women than for White women. African American women are, throughout the published literature, at a higher risk for preterm delivery. In the year 2001, the United States preterm delivery rates among Black and White women were 17.5 and 10.8 per 100 live births, respectively (Mustillo, et al., 2004). This gap persists, even after consideration for socioeconomic status, and other known risk factors. Collins et al investigated the causal mechanisms of this association. When other risk factors, such as socioeconomic condition, levels of support, cigarette smoking, alcohol and illicit drug use were excluded, they reported that African American mothers with very low birth weight infants, less than 1500g, were twice as likely to report experiences of racial discrimination during pregnancy than women who had infants of normal birth weight (more than 2500g) (Collins, et al., 2000). This elevated rate may account for the difference in the pre-term birth rate between the USA and other countries.

Subsequent studies supported this finding. In a study comparing African American women who delivered low birth weight infants, who were all preterm, and matched controls, with normal birth weight infants, it was concluded that "lifelong accumulated experiences of racial discrimination experienced by African American women constitute an independent risk factor for preterm delivery" (Collins, et al., 2004).

Mustillo and colleagues carried out a 10 year prospective study on a large cohort of African American and White women who gave birth to live infants at 20 weeks gestation or longer. Firstly, they found that race was a risk factor for preterm birth. Black women were 2.5 times more likely to have a preterm delivery than White women. Those reporting racial discrimination in 3 or more situations, were 3.1 times at increased risk of preterm birth. Second, women who had experienced lifetime discrimination were almost five times more likely to deliver a low birth weight infant, (less than 2500g) than those who had not experienced any racism (Mustillo, et al., 2004). These reports suggest that lifetime experiences of racism, as a psychosocial stressor, may significantly contribute to the racial and ethnic disparities in the rates of both preterm birth and low birth weight.

2.9 Assisted reproduction

Worldwide, more than 10% of couples are infertile (Nelson & Lawlor, 2011). Until recently very little could be done to help infertile or subfertile couples. Then, in July 1978, the world's first successful in vitro fertilization (IVF) baby was born. Since then, 4 million babies have been born through in vitro fertilization (Nelson & Lawlor 2011).

Infertile couples that conceive following IVF with or without intra-cytoplasmic sperm injection (ICSI) are at an increased risk for obstetrical and perinatal complications, most notably, preterm delivery and low birth weight (Basso & Baird, 2003). Singleton pregnancies achieved by assisted reproduction are at higher risk for adverse perinatal outcomes than spontaneous singleton pregnancies in fertile couples. Another significant risk of assisted reproduction is multiple gestations. Although the majority of twinning that occurs with assisted reproduction are dichorionic, the incidence of monochorionic twinning following assisted reproduction is 4-5 times that of normally conceived twins: 1.88% versus 0.4%, respectively (Alikani, et al., 2003). Aspects of assisted reproductive techniques, which increases the risk of preterm birth include, assisted hatching (2.35% versus 1.58% with no assisted hatching) and day 5 or day 6 blastocyst transfer (1.5% versus 0.2% in embryos transferred on day 2) (Alikani, 2003, Wright, 2004). This carries with it an increase in poor perinatal outcome. Risks of multiple pregnancies include higher rates of preterm birth and low birth weight with its associated perinatal mortality (Allen et al., 2006).

Nelson and Lawlor carried out a study to evaluate the factors that influence the success of assisted reproductive treatment. Among their findings, they discovered that there was a marked increase in the risk of preterm birth, if oocyte donation for female factor infertility was required. They also found that other maternal characteristics, especially maternal age and cervical causes of infertility are strongly associated with the risk of preterm delivery in singleton live births resulting from IVF (Nelson & Lawlor, 2011).

It remains uncertain if the increased risks of preterm birth associated with assisted reproduction are attributable to the underlying infertility, characteristics of the infertile couple, or possible adverse effects of the assisted reproductive treatments (Allen et al., 2006; Basso & Baird, 2003). The fact that infertile women who require assisted reproduction are older and are more likely to have an underlying chronic illness may also explain a patient-related increase in preterm birth (Blickstein, 2006). However, treatment bias, such as iatrogenic preterm birth, cannot be excluded.

2.10 Body Mass Index

Maternal body mass index (BMI), calculated as the weight (kg) divided by the height (m^2), is hypothesized to play a significant role in the aetiology of preterm birth. Evidence suggests that a low pre-pregnancy weight is associated with an increased risk of preterm birth (Zhong, 2010). Al-Eissa, & Ba'Aqeel, 1994 carried out a case control study in Saudi, to determine the risk factors that were associated with preterm birth. Their findings included a significant correlation between a maternal BMI of less than 23 and an increased risk for preterm delivery (Al- Eissa, & Ba'Aqeel, 1994). This evidence is further supported by various other studies, most notable The Preterm Prediction Study, where it was reported that a maternal BMI of less than 19.8 was strongly associated with an increased risk of very preterm birth less than 32 weeks gestation, with a relative risk of 2.5 (Goldenberg et al., 1998).

The incidence of obesity is escalating worldwide, and has become the focus of initiatives to preclude its occurrence and reduce the associated adverse health consequences. Pregnant women who are obese are at an increased risk for certain complications during pregnancy, labour and delivery and in the post partum period. These include an increased risk of malformations, including neural tube defects, shoulder dystocia and other birth traumas, endometritis and caesarean wound infection, in comparison to non-obese women (Magann, et al., 2010). Pre-pregnancy obesity is implicated in the aetiology of preterm birth by increasing the risk of PPROM. The risk of spontaneous preterm birth in obese mothers at less than 37 weeks gestation, without PPROM is reduced: 6.2% versus 11.2% in non-obese mothers (Zhong, 2010, Hendler, 2005). This finding is supported by more recent studies on the subject with obese women in early pregnancy being more likely to have post term babies, than their non-obese controls (Khashan, & Kenny, 2009, Magann, et al., 2010). However, indicated preterm delivery for congenital defects, large for gestational age, gestational diabetes, preeclampsia, and stillbirth, contributes significantly to the proportion of preterm birth rates in obese women (Hendler, et al., 2005).

2.11 Maternal age

The importance of maternal age, which has been widely reported to influence pregnancy outcomes and therefore duration, is escalating. This is due to the increasing frequency in the last 20 years of mothers bearing children at advancing ages. Women under 16 and those above 35 have a 2 to 4 percent higher rate of preterm birth compared with those between 21 and 24 years of age.

Several studies have examined the relationship between advancing maternal age and preterm delivery, with preterm births occurring in 8% of mothers more than 35 years compared to less than 4% of births among mothers younger than 35 years (Martius, 1998, & Astolfi, 1999). This finding has been attributed to the hormonal factors associated with advancing maternal age. However, there is insufficient evidence to determine if advancing maternal age is an independent and direct risk factor for preterm birth.

Teenage mothers also carry an increased risk of adverse pregnancy outcomes including an increased risk of delivering earlier than mothers between 20 to 39 years old. They are also more likely to have higher rates of extreme prematurity (Shrim, 2011). This high proportion of preterm births in young mothers may be indicative of unfavourable socio-economic situations. However, it is important to remember that gestational age may be more frequently underestimated in the poorly educated or very young mothers.

2.12 Infections

Infections and associated inflammation are important initiators of the preterm birth pathways. This is suggested by the repeated discovery of positive bacterial cultures from the placentas or membranes of a high proportion of patients with preterm birth (Salafia, 1991). 25% of all preterm births occur in mothers with bacterial colonization of the uterus (Romero, et al., 2007). Other studies have shown that bacteria, which cause placental infection, are capable of producing prostagandins, which disrupts uterine quiescence, causing cervical softening and preterm birth (Bejar, 1981). In addition, vaginal infection and associated inflammation, causes an inflammatory response with cytokines, which cause a further increase in prostaglandin levels (Srinivasan, et al., 2009).

Raised levels of neutrophils and a raised pH of more than 5, was shown to be significantly associated with preterm birth. There is an inverse relationship between neutrophilia and preterm birth, with the strength of the association increasing as the gestational age at delivery decreases (Sinham, 2003). Intrauterine infection is a particularly important risk factor for adverse neurodevelopmental outcomes after PPROM. The colonization of the placenta and membranes can arise directly from the genito-urinary tract with sexually transmitted infections or from haematogenous spread with systemic infections.

2.12.1 Sexually transmitted infections

In evaluating the risk of spontaneous preterm birth associated with genitourinary tract infections, Andrews, et al., carried out a case control study in The Preterm Prediction Study. They found that women with Chlamydia trachomatis infection were more likely to have a short cervix less than 25mm, than uninfected controls (33% versus 17.9% respectively). They also noted that infection with C. trachomatis at 24 weeks gestation predisposed the mothers to a risk of preterm delivery 2 times and 3 times that of the uninfected controls at less than 37 weeks' and less than 35 weeks' gestation respectively (Andrews, et al., 2000). Andrews et al also published a secondary analysis in 2006 on the relationship between mid-pregnancy genitourinary tract infection with Chlamydia and its association with subsequent preterm birth, refuting their primary results regarding an increased risk in Chlamydia infected mothers and preterm birth (Andrews, et al., 2006). Subsequent research in the area has resulted in conflicting results. It therefore remains uncertain if an association exists between sexually transmitted infections and preterm birth. There is some indication that it is the relative load of bacteria, or the specific species of bacterium, rather than its presence *per se*, that predisposes to preterm birth.

2.12.2 Periodontal disease

Recent evidence suggests that infections remote from the fetal site may also be causative. Bacteria are capable of entering the uterine cavity by haematogenous spread. Periodontal disease, a chronic low-grade infection, has been repeatedly implicated in the causation of preterm birth. Oral and vaginal sites are comparable in their bacterial microbiology. Mothers with periodontitis and bacterial vaginosis also share similar social and socio-demographic risk factors, suggesting a common pathophysiology (Srinivasan, et al., 2009).

Low levels of infections and disturbances of the bacterial flora in the mouth have been shown to be enough to initiate preterm birth via the production of pro-inflammatory cytokines in the uterus (Romero, et al., 2007).
Offenbacher and colleagues, in the OCAP (Oral Conditions and Pregnancy) study, investigated obstetric outcomes in women with periodontal disease. Their results illustrate a preterm birth incidence of 28.6% in women with moderate to severe periodontal disease compared to 11.2% among women with good oral health (Offenbacher, et al., 2006). Several other studies report an inverse relationship between severe or generalized periodontal disease and decreasing gestational age at delivery, with an odds ratio of 4.45 for preterm delivery less than 37 weeks, increasing to an odds ratio of 7.07 for delivery before 32 weeks gestation (Jeffcoat, et al., 2001).
As regards antenatal treatment of periodontal disease, Offenbacher and colleagues carried out a randomized controlled trial, the Maternal Oral Therapy to Reduce Obstetric Risk (MOTOR) study, to evaluate the effect of non-surgical treatment of periodontal disease on preterm birth rates. They found that treatment of women with periodontal disease had minimal improved benefit on gestational age at delivery of less than 37, 35 or 32 weeks, 13.1% versus 11.5% in non-treated controls (Offenbacher, et al, 2009). This is in contrast to the recent Australian meta-analysis of 10 randomized trials by George et al 2011, which found that antenatal periodontal treatment significantly lowered preterm birth and low birth weight rates (George, et al., 2011).
Given the mounting evidence and continued speculation regarding the effect of periodontal disease and treatment on preterm birth, every opportunity should be taken to advise mothers about the importance of good oral health preconceptually and prevention of periodontal disease.

2.13 Fetal factors

2.13.1 Congenital abnormalities

The presence of a major congenital abnormality greatly increases the risk of preterm delivery, 3.8-fold increased risk compared with newborns without congenital malformations (Mohangoo et al., 2010). It is also associated with the presence of other risk factors that predispose to preterm birth, with pregnancies with multiple malformations at the highest risk of preterm birth. A study carried out in Washington to evaluate the relative risk of preterm birth associated with major congenital abnormalities quoted a preterm birth prevalence of 11.5% in pregnancies complicated by all congenital abnormalities (Purisch, et al., 2008). The most lethal of these, congenital cardiovascular malformations, is associated with an increased incidence of preterm birth, present in 12.5 per 1000 cases of preterm birth, in comparison with 5.1 per 1000 cases in term infants (Tanner, et al., 2005). The highest risk of preterm birth was associated with infants with congenital abnormalities of the central nervous system, respiratory system and infants with chromosomal anomalies (Mohangoo et al., 2010).

2.13.2 Intrauterine growth restriction

Intrauterine growth restriction (IUGR), which is classified as a fetal weight below a certain centile for gestational age is associated with an increased incidence of preterm birth. IUGR is defined as a fetus with an estimated weight at below the 3rd, 5th, or 10th centile for gestational age according to population matched centile charts. It is obvious that the higher

the threshold for classifying a fetus as growth restricted, the more likely it is that the fetus is a constitutionally small for gestational age fetus. The greatest risk of adverse perinatal outcome with growth restricted fetuses are those with an estimated fetal weight below the 3rd centile, with a 10 fold increased risk of neonatal death, than normally grown babies, 26th - 75th percentile or weight (McIntire, et al., 1999).
It is hypothesized that spontaneous preterm labour and birth in growth-restricted fetuses is an adaptive response of the fetus to a hostile intrauterine environment. A European study evaluating the relationship between small for gestational age fetuses and preterm birth, reports an incidence for indicated preterm delivery of more than 40% for small for gestational age fetuses, in comparison to 10.7% of control normally grown fetuses. Not surprisingly, the relationship between growth restriction and preterm delivery is stronger the earlier the gestation (Zeitlin, et al., 2000).

2.13.3 Fetal gender

It has been long noticed that female fetuses have a better perinatal survival than male fetuses. A study analyzing the relationship between fetal gender and preterm births confirmed this stating that male fetuses are at an increased risk of being born preterm than female fetuses, in both singleton and twin pregnancies (Cooperstock and Campbell, 1996). This finding was consistent with other studies on the subject, with male babies at higher risk of being delivered at earlier gestations than female babies, 4.4% versus 4.0% (Astolfi, 1999, Hall and Carr-Hill, 1982). Speculation exists regarding the male fetal hormonal input into the onset of labour, or the genetic disadvantage of the male fetus, evidenced by the excessive male sex percentage in adverse pregnancy outcomes (Astolfi, 1999). However, despite numerous studies on the mechanisms of preterm labour influenced by fetal gender, an explanation for this remains uncertain.

2.14 Others

The decision to undergo abdominal surgery during pregnancy is a difficult one. The risk and benefits of treating the surgical condition must be weighed up against the risk of adverse pregnancy outcomes, including pregnancy loss and preterm delivery. Abdominal surgery during the first and second trimester of pregnancy is not associated with a significant preterm birth risk, but this risk becomes of significance in the third trimester of pregnancy (Visser, et al., 2001).
A short inter-pregnancy interval appears to be a risk factor for adverse perinatal outcomes, including preterm birth. The optimal inter-pregnancy interval is between 18 to 23 months, with increasing risk the shorter the interval. Infants conceived at less than 6 months intervals, had an odds ratio of 1.4 for preterm birth (Zhu, et al., 1999).

3. Future research on risk factors

Research into the risk factors attributable to preterm birth is ongoing, with international collaboration. The SCOPE (Screening for Pregnancy Endpoints) study is an international prospective study of pregnancy outcomes. Its 3 main objectives are to distinguish women in early pregnancy at risk of developing pregnancy related complications, identify novel markers that predict each complication, and develop tests that can aid in rating individual risk. Early identification of at risk women, prediction of disease and prompt intervention provides the opportunity to dramatically improve maternal and infant health.

The SCOPE study is further supported by the PREHOT and PREBIC studies to contribute to an increased understanding of preterm birth. Currently there are no dependable or replicable methods available to detect women at high risk of preterm birth. The Preterm birth and healthy outcome team (PREHOT), using the information from genes works under 3 themes: 1. Better prediction of preterm birth, 2. Development and testing of interventions to reduce the rate of preterm birth and 3. Examination of outcomes associated with follow up interventions. The Preterm Birth International Collaborative (PREBIC) initiative aims to improve pregnancy and birth outcomes and optimize infant health to assure optimal adult health. It too, is an international initiative investigating the causes and prevention of preterm birth and low birth weight. As with the previous 2 studies, PREBIC also focuses on use of biomarkers to identify those patients at increased risk of preterm birth and formulate intervention strategies to prevent and manage those pregnancies at increased risk for indicated preterm delivery.

4. Conclusion

Preterm birth and low birth weight remain the most important predictors of perinatal morbidity and mortality among otherwise healthy infants. Despite the increasing survival of preterm infants due to the improvement in skills and technologies used in their management, the incidence of preterm birth continues to increase globally. Many risk factors have been proven to be causative, while others remain under speculation needing ongoing research. Previous history of preterm birth remains by far the most accurate predictor of risk for subsequent preterm delivery. Many of the risk factors that predispose to this condition, if not correctly identified and adequately treated persist, and contribute to the rising incidence of preterm birth. It is important to note that many preterm births occur in women with no prior identifiable risk factors, and a precise mechanism cannot be determined.

Successful reduction of the perinatal morbidity and mortality associated with prematurity requires the implementation of effective risk identification and behavioural modification programs such as the SCOPE study. Every opportunity has to be grasped by health care providers to assess modifiable risk factors, and encourage mothers to avoid adverse health behaviours, such as smoking and illicit drug use. The importance of pre pregnancy optimal weight attainment, and good oral hygiene is to be reinforced and the opportunity for STI screening sought.

Finally, identification and timely referral for specialized obstetrical evaluation and management of these high risk women pre-conceptually or in early pregnancy, is important in reducing the morbidity, mortality, psychological trauma and expense associated with preterm birth. Data mining in ongoing prospective trials such as SCOPE, PREHOT and PREBIC may reveal novel clinical risk factors and lead to the development of clinical risk algorithms.

5. References

Aharoni, A., Reiter, A., Golan, D., Paltiely, Y., & Sharf, M. (1988). Patterns of growth of uterine leiomyomas during pregnancy. *British Journal of Obstetrics and Gynaecology.* Vol. 95, No. 5, (May 1988), pp. 510-3.

Albertsen, K., Andersen, AMN., Olsen, J., Grønbæ, M. (2004). Alcohol consumption during pregnancy and the risk of preterm delivery. *American Journal of Epidemiology.* Vol. 159, No. 2, (July 2003), pp. 155-161.

Al-Eissa, YA., & Ba'Aqeel, HS. (1994). Risk factors for spontaneous preterm birth in a Saudi population. *European Journal of Obstetrics & Gynecology and Reproductive Biology.* Vol. 57, No. 1, (Oct 1994), pp. 19-24

Alexander, JM., & Cox, SM. (1996). Clinical course of premature rupture of the membranes. *Seminars in Perinatology.* Vol. 20, No. 5, (Oct 1996), pp. 369-74.

Alikani, M., Cekleniak, NA., Walters, E., & Cohen, J. (2003). Monozygotic twinning following assisted conception: an analysis of 81 consecutive cases. *Human Reproduction.* Vol. 18, No. 9, (Sep 2003), pp 1937-43.

Allen, MC. (2008). Neurodevelopmental outcomes of preterm infants. *Current Opinion in Neurology.* Vol. 21, No. 2, (Apr 2008), pp 123-8.

Allen, VM., Wilson, RD., & Cheung, A. (2006) Pregnancy outcomes after assisted reproductive technology. *Journal of Obstetrics and Gynaecology of Canada.* Vol. 28, No. 3, (Mar 2006), pp. 220-50.

Ananth, CV., Peltier, MR., Chavez, MR., Kirby, RS., Getahun, D., & Vintzileos, AM. (2007). Recurrence of ischemic placental disease. *Obstetrics and Gynaecology.* Vol. 110, No. 1, (Jul 2007), pp. 128-33.

Andrews, WW., Goldenburg, RL., Mercer, B., Iams, J., Meis, P., Moawad, A., Das, A., Vandorsten, JP., Caritis, SN., Thurnau, G., Miodovnik, M., Roberts, J., & McNellis, D. (2000). The Preterm Prediction Study: association of Second-trimester genitourinary chlamydia infection with subsequent spontaneous preterm birth. *American Journal of Obstetrics and Gynaecology.* Vol. 183, No. 3, (Sept 2000), pp. 662-8.

Andrews, WW., Klebanoff, MA., Thom, EA., Hauth, JC., Carey, JC., Meiss, PJ., Caritis, SN., Leveno, KJ., Wapner, RJ., Varner, MW., Iams, JD., Moawad, A., Miodovnik, M., Sibai, B., Dombrowski, M., Langer, O., & O'Sullivan, MJ. (2006). Mid-pregnancy genitourinary tract infection with Chlamydia trachomatis: association with subsequent preterm delivery in women with bacterial vaginosis and Trichomonas vaginalis. *American Journal of Obstetrics and Gynaecology.* Vol. 194, No. 2, (Feb 2006), pp. 493-500.

Astolfi, P., & Zonta, LA. (1999). Risks of preterm delivery and association with maternal age, birth order and fetal gender. *Human Reproduction.* Vol. 14, No. 11, (Nov 1999), pp. 2891-2894.

Barigye, O., Pasquini, L., Galea, P., Chambers, H., Chappell, L., Fisk, NM. (2005). High risk of unexpected late fetal death in monochorionic twins despite intensive ultrasound surveillance: a cohort study. *PLoS Medicine.* Vol. 2, No. 6, (Jun 2005), pp. e172.

Barker, DJ., Osmond, C., Simmonds, SJ., & Weild, A. (1993). The relationship of small head circumference and thinness at birth to death from cardiovascular disease in adult life. *British Medical Journal.* Vol. 306, No. 6875, (Feb 1993).

Basso, O., & Baird, DD. (2003). Infertility and preterm delivery, birthweight, and Caesarean section: a study within the Danish National Birth Cohort. *Human Reproduction.* Vol. 18, No. 11, pp. 2478-2484

Behrman, RE., & Butler, SA. (2007) *Preterm birth: Causes, consequences, and prevention.* National Academic Press, ISBN, Washington, DC.

Bejar, R., Curbelo, V., Davis, C., & Gluck, l. (1981). Premature labour. II. Bacterial sources of phospholipase. *Obstetrics and Gynaecology.* Vol. 57, No. 4, (April 1981), pp. 479-82.

Beloosesky, R., & Ross, MG. (2010). Polyhydarmnios. *UpToDate*. Vol. 19, No. 1, (Nov 2010). Available from http://www.uptodate.com/contents/polyhydramnios?source=search_result&selectedTitle=1%7E95

Berkowitz, GS., Herlap, S., Beck, GJ., Freeman, DH., & Baras, M. (1983). Early gestational bleeding and pregnancy outcome: a multivariable analysis. *International Journal of Epidemiology*. Vol. 12, No. 2, (Jun 1983), pp. 165-73.

Blickstein, I. (2006). Does assisted reproduction technology, per se, increase the risk of preterm birth? *British Journal of Obstetrics and Gynaecology*. Vol. 113, No. 3, (Dec 2006), pp. 68-71

Bloom, SL., Yost, NP., McIntire, DD., & Leveno, KJ. (2001). Recurrence of preterm birth in singleton and twin pregnancies. *Obstetrics and Gynaecology*. Vol. 98, No. 3, (2001), pp. 379.

Bundgaard, A., Andersen, BR., Rode, L., Lebech, M., & Tabor, A. (2007). Prevalence of polyhydramnios at a Danish hospital- a population based study. *Acta Obstetricia et Gynaecologica Scandinavica*. Vol. 86, No. 12, (Aug 2007), pp. 1427-31.

Chan, CC., & To, WW. (1999). Antepartum hemorrhage of unknown origin- what is its clinical significance. *Acta Obstetricia et Gynaecologica Scandinavica*. Vol. 78, No. 3, (Mar 1999) pp. 186-90.

Collins, JW., David, R., Symons, R., Handler, A., Wall, S., & Dwyer, L. (2000). Low-Income African-American Mothers' Perception of Exposure to Racial Discrimination and Infant Birth Weight. *Epidemiology*. Vol. 11, No. 3, (May 2000), pp. 337-339.

Collins, JW., David, RJ., Handler, A., Wall, S., & Andes, S. (2004)Very Low Birthweight in African America Infants: The role of Maternal Exposure to Interpersonal Racial Discrimination. *American Journal of Public Health*. Vol. 94, No. 12, (Dec 2004), pp. 2132-2138.

Cooney, MJ., Benson, CB., Doubilet, PM. (1998). Outcome of pregnancies in women with uterine duplication anomalies. *Journal of Clinical Ultrasound*. Vol. 26, No. 1, (Jan 1998), pp. 3-6.

Cooperstock, M., & Campbell, J. (1996). Excess males in preterm birth: interactions with gestational age, race, and multiple birth. *Obstetrics and Gynaecology*. Vol. 88, No. 2, (Aug 1996), pp. 189-93.

Damus, K., & Petrini, JR. (2007) Cost of Hospitalisation for Preterm and Low Birth Weight Infants in the United States. *Paediatrics*. Vol. 120, No. 1, (July 2007), pp. 1-9.

Delobel-Ayoub, M., Arnaud, C., White-Koning, M., Casper, C., Pierrat, V., Garel, M., Burguet, A., Roze,

Finer, LB., & Henshaw, SK. (2003). Abortion incidence and services in the United States in 2000. *Perspectives on Sexual and Reproductive Health*. Vol. 35, No. 1, (Jan 2003), pp. 6-15.

Gadner, MO., Goldenberg, RL., Cliver, SP., Tucker, JM., Nelson, KG., & Copper, RL. (1995). The origin and outcome of preterm twin pregnancies. *Obstetrics and Gynaecology*. Vol. 85, No. 4, (April 1995), pp. 553-7.

George, A., Shamim, S., Johnson, M., Ajwani, S., Bhole, S., Blinkhorn, A., Ellis, S., & Andrews, K. (2011). Periodontal treatment during pregnancy and birth outcomes: a meta-analysis of randomized trials. *International Journal of Evidence Based Healthcare*. Vol. 9, No. 2, (Jun 2011), pp. 122-47.

Gold, EB., Tomich, E. (1994) Occupational hazards to fertility and pregnancy outcome. *Occupational medicine*. Vol. 9, No. 3 (Jul-Sep 1994), pp. 435-69.NHS: The Health and Social Care Information Centre. Stastistics on smoking, England 2006.

Goldenberg, RL., Culhane, JF., Iams, JD., & Romero, R. (2008). Epidemiology and causes of preterm birth. *Lancet.* Vol. 371, No. 9606 (Jan 2008), pp 75-84

Goldenberg, RL., Iams, JD., Mercer, BM., Meis, PJ., Moawad, AH., Copper, RL., Das, A., Thom, E., Johnson, F.,

Gouin, K., Murphy, K., & Shah, PS. (2011) Effects of cocaine use during pregnancy on low birthweight and preterm birth: systematic review and metanalysis. *American Journal of Obstetrics and Gynaecology.* Vol. 204, No. 4, (Jan 2011), pp. 340.e1-340.e12

Hall, MH, & Carr-Hill, R. (1982). Impact of sex ratio on onset and management of labour. *British Medical Journal (Clinical Research Edition).* Vol. 285, No. 6339, (Aug 1982), pp. 401-3.

Harger, JH., Hsing, AW., Tuomala, RE., Gibbs, RS., Mead, PB., Eschenbach, DA., Knox, GE., & Polk, BF. (1990). Risk factors for preterm premature rupture of fatal membranes: a multicenter case-control study. *American Journal of Obstetrics and Gynaecology.* Vol. 163, No. 1, (July 1990), pp. 130-7.

Hatch, EE., Herbst, AL., Hoover, RN., Noller, KL., Adam, E., Kaufmann, RH., Palmer, JR., Titus-Ernstoff, L.,

Hauth, JC. (2006). Spontaneous preterm labour and premature rupture of membranes at late preterm gestations: to deliver or not to deliver. *Seminars in Perinatology.* Vol. 30, No. 2, (Apr 2006), pp. 98-102.

Hendler, I., Goldenberg, RL., Mercer, BM., Iams, JD., Meis, PJ., Moawad, AH., MacPherson, CA., Caritis, SN.,

Herbst, AL., Ulfelder, H., Poskanzer, DC. (1971). Adenocarcinoma of the vagina. Association of maternal stilbestrol therapy with tumor appearance in young women. *New England Journal of Medicine.* Vol. 284, No. 15, (Apr 1971), pp. 878-81.

Herbst. AL., Hoover, RN. (2007). Cancer risk in women prenatally exposed to diethylstilbestrol. *International Journal of Cancer.* Vol. 121, No. 2, (Jul 2007), pp. 356-60.

Hill, LM., Breckle, R., Thomas, ML., & Fries, JK. (1987). Polyhydramnios: ultrasonically detected prevalence and neonatal outcome. *Obstetrics and Gynaecology.* Vol 69, No. 1, (Jan 1987), pp. 21-5.

Hyer, M., Harte, P., Robboy, SJ. (2001). Incidence of squamous neoplasia of the cervix and vagina in women exposed prenatally to diethylstilbestrol (Unites States). *Cancer Causes and Control.* Vol. 12, No. 9, (Nov 2001), pp. 837-45.

Iams, JD, Goldenberg, RL., Mercer, BM., Moawad, A., Thom, E., Meis, PJ., McNeills, D., Caritis, SN., Miodovnik, M., Thurnau, GR., Bottoms, SE., & Roberts, JM. (1998). The Preterm Prediction Study: recurrence risk of spontaneous preterm birth. National Institute of Child Health and Human Development Maternal-Fetal Medicine Units Networks. *American Journal of Obstetrics and Gynaecologists.* Vol. 178, No. 5, (May 1998), pp. 1035-40.

Jakobsson, M., Gissler, M., & Tapper, AM. (2009). Loop electrosurgical excision procedure and the risk for preterm birth. *Obstetrics and Gynaecology.* Vol. 114, No. 3, (Sept 2009), pp. 504.

JC., Matis, J., Picaud, JC., Kaminski, M., & Larroque, B. EPIPAGE Study Group. (2009). Behavioral problems and cognitive performance at 5 years of age after very preterm birth: the EPIPAGE Study. *Pediatrics.* Vol. 123, No. 6, (Jun 2009), pp. 1485-92.

Jeffcoat, MK., Geurs, NC., Reddy, MS., Cliver, SP., Goldenberg, RL., & Hauth, JC. (2001). Periodontal infection and preterm birth: results of a prospective study. *Journal of the American Dental Association.* Vol. 132, No. 7, (Jul 2001), pp. 875-80.

Kaufman, RH., Adam, E., Hatch, EE., Noller, K., Herbst, AL., Palmer, JR., & Hoover, RN. (2000). Continued follow-up of pregnancy outcomes in diethylstilbestrol-exposed offspring. *Obstetrics and Gynaecology.* Vol. 96, No. 4, (Oct 2000), pp. 483-9.

Khashan, AS, & Kenny, LC. (2009). The effects of maternal body mass index on pregnancy outcome. *The European Journal Of Epidemiology.* Vol. 24, No. 11, (Aug 2009), pp. 697-705.

Khashan, AS., McNamee, R., Abel, KM., Kenny, LC., Pedersen, MG., Webb, RT., & Baker, PN. (2008). Rates of preterm birth following antenatal maternal exposure to severe life events: a population-based cohort study. *Journal of Human Reproduction.* Vol. 24, No. 2, (Feb 2009), pp 429-437.

Krampl, E., & Klein, K. (2007). Prematurity in multiple pregnancies. *Gynakologisch-Geburtshilfliche Rundschau.* Vol. 47, No. 2, (2007), pp. 64-9.

Kristensen, J., Langhoff-Roos, J., Kristensen, FB., Witrup, M., & Bock, JE. (1994). Increased risk of preterm delivery in women with earlier conization. *Ugeskr Laeger.* Vol. 156, No. 24, (Jun 1994), pp. 3632-5.

Lee, YM., Cleary-Goldman, J., D'Alton, ME. (2006). The impact of multiple gestations on late preterm (near-term) births. *Clinics in Perinatology.* Vol. 33, No. 4, (Dec 2006), pp. 777-92.

Lee, YM., Wylie, BJ., Simpson, LL., & D'Alton, ME. (2008). Twin chorionicity and the risk of stillbirth. *Obstetrics and Gynaecology.* Vol 111, No. 2 Pt 1, (Feb 2008), pp. 301-8

Leung, TY., Chan, LW., Tam, WH., Leung, TN., & Lau, TK. (2001). Risk and prediction of preterm delivery in pregnancies complicated by antepartum hemorrhage of unknown origin before 34 weeks. *Gynaecologic and Obstetric Investigation.* Vol. 52, No. 4, pp. 227-31.

Lev-Toaff, AS., Coleman, BG., Arger, PH., Mintz, MC., Arenson, RL., & Toaff, ME. (1987). Leiomyomas in pregnancy: sonographic study. *Radiology.* Vol 164, No. 2, (Aug 1987), pp. 375-80.

Li, DK. (1999). Changing paternity and the risk of preterm delivery in the subsequent pregnancy. *Epidemiology.* Vol. 10, No. 2, (Mar 1999), pp. 148-52.

Lockwood, CJ., Paidas, M., Murk, WK., Kayisli, UA., Gopinath, A., Krikun, G., Huang, SJ., & Schatz, F. (2009). Involvement of human decidual cell-expressed tissue factor in uterine hemostasis and abruption. *Thrombosis Research.* Vol. 124, No. 5, (Nov 2009), pp. 516-520.

Lockwood, CJ., Ramin, SM., & Barss, VA. (2011). Overview of preterm labour and delivery. *UpToDate.* Vol. 19, No. 1, (Jan 2011).

MacDorman, MF., & Mathews, TJ. (2010). Behind International rankings of infant mortality: How the United States compares with Europe. *International Journal of Health Services.* Vol. 40, No. 4, (2010), pp 557-88

Magann, EF., Doherty, DA., Chauhan, SP., Klimpel, JM., Morrison, JC. (2010). Pregnancy, obesity and gestational weight gain, and parity as predictors of peripartum complications. *Archives of Gynaecology and Obstetrics.* Nov 2010.

Martiusa, JA., Stecka, T., Oehlerb, MK., & Wulfa, KH. (1998) Risk factors associated with preterm (<37+0 weeks) and early preterm birth (<32+0 weeks): univariate and multivariate analysis of 106 345 singleton births from the 1994 statewide perinatal survey of Bavaria. *European Journal of Obstetrics and Gynaecology and Reproductive Biology.* Vol. 80, No. 2. (Oct 1998), pp. 183-189.

Mathews, TJ., Menacker, F., & MacDorman, MF. (2004). Infant mortality statistics from the 2002 period: linked birth/ infant death data set. *National Vital Statistics Rep.* Vol. 53, No. 10, (Nov 2004), pp. 1-29.

Mathews, TJ., Menacker, F., & MacDorman, MF. (2004). Infant mortality statistics from the 2002 period: linked birth/ infant death data set. *National Vital Statistics Rep.* Vol. 53, No. 10, (Nov 2004), pp. 1-29.

McIntire, DD., Bloom, SL., Casey, BM., Leveno, KJ. (1999). Birth weight in relation to morbidity and mortality among newborn infants. *New England Journal of Medicine.* Vol 340, No. 16, (Apr 1999), pp. 1234-8.

McNellis, D., Miodovnik, M., Van Dorsten, JP., Caritis, SN., Thurnau, GR., & Bottoms, SF. (1998). The preterm prediction study: the value of new vs standard risk factors in predicting early and all spontaneous preterm births. NICHD MFMU Network. *American Journal of Public Health.* Vol. 88, No. 2, (Feb 1998), pp. 223-238

Miodovnik, M., Menard, KM., Thurnau, GR., & Sorokin, Y. (2005). The Preterm Prediction Study: association between maternal body mass index and indicated preterm birth. *American Journal of Obstetrics and Gynaecology.* Vol. 192, No. 3, (March 2005), pp. 882-6.

Mohangoo, A., Lanting, C., Bennebroek, J., Verloove-Vanhorick, P., & Buitendijk, S. (2010). Contribution of Congenital Anomalies to Preterm Birth risk in the Netherlands:457. *Pediatric Research.* (Nov 2010), pp. 234-5.

Moutquin, JM. (2003). Classification and heterogeneity of preterm birth. *British Journal of Obstetrics and Gynaecology.* Vol. 110, No. 20, (Apr 2003), pp. 30-3.

Mustillo, S., Krieger, N., Gunderson, EP., Sidney, S., McCreath, H., & Kiefe, CI. (2004) Self-Reported Experiences of Racial Discrimination and Black-White Differences in Preterm and Low-birthweight Deliveries: The CARDIA Study. *American Journal of Public Health.* Vol. 94, No. 12, (Dec 2004), pp. 2125-2131.

Mutambudzi, M., Meyer, JD., Warren, N., & Reisine, S. (2011). Effects of psychosocial characteristics of work on pregnancy outcomes: a critical review. *Women Health.* Vol. 51, No. 1, (May 2011), pp. 279-97.

Nelson, SM., & Lawlor, DA. (2011). Predicting Live Birth, Preterm Delivery, and Low Birth Weight in Infants Born from In Vitro Fertilisation: A Prospective Study of 144,018 Treatment Cycles. *Public Library of Science Medicine.* Vol. 8, No. 1, (Jan 2011), e1000386.

Offenbacher, S., Beck, JD., Jared, HL., Mauriello, SM., Mendoza, LC., Couper, DJ., Stewart, DD., Murtha, AP., Cochran, DL., Dudley, DJ., Reddy, MS., Geurs, NC., & Hauth, JC. The Maternal Oral Therapy to Reduce Obstetric Risk (MOTOR) Investigators. (2009). Effects of Periodontal Therapy on Rate of Preterm Delivery: A randomized controlled trial. *Obstetrics and Gynaecology. Vol.* 114, No. 3, (Sep 2009), pp. 551-9.

Ou, CW., Orsino, A., & Lye. SJ. (1997). Expression of connexin-43 and connexin-26 in the rat myometrium during pregnancy and labor is differentially regulated by mechanical and hormonal signals. *Endocrinology.* Vol. 138, No. 12, (1997), pp. 5398.

Ouyang, DW., & Norwitz, ER. (2011). Pregnancy in women with uterine leiomyomas. *UpToDate.* Vol. 19, No. 1, (Jan 2011). Available from http://www.uptodate.com/contents/pregnancy-in-women-with-uterine-leiomyomas-fibroids?source=search_result&selectedTitle=6%7E150

Ouyang, DW., Economy, KE., & Norwitz, ER. (2006). Obstetric complications of fibroids. *Obstetric and Gynaecology Clinics of North America.* Vol. 33, No. 1, (Mar 2006), pp. 153-69.

Petrozella, LN., Dashe, JS., McIntire, DD., & Leveno, KJ. (2011). Clinical significance of borderline amniotic fluid index and oligohydramnios in preterm pregnancy. *Obstetrics and Gynaecology.* Vol. 117, No. 2 Pt1, (Feb 2011), pp. 338-42.

Plunkett, J., Borecki, I., Morgan, T., Stamilio, D., & Muglia, LJ. Population based estimate of sibling risk for preterm birth, preterm premature rupture of membranes, placental abruption and pre-eclampsia. (2008). *BMC Genetics.* Vol. 9, No. 44. (Jul 2008), pp. 9-44.

Purisch, SE., DeFranco, EA., Muglia, LJ., Odibo, AO., & Stamilo, DM. (2008). Preterm birth in pregnancies complicated by major congenital malformations: a population-based study. *American Journal of Obstetrics and Gynaecology.* Vol. 199, No. 3, (Sep 2008), pp. 287.

Rasmussen, KL., & Knudsen, HJ. (1994). Effect of uterine fibromas on pregnancy. *Ugeskr Laeger.* Vol. 156, No. 51, (Dec 1994), pp. 7668-70.

Reichman, D., Laufer, MR., Robinson, BK. (2009). Pregnancy outcomes in unicornuate uteri: a review. *Fertility and Sterility.* Vol. 91, No. 5, (May 2009), pp. 1886-94.

Robinson, JN., & Norwitz, ER. (2011). Risk factors for preterm birth. *UpToDate.* Vol. 19, No. 1, (Jan 2011).

Romero, R., Gotsch, F., Pineles, B., & Kusanovic, JP. (2007). Inflammation in pregnancy: its role in reproductive physiology, obstetrical complications, and fetal injury. *Nutrition Reviews.* Vol. 65, No. 12 pt 2, (Dec 2007), pp. 194-202.

Rouse, BA. (1991). Trends in Cocaine Use in the General Population, In: *The Epidemiology of Cocaine Use and Abuse,*

Royal College of Obstetricians and Gynaecologists. Green-top guideline. No. 44. Preterm prelabour rupture of membranes. (Nov 2006).

Russell, RB., Green, NS., Steiner, CA., Meikle, S., Howse, JL., Poschman, K., Dias, T., Potetz, L., Davidoff, MJ.,

Salafia, CM., López-Zeno, JA., Sherer, DM., Whittington, SS., Minior, VK., & Vintzileos, AM. (1995). Histologic evidence of old intrauterine bleeding is more frequent in prematurity. *American Journal of Obstetrics and Gynaecology.* Vol. 173, No. 4, (Oct 1995), pp. 1065-70.

Salafia, CM., Vogel, CA., Vintzileos, AM., Bantham, KF., Pezzullo, J., & Silerman, L. (1991). Placental pathologic findings in preterm birth. *American Journal of Obstetrics and Gynaecology.* Vol. 165, No. 4, (Oct 1991), pp. 934-8

Schober, S., Schade, C., pp. 5-18, DHHS publications, Available from http://docs.google.com/viewer?a=v&q=cache:whBTq7xRtHUJ:archives.drugabuse.gov/pdf/monographs/110.pdf+epidemiology+of+cocaine+use

Shah, PS., & Zao, J. (2009). Induced termination of pregnancy and low birthweight and preterm birth: a systematic review and meta-analysis. *British Journal of Obstetrics and Gynaecology.* Vol. 116, No. 11, (Oct 2009), pp. 1425-42.

Shanbhag, S., Clark, H., Timmaraju, V., Bhattacharya, S., & Criuckshank, M. (2009). Pregnancy outcome after treatment for cervical intraepithelial neoplasia. *Obstetrics and Gynaecology.* Vol. 114, No. 4, (Oct 2009), pp. 727-35.

Shrim, A., Ates, S., Mallozzi, A., Brown, R., Ponette, V., Levin, I., Shehata, F., & Almog, B. (2011). Is young maternal age really a risk factor for adverse pregnancy outcome in a Canadian tertiary referral hospital. *Journal of Peadiatric Adolescence and Gynaecology.* (May 2011)

Sinham, HN., Caritis, SN., Krohn, MA., & Hillier, SL. Elevated vaginal pH and neutrophils are associated strongly with early spontaneous preterm birth. *American Journal of Obstetrics and Gynaecology.* Vol. 189, No. 4, (Oct 2003), pp1150-4.

Srinivasan, U., Misra, D., Marazita, ML., & Foxman, B. (2009). Vaginal and oral microbes, host genotype and preterm birth. *Medical Hypotheis.* Vol. 73, (June 2009), pp. 963-75.

Strobelt, N., Ghidini, A., Cavallone, M., Pensabene, I., Ceruti, P., & Vergani, P. (1994). Natural history of uterine leiomyomas in pregnancy. *Journal of Ultrasound in Medicine.* Vol. 13, No. 5, (May 1994), pp. 399-401.

Tanner, K., Sabrine, N., & Wren, C. (2005). Cardiovascular malformations among preterm infants. *Paediatrics.* Vol. 116, No. 6, (Dec 2005), pp. 833-8.

Troisi, R., Hatch, EE., Titus-Ernstoff, L., Hyer, M., Palmer, JR., Robboy SJ., Stronhsnitter, WC., Kaufman, R.,

Vintzileos, AM. (2008). Ischemic placental disease is the main cause for indicated preterm births. *The Female Patient.* Vol. 33, No. 12, (2008), pp. 53-67.

Visser, BC., Glasgow, RE, Mulvihill, KK., & Mulvihill, SJ. (2001). Safety and timing of nonobstetric surgery in pregnancy. *Digestive Surgery.* Vol. 18, No. 5, (2001), 409-17.

Weaver K., Campbell, R., Mermelstein, R., & Wakschlag, L. (2007). Pregnancy Smoking in context: The influence of Multiple levels of stress. *Oxford Journals.* Vol. 10, No 6, (Sept 2007), pp. 10665-1073.

Weiss, G., Goldsmith, LT., Hagen, S., & Lederer, K. (1993). Elevated first-trimester serum relaxin concentrations in pregnant women following ovarian stimulation predict prematurity risk and preterm delivery. *Obstetric and Gynaecology.* Vol. 82, No. 5, (Nov 1993), pp. 821-8.

Wilcox,AJ., Skjaerven, R., & Lie, RT. (2008). Familial patterns of preterm delivery: maternal and fetal contributions. *American Journal of Epidemiology.* Vol. 167, No. 4, (Feb 2008), pp. 474-9.

Williams, MA., Mittendorf, R., Lieberman, E., & Monson, RR. (1991). Adverse infant outcomes associated with first trimester vaginal bleeding. *Obstetrics and Gynaecology.* Vol. 78, No. 1, (Jul 1991), pp. 14-8.

Wright, V., Schieve, LA., Vahratian, A., & Reynolds, MA. (2004). Monozygotic twinning associated with day 5 embryo transfer in pregnancies conceived after IVF. *Human Reproduction.* Vol. 19, No. 8, (May 2004), pp. 1831-36.

Zeitlin, J., Ancel, PY., Saurel-Cubizolles, MJ., & Papiernik, E. (2000). The relationship between intrauterine growth restriction and preterm delivery: an empirical approach using data from a European case-control study. *British Journal of Obstetrics and Gynaecology.* Vol. 107, No. 6, (Jun 2000), pp. 750-8.

Zhong, Y., Cahill, AG., Macones, GA., Zhu, F., & Odibo, AO. (2010). The association of prepregnancy maternal body mass index and preterm delivery. *American Journal of Perinatology.* Vol. 27, No. 4, (April 2010), pp. 293-8.

Zhu, BP., Rolfs, RT., Nangle, BE., & Horan, JM. (1999). Effect of the interval between pregnancies on perinatal outcomes. *New England Journal of Medicine.* Vol.340, No. 8, (Feb 1999), pp. 589-94.

4

Psychobiological Stress and Preterm Birth

Curt A. Sandman[1], Elysia P. Davis[1,2] and Laura M. Glynn[1,3]
[1]*Department of Psychiatry and Human Behavior University of California, Irvine,*
[2]*Department of Pediatrics University of California, Irvine,*
[3]*Crean School of Health and Life Sciences Chapman University,*
USA

1. Introduction

Despite current research progress, preterm birth (delivery before 37 weeks gestation) remains a significant problem in maternal-child health because of its high prevalence rate and association with severe adverse health consequences (March of Dimes, 2009; Goldenberg et al., 2000; Sibai et al., 2005; Ventura et al., 2000). Globally, an estimated 13 million babies are born preterm each year representing a 9.6% prevalence of preterm birth (March of Dimes, 2009). The incidence and consequences of preterm birth (PTB) are particularly high and harsh in Africa and Asia where over 11 million (85%) of all preterm births occur. Preterm birth is the leading cause of infant morbidity and mortality. About one million deaths in the first month of life (or 28 percent of total newborn deaths) are attributable to preterm birth.

In the United States (US) preterm birth occurs in 10-15% of all pregnancies and the rate has increased by 35% in the past 25 years (March of Dimes, 2009; Institute of Medicine, 2006). There is a significantly higher rate of preterm birth among African-American women (17.8%) compared to Caucasian women (8.8%) (Institute of Medicine, 2006). In the US, preterm births are associated with 75% of perinatal mortality (Adams & Barfield, 2008; Nathanielsz, 1995; Novy et al., 1995). Long term follow-up indicates that between one-third to one-fifth of preterm children have moderate to severe sensory handicaps by age two (including cerebral palsy, mental retardation, epilepsy, blindness or deafness) (Escobar et al., 1991; Kramer, 2009; Kuban & Leviton, 1994). Because of this the economic consequences of PTB are of similar magnitude as smoking, alcohol abuse and AIDS (Novy et al., 1995). An Institute of Medicine (2006) report estimated the cost of PTB to be $26.2 billion in 2005 with daily NICU costs exceeding $3,500 per infant, and it is not unusual for costs to top $1 million for a prolonged stay (Catlin, 2006). Despite the magnitude of this problem, the etiology of preterm birth remains poorly understood.

The precise mechanisms by which human parturition is initiated spontaneously, either at term or preterm, are not well understood (Kramer et al., 2009). It is established that microbial colonization and inflammation in the maternal genital tract is one cause of preterm birth (Gibbs et al., 1992) and account for the majority of preterm births between 21 and 24 weeks. As gestation progresses to 33 weeks, however, the incidence of preterm birth due to infection drops below 10%. Thus, in the large majority of preterm births there is no known etiological agent. While the exact causes of preterm labor are not known, they may include behavioral, environmental, biological and psychosocial factors, medical conditions and genetics. As described above, there are striking racial-ethnic and socioeconomic differences in preterm birth rates that are largely unexplained (Kramer & Hogue, 2009; Institute of Medicine, 2006). At the physiological level, it is clear that many factors are involved in the onset of labor, including hormonal metabolism and structural changes to the uterus and myometrium (Petraglia et al., 1996) but the effects and interactions among these factors are not fully understood (Challis, 1994). Research from our group (Wadhwa et al., 2004; Sandman et al., 2006; Sandman et al., 1995, 1999b; Wadhwa et al., 1996; Wadhwa et al., 2004; Wadhwa et al., 1998) and many others (Braastad, 1998; Lindsay & Nieman, 2005; Makrigiannakis et al., 2007; Neumann et al., 1998) indicates that a primary pathway of the effects of stress on the human fetus is the HPA stress axis. This review will focus on the role that stress plays in determining preterm birth.

2. Stress: Definitions

In physics, stress historically was defined as the degree of distortion in a malleable metal when it is subjected to an external load. A similar concept of systemic stress was introduced to the life sciences by Hans Selye in the 1930s. He defined stress as "the non-specific response of the body to any demand for change" (Selye, 1936). In connecting stress to disease states, Selye emphasized the non-specificity of stressful events--it could be heat, cold, exercise, bacterial infection, and a host of other agents (Selye, 1959). Selye refined and broadened his initial definition over the years by adding to the concept the idea that stress included an inadequate physiological response to any demand that resulted in "wear and tear on the body" (Selye, 1956). He recognized that individuals adapted to, and developed defenses against, stress (Selye, 1955). His General Adaptation Syndrome was characterized by an *alarm* reaction or shock phase, a stage of *resistance* and finally, if defenses fail, an *exhaustion* stage placing the organism at risk for ill health.

2.1 Endocrine stress system

Systemic stress activates the expression of the master stress hypothalamic (H) hormone, corticotrophic releasing hormone (CRH), which stimulates the cascade of events preparing the organism for "fight or flight". CRH, a 41-amino acid neuropeptide, is synthesized primarily in the paraventricular nucleus of the hypothalamus and has a major role in regulating pituitary (P)-adrenal (A) function and the physiological response to stress (Chrousos, 1992; Vale et al., 1981). CRH stimulates the synthesis of a bioinactive 31K dalton prohormone, proopiomelanocortin (POMC) in the pituitary which is converted by enzymes into adrenocorticotrophic hormone, ACTH and other active peptides. ACTH enters the blood stream and elicits secretion of glucocorticoids (cortisol in humans) from the adrenal gland. There is negative feedback between the adrenal gland and both the hypothalamus and pituitary gland that shuts down the stress response under normal conditions. In addition, cortisol crosses the blood-brain barrier and activates specific receptors in limbic brain structures and in the cortex. The limbic structures, especially the hippocampus, prefrontal cortex (PFC) and amygdala have both excitatory and inhibitory connections with the HPA axis (Avishai-Eliner et al., 2002).

The amygdala activates the HPA axis. Stimulation of the amygdala promotes synthesis and release of CRH from the hypothalamus and begins the sequence of events which ultimately results in corticosteroid biosynthesis and secretion in the adrenal gland. In contrast to the amygdala, the hippocampus is involved in terminating the HPA axis responses to stress. Hippocampal lesions are associated with basal hypersecretion of glucocorticoids (Knigge &

Hays, 1963), enhanced basal CRH mRNA expression (Herman et al., 1995; Herman et al., 1989), increased ACTH secretion in paraventricular nucleus (PVN) and prolonged corticosterone and ACTH release following exposure to a variety of stressors (Herman et al., 1998; Nettles et al., 2000). Like the hippocampus, the prefrontal cortex also plays an important role in negative feedback regulation of the HPA axis (Meaney et al., 1996). Studies in rats (Bagley & Moghaddam, 1997; Feldman & Conforti, 1985; Moghaddam, 1993) and humans (Murros et al., 1993; Shimizu et al., 1997) show that the PFC is a significant target for the negative-feedback actions of circulating corticosteroids. Direct implants of corticosterone into the medial prefrontal region decrease stress-induced ACTH and corticosterone secretion following acute or repeated restraint (Akana et al., 2001; Diorio et al., 1993). Administration of CRH enhances CRF1 RNA expression throughout the medial prefrontal cortex. There is evidence that the CRH peptide interacts with CRH neurons in the PFC to inhibit the hypothalamic–pituitary adrenal axis via indirect pathways reducing CRH release from the PVN (Brunson et al., 2002).

2.2 Psychological stress

In our work we adopt an umbrella concept (Lazarus, 1966, 1968) to characterize prenatal stress. This view includes both stress exposures and responses under the same framework of prenatal stress. The overarching concept is divided into stressors (environmental exposures) and responses. Exposures include new, intense or rapidly changing conditions, or conversely, absence of expected stimulation, fatigue, boredom and even misperceptions. Responses include biological, emotional, cognitive, and behavioral reactions. A further theoretical component is cognitive appraisals of stress, which operate as a critical mediator between stressors and responses in human research (Lazarus & Folkman, 1984).

3. Stress and pregnancy

3.1 Endocrine stress system during pregnancy

The endocrine stress or "fight or flight" system is profoundly altered during human pregnancy. The pituitary gland doubles in size and the output of pituitary peptides increases severalfold as gestation progresses. But it is the growth and development of a new organ, the placenta, in primates that is primarily responsible for the profound changes in the stress circuit (Figure 1). CRH immunoreactivity in the plasma of non-pregnant women is very low or undetectable. The human placenta and amniotic membrane expresses the genes for the major stress hormones, CRH (hCRHmRNA) and POMC by the seventh week of gestation. All of the HPA and placental stress hormones increase as pregnancy advances, but the exponential increase in placental CRH in maternal plasma is especially dramatic, reaching levels observed only in the hypothalamic portal system during physiological stress (Lowry, 1993). The levels of hCRHmRNA increase more than 20-fold in the five weeks preceding delivery (Frim et al., 1988) resulting in a significant elevation in maternal CRH plasma concentrations during the second half of pregnancy. Levels rise exponentially as pregnancy advances, peaking during labor, and falling to very low or undetectable levels within 24 hours after delivery (Campbell et al., 1987; Chan et al., 1993; Goland et al., 1992; Sasaki et al., 1987; Wolfe et al., 1988). Placental CRH is identical to hypothalamic CRH in structure, immunoreactivity and bioactivity (Petraglia et al., 1989; Sasaki et al., 1988). However, in contrast to the inhibitory influence on the promoter region of the CRH gene in the hypothalamus,

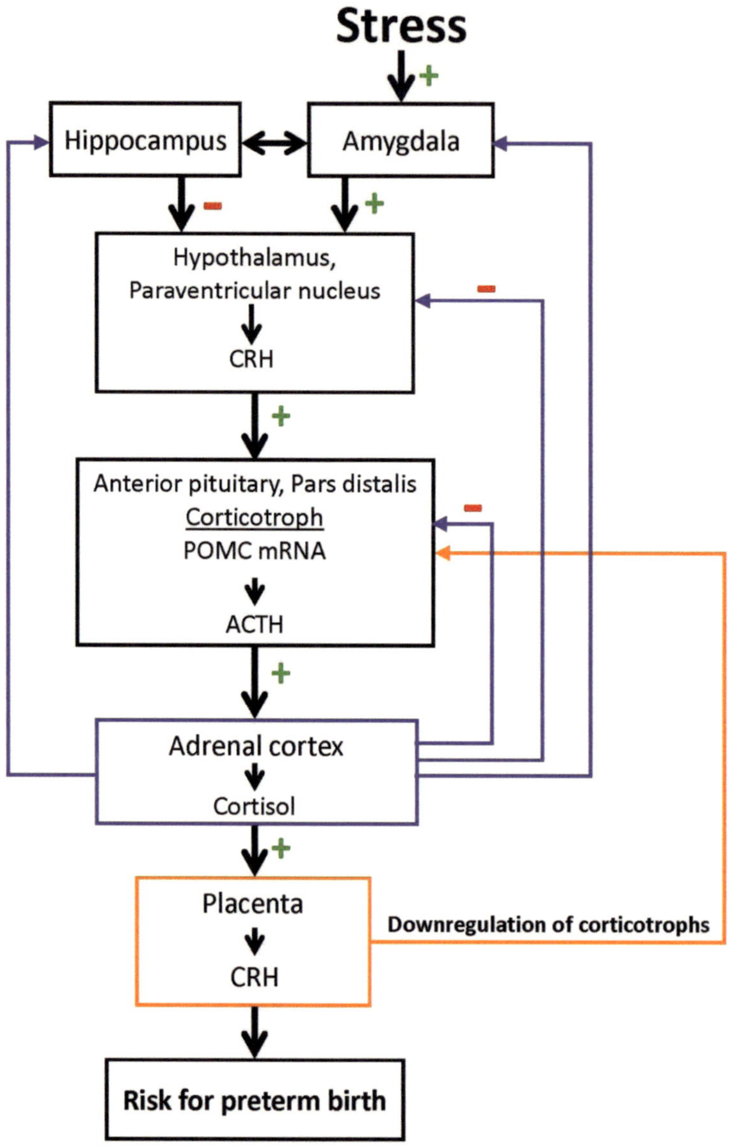

Fig. 1. The regulation of the HPA axis changes dramatically over the course of gestation with profound implications for the mother and the fetus. One of the most significant changes during pregnancy is the development of the placenta, a fetal organ with significant endocrine properties. During pregnancy CRH is released from the placenta into both the maternal and fetal compartments. In contrast to the negative feedback regulation of hypothalamic CRH, cortisol *increases* the production of CRH from the placenta. Placental CRH (pCRH) concentrations rise exponentially over the course of gestation. Rapid acceleration of CRH, especially between weeks 25 and 30 GA increase the risk of shortened gestation.

maternal stress signals (cortisol) from the adrenal glands activate the promoter region in the placenta and stimulate the expression of hCRHmRNA establishing a positive feedback loop that allows for the simultaneous increase of CRH, ACTH and cortisol over the course of gestation. The difference in behavior of the CRH gene in the placenta and hypothalamus is due to the expression of different transcription factors, co-activators and co-repressors in these two tissues (King et al., 2002). The increase of CRH especially over the latter part of human gestation plays a fundamental role in the organization of the fetal nervous system (Sandman et al., 1999b), influencing the timing of the onset of spontaneous labor and delivery (McLean et al., 1995; Sandman et al., 2006; Smith et al., 2002; Smith & Nicholson, 2007; Tyson et al., 2009) and in maternal adaptation during pregnancy, including dampening psychological stress (Glynn & Sandman, in press).

3.2 Alterations in stress responding during pregnancy

The dramatic maternal endocrine alterations that accompany pregnancy have implications not only for the maintenance of gestation, successful parturition and optimal fetal/infant/child development, but also have ramifications for the maternal brain and behavior. HPA axis, blood pressure, heart rate and catecholamine responses to stress are *dampened* as pregnancy progresses (de Weerth & Buitelaar, 2005). These changes in physiological responding are mirrored by changes in psychological responding. Exposures to stress are found to be less distressing when they occur later in pregnancy compared to when they occur early in pregnancy or in the non-pregnant state (Glynn et al., 2008; Glynn et al., 2004). The changes in stress responding as gestation advances may be adaptive and promote survival (Glynn et al., 2008). Specifically, down-regulated psychological and physiological maternal stress responding provides protection for mother and fetus from the effects of adversity as pregnancy progresses toward term. For instance, stress experienced early in gestation, but not later, is associated with preterm birth (Glynn et al., 2004; Lederman et al., 2004). Moreover, women who fail to show the expected decrease in generalized stress and anxiety or dampening in the cortisol awakening response during pregnancy are at increased risk for preterm delivery (Buss et al., 2009b; Glynn et al., 2008).

4. Risk for preterm birth

Because each developing organism plays an active role in its own construction, the embryo and the fetus must acquire information about the environment that guide its development. The human placenta is both a sensory and effector organ that incorporates and transduces information from its maternal host environment into the fetal developmental program. The fetal/placental unit's early detection of stress signals from the maternal environment "informs" the fetus that there may be a threat to survival. If the nature of the environment is perceived to be stressful or hostile, it may promote developmental trajectories that ensure survival. Compelling evidence from the desert-dwelling Western spadefoot toad illustrates this conserved function (Boorse & Denver, 2002; Denver, 1997, 1999; Seasholtz et al., 2002). This toad lays its eggs in pools of desert rainwater. Tadpoles exposed to rapidly evaporating pools, accelerate their metamorphosis to escape imminent peril. This highly adaptive function allows the tadpole to reach maturity before the life-sustaining environment desiccates. If stress hormones are blocked during environmental desiccation, then the rate of development is arrested and the tadpole's survival is compromised. Survival under these circumstances, however, is associated with long-term costs. Tadpoles that survived by accelerating their development were smaller than normal at emergence as toads and had reduced capacity to forage for food and to mate (Denver, 1997; John-Adler & Morin, 1990; Newman, 1989; Smith, 1987).

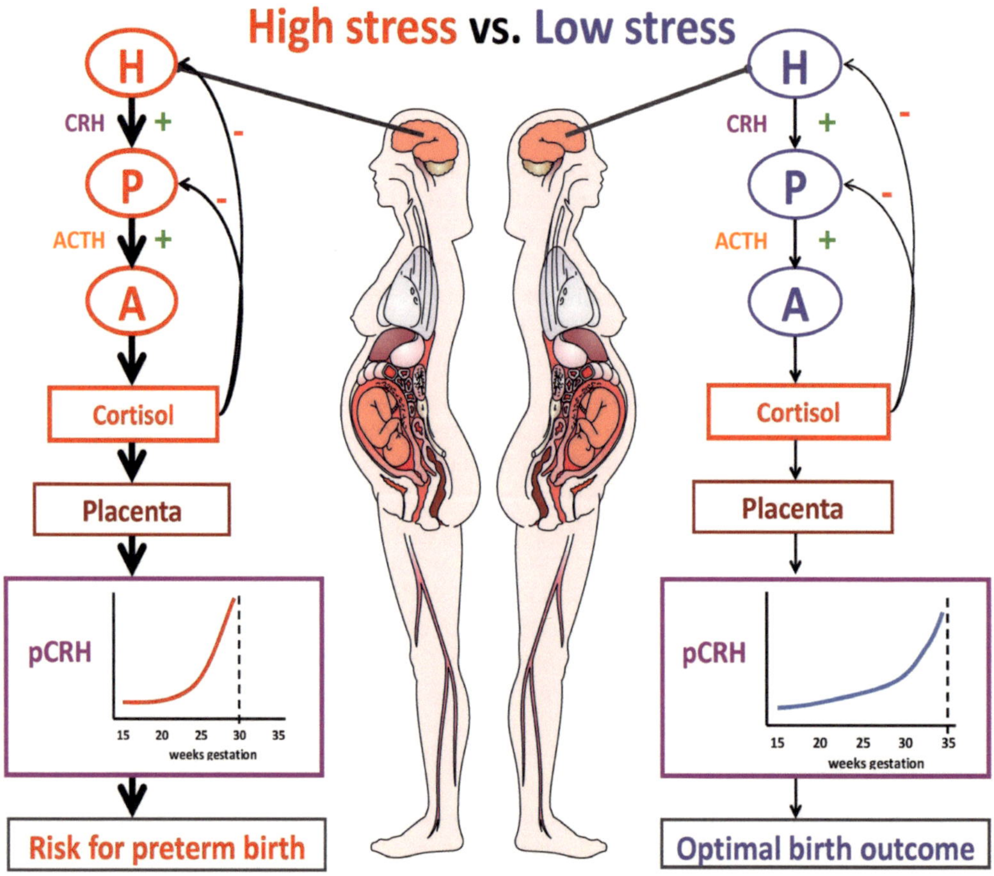

Fig. 2. The BLUE panel shows the normal activity of the HPA axis during pregnancy. One of the most significant changes during pregnancy is the development of the placenta, a fetal organ with significant endocrine properties. CRH is released from the placenta into both the maternal and fetal compartments. In contrast to the negative feedback regulation of hypothalamic CRH, cortisol *increases* the production of CRH from the placenta. Placental CRH (pCRH) concentrations rise exponentially over the course of gestation. The RED panel illustrates (by the thicker lines) that the normal changes are exaggerated under conditions of high stress that results in accelerated release of CRH and increasing the risk for preterm birth. H=Hypothalamus; P= pituitary; A=adrenal cortex

4.1 Endocrine risk

There is substantial *in vitro* and *in vivo* findings indicating that the placenta detects and responds to a variety of maternal physiological and psychological stress signals. The human placenta integrates numerous sources of maternal stress signals, including cortisol, and responds with a dose-dependent release of CRH. The surge in CRH is produced by syncytial cells which can be created *in vitro* by fusion of purified cytotrophoblast cells (Petraglia et al., 1989). The exponential increase in CRH observed during the course of human pregnancy can be reproduced using a model which incorporates positive feed forward between cortisol and CRH (Emanuel et al., 1994). In contrast to the inhibition of hypothalamic CRH, cortisol stimulates the release of CRH from the placenta. The postitive relation between cortisol and CRH release from the placenta is similar to the positive effect of cortisol observed in the amygdala (Schulkin, 1999). Using transfections of CRH promoter constructs, the stimulatory mechanism has been partially explained. In placental tissue, glucocorticoids stimulate CRH gene expression by interacting with proteins that bind to the cAMP response site of the CRH promoter (Cheng et al., 2000).

Evidence suggests that the normal trajectory of placental CRH production over the course of gestation may be accelerated by an adverse intrauterine environment characterized by physiological stress. For example, elevated placental CRH has been observed in pregnancies complicated by pre-eclampsia, reduced utero-placental perfusion, intrauterine infection, and in cases where fetal distress has led to elective preterm delivery (Giles et al., 1996). A series of *in vitro* studies (Petraglia et al., 1987; Petraglia et al., 1989; Petraglia et al., 1990) have shown that CRH is released from cultured human placental cells in a dose-response manner in response to *all* the major biological effectors of stress, including cortisol, catecholamines, and pro-inflammatory cytokines. We have shown that elevated levels of maternal cortisol early in gestation are associated with a more rapid rise in placental CRH concentrations (Sandman et al., 2006). Not only is placental CRH responsive to stress related increases in maternal cortisol, but the administration of synthetic glucocorticoids for fetal lung maturation to pregnant women at risk for preterm delivery is similarly associated with significant increases in circulating placental CRH. Placental CRH concentrations increase 1.5 fold within 12 hours in response to the administration of synthetic glucocorticoids such as betamethasone (Korebrits et al., 1998; Marinoni et al., 1998). Further, placental CRH concentrations remain elevated for at least one week after a single course of treatment. These finding are consistent with the report of decreased gestational length among women administered corticosteroids during their first trimester (Gur et al., 2004) probably by stimulating synthesis and release of placental CRH.

The placental detection of stress or adversity may prime or advance the "placental clock" by activating the promoter region of the CRH gene and increase the placental synthesis of CRH. The rapid increase in circulating CRH begins the cascade of events influencing myometria (Tyson et al., 2009) and in extreme cases, precipitating preterm birth. Placental CRH has been shown to increase the placental production of estrogens and to inhibit the synthesis of progesterone (Yang et al., 2006; You et al., 2006). Placental CRH is additionally released into the fetal compartment where it stimulates the fetal adrenal gland to release dehydroepiandrosterone sulfate (DHEAS) an obligate precursor for placental estriol production (Smith et al., 1998). Alterations in the production of progesterone and estriol may be one pathway by which placental CRH regulates the timing of delivery (Smith et al., 2009). Data indicate that it is the trajectory of placental CRH production over gestation, rather than the absolute hormone concentration that best predicts preterm delivery, suggesting that target cells are highly responsive to relative changes in placental CRH concentrations. The effects of HPA and placental axis hormones on gestational length are modulated by the activities of binding proteins and enzymes. For example, concurrent with increases in circulating levels of placental CRH, a CRH-binding protein (CRH-BP) is produced in the liver and also in the trophoblast and intrauterine tissues during pregnancy, and binds to circulating CRH, reducing its biological action (Orth & Mount, 1987; Petraglia, et al., 1996; Petraglia et al., 1993). In contrast to the exponentially increasing levels of circulating CRH over the course of gestation, CRH-BP levels, which are constant in the first, second, and early third trimester and are not significantly different from non-pregnant levels, fall by approximately 30% as birth approaches (Linton et al., 1993). The net effect of these changes in levels of CRH and CRH-BP is a sharp increase in the availability of free and bioactive CRH during this last part of gestation. There is some evidence that women who deliver preterm have lower levels of CRH-BP (Hobel et al., 1999). Maternal plasma cortisol binding globulin (CBG) levels also change across pregnancy. CBG is stimulated by estrogen and these levels increase progressively with advancing gestation until the end of gestation when there is a significant decline in CBG leading to an increase in bioactive cortisol (Ho et al., 2007). The activity of placental 11β-HSD2 (which oxidizes cortisol into its inactive form, cortisone) (Sun et al., 1999) increases as gestation progresses before falling precipitously near term. Both the decrease in CBG and the decrease in activity of placental 11β-HSD2 increase fetal exposure to maternal cortisol ensuring maturation of the fetal lungs, CNS and other organ systems in full term births (Ma et al., 2003; Murphy & Clifton, 2003).

The association between maternal plasma concentrations of CRH and preterm labor/delivery has been examined in many published studies (Markovic et al., 2007). During pregnancy, maternal stress threatens the fetal nervous system (Coe et al., 2003; Insel et al., 1990; Poland et al., 1999; Sanchez et al., 1993; Sandman et al., 2003; Sandman et al., 1999a; Sandman et al., 1999b; Weinstock, 1996) and shortens the length of gestation (Campbell et al., 1987; McLean et al., 1995; Wadhwa et al., 2004; Wadhwa et al., 1998; Wadhwa et al., 1993; Warren et al., 1992; Wolfe et al., 1988). The general findings are that plasma CRH concentrations of women in preterm labor are significantly higher than those of gestational-age matched controls and the rate of change of CRH over gestation is accelerated in women destined to deliver early. Studies measuring CRH at a single point during gestation produce equivocal findings because there are wide individual differences that can only be assessed with longitudinal designs (Sibai et al., 2005) and because it is the trajectory of placental CRH production over gestation that best predicts preterm birth (Smith et al., 2009). The most convincing early support for the role of CRH in the timing of human delivery was demonstrated by McLean et al (1995). In a prospective, longitudinal study, CRH levels were assessed between one and four times from 16-20 weeks gestation to term. Plasma CRH levels at 18-20 weeks gestation were significantly higher in women delivering preterm (N=24) than at term (N=308), and were significantly lower in women delivering post-term (N=29). These findings demonstrated that patterns of plasma CRH are associated with the timing of delivery, both early and late, and may be established as early as the beginning of the second trimester of gestation.

4.2 Psychological risk

Early work examining psychological risk was plagued by methodological issues rendering a definitive answer about the role of psychological stress in preterm birth difficult to assess. An early careful review by Savitz & Pastore (1999) of 20 of the more rigorous studies, stated that it was difficult to draw conclusions due to methodological limitations. Study designs until that time had been a mix of retrospective and case-control studies, with relatively few prospective studies and approximately half of the studies reviewed found associations of stress and length of gestation. However, more recent work with more methodologically sound approaches, including reports from our own group (Campos et al., 2008; Dominguez et al., 2008; Glynn et al., 2008; Glynn et al., 2001; Hilmert et al., 2008; Rini et al., 1999; Wadhwa et al., 1993) have consistently demonstrated significant associations between prenatal stress and adverse birth outcomes. In a recent comprehensive review, Dunkel Schetter and Glynn (2011) concluded that prenatal stress represents a significant risk for preterm birth or shortened gestation. However the findings also indicated that stress was not a unitary construct and some characterizations of stress were stronger predictors of birth outcome than others. For instance, of the fourteen studies of exposure to stressful life events during pregnancy, eight found a significant influence on the risk for shortened gestation, and another form of episodic stress, catastrophes, also were consistently identified as risk factors. High levels of chronic forms of stress (chronic strain, perceived racism, and neighborhood or community stressors) showed consistent links with decreased gestational length. Inconsistent and very modest effects are detected with instruments targeting appraised or perceived stress (all twelve studies used Cohen's Perceived Stress Scale [Cohen et al., 1983], and only four found an association). Similarly, depression is not a reliable predictor of shortened gestation. Perhaps the most compelling pattern was the finding that anxiety related to pregnancy outcomes, mostly reflecting fears, concerns and beliefs, significantly shortened gestation in ten of eleven studies.

Viewed collectively, the evidence is quite clear that stress conceived of as a general multidimensional concept contributes to the etiology of preterm birth. There are at least three emerging themes, however, that dictate future directions and refinement of models examining the role of stress in preterm birth. First, some conceptions or dimensions of stress now are emerging as more potent predictors than others, suggesting a need for further theoretical specificity. By far the most consistent results are found for pregnancy-related stress and anxiety, and a close second is major life events. Also notable are chronic strains, catastrophes, community stressors, and racism, but these literatures still are in the early stages. Second, the predictable changes in maternal stress responding (both psychological and physiological) represent a critical moderating variable (Glynn, 2010). Normative changes in stress responding have important implications both for the impact of exposures to stress and also for interpreting the relations between stress, measured at different points in gestation, and adverse outcomes. It is worth noting that from a methodological standpoint, it is difficult if not impossible, to understand timing without prospective, longitudinal study designs. Last, an additional moderating variable worth considering relates to ethnic and cultural differences. Some stress concepts do not generalize well across ethnic, cultural and foreign populations and some dimensions of stress apply only to specific groups. For example, lifetime exposures to racism are predictive of restricted fetal growth, but only among African American women (Dominquez et al., 2008). Similarly, anxiety in pregnancy has been shown to characterize Latina women in particular, especially new and unacculturated immigrants from countries with poor medical care (Rini et al., 1999; Zambrana et al., 1997). Adding further complexity to this issue is the fact that the relevance of biological mediators and the physiological pathways to preterm birth may differ depending on race/ethnicity. For example, the threshold of CRH exposure that is associated with preterm birth is lower among African American women (Holzman et al., 2001), and others have shown that elevated prenatal cortisol is more likely to be associated with an accelerated CRH trajectory in African American and Latina women than among white women (Glynn et al., 2007). Even more recently it was shown that among Latinas, perceived discrimination is associated with elevated prenatal cortisol trajectories, which predict reduced fetal growth, but this is not the case for non-Hispanic white women (Glynn, 2011). These findings highlight the importance of developing population-specific concepts and measures of stress. In addition, stress concepts and measures that generalize well over ethnic, cultural, and international populations are needed. The emergence of pregnancy-specific validated measures of stress and anxiety represents a promising avenue to achieve this goal (Huizink et al., 2004; Lobel et al., 2008).

In recent years, many more studies have been published on this topic, often with prospective designs, large sample sizes, and appropriate controls. Recent reviews concur that the evidence regarding stress as a significant independent risk factor for spontaneous preterm labor and delivery is now clearer (Beydoun & Saftlas, 2008; Institute of Medicine, 2006). Beydoun and Saflas (2008) report that nine of eleven studies between 2000 and 2006 found significant effects of prenatal maternal stress on length of gestation or risk of preterm labor or birth, although not all studies adjusted for appropriate control variables.

5. Our approach

Our research team has been exploring the effects of stress and specifically the HPA axis on developmental processes for over 30 years (Glynn & Sandman, in press; Sandman & Davis, 2010; Sandman et al., 2011a; Sandman et al., 2011b). The initial studies were among the first to describe the long lasting (perhaps permanent and programming) effects of neonatal exposure to ACTH on the brain and behavior of rats (Beckwith et al., 1977; Champney et al., 1976; Sandman & O'Halloran, 1986). In another comprehensive project, we discovered that *in utero* exposure of rats to high levels of beta endorphin (BE) delayed developmental milestones, permanently altered pain threshold, exploration, and both active and passive avoidance responding (Sandman & Kastin, 1981). We found that fetal exposure to BE increased the expression of opioids (Moldow et al., 1981) and down-regulated dopamine (D_2) receptors (Sandman & Yessaian, 1986) in the brains of these animals as adults. During the past 15+ years our group has been examining the effects of stress and activation of the HPA/placental axis on birth outcomes and on the human fetus. As described below, our findings contribute to the growing acceptance that maternal stress is a risk factor for adverse outcomes. Our studies also have made significant contributions to understanding the mechanisms of the effects of stress on gestational length. Other findings were the first to indicate that very high levels of CRH are associated with both preterm delivery and infants who are small for gestational age. Moreover, we discovered that very low levels of CRH were associated with post-term birth adding strong support to the suggestion that CRH primed a "placental clock" controlling the timing of delivery. We published evidence that a maternal stress message early in pregnancy may prime a subsequent fetal/placental CRH response and increase the risk for preterm birth and that racial/ethnic differences may exist in this priming process (Glynn et al., 2007). Other studies from our project were the first to show that elevated levels of CRH in the maternal circulation influences the human fetal nervous system and fetal exposure to elevated levels of CRH persist into infancy and childhood.

5.1 Assessment

We have developed a prospective protocol for the assessment of prenatal exposure to maternal stress and stress hormones on fetal, infant and child development (Figure 3). Maternal psychosocial and biological stress measures are collected at five gestational intervals beginning between 14 and 16 weeks. Maternal/fetal dyads are assessed at 15, 20, 25, 31 and 36 weeks of gestation. At ~25, ~31 and ~36 gestational weeks, fetal neurodevelopment is evaluated with a measure of startle and habituation. At delivery, information on length of gestation and birth weight is abstracted from medical records. Infant assessments begin 24 hours post delivery with the collection of cortisol and behavioral responses to the painful stress of the heel-stick procedure and measures of neonatal neuromuscular maturity. Infant cognitive, neuromotor development, stress and emotional regulation are evaluated at 3, 6, 12 and 24 months of age. Maternal psychosocial stress and demographic information is collected in parallel with infant assessments. Child neurodevelopment is assessed with cognitive tests, measures of adjustment and brain imaging.

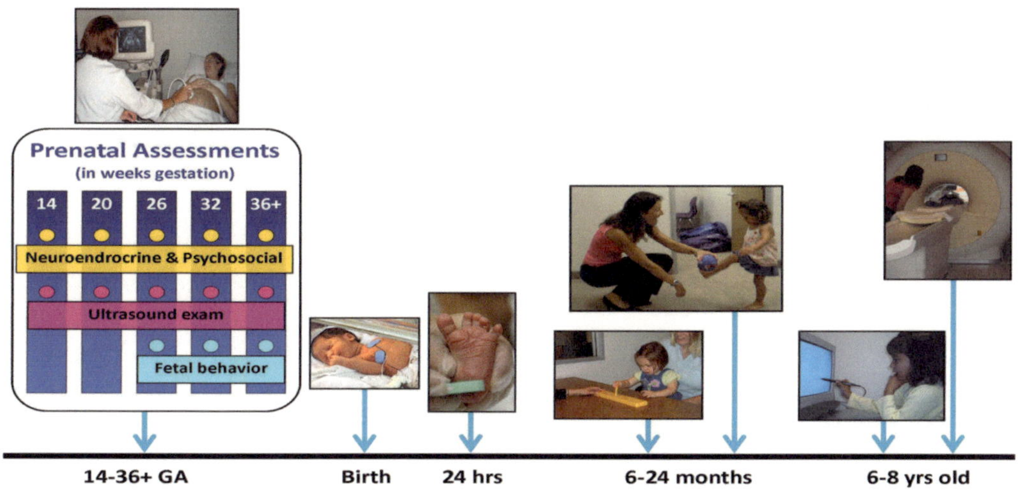

Fig. 3. Schematic representation of the psychobiological stress model that guides our research program. Multiple endocrine and psychological assessments are made during gestation and mother and infant are followed from birth to late childhood.

Over 800 adult women have participated in our studies of prenatal psychobiological stress. The majority of our women are married and high school educated. Our sample is racially/ethnically diverse with a small majority that is White/Non-Hispanic. All subjects presented with a singleton intrauterine pregnancy, a normal uterus and cervix and for the majority the current pregnancy is their first. A comprehensive structured medical interview and thorough chart review is conducted to exclude subjects if they present with prior or present obstetric risk conditions including systemic maternal disease (cancer, cardiac disease, seizure history, autoimmune diseases and blood disorders), placental or cord abnormalities, uterine anomalies, infection, congenital malformations or chromosomal abnormalities determined in the first trimester. Women also are excluded if they present with any condition that could disregulate neuroendocrine function such as endocrine, hepatic or renal disorders or the use of corticosteroid medications. Interviews assessed health behaviors to exclude women who smoked or consumed alcohol or drugs of abuse six months before and during the index pregnancy. A clinical ultrasound performed early in gestation (15 or 20 weeks) confirms gestational age. Blood is collected at each interval for assessment of neuroendocrine profiles. To control possible circadian influences, subjects are evaluated each session between 14:00 and 16:00. Women were followed to term and birth outcome information is abstracted from medical charts.

5.2 Findings

In addition to the well known increase in infant and toddler mortality and morbidity associated with preterm birth, there are other longer term risks associated with abbreviated gestation. Retrospective studies have concluded that fetuses born early or small for gestational age are at greater subsequent risk for later cardiovascular disease, hypertension, hyperlipidemia, insulin resistance, non-insulin dependent diabetes mellitus, obesity, higher serum cholesterol concentrations, shortened life span, and other poor health outcomes (Barker et al., 1993; Barker, 1998; McCormack et al., 2003; Richards et al., 2001; Roseboom et al., 2000). Our program of research is guided by the assumption that birth phenotype itself (that is preterm birth) is not the only source of risk but instead reflects adverse *in utero* exposures that influence fetal development and contribute to poor birth outcomes. These influences on the fetus have been described as "programming" (Barker, 1998). Thus, findings from our prospective studies of early human development, consistent with our assumptions and the assessment protocol in Figure 3, include the effects of endocrine and psychological stress on the fetus, birth outcome and subsequent development.

5.2.1 Findings: Endocrine stress

5.2.1.1 Fetal behavior

Measures of fetal responses to external stimulation have been used in our projects to directly assess the developmental consequences of exposure to psychobiological stress (Sandman et al., 1997). We discovered that fetuses of women with elevated pCRH during the third trimester were less responsive to the presence of a novel stimulus (Sandman et al., 1999b). In a subsequent study we reported that fetal heart rate habituation was delayed when fetuses were exposed to over-expression of maternal endogenous BE (Sandman et al., 2003). To evaluate programming influences on the fetus, we assessed the consequences of gestational stress during the early second trimester on fetal behavior in the early third trimester. We found that low CRH at 15 gestational weeks, but not later, predicted a more mature fetal heart rate pattern at 25 gestational weeks (Class et al., 2008). This is evidence that endocrine stress exerted influence, on the developing nervous system and that these effects may influence directly or indirectly, birth outcome (Sandman et al., 2011a; Sandman et al., 2011b).

5.2.1.2 Birth outcome

In our initial prenatal endocrine study of gestational length we found that early third trimester levels of maternal CRH were inversely and significantly correlated with gestational age at delivery after adjusting for biomedical correlates of outcome including parity and antepartum medical risk (Wadhwa et al., 1998). Moreover, subjects who delivered preterm had significantly higher levels of CRH in the early third trimester of gestation than those who delivered at term. These results were the first to suggest that this association was independent of the effects of antepartum medical risk on the timing of delivery and supported the premise that placental CRH was implicated in the normal physiology of human parturition. Moreover, these findings supported the sparse literature that premature or accelerated activation of the maternal-placental-fetal neuroendocrine axis was associated with earlier delivery.

We confirmed and extended these findings in a sample of 232 pregnant women at approximately 32 weeks gestation (Wadhwa et al., 2004). Women who delivered preterm had significantly higher CRH levels at 32 weeks gestation than those who delivered at term (215.0 ± 31.5 vs. 139.6 ± 11.7 pg/ml $\pm$SEM), respectively. Conversely women who delivered *post-term* had significantly lower CRH levels at 32 weeks gestation than those who delivered at term (62.0 ± 11.4 vs. 139.6 ± 11.7 pg/ml $\pm$SEM). We also reported that women who delivered growth-restricted infants (SGA) had significantly higher CRH levels at 32 weeks gestation than those who delivered average or large for gestational age infants. Both of these effects on gestational age and birth weight were independent from medical risk. These findings are the first to indicate that fetal growth restriction is associated with elevated CRH. Moreover, extremely elevated maternal levels of the stress hormone were associated with both early birth and growth restriction. Infants with both of these outcomes have been found to have highly significant risk for motor, sensory and cognitive handicaps and may be at "double biological jeopardy" for developmental complications.

In a recent study of 203 pregnant women the HPA and placental stress axis was evaluated by assessing levels of BE, ACTH, cortisol and CRH at regular intervals from 15 to 36 weeks gestation (Sandman et al., 2006). Consistent with our previous studies, placental CRH levels in women destined to deliver preterm (before 37 weeks) had faster rates of increase and significantly higher levels of CRH confined to the beginning of the early third trimester than women who subsequently delivered at term (Figure 2).

Maternal levels of cortisol, ACTH and BE also increased significantly with advancing gestation. The two-fold increases in maternal ACTH and BE and the three-fold increase in maternal cortisol were considerably less than the twenty-five fold increase in *placental* CRH through 31 weeks of gestation. Of these *maternal* measures, only cortisol distinguished women delivering term and preterm. This was the first evidence that levels of cortisol are higher as early as 15 weeks in women who subsequently delivered preterm compared with women delivering after 37 weeks. However, statistical models that accounted for the independent and shared variance of CRH and cortisol indicated that only CRH between 26 and 31 weeks gestation predicted gestational length.

Because CRH level at 31 weeks was the best predictor both of preterm birth and gestational length, a model to predict its precipitous rise during gestation was constructed using all endocrine stress markers collected from the beginning of the second trimester (15 weeks) through week 26 of gestation. The prediction of CRH levels at 31 weeks using all the endocrine markers was highly significant but the single best and highly significant independent predictor of third trimester CRH was cortisol at 15 weeks gestation. Our longitudinal study of human pregnancy provided evidence that the earliest, and perhaps critical, period for the effects of CRH on gestational length was the interval between weeks 26 and 31. The rate of increase during this interval is faster and the level of CRH at 31 weeks is higher in women destined to deliver preterm. Serial sampling of maternal plasma provides no support for the possibility that CRH earlier in pregnancy influenced gestational length. New findings from this study indicated that a plausible stress-related endocrine signal, elevated cortisol from the mother very early in pregnancy, predicts the precocious rise in CRH leading to an abbreviated gestation. The pattern of findings supports the argument that the effect of elevated cortisol early in pregnancy on gestational length reflects a priming or programming (Barker, 1998; McLean et al., 1995; McLean & Smith, 2001) effect on the eventual fetal/placental CRH response.

A recent study further assessed the association of prenatal levels of cortisol with gestational length using a naturally occurring circadian challenge, the cortisol awakening response (CAR) (Buss et al., 2009b). Complete data from a home-based awakening cortisol response were obtained from 51 women early (~17 weeks gestation) and late (~31 weeks gestation). The CAR progressively declined over the course of gestation. A larger CAR in late pregnancy and reduced attenuation of the CAR from early to late gestation were associated with shorter gestational length. Thus, women who exhibited high HPA responsiveness in late gestation and showed reduced dampening of the CAR over gestation were at an increased risk to deliver early.

5.2.1.3 Neonatal and infant outcomes

In a study from our group (Ellman et al., 2008) the New Ballard Maturation Score was used to assess physical and neuromuscular maturation of 158 newborns within 24 hours after birth. Specifically, the neuromuscular and physical characteristics of the newborn were rated and consisted of measures of muscle tone, distinct posture, and angles of resistance in key muscle groups. The results of this study provided evidence that fetal exposure to increases in levels of maternal cortisol at 15 and at 19 weeks gestation and increases in levels of pCRH at 31 weeks gestation were associated with significant decreases in newborn physical and neuromuscular maturation. These effects were observed after adjusting for length of gestation, indicating that fetal exposure to stress hormones programs neonatal neuromuscular maturation independent of gestational age.

Prenatal exposure to maternal stress hormones similarly programs the development of the fetal HPA axis with consequences for neonatal functioning. Recently we reported (Davis et al., 2011b) in a sample of 116 mothers and their healthy full term infants assessed at five gestational intervals and at 24 hours after birth, that prenatal maternal cortisol and psychosocial stress each exerted influences on neonatal stress regulation and these influences were dependent upon the gestational period during which the fetus was exposed. Specifically elevated maternal cortisol early in gestation was associated with slower neonatal behavioral recovery from the painful stress of a heel-stick procedure. Elevated maternal cortisol during the second half of gestation was associated with a larger and more prolonged neonatal cortisol response to stress. The data from this study are consistent with evidence that prenatal exposure to synthetic glucocorticoids during the late second and early third trimester is associated with an amplified cortisol response to stress among healthy full term neonates (Davis et al., 2011c). Together, these data provide evidence that gestational exposure to excess glucocorticoids alters the developmental trajectory of the fetal

HPA axis with consequences for postnatal stress regulation. Alterations to neurological systems at different times during fetal development resulting from prenatal exposures may determine the neonate's ability to respond behaviorally and physiologically to stressors in the postnatal environment. It is plausible that neonates who are more reactive may carry a greater risk for developmental and other health risks independent from birth outcome.

In a sample of over 200 mother child pairs we have shown that elevations in both maternal and placental hormones are associated with fearful infant temperament after controlling for the influence of postpartum maternal state. Specifically, elevated placental CRH at 25 gestational weeks and elevated maternal cortisol during the third trimester independently predicted fearful temperament (Davis et al., 2005; Davis et al., 2007). The increased report of fearful temperament observed in infants exposed to elevated cortisol and placental CRH may have implications for subsequent behavioral problems. The temperament measure included in these studies assesses infants' reactivity to novel stimuli. Infants who are easily aroused by varied stimulation are more likely to become behaviorally inhibited as young children (Kagan et al., 1998; Pfeifer et al., 2002). Furthermore, difficulty adapting to the presentation of novel sensory stimuli in infancy is predictive of later behavioral problems such as adolescent social anxiety (Schwartz et al., 1999).

In a large study (125 subjects) with repeated evaluations at five prenatal intervals and three intervals during infancy we reported that fetal exposure to cortisol early in pregnancy resulted in significantly lower scores on measures of mental development at 12 months of age (Davis & Sandman, 2010). Conversely, elevated maternal cortisol late in gestation was associated with significantly higher scores on measures of mental development. These findings linking cortisol to infant cognitive development are consistent with its function in the maturation of the human fetus. The fetus is partially protected from maternal cortisol because it is oxidized and inactivated by 11β-HSD2. However, because 11β-HSD2 is only a partial barrier, excessive synthesis and release of maternal cortisol exposes the fetus to concentrations that may have detrimental neurological consequences. As pregnancy advances toward term, fetal exposure to elevated cortisol is necessary for maturation of the fetal nervous system and lungs. Fetal exposure to cortisol during the third trimester is facilitated by the sharp drop in 11β-HSD2 which allows a greater proportion of maternal cortisol to cross the placental barrier (Giannopoulos et al., 1982; Murphy et al., 2006).

5.2.2 Findings: Psychological stress

5.2.2.1 Birth outcomes

In our initial study of the association between psychological stress and birth outcome, ninety women were self-administered questionnaires to obtain measures of prenatal psychosocial stress, sociodemographic factors, and health practices (Wadhwa et al., 1993). Independent of biomedical risk, life event stress and pregnancy anxiety significantly predicted infant birth weight and gestational age at birth, respectively. Each unit increase of prenatal Life Event Stress (from a possible sample range of 14.7 units of Life Event Stress) was associated with a 55.03 gram decrease in infant birth weight, and with a 1.32 times increase in the likelihood of occurrence of low birth weight (< 2500 g). Each unit increase of prenatal Pregnancy Anxiety (from a possible sample range of 5 units of Pregnancy Anxiety) was associated with a 3 day decrease in gestational age at birth.

In a diverse sample of 230 women we examined the effects of stress and personal resources (self-esteem, optimism, etc) and sociocultural factors on birth outcomes (Rini et al, 1999).

Resources and prenatal stress had independent influences on outcomes. Greater personal resources were related to higher birth weight babies and women who reported more prenatal stress had shorter gestations.

Our model of the effects of stress in pregnancy (Sandman et al., 1999a) predicts that stress early during gestation has greater consequences on outcomes than stress that is closer to term. To explore this possibility, we focused on the acute effects of a 6.8 earthquake that occurred during our study (Glynn et al., 2001). We identified forty women in our project who had experienced this uncontrollable stressful event while pregnant. We discovered that the ratings of stress were highest if the earthquake occurred during first trimester and lowest if it occurred during third trimester. Consistent with predictions from our model, the timing of the earthquake also was related to gestational age at birth. The earlier during pregnancy the stress occurred, the earlier the delivery occurred. The relation between the timing of stress and gestational age remained unchanged when taking into account medical risk, maternal age, marital status, race, and parity. These findings suggest both that stress, and when stress occurs are critical factors in determining its impact on birth outcomes.

Timing effects and length of gestation were explored by our group (Glynn et al., 2008) in a more recent study of 415 pregnant women in whom prenatal stress assessed at 18–20 and 30–32 weeks gestation. At neither assessment did levels of anxiety or perceived stress predict gestational length. However, patterns of anxiety and stress were associated with gestational length. Although the majority of women who delivered at term exhibited declines in stress and anxiety over the course of gestation as expected, those who delivered preterm exhibited increases. The elevated risk for preterm delivery associated with an increase in stress or anxiety persisted when adjusting for obstetric risk, pregnancy related anxiety, ethnicity, parity, and prenatal life events. These findings suggest that women who do not show the expected or normative decline in stress responding are at increased risk for early delivery, an assumption that was confirmed by the findings from the study examining changes in the CAR across gestation described above (Buss et al., 2009c).

5.2.2.2 Infant and child outcomes

We have shown that prenatal measures of maternal psychological stress are associated with infant and child behavioral regulation and temperament. Elevated gestational anxiety and depression were associated with slower behavioral recovery from the painful stress of the heel-stick blood draw at 24 hours of age (Davis et al., 2011b). These measures of psychological distress were additionally predictive of more fearful and reactive temperament during early infancy (Davis 2007; Davis et al., 2004). More recently we have shown that pregnancy specific anxiety (PSA) is associated with negative child temperament at 3 months and 2-years of age (Blair et al., in press; Sandman et al., 2011a). Furthermore, pregnancy specific anxiety is a more potent predictor of child temperament as compared to general anxiety. These findings underscore the growing recognition that PSA may be a particularly potent influence on adverse birth and infant outcomes.

In the study of the effects of exposure to maternal cortisol on infant cognition described above, we also assessed the influence of maternal stress and anxiety on mental development (Davis & Sandman, 2010). Our results for PSA were similar as they were for cortisol; high levels of anxiety early in pregnancy (~15 weeks gestation) were associated with poorest performance on tests of cognition at one year of age. Despite the similar effects of maternal cortisol and anxiety on infant cognition, these two measures of prenatal stress were not related and exerted independent effects on developmental outcomes. The consequences for the infant were confined to cognitive outcomes. Motor performance was unaffected by either exposure to cortisol or maternal anxiety.

Low birth weight and preterm birth have been related to reductions in regional brain volumes (Abernethy et al., 2002; Beauchamp et al., 2008; Buss et al., 2007; Nosarti et al., 2002; Peterson et al., 2000). However, because adverse birth outcomes may be markers of *in utero* stress exposure, it has been difficult to separate the effects of fetal stress exposures on brain morphology from perinatal complications. Recently, our group published the first study to show that fetal exposure to PSA was related to specific changes in brain morphology at six to nine years of age independent of birth phenotype (Buss et al., 2010). Specifically, serial assessment of PSA in 35 women was conducted at 19, 25 and 31 weeks gestation and then their children were followed up with structural MRI at 6-9 years of age. We found that elevated PSA early in gestation but not other times was associated with gray matter volume reductions in the prefrontal cortex, the premotor cortex, the medial temporal lobe, the lateral temporal cortex, the postcentral gyrus as well as the cerebellum extending to the middle occipital gyrus and the fusiform gyrus. These brain regions are associated with a variety of cognitive functions. Specifically, the prefrontal cortex is involved in executive cognitive functions such as reasoning, planning, attention, working memory, and some aspects of language. We found that the reduction in brain volumes in children exposed to elevated PSA early in gestation (Buss et al., 2010) primarily were observed in girls (Sandman et al., 2011a). These are the first prospective studies in healthy children to show that fetal exposure to maternal anxiety is related to distinctive patterns of structural brain development.

6. Conclusions

Fetal exposure to endocrine and psychological stress profoundly influences the developing human fetus and birth outcome and with consequences that persist into childhood. It is important to acknowledge the independent and joint influences of psychosocial and endocrine stress on development. The human placenta integrates numerous sources of maternal stress signals and responds with a dose-dependent release of stress hormones. As we reviewed here, placental CRH concentrations are observed in pregnancies characterized by high levels of maternal stress and those complicated by pre-eclampsia, reduced utero-placental perfusion, intrauterine infection, and in cases where fetal distress has led to elective preterm delivery. However, because the HPA and placental system is responsive to *both* psychosocial and physiological stress, these two sources can exert independent influences on the fetus and birth outcome. Thus, maternal psychosocial stress does not exclusively determine fetal exposure to biological stress signals and elevated levels of stress hormones do not necessarily reflect the experience of increased maternal stress. The evidence indicates that both biological and psychosocial sources of stress, especially pregnancy specific stress, have significant influences on the fetus and birth outcomes with long term consequences in the infant and child. Moreover, several studies reported in this review found that pregnancy specific anxiety was a stronger predictor of various outcomes than generalized anxiety. The experience of pregnancy presents unique fears and concerns and these dimensions are captured by items that are included in our measures (e.g., *"I am fearful regarding the health of my baby;" "I am concerned or worried about losing my baby;" "I am concerned or worried about developing medical problems during my pregnancy").*

There are plausible routes of maternal biological stress influencing birth outcome and the fetal nervous system. One possible endocrine route discussed here posits that the placental detection of stress or adversity primes or advances the "placental clock" by activating the promoter region of the CRH gene and increases the placental synthesis of CRH. The rapid increase in circulating CRH begins the cascade of events influencing myometria (Tyson et al., 2009) and may precipitate preterm birth. As such, fetal exposure to pCRH may be a final common pathway for the "programming" effects of some stressors on birth outcome and the developing fetus. The precise mechanism by which the pregnant woman communicates her psychological state of stress or adversity to her fetus and influences birth outcome, however, is less clear. As discussed here fetal exposure to stress hormones alone is not the mechanism of communication. We did not discuss other possible pathways, such as vascular or immunological, or even other endocrine systems, but these are areas that deserve further study.

One new area of research that we only briefly acknowledged was sex differences in birth and developmental outcomes. We have reported that (i) female fetuses displayed more mature responses than males at 31 and 36 gestational weeks (Buss et al., 2009a), (ii) delayed neuromotor development associated with fetal exposure to cortisol early in gestation and CRH late in gestation was confined to males (Ellman et al., 2008) and (iii) the reduction in brain volumes in children exposed to elevated PSA early in gestation primarily were observed in girls (Sandman et al., 2011a). These findings are consistent with findings of sex specific trajectories of fetal development and the sexually dimorphic risk of neurological impairment associated with neonatal complications (Kesler et al., 2008).

There is evidence that sexually specific patterns are formed very early in development and are reflected in the function and response to stress of the placenta. Clifton (2010) has argued that sexually dimorphic placental sensitivity to signals of adversity (elevated glucocorticoids) results in different patterns of response and in particular in different patterns of growth. Male fetuses, Clifton suggests, do not alter their patterns of development in response to adversity and continue to grow despite reduced resources. Because the male fetus has not adjusted to the initial adversity and has not conserved its resources, it is more susceptible to later stress with increases in morbidity and mortality. In contrast, the female placenta responds or adjusts to an adverse maternal environment in multiple ways resulting in reduced growth. If exposed to stress that reduces nutrients and resources later in gestation, the female fetus has conserved its energy needs which increases the probability of survival. By this mechanism, sexually specific patterns of response to stress may be determined very early in fetal development.

7. Future perspectives

Despite the fact that this area of research is in its embryonic stage, the findings have created a paradigm shift. It is now essential to consider fetal experience (or exposure) and birth outcomes in order to fully understand human development. There are several areas of research that must continue to evolve. First, a more comprehensive understanding of the fetal experience is critical. This review focused on stress-related exposures and primarily endocrine and psychological markers. However there is growing interest in vascular and immune exposures that exert both independent and additive influences on fetal health and developmental outcomes. It is important that the field of fetal neurology/psychology explores the mechanisms of communication of stress and adversity between the host (mother) and the fetus. The precise mechanisms of communication are largely unknown and in some cases the most plausible candidates have been ruled out. New results from our studies indicate that fetuses receive neurodevelopmental benefit from longer gestation even after 37 weeks (Davis et al., 2011a). Neurodevelopment was evaluated with structural magnetic resonance imaging in 100 healthy right-handed 6- to 10-year-old children born between 28 and 41 gestational weeks with a stable neonatal course. We found that longer duration of gestation was associated with region-specific increases in gray matter brain density. Further, the benefit of longer gestation for brain development was present even in children born after 37 weeks. The significant linear association between gestational age at birth and brain development in young children challenges the commonly held assumption of a "non-linear" developmental course that defines fetal maturity as occurring at 37 gestational weeks. Our findings emphasize that there is a benefit for the developing brain of increased gestational length throughout the course of fetal development. In addition to providing new information about the importance of longer gestation beyond 37 gestational weeks for brain development, this finding has implications for medical decisions involving assisted deliveries. The decision about when to deliver a fetus, especially after 37 weeks, rarely involves concerns about the fetal nervous system. The findings reported here suggest that the neurological maturity of the fetus should enter the decision algorithm because even modest increases in gestational length have significant and long-lasting influences on the structure and function of the nervous system.

8. Acknowledgments

The research reported here was supported by awards from the National Institutes of Health: NS-41298, HD-51852 and HD-28413 to CAS, HD-50662 and HD-65823 to EPD and HD-40967 to LMG. The assistance of Cheryl Crippen, Megan Blair, Christina Canino, Natalie Hernandez, Kendra Leak and Christine Cordova is gratefully acknowledged. The authors are especially grateful to the families who participated in these studies.

9. References

Abernethy, L. J., Palaniappan, M., & Cooke, R. W. (2002). Quantitative magnetic resonance imaging of the brain in survivors of very low birth weight. *Arch Dis Child Fetal Neonatal Ed, 87*(4), 279-283.

Adams, M. M., & Barfield, W. D. (2008). The future of very preterm infants: learning from the past. *Jama, 299*(12), 1477-1478.

Akana, S. F., Chu, A., Soriano, L., & Dallman, M. F. (2001). Corticosterone exerts site-specific and state-dependent effects in prefrontal cortex and amygdala on regulation of adrenocorticotropic hormone, insulin and fat depots. *J Neuroendocrinol, 13*(7), 625-637.

Avishai-Eliner, S., Brunson, K. L., Sandman, C. A., & Baram, T. Z. (2002). Stressed-out, or in (utero)? *Trends Neurosci, 25*(10), 518-524.

Bagley, J., & Moghaddam, B. (1997). Temporal dynamics of glutamate efflux in the prefrontal cortex and in the hippocampus following repeated stress: effects of pretreatment with saline or diazepam. *Neuroscience, 77*, 65-73.

Barker, D. J., Osmond, C., Simmonds, S. J., & Wield, G. A. (1993). The relation of small head circumference and thinness at birth to death from cardiovascular disease in adult life. *BMJ, 306*(6875), 422-426.

Barker, D. J. P. (1998). *Mothers, babies and health in later life*. Edinburgh: Churchill Livingston.

Beauchamp, M. H., Thompson, D. K., Howard, K., Doyle, L. W., Egan, G. F., Inder, T. E., & Anderson, P. J. (2008). Preterm infant hippocampal volumes correlate with later working memory deficits. *Brain, 131*(Pt 11), 2986-2994.

Beckwith, B. E., Sandman, C. A., Hothersall, D., & Kastin, A. J. (1977). Influence of neonatal injections of alpha-MSH on learning, memory and attention in rats. *Physiol Behav, 18*(1), 63-71.

Beydoun, H., & Saftlas, A. F. (2008). Physical and mental health outcomes of prenatal maternal stress in human and animal studies: a review of recent evidence. *Paediatr Perinat Epidemiol, 22*(5), 438-466.

Blair, M., Glynn, L. M., Sandman, C. A., & Davis, E. P. (in press). Prenatal maternal anxiety and early childhood temperament. *Stress.*

Boorse, G. C., & Denver, R. J. (2002). Acceleration of Ambystoma tigrinum metamorphosis by corticotropin-releasing hormone. *Journal of Experimental Zoology, 293*(1), 94-98.

Braastad, B. O. (1998). Effects of prenatal stress on behaviour of offspring in laboratory and farmed animals. *Applied Animal Behaviour Science, 61*, 159-180.

Brunson, K. L., Grigoriadis, D. E., Lorang, M. T., & Baram, T. Z. (2002). Corticotropin-releasing hormone (CRH) downregulates the function of its receptor (CRF1) and induces CRF1 expression in hippocampal and cortical regions of the immature rat brain. *Exp Neurol, 176*(1), 75-86.

Buss, C., Davis, E. P., Class, Q. A., Gierczak, M., Pattillo, C., Glynn, L. M., & Sandman, C. A. (2009a). Maturation of the human fetal startle response: evidence for sex-specific maturation of the human fetus. *Early Human Development, 85*(10), 633-638.

Buss, C., Davis, E. P., Muftuler, L. T., Head, K., & Sandman, C. A. (2010). High pregnancy anxiety during mid-gestation is associated with decreased gray matter density in 6-9-year-old children. *Psychoneuroendocrinology, 35*(1), 141-153.

Buss, C., Entringer, S., Reyes, J. F., Chicz-DeMet, A., Sandman, C. A., Waffarn, F., & Wadhwa, P. D. (2009b). The maternal cortisol awakening response in human pregnancy is associated with the length of gestation. *Am J Obstet Gynecol, 201*(4), 398 e391-398.

Buss, C., Entringer, S., Reyes, J. F., Chicz-Demet, A., Sandman, C. A., Waffarn, F., & Wadhwa, P. D. (2009c). The maternal cortisol awakening response in human pregnancy is associated with the length of gestation. *Am J Obstet Gynecol.*

Buss, C., Lord, C., Wadiwalla, M., Hellhammer, D. H., Lupien, S. J., Meaney, M. J., & Pruessner, J. C. (2007). Maternal care modeulates the relationship between prenatal risk and hippocampal volume in women but not in men. *Journal of Neuroscience, 27*(10), 2592-2595.

Campbell, E. A., Linton, E. A., Wolfe, C. D., Scraggs, P. R., Jones, M. T., & Lowry, P. J. (1987). Plasma corticotropin-releasing hormone concentrations during pregnancy and parturition. *J Clin Endocrinol Metab, 64*(5), 1054-1059.

Campos, B., Schetter, C. D., Abdou, C. M., Hobel, C. J., Glynn, L. M., & Sandman, C. A. (2008). Familialism, social support, and stress: positive implications for pregnant Latinas. *Cultur Divers Ethnic Minor Psychol, 14*(2), 155-162.

Catlin, A. (2006). Extremely long hospitalizations of newborns in the United States: data, descriptions, dilemmas. *J Perinatol, 26*(12), 742-748.
Challis, J. R. (1994). Characteristics of parturition. In R. K. r. Creasy, R. (Ed.), *Maternal Fetal Medicine: Principles and Practice* (3rd ed.).
Champney, T. F., Sahley, T. L., & Sandman, C. A. (1976). Effects of neonatal cerebral ventricular injection of ACTH 4-9 and subsequent adult injections on learning in male and female albino rats. *Pharmacol Biochem Behav, 5*(Suppl 1), 3-9.
Chan, E. C., Smith, R., Lewin, T., Brinsmead, M. W., Zhang, H. P., Cubis, J., Thornton, K., & Hurt, D. (1993). Plasma corticotropin-releasing hormone, beta-endorphin and cortisol inter-relationships during human pregnancy. *Acta Endocrinol (Copenh), 128*(4), 339-344.
Cheng, Y. H., Nicholson, R. C., King, B., Chan, E. C., Fitter, J. T., & Smith, R. (2000). Glucocorticoid stimulation of corticotropin-releasing hormone gene expression requires a cyclic adenosine 3',5'-monophosphate regulatory element in human primary placental cytotrophoblast cells. *J Clin Endocrinol Metab, 85*(5), 1937-1945.
Chrousos, G. P. (1992). Regulation and dysregulation of the hypothalamic-pituitary-adrenal axis. The corticotropin-releasing hormone perspective. *Endocrinol Metab Clin North Am, 21*(4), 833-858.
Class, Q. A., Buss, C., Davis, E. P., Gierczak, M., Pattillo, C., Chicz-DeMet, A., & Sandman, C. A. (2008). Low levels of corticotropin-releasing hormone during early pregnancy are associated with precocious maturation of the human fetus. *Developmental Neuroscience, 30*(6), 419-426.
Clifton, V. L. (2010). Review: Sex and the human placenta: mediating differential strategies of fetal growth and survival. *Placenta, 31 Supplement 1*, S33-39.
Coe, C. L., Kramer, M., Czeh, B., Gould, E., Reeves, A. J., Kirschbaum, C., & Fuchs, E. (2003). Prenatal stress diminishes neurogenesis in the dentate gyrus of juvenile rhesus monkeys. *Biological Psychiatry, 54*, 1025-1034.
Cohen, S., Kamarck, T., & Mermelstein, R. (1983). A global measure of perceived stress. *Journal of Health and Social Behavior, 24*, 385-396.
Davis, E. P. (2007). *Prenatal exposure to maternal stress hormones influences human infant development*. Paper presented at the International Society for Developmental Psychobiology.
Davis, E. P., Buss, C., Muftuler, L. T., Head, K., Hasso, A., Wing, D. A., Hobel, C., & Sandman, C. A. (2011a). Children's Brain Development Benefits from Longer Gestation. *Front Psychol, 2*, 1.
Davis, E. P., Glynn, L. M., Dunkel Schetter, C., Hobel, C., Chicz-De Met, A., & Sandman, C. A. (2005). Maternal plasma corticotropin-releasing hormone levels during pregnancy are associated with infant temperament. *Developmental Neuroscience, 27*(5), 299-305.
Davis, E. P., Glynn, L. M., Dunkel Schetter, C., Hobel, C., Chicz-DeMet, A., & Sandman, C., A. (2007). Prenatal exposure to maternal depression and cortisol influences infant temperament. *Journal of the American Academy of Child and Adolescent Psychiatry, 46*(6), 737-746.
Davis, E. P., Glynn, L. M., Waffarn, F., & Sandman, C. A. (2011b). Prenatal maternal stress programs infant stress regulation. *J Child Psychol Psychiatry, 52*(2), 119-129.

Davis, E. P., & Sandman, C. A. (2010). The timing of prenatal exposure to maternal cortisol and psychosocial stress is associated with human infant cognitive development. *Child Development, 81*(1), 131–148.

Davis, E. P., Snidman, N., Wadhwa, P. D., Dunkel Schetter, C., Glynn, L., & Sandman, C. A. (2004). Prenatal maternal anxiety and depression predict negative behavioral reactivity in infancy. *Infancy, 6*(3), 319-331.

Davis, E. P., Waffarn, F., & Sandman, C. A. (2011c). Prenatal treatment with glucocorticoids sensitizes the hpa axis response to stress among full-term infants. *Dev Psychobiol, 53*(2), 175-183.

de Weerth, C., & Buitelaar, J. K. (2005). Physiological stress reactivity in human pregnancy - a review. *Neuroscience and Biobehavioral Reviews, 29*, 295-312.

Denver, R. J. (1997). Environmental stress as a developmental cue: corticotropin-releasing hormone is a proximate mediator of adaptive phenotypic plasticity in amphibian metamorphosis. *Hormones and Behavior, 31*(2), 169-179.

Denver, R. J. (1999). Evolution of the corticotropin-releasing hormone signaling system and its role in stress-induced phenotypic plasticity. *Annals of the New York Academy of Sciences, 897*, 46-53.

Diorio, D., Viau, V., & Meaney, M. J. (1993). The role of the medial prefrontal cortex (cingulate gyrus) in the regulation of hypothalamic-pituitary-adrenal responses to stress. *J Neurosci, 13*(9), 3839-3847.

Dominguez, T. P., Dunkel-Schetter, C., Glynn, L. M., Hobel, C., & Sandman, C. A. (2008). Racial differences in birth outcomes: the role of general, pregnancy, and racism stress. *Health Psychol, 27*(2), 194-203.

Dominquez, T. P., Dunkel-Schetter, C., Glynn, L. M., Hobel, C. J., & Sandman, C. A. (2008). Racial differences in birth outcomes: the role of general, pregnancy, and racism stress. *Health Psychology, 27*, 194-203.

Dunkel Schetter, C., & Glynn, L. M. (2011). Stress in pregnancy: empirical evidence and theoretical issues to guide interdisciplinary research. In R. J. Contrada & A. Baum (Eds.), *The handbook of stress science: biology, psychology and health*. New York: Springer Publishing Company.

Ellman, L. M., Dunkel-Schetter, C., Hobel, C. J., Chicz-DeMet, A., Glynn, L. M., & Sandman, C. A. (2008). Timing of fetal exposure to stress hormones: Effects on newborn physical and neuromuscular maturation. *Developmental Psychobiology, 50*, 232-241.

Emanuel, R. L., Robinson, B. G., Seely, E. W., Graves, S. W., Kohane, I., Saltzman, D., Barbieri, R., & Majzoub, J. A. (1994). Corticotrophin releasing hormone levels in human plasma and amniotic fluid during gestation. *Clin Endocrinol (Oxf), 40*(2), 257-262.

Escobar, G. J., Littenberg, B., & Petitti, D. B. (1991). Outcome among surviving very low birthweight infants: a meta-analysis. *Arch Dis Child, 66*(2), 204-211.

Feldman, S., & Conforti, N. (1985). Modifications of adrenocortical responses following frontal cortex stimulation in rats with hypothalamic differentiations and medial forebrain bundle lesions. *Neuroscience, 15*, 1045-1047.

Frim, D. M., Emanuel, R. L., Robinson, B. G., Smas, C. M., Adler, G. K., & Majzoub, J. A. (1988). Characterization and gestational regulation of corticotropin-releasing hormone messenger RNA in human placenta. *J Clin Invest, 82*(1), 287-292.

Giannopoulos, G., Jackson, K., & Tulchinsky, D. (1982). Glucocorticoid metabolism in human placenta, decidua, myometrium and fetal membranes. *J Steroid Biochem, 17*(4), 371-374.

Gibbs, R. S., Romero, R., Hillier, S. L., Eschenbach, D. A., & Sweet, R. L. (1992). A review of premature birth and subclinical infection. *Am J Obstet Gynecol, 166*(5), 1515-1528.

Giles, W. B., McLean, M., Davies, J. J., & Smith, R. (1996). Abnormal umbilical artery doppler waveforms and cord blood corticotropin-releasing hormone. *Obstet and Gynecol, 87*, 107-111.

Glynn, L. M. (2010). Implications of maternal programming for fetal neurodevelopment. In A. Zimmerman & S. Connors (Eds.), *Maternal influences on fetal neurodevelopment* (pp. 33-54). New Jersey: Springer Science+Business Media, LLC.

Glynn, L. M. (2011). Perceived discrimination predicts prenatal stress hormone trajectories among pregnant latina women. *Annals of Behavioral Medicine, 41*, s56.

Glynn, L. M., & Sandman, C. A. (in press). Prenatal origins of neurological development: a critical period for fetus and mother. *Current Directions in Psychological Science.*

Glynn, L. M., Schetter, C. D., Chicz-DeMet, A., Hobel, C. J., & Sandman, C. A. (2007). Ethnic differences in adrenocorticotropic hormone, cortisol and corticotropin-releasing hormone during pregnancy. *Peptides, 28*(6), 1155-1161.

Glynn, L. M., Schetter, C. D., Hobel, C. J., & Sandman, C. A. (2008). Pattern of perceived stress and anxiety in pregnancy predicts preterm birth. *Health Psychology, 27*(1), 43-51.

Glynn, L. M., Schetter, C. D., Wadhwa, P. D., & Sandman, C. A. (2004). Pregnancy affects appraisal of negative life events. *Journal of Psychosomatic Research, 56*(1), 47-52.

Glynn, L. M., Wadhwa, P. D., Dunkel-Schetter, C., Chicz-Demet, A., & Sandman, C. A. (2001). When stress happens matters: effects of earthquake timing on stress responsivity in pregnancy. *American Journal of Obstetrics & Gynecology, 184*(4), 637-642.

Goland, R. S., Conwell, I. M., Warren, W. B., & Wardlaw, S. L. (1992). Placental corticotropin-releasing hormone and pituitary-adrenal function during pregnancy. *Neuroendocrinology, 56*(5), 742-749.

Goldenberg, R. L., Hauth, J. C., & Andrews, W. W. (2000). Mechanisms of disease: intrauterine infection and preterm delivery. *New England Journal of Medicine, 342*, 1500-1507.

Gur, C., Orna Diav-Citrin, O., Shechtman, S., Arnon, J., & Ornoy, A. (2004). Pregnancy outcome after first trimester exposure to corticosteroids: a prospective controlled study. *Reproductive Toxicology, 18*, 93-101.

Herman, J. P., Cullinan, W. E., Morano, M. I., Akil, H., & Watson, S. J. (1995). Contribution of the ventral subiculum to inhibitory regulation of the hypothalamo-pituitary-adrenocortical axis. *J Neuroendocrinol, 7*(6), 475-482.

Herman, J. P., Dolgas, C. M., & Carlson, S. L. (1998). Ventral subiculum regulates hypothalamo-pituitary-adrenocortical and behavioural responses to cognitive stressors. *Neuroscience, 86*(2), 449-459.

Herman, J. P., Schafer, M. K., Young, E. A., Thompson, R., Douglass, J., Akil, H., & Watson, S. J. (1989). Evidence for hippocampal regulation of neuroendocrine neurons of the hypothalamo-pituitary-adrenocortical axis. *J Neurosci, 9*(9), 3072-3082.

Hilmert, C. J., Schetter, C. D., Dominguez, T. P., Abdou, C., Hobel, C. J., Glynn, L., & Sandman, C. (2008). Stress and blood pressure during pregnancy: racial differences and associations with birthweight. *Psychosom Med, 70*(1), 57-64.

Ho, J. T., Lewis, J. G., & O'loughlin, P. (2007). Reduced maternal corticosteroid-binding globulin and cortisol levels in pre-eclampsia and gamete recipient pregnancies. *Clin Endocrinol (Oxf), 66*(6), 869-877.

Hobel, C. J., Dunkel-Schetter, C., Roesch, S. C., Castro, L. C., & Arora, C. P. (1999). Maternal plasma corticotropin-releasing hormone associated with stress at 20 weeks gestation in pregnancies ending in preterm delivery. *American Journal of Obstetrics and Gynecology, 180*(1 Pt 3), 257-263.

Holzman, C., Jetton, J., Siler-Khodr, T., Fisher, R., & Rip, T. (2001). Second trimester corticotropin-releasing hormone levels in relation to preterm delivery and ethnicity. *Obstetrics and Gynecology, 97*, 657-663.

Huizink, A. C., Mulder, E. J., Robles de Medina, P. G., Visser, G. H., & Buitelaar, J. K. (2004). Is pregnancy anxiety a distinctive syndrome? *Early Human Development, 79*, 81-91.

Insel, T. R., Kinsley, C. H., Mann, P. E., & Bridges, R. S. (1990). Prenatal stress has long-term effects on brain opiate receptors. *Brain Res, 511*(1), 93-97.

Institute of Medicine (2006). *Preterm birth: Causes, consequences, and prevention.* Washington, D.C.: National Academies Press.

John-Adler, H. B., & Morin, P. J. (1990). Effects of larval density on jumping ability and stamina in newly metamorphosed Bufo-Woodhousi-fowleri. *Copeia*, 856-860.

Kagan, J., Snidman, N., & Arcus, D. (1998). Childhood derivatives of high and low reactivity in infancy. *Child Development, 69*(6), 1483-1493.

Kesler, S. R., Reiss, A. L., Vohr, B., Watson, C., Schneider, K. C., Katz, K. H., Maller-Kesselman, J., Silbereis, J., Constable, R. T., Makuch, R. W., & Ment, L. R. (2008). Brain volume reductions within multiple cognitive systems in male preterm children at age twelve. *Journal of Pediatrics, 152*(4), 513-520, 520 e511.

King, B. R., Smith, R., & Nicholson, R. C. (2002). Novel glucocorticoid and cAMP interactions on the CRH gene promoter. *Mol Cell Endocrinol, 194*(1-2), 19-28.

Knigge, K. M., & Hays, M. (1963). Evidence of Inhibitive Role of Hippocampus in Neural Regulation of Acth Release. *Proc Soc Exp Biol Med, 114*, 67-69.

Korebrits, C., Yu, D. H., Ramirez, M. M., Marinoni, E., Bocking, A. D., & Challis, J. R. (1998). Antenatal glucocorticoid administration increases corticotrophin-releasing hormone in maternal plasma. *British Journal of Obstetrics and Gynecology, 105*(5), 556-561.

Kramer, M. R., & Hogue, C. R. (2009). What causes racial disparities in very preterm birth? A biosocial perspective. *Epidemiol Rev, 31*, 84-98.

Kramer, M. S. (2009). Late preterm birth: appreciable risks, rising incidence. *J Pediatr, 154*(2), 159-160.

Kramer, M. S., Lydon, J., Seguin, L., Goulet, L., Kahn, S. R., McNamara, H., Genest, J., Dassa, C., Chen, M. F., Sharma, S., Meaney, M. J., Thomson, S., Van Uum, S., Koren, G., Dahhou, M., Lamoureux, J., & Platt, R. W. (2009). Stress pathways to spontaneous preterm birth: the role of stressors, psychological distress, and stress hormones. *Am J Epidemiol, 169*(11), 1319-1326.

Kuban, K. C., & Leviton, A. (1994). Cerebral palsy. *N Engl J Med, 330*(3), 188-195.

Lazarus, R. S. (1966). *Psychological Stress and the Coping Process.* New York: McGraw-Hill.

Lazarus, R. S. (1968). Emotions and adaptation: conceptual and empirical relations *Nebraska Symposium on Motivation*. Lincoln: University of Nebraska Press.

Lazarus, R. S., & Folkman, S. (1984). *Stress, Appraisal, and Coping*. New York: Springer Publishing Company, Inc.

Lederman, S. A., Rauh, V., Weiss, L., Stein, J. L., Hoepner, L. A., Becker, M., & Perera, F. P. (2004). The effects of the World Trade Center event on birth outcomes among term deliveries at three lower Manhatten hospitals. *Environmental Health Perspectives, 112*, 1772-1778.

Lindsay, J. R., & Nieman, L. K. (2005). The hypothalamic-pituitary-adrenal axis in pregnancy: challenges in disease detection and treatment. *Endocr Rev, 26*(6), 775-799.

Linton, E. A., Perkins, A. V., Woods, R. J., Eben, F., Wolfe, C. D., Behan, D. P., Potter, E., Vale, W. W., & Lowry, P. J. (1993). Corticotropin releasing hormone-binding protein (CRH-BP): plasma levels decrease during the third trimester of normal human pregnancy. *J Clin Endocrinol Metab, 76*(1), 260-262.

Lobel, M., Cannella, D. L., Graham, J. E., DeVincent, C., Schneider, J., & Meyer, B. A. (2008). Pregnancy-specific stress, prenatal health behaviors, and birth outcomes. *Health Psychology, 27*, 604-615.

Lowry, P. J. (1993). Corticotropin-releasing factor and its binding protein in human plasma. *Ciba Found Symp, 172*, 108-115; discussion 115-128.

Ma, X. H., Wu, W. X., & Nathanielsz, P. W. (2003). Gestation-related and betamethasone-induced changes in 11beta-hydroxysteroid dehydrogenase types 1 and 2 in the baboon placenta. *Am J Obstet Gynecol, 188*(1), 13-21.

March of Dimes (2009). *White paper on preterm birth: the global and regional toll*. White Plains, N.Y.: March of Dimes Foundation.

Makrigiannakis, A., Semmler, M., Briese, V., Eckerle, H., Minas, V., Mylonas, I., Friese, K., & Jeschke, U. (2007). Maternal serum corticotropin-releasing hormone and ACTH levels as predictive markers of premature labor. *Int J Gynaecol Obstet, 97*(2), 115-119.

Marinoni, E., Korebrits, C., Di Lorio, R., Cosmi, E. V., & Challis, J. R. (1998). Effect of betamethasone in vivo on placental corticotropin-releasing hormone in human pregnancy. *American Journal of Obstetrics and Gynecology, 178*(4), 770-778.

Markovic, D., Vatish, M., Gu, M., Slater, D., Newton, R., Lehnert, H., & Grammatopoulos, D. K. (2007). The onset of labor alters corticotropin-releasing hormone type 1 receptor variant expression in human myometrium: putative role of interleukin-1beta. *Endocrinology, 148*(7), 3205-3213.

McCormack, V. A., Dos Santos Silva, I., De Stavola, B. L., Mohsen, R., Leon, D. A., & Lithell, H. O. (2003). Fetal growth and subsequent risk of breast cancer: Results from long term follow up of Swedish cohort. *British Medical Journal, 326*(7383), 248.

McLean, M., Bisits, A., Davies, J., Woods, R., Lowry, P., & Smith, R. (1995). A placental clock controlling the length of human pregnancy. *Nature Medicine, 1*, 460-463.

McLean, M., & Smith, R. (2001). Corticotrophin-releasing hormone and human parturition. *Reproduction, 121*(4), 493-501.

Meaney, M. J., Diorio, J., Francis, D., Widdowson, J., LaPlante, P., Caldji, C., Sharma, S., Seckl, J. R., & Plotsky, P. M. (1996). Early environmental regulation of forebrain glucocorticoid receptor gene expression: implications for adrenocortical responses to stress. *Dev Neurosci, 18*(1-2), 49-72.

Moghaddam, B. (1993). Stress preferentially increases extraneuronal levels of excitatory amino acids in the prefrontal cortex: Comparison to hippocampus and basal ganglia. *Journal of Neurochemistry, 60*(1650-1657).

Moldow, R. L., Kastin, A. J., Hollander, C. S., Coy, D. H., & Sandman, C. A. (1981). Brain beta-endorphin-like immunoreactivity in adult rats given beta-endorphin neonatally. *Brain Res Bull, 7*(6), 683-686.

Murphy, V. E., & Clifton, V. L. (2003). Alterations in human placental 11beta-hydroxysteroid dehydrogenase type 1 and 2 with gestational age and labour. *Placenta, 24*(7), 739-744.

Murphy, V. E., Smith, R., Giles, W. B., & Clifton, V. L. (2006). Endocrine regulation of human fetal growth: The role of the mother, placenta, and fetus. *Endocrine Reviews, 27*(2), 141-169.

Murros, K., Fogelholm, R., Kettunen, S., & Vurela, A. L. (1993). Serum cortisol and outcome of ischemic brain infarctions. *Journal of the Neurological Sciences, 116*, 12-17.

Nathanielsz, P. W. (1995). The role of basic science in preventing low birth weight. *Future Child, 5*(1), 57-70.

Nettles, K. W., Pesold, C., & Goldman, M. B. (2000). Influence of the ventral hippocampal formation on plasma vasopressin, hypothalamic-pituitary-adrenal axis, and behavioral responses to novel acoustic stress. *Brain Res, 858*(1), 181-190.

Neumann, I. D., Wigger, A., Liebsch, G., Holsboer, F., & Landgraf, R. (1998). Increased basal activity of the hypothalamo-pituitary-adrenal axis during pregnancy in rats bred for high anxiety-related behaviour. *Psychoneuroendocrinology, 23*(5), 449-463.

Newman, R. A. (1989). Developmental plasticity of Scaphiopus coouchii tadpoles in an unpredictable environment. *Ecology, 70*, 1775-1787.

Nosarti, C., Al-Asady, M. H., Frangou, S., Stewart, A. L., Rifkin, L., & Murray, R. M. (2002). Adolescents who were born very preterm have decreased brain volumes. *Brain, 125*(Pt 7), 1616-1623.

Novy, M. J., McGregor, J. A., & Iams, J. D. (1995). New perspectives on the prevention of extreme prematurity. *Clin Obstet Gynecol, 38*(4), 790-808.

Orth, D. N., & Mount, C. D. (1987). Specific high-affinity binding protein for human corticotropin-releasing hormone in normal human plasma. *Biochem Biophys Res Commun, 143*(2), 411-417.

Peterson, B. S., Vohr, B., Staib, L. H., Cannistraci, C. J., Dolberg, A., Schneider, K. C., Katz, K. H., Westerveld, M., Sparrow, S., Anderson, A. W., Duncan, C. C., Makuch, R. W., Gore, J. C., & Ment, L. R. (2000). Regional brain volume abnormalities and long-term cognitive outcome in preterm infants. *Journal of the American Medical Association, 284*(15), 1939-1947.

Petraglia, F., Florio, P., Nappi, C., & Genazzani, A. R. (1996). Peptide signaling in human placenta and membranes: autocrine, paracrine, and endocrine mechanisms. *Endocr Rev, 17*(2), 156-186.

Petraglia, F., Potter, E., Cameron, V. A., Sutton, S., Behan, D. P., Woods, R. J., Sawchenko, P. E., Lowry, P. J., & Vale, W. (1993). Corticotropin-releasing factor-binding protein is produced by human placenta and intrauterine tissues. *J Clin Endocrinol Metab, 77*(4), 919-924.

Petraglia, F., Sawchenko, P. E., Rivier, J., & Vale, W. (1987). Evidence for local stimulation of ACTH secretion by corticotropin-releasing factor in human placenta. *Nature, 328*(6132), 717-719.

Petraglia, F., Sutton, S., & Vale, W. (1989). Neurotransmitters and peptides modulate the release of immunoreactive corticotropin-releasing factor from cultured human placental cells. *Am J Obstet Gynecol, 160*(1), 247-251.

Petraglia, F., Volpe, A., Genazzani, A. R., Rivier, J., Sawchenko, P. E., & Vale, W. (1990). Neuroendocrinology of the human placenta. *Frontiers in Neuroendocrinology, 11*, 6-37.

Pfeifer, M., Goldsmith, H. H., Davidson, R. J., & Rickman, M. (2002). Continuity and change in inhibited and uninhibited children. *Child Dev, 73*(5), 1474-1485.

Poland, R. E., Cloak, C., Lutchmansingh, P. J., McCracken, J. T., Chang, L., & Ernst, T. (1999). Brain N-acetyl aspartate concentrations measured by H MRS are reduced in adult male rats subjected to perinatal stress: preliminary observations and hypothetical implications for neurodevelopmental disorders. *J Psychiatr Res, 33*(1), 41-51.

Richards, M., Hardy, R., Kuh, D., & Wadsworth, M. E. (2001). Birth weight and cognitive function in the British 1946 birth cohort: longitudinal population based study. *British Medical Journal, 322*, 199-203.

Rini, C. K., Dunkel-Schetter, C., Wadhwa, P. D., & Sandman, C. A. (1999). Psychological adaptation and birth outcomes: the role of personal resources, stress, and sociocultural context in pregnancy. *Health Psychology, 18*(4), 333-345.

Roseboom, T., van der Meulen, J., Osmond, C., Barker, D., Ravelli, A., Schroeder-Tanka, J., van Montfrans, G., Michels, R., & Bleker, O. (2000). Coronary heart disease after prenatal exposure to the Dutch famine, 1944-45. *Heart, 84*(6), 595-598.

Sanchez, M. D., Milanes, M. V., Fuente, T., & Laorden, M. L. (1993). The beta-endorphin response to prenatal stress during postnatal development in the rat. *Brain Res Dev Brain Res, 74*(1), 142-145.

Sandman, C., A., Glynn, L., Wadhwa, P. D., Chicz-DeMet, A., Porto, M., & Garite, T. (2003). Maternal hypothalamic-pituitary-adrenal disregulation during the third trimester influences human fetal responses. *Developmental Neuroscience, 25*, 41-49.

Sandman, C. A., & Davis, E. P. (2010). Gestational stress influences cognition and behavior. *Future Neurology, 5*(5), 675-690.

Sandman, C. A., Davis, E. P., Buss, C., & Glynn, L. M. (2011a). Exposure to Prenatal Psychobiological Stress Exerts Programming Influences on the Mother and Her Fetus. *Neuroendocrinology.*

Sandman, C. A., Davis, E. P., Buss, C., & Glynn, L. M. (2011b). Prenatal programming of human neurological function. *International Journal of Peptides, 2011*, 1-9.

Sandman, C. A., Glynn, L., Schetter, C. D., Wadhwa, P., Garite, T., Chicz-DeMet, A., & Hobel, C. (2006). Elevated maternal cortisol early in pregnancy predicts third trimester levels of placental corticotropin releasing hormone (CRH): priming the placental clock. *Peptides, 27*(6), 1457-1463.

Sandman, C. A., & Kastin, A. J. (1981). Intraventricular administration of MSH induces hyperalgesia in rats. *Peptides, 2*(2), 231-233.

Sandman, C. A., & O'Halloran, J. P. (1986). Pro-opiomelanocortin, learning, memory and attention. In D. DeWied, W. H. Gispen & T. B. van Wimersma Greidanus (Eds.), *Encyclopedia on Pharmacology and Therapeutics* (pp. 397-420): Pergamon Press.

Sandman, C. A., Wadhwa, P., Glynn, L., Chicz-Demet, A., Porto, M., & Garite, T. J. (1999a). Corticotrophin-releasing hormone and fetal responses in human pregnancy. *Ann N Y Acad Sci, 897*, 66-75.

Sandman, C. A., Wadhwa, P. D., Chicz-DeMet, A., Dunkel-Schetter, C., & Porto, M. (1997). Maternal stress, HPA activity, and fetal/infant outcome. *Annals of the New York Academy of Sciences, 814*, 266-275.

Sandman, C. A., Wadhwa, P. D., Chicz-DeMet, A., Porto, M., & Garite, T. J. (1999b). Maternal corticotropin-releasing hormone and habituation in the human fetus. *Developmental Psychobiology, 34*(3), 163-173.

Sandman, C. A., & Yessaian, N. (1986). Persisting subsensitivity of the striatal dopamine system after fetal exposure to beta-endorphin. *Life Sci, 39*(19), 1755-1763.

Sasaki, A., Shinkawa, O., Margioris, A. N., Liotta, A. S., Sato, S., Murakami, O., Go, M., Shimizu, Y., Hanew, K., & Yoshinaga, K. (1987). Immunoreactive corticotropin-releasing hormone in human plasma during pregnancy, labor, and delivery. *J Clin Endocrinol Metab, 64*(2), 224-229.

Sasaki, A., Tempst, P., Liotta, A. S., Margioris, A. N., Hood, L. E., Kent, S. B., Sato, S., Shinkawa, O., Yoshinaga, K., & Krieger, D. T. (1988). Isolation and characterization of a corticotropin-releasing hormone-like peptide from human placenta. *J Clin Endocrinol Metab, 67*(4), 768-773.

Savitz, D. A., & Pastore, L. M. (1999). Causes of prematurity *Prenatal Care: Effectiveness and Implementation* (pp. 63-104). Cambridge: Cambridge University Press.

Schulkin, J. (1999). Corticotropin-releasing hormone signals adversity in both the placenta and the brain: regulation by glucocorticoids and allostatic overload. *J Endocrinol, 161*(3), 349-356.

Schwartz, C. E., Snidman, N., & Kagan, J. (1999). Adolescent social anxiety as an outcome of inhibited temperament in childhood. *Journal of the American Academy of Child and Adolescent Psychiatry, 38*(8), 1008-1015.

Seasholtz, A. F., Valverde, R. A., & Denver, R. J. (2002). Corticotropin-releasing hormone-binding protein: biochemistry and function from fishes to mammals. *J Endocrinol, 175*(1), 89-97.

Selye, H. (1936). A syndrome produced by diverse nocuous agents. *Nature, 138*, 32.

Selye, H. (1955). Stress and disease. *Science, 122*(3171), 625-631.

Selye, H. (1956). *The Stress of Life*. New York: McGraw-Hill.

Selye, H. (1959). Perspectives in stress research. *Perspect Biol Med, 2*(4), 403-416.

Shimizu, E., Kodama, K., Sakamoto, T., Komatsu, N., Yamanouchi, N., Okada, S., & Sato, T. (1997). Recovery from neuroendocrinological abnormalities and frontal hypoperfusion after remission in a case with rapid cycling bipolar disorder. *Psychol Clin Neurosci, 51*, 207-212.

Sibai, B., Meis, P. J., Klebanoff, M., Dombrowski, M. P., Weiner, S. J., Moawad, A. H., Northen, A., Iams, J. D., Varner, M. W., Caritis, S. N., O'Sullivan, M. J., Miodovnik, M., Leveno, K. J., Conway, D., Wapner, R. J., Carpenter, M., Mercer, B., Ramin, S. M., Thorp, J. M., Jr., Peaceman, A. M., & Gabbe, S. (2005). Plasma CRH measurement at 16 to 20 weeks' gestation does not predict preterm delivery in women at high-risk for preterm delivery. *Am J Obstet Gynecol, 193*(3 Pt 2), 1181-1186.

Smith, D. C. (1987). Adult recruitment in chorus frogs: Effects of size and date at metamorphosis. *Ecology, 68*, 344-350.

Smith, R., Mesiano, S., Chan, E. C., Brown, S., & Jaffe, R. B. (1998). Corticotropin-releasing hormone directly and preferentially stimulates dehydroepiandrosterone sulfate secretion by human fetal adrenal cortical cells. *J Clin Endocrinol Metab, 83*(8), 2916-2920.

Smith, R., Mesiano, S., & McGrath, S. (2002). Hormone trajectories leading to human birth. *Regul Pept, 108*(2-3), 159-164.

Smith, R., & Nicholson, R. C. (2007). Corticotrophin releasing hormone and the timing of birth. *Front Biosci, 12*, 912-918.

Smith, R., Smith, J. I., Shen, X., Engel, P. J., Bowman, M. E., McGrath, S. A., Bisits, A. M., McElduff, P., Giles, W. B., & Smith, D. W. (2009). Patterns of plasma corticotropin-releasing hormone, progesterone, estradiol, and estriol change and the onset of human labor. *J Clin Endocrinol Metab, 94*(6), 2066-2074.

Sun, K., Adamson, S. L., Yang, K., & Challis, J. R. (1999). Interconversion of cortisol and cortisone by 11beta-hydroxysteroid dehydrogenases type 1 and 2 in the perfused human placenta. *Placenta, 20*(1), 13-19.

Tyson, E. K., Smith, R., & Read, M. (2009). Evidence that corticotropin-releasing hormone modulates myometrial contractility during human pregnancy. *Endocrinology, 150*(12), 5617-5625.

Vale, W., Spiess, J., Rivier, C., & Rivier, J. (1981). Characterization of a 41-residue ovine hypothalamic peptide that stimulates secretion of corticotropin and beta-endorphin. *Science, 213*(4514), 1394-1397.

Ventura, S. J., Martin, J. A., Curtin, S. C., Mathews, T. J., & Park, M. M. (2000). Births: final data for 1998. *Natl Vital Stat Rep, 48*(3), 1-100.

Wadhwa, P. D., Garite, T. J., Porto, M., Glynn, L., Chicz-DeMet, A., Dunkel-Schetter, C., & Sandman, C. A. (2004). Placental corticotropin-releasing hormone (CRH), spontaneous preterm birth, and fetal growth restriction: a prospective investigation. *Am J Obstet Gynecol, 191*(4), 1063-1069.

Wadhwa, P. D., Porto, M., Garite, T. J., Chicz-DeMet, A., & Sandman, C. A. (1998). Maternal corticotropin-releasing hormone levels in the early third trimester predict length of gestation in human pregnancy. *Am J Obstet Gynecol, 179*(4), 1079-1085.

Wadhwa, P. D., Sandman, C. A., Porto, M., Dunkel Schetter, C., & Garite, T. J. (1993). The association between prenatal stress and infant birth weight and gestational age at birth: A prospective investigation. *American Journal of Obstetrics and Gynecology, 169*, 858-865.

Warren, W. B., Patrick, S. L., & Goland, R. S. (1992). Elevated maternal plasma corticotropin-releasing hormone levels in pregnancies complicated by preterm labor. *Am J Obstet Gynecol, 166*(4), 1198-1204; discussion 1204-1197.

Weinstock, M. (1996). Does prenatal stress impair coping and regulation of the hypothalamic-pituitary-adrenal axis? *Neuroscience and Biobehavioral Reviews, 21*(1), 1-10.

Wolfe, C. D., Patel, S. P., Linton, E. A., Campbell, E. A., Anderson, J., Dornhorst, A., Lowry, P. J., & Jones, M. T. (1988). Plasma corticotrophin-releasing factor (CRF) in abnormal pregnancy. *Br J Obstet Gynaecol, 95*(10), 1003-1006.

Yang, R., You, X., Tang, X., Gao, L., & Ni, X. (2006). Corticotropin-releasing hormone inhibits progesterone production in cultured human placental trophoblasts. *J Mol Endocrinol, 37*(3), 533-540.

You, X., Yang, R., Tang, X., Gao, L., & Ni, X. (2006). Corticotropin-releasing hormone stimulates estrogen biosynthesis in cultured human placental trophoblasts. *Biol Reprod, 74*(6), 1067-1072.

Zambrana, R. E., Scrimshaw, S. C., Collins, N., & Dunkel-Schetter, C. (1997). Prenatal health behaviors and psychosocial risk factros in pregnant women of Mexican origin: the role of acculturation. *American Journal of Public Health, 87*, 1022-1026.

5

Oxidative Stress and Antioxidants: Preterm Birth and Preterm Infants

Robert A. Knuppel[1], Mohamed I. Hassan[1], James J. McDermott[2], J. Martin Tucker[3] and John C. Morrison[3]
[1]*Departments of Obstetrics and Gynecology and Newborn Medicine, DuBois Regional Medical Center, DuBois, PA,*
[2]*Glen Allen, VA,*
[3]*Department of OB/GYN, University of Mississippi Medical Center, Jackson, Mississippi, USA*

1. Introduction

1.1 General

It is agreed by all physicians that preterm labor is comprised of regular uterine contractions, usually <5 minutes apart, that results in cervical change occurring before the 37th week of pregnancy. (Elliott, 2011) Often times, preterm labor can be successfully treated with tocolytic drugs, but when such treatment results in early delivery particularly (<32 weeks) it is devastating for the family, the physician, and society in general. According to statistics in the United States preterm birth occurred in 12.6% of deliveries in 2007. (Goldenberg, 2008) Indeed, up to 75% of all perinatal mortality and half of the neurologic disadvantaged children can be traced to simply delivering before term. Adequate nutritional status of women before becoming pregnant, during the pregnancy, and after delivery, reduces adverse outcomes for both mother and baby. (Kontic & Vucinic, 2006) The absence of appropriate micronutrients lead to maternal complications such as preterm labor (PTL), iron deficiency anemia, preterm premature rupture of the membranes (PPROM), preeclampsia, intrauterine growth restriction (IUGR), as well as small for gestational (SGA) infants, and congenital malformations. (Scholl, 2008) Oxidative stress has been implicated in the development and pathogenesis of a number of diseases in neonates and especially those delivered prematurely. Newborns, and in particular preterm neonates, have less protection against and are very susceptible to free radical oxidative damage. (Saugstad, 2003)

Good nutrition is vital to the health of the mother and baby. Unfortunately, the typical American diet exceeds the recommended daily allowance of meat, grains, and fats by approximately 20% and is as much as 40-60% deficient in dairy, fruit, and vegetables. (Kaiser & Allen, 2002). Pregnancy involves rapidly dividing cells, not only in the fetus, newborn and placenta, but also in the maternal compartment (such as red cell mass and the growing uterus). Pregnancy is one state where there is almost certainly a need for additional antioxidants to combat this stress. (Kaiser & Allen, 2002) Oxidative stress during pregnancy yields free radicals and other oxidative molecules exceeding the available antioxidant buffering capacity in the mother and growing fetus. This results in cellular damage, which is associated not only with PTL and delivery, but also preeclampsia, PPROM and IUGR as well as several serious post delivery issues for the premature infant. (Joshi et al., 2008) If not buffered, the excess of free radicals attack the endothelial lining cells of blood vessels and many organ systems by acquiring electrons from nucleic acids, lipids, proteins and carbohydrates, thus denaturing DNA in these cells. (Burton & Jauniaux, 2010) Free radicals may affect normal placental growth and cause abortions or stillbirths, while at the same time resulting in a number of chromosomal abnormalities. (Stein et al., 2008) Oxidative stress can also cause preeclampsia by disrupting the body's vasodilatation signaling process, allowing maternal blood pressure to rise, and disrupting placental blood flow. (Buhimschi et al., 2003) Oxidative stress is also related to alterations in the genetic metabolic detoxification through the cytochrome P450 1A1 gene as well as others. (Agarwal et al., 2005) When these genes are over expressed in an environment of excess radicals PTL results, which can lead to early delivery. This chapter will highlight the conditions and diseases of the mother, fetus, placenta as well as the newborn and discuss studies how micronutrients supplementation may help restore balance to the oxidative pathways.

1.2 Oxidative stress

Oxidative stress occurs when the rate of free radical production exceeds the rate of removal (or buffering) by the cellular defense mechanisms. (Burton & Jauniaux, 2010) As mentioned previously, oxidative stress has been associated with PTL and early deliveries as well as preeclampsia, PPROM and IUGR as well as many conditions and diseases in the preterm infant. (Buhimschi et al., 2003; O'Donovan & Fernandes, 2004) As shown on Figure 1, the reactive oxygen and nitrogen species will cause cytotoxic damage to proteins, lipids or DNA, unless the enzymatic and nonenzymatic antioxidants are able to balance their adverse effects. Free radicals works in many ways, for example, iron-mediated formation of ROS leading to DNA and lipid damage appears to result from an exaggeration of the normal function of iron; which is to transport oxygen to tissues, resulting in iron-induced free radical damage to cellular DNA. Free radicals are released by macrophage and neutrophil activation associated with infection and inflammation. The free radicals of interest are frequently referred to as Reactive Oxygen Species (ROS) because the most biologically important free radicals are predominantly derived from oxygen (oxygen free radicals). (Saugstad, 1996) ROS is a collective concept that includes not only superoxide anion and hydroxyl radicals but also radicals such hydrogen peroxide, which is derived from molecular oxygen (Fig. 1). ROS may be generated by different mechanisms, such as the normal electron transport chain in mitochondria and fatty acids, prostaglandin metabolism, ischemia-reperfusion, hypoxia, hyperoxia, neutrophil and macrophage activation (inflammation), the endothelial cell hypoxanthine-xanthine oxidase system (adenosine triphosphate degradation), increased free circulating transition metals, and the Fenton reaction (ferrous to ferric iron). (Shoji & Koletzko, 2007) Reactive Nitrogen Species (RNS) also damage cellular DNA and also disrupt nitric oxide signaling which controls vasodilatation (Fig. 1) Both ROS and RNS are simply molecules that have been charged with extra electron and therefore are very unstable. (Agarwal et al., 2005)

As the placenta is growing, fetus and mother require increased blood flow as pregnancy progresses and damage to the endothelial cell lining of the blood vessel wall is particularly serious. For example, as shown in a cartoon (Figure 2a), blood vessels normally use nitric oxide (NO) signaling to initiate vasodilatation. There are circumferential muscle cells around the blood vessel wall that control additional blood flow by dilating the vessel itself. Figure 2b, notes that vasodilatation (by relaxing the muscle cells in the vessel wall) leads to increased blood flow needed for the growing uterus and fetus. (Edemann & Schiffrin, 2004) Excessive free radicals in the blood will disrupt the ability for the vasodilatation signaling process (Fig. 2a); thus, vasoconstriction occurs leading to diminished blood flow to the uterus and placenta, which can result in PTL, preeclampsia and/or IUGR. (Stein et al., 2008) Severe oxidative stress may trigger chromosomal abnormalities that may lead to fetal demise. Oxidative stress can also effect the process in reverse by decreasing the body's ability to detoxify oxygen radicals. (Blondi et al., 2005) For example, the Cytochrome P450 A1A gene (CYP1A1), Glutathione S-transferases μ1 (GST m1), and 01 (GSTT1) all can interfere with the detoxification process. The ROS can also trigger a cascade of fatty acids (such as arachidonic acid) which lead to preterm contractions, cervical dilatation and birth before 37 weeks as well as inciting vasoconstriction leading to preeclampsia and IUGR. (Joshi et al., 2008) The key treatment process is to balance the impact of free oxygen and nitrogen radicals by supplying antioxidants from the diet and/or by micronutrient supplementation.

2. Maternal/fetal antioxidant issues

As previously noted, pregnancy itself places a burden of excess and unstable radicals on maternal tissues as well as those of the developing fetus and placenta. The subsequent inability to vasodilate (or direct vasoconstriction) caused by these reactive species result in diminished blood flow and can lead to PTL, PPROM, preeclampsia, and primary IUGR (or secondary due to the preeclampsia). There have been many strategies to address this excess of oxidative radicals over the last 20 years, particularly supplementation of one or two micronutrients in the hopes of reducing these serious maternal/fetal disorders. Such therapy is directed at decreasing the numbers of reactive oxygen/nitrogen species by supplementing vitamins A, C or E in hopes of reducing vasoconstriction and/or organ damage. Clinically, the hypothesis is that if vasoconstriction is reduced there would be less early deliveries both from PTL and PPROM as well as from indicated deliveries due to preeclampsia and severe fetal growth restriction.

2.1 Preterm birth/preterm premature rupture of the membranes

Recently Kramer et al., (2009) illustrated the linkage between antioxidant vitamins and spontaneous preterm birth. In this case control study blood samples were taken from a large prospective multicenter cohort (n=5337) at 24-26 weeks' gestation. Aliquots were analyzed in women with spontaneous preterm birth (n-207), and compared with two term controls per case (n=443). They were analyzed for carotenoids, retinol and tocopherols as well as long chain fatty acids. The findings revealed that high plasma concentrations of alpha and beta-carotene as well as lycopene were all associated with reductions in spontaneous preterm birth with a positive dose response across all groups. In the United States the majority of dietary alpha-carotene and nearly 40% beta-carotene is supplied by carrots,

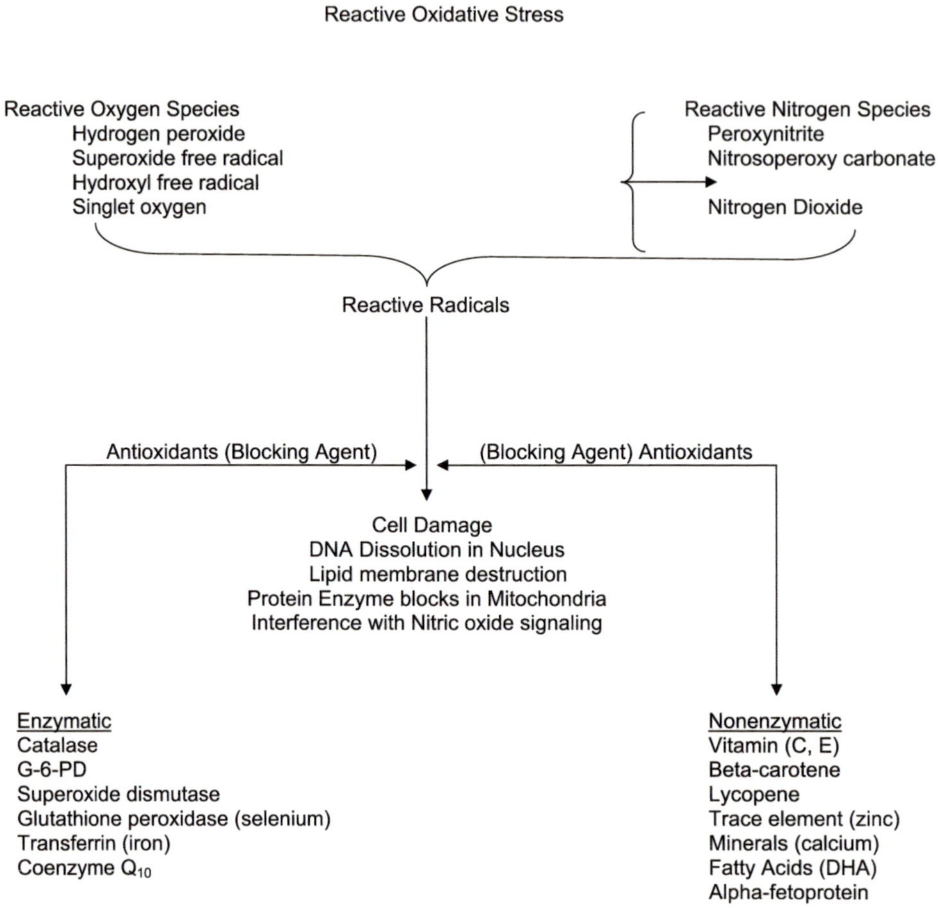

Fig. 1. Oxidative stress and various antioxidants.

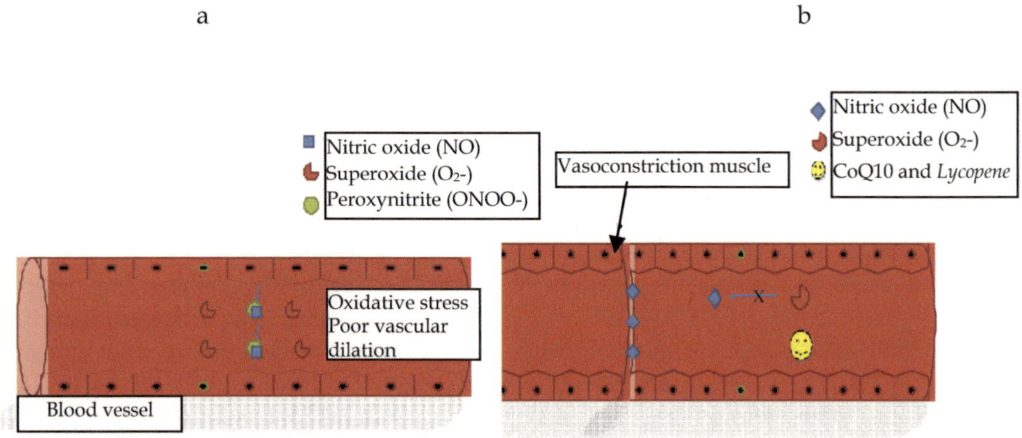

Fig. 2. A: Effect of free radicals on vascular endothelium; B: Effect of antioxidants blocking free radicals to allow normal vasodilation.

whereas almost all the lycopene (80%) is provided by tomato and tomato products; two sources low in the normal diet. (Clinton SK, 1998) Therefore, there appears to be a need for supplementation as many women studied in this and other investigations have low plasma levels of carotenoids and lycopene.

Lycopene is a cyclic carotenoid with 11 conjugated double bonds and is found in relative few foods; therefore, requires supplementation during pregnancy. (Clinton SK, 1998) It has long been known that low levels of this carotenoid has been associated with cancers of the digestive tract, cervix, breast, skin, bladder, prostate, as well as cardiovascular diseases. (Helzlsouer, 1989) The oxidative pathways connecting low lycopene to preterm birth and PPROM have not been fully studied, but have been linked by several investigators. (Luo et al., 2006; Masters et al., 2007) Lycopene has been linked to a decrease in preterm birth by Sharma et al., (2002) who entered 251 primagravida women in a prospective randomized control trial in the second trimester. One hundred sixteen women received lycopene (2mg twice daily) while 135 women received placebo (both until delivery). Gestational age as well as mean birth weight were significantly higher in the active treatment group. The results also showed that preeclampsia (8.6% versus 17.7%), as well as IUGR (12% versus 23.7%), were lower among lycopene treated patients. The high number of double bonds in the lycopene structure is hypothesized to be responsible for the very potent antioxidant effects noted in this study. Compared with other carotenoids such as vitamin C and E, lycopene appears to be a more potent antioxidant particularly with complications such as PTL, and PPROM.

2.2 Antioxidants and preeclampsia

As noted above, lycopene was shown by Sharma et al., (2002) to reduce the incidence of PTL and preeclampsia compared to placebo treated patients. Similarly, there appears to be new interest in coenzyme Q10 (CoQ10) which is a vitamin like 1, 4-benzoquinone that, like lycopene, has a very potent antioxidant action. CoQ10 is an essential component of oxidative phosphorylation at the mitochondrial level, which helps stabilize cell membranes by acting as an antioxidant. (Crane, 1997) CoQ10 plays a well known preventive role in cardiovascular disease, cancer, as well as muscular and mitochondrial disorders. (Langsjoen et al., 1994; Folker et al., 1997; Bresolin et al., 1988) In 2003, Teran EP et al., hypothesized, because of the antihypertensive effect of CoQ10, that it might be helpful in reducing maternal preeclampsia. Teran studied a small number of normal pregnant women, non-pregnant women, and pregnant women with preeclampsia. He found that plasma levels of CoQ10 were significantly higher in normal pregnant women in comparison to non-pregnant women. However, CoQ10 levels were noted to be even lower in women with preeclampsia compared to the non-pregnant state. Pregnant women with preeclampsia had approximately ½ of the levels of CoQ10 as compared to normal pregnant women. Teran's group hypothesized that coenzyme Q10 could help regulate nitric oxide vasodilation and possible lead to less preeclampsia as well as IUGR and thus indirectly lead to less preterm birth. More recently the same investigators (Teran et al., 2009) conducted a randomized control trial with 197 women of whom 47 developed preeclampsia. The treatment group took 100mg of CoQ10 twice per day versus placebo in control women. Of the 47 women who developed preeclampsia, 30 (25.6%) were in the control group compared to only 17 (14.4%) in the CoQ10 group ($p=0.03$, RR 0.56 CI 0.33-0.96). Again, larger babies and less

IUGR were noted amongst CoQ10 treated patients. The results indicated that CoQ10 protection of the essential components of mitochondrial complexes as well as its protective effect on vascular endothelium in the placenta might be responsible for these positive findings. Tiano et al., work (2007) also mirrors this conclusion.

More recently Boutet et al., (2009) supported the protective effect hypothesis by showing a rise in glutathione peroxidase (an antioxidant) in those given lycopene and CoQ_{10}. This was particularly true in preeclampsia and demonstrates that both the fetus and mother are affected during preeclampsia. They showed that glutathione peroxidase controls lipid peroxidation in cell membranes which is also a function of lycopene and CoQ_{10}. As shown on Figure 2b, the lycopene and CoQ_{10} also degrade superoxide, thus preventing depletion of nitric oxide in the blood. This allows successful vasodilatation particularly in the placenta as well as the maternal organs. In turn, this could clinically lead to a reduction in preterm birth due to PTL and/or preeclampsia. (Endermann & Schiffrin, 2004). IUGR and PPROM could also be reduced. Landmesser et al., (2000) also showed that CoQ_{10} increased levels of extracellular superoxide dismutase (SOD), a major antioxidant enzyme system of endothelial cells lining vessel walls, which scavenge oxygen radicals and allow endothelial dependent dilation to occur in the conduit arteries. In this randomized study (Landmesser et al., 2000), CoQ_{10} supplementation versus placebo, increased superoxide dismutase and led to relaxation of the arteries. In addition, VO_2 and O_2 pulse pressure was greater in placebo treated patients, rather than those receiving CoQ_{10}.

In summary, the dietary supplements CoQ_{10} and lycopene prevents a wide range of radicals from degrading nitric oxide and damaging various organs. With better balance the nitric oxide is able to signal vasodilatation where needed, such as an increase in uterine blood flow during pregnancy to establish the placenta. Clinically, this could lead to a decrease in preeclampsia, IUGR, PTL, and PPROM.

2.3 Vitamin C and E

CoQ10 and lycopene have demonstrated very positive effects relative to reducing and perhaps preventing preeclampsia. However, other known antioxidants such as vitamin C and E have not been proven to be effective in published studies. For example, Poston et al., (2006) performed a randomized placebo control trial involving 2410 patients at high risk for preeclampsia from 25 hospitals. They supplemented 1000mg vitamin C and 400 IU vitamin E versus placebo from the second trimester of pregnancy until delivery. They studied the incidence of low birth weight, small for gestational age infants, and preeclampsia. The incidence of small for gestational age infants and maternal preeclampsia were identical and paradoxically the numbers of low birth weight infants were higher in the treatment group than in the control group (28% vs. 24%). Similarly, Xu et al., (2010) studied the supplementation of the same vitamins in 27 centers vs. placebo amongst 2363 women. They found no reduction in preeclampsia, but surprisingly a small, non-significant increase, in the number of growth restricted babies and perinatal death. Current studies to address these conflicting results are underway.

2.4 Omega-3 fatty acids (Docosahexaenoic Acid-DHA)

The supplementation of various omega-3 fatty acids, which have been shown to have a positive effect on the development of the fetal central nervous system and retina, has also been correlated with a greater gestational age at birth. (Gallagher, 2004) There are over 20 fatty acids, but only the omega-3 and omega-6 polyunsaturated fatty acids cannot be manufactured by the body; thus they must be accumulated by the fetus from placental transport. (Bell 1997) The omega-3 fatty acids are essentially derived from linolenic acid and they produce eicosanoids which have anti-inflammatory and immunosuppressant properties. In contrast, omega-6 fatty acids promote inflammation and blood clotting (Adam et al., 2003). In large amounts omega-6 fatty acids lead to production of arachidonic acid (prostaglandins), which stimulate the preterm labor cascade, weaken fetal membranes and reduce placental blood flow. Unfortunately, in the typical United States diet there is a ratio of 20:1 of omega-6 versus omega-3, when the ratio should be between 1:1 and 4:1. A recent review by Greenberg et al., (2008) offers a nice description of how to meet omega-3 fatty acid needs during pregnancy. Basically, these methods involve increasing the amount of fish in the diet (two servings per week), which results in omega-3 fatty acid levels of 100-250mg per day of DHA.

It has been shown the intake of fresh fish increases birth weight by prolonging gestation. (Olsen et al., 1995) The same investigators showed that fish oil supplementation had the same affect (Olsen, 2000). In one study, five Australian maternity hospitals enrolled 2399 women <21 weeks' of gestation to determine if taking fish oil in the latter half of pregnancy reduced maternal depressive symptoms and improved developmental outcomes in the offspring. (Makrides, 2010) While there was no reduction of postpartum depression symptoms, the treated patients had a lower incidence of both preterm birth and low birth weight infants, which resulted in fewer admissions to the neonatal intensive care unit and a 67% reduction in infant death. (Makrides, 2009) In an accompanying editorial, Oken & Belfort, (2009), suggest supplementing 100-200mg of DHA in addition to diet, which seems to be appropriate. Unfortunately, one need only remember as a child, taking cod liver oil, to know that fish oil supplementation is accompanied by halitosis, gastric upset, and in some cases nausea and vomiting, thus limiting patient compliance. As previously mentioned, most women normally do not consume enough fresh fish to meet the daily requirement and therefore, DHA supplementation is important.

More palatable supplementations are available to increase DHA in the diet. Omega-3 fatty acids have been found in algeal sources which are equivalent to the DHA levels found in fresh fish. (Arterburn et al., 2007; Arterburn, 2008) Indeed these algeal supplements containing DHA have been found to raise the plasma erythrocyte omega-3 fatty acid levels. (Otto, 2000) More recently Hawthorne et al., (2007) revealed that supplementation of this form of DHA in orange juice significantly improved the plasma phospholipid levels in children. (Hawthorne, 2007) Similarly, Smuts, (2003) revealed that supplementation of algeal DHA in eggs resulted in an extension of gestational age in the treated groups in a randomized clinical study. In summary, supplementation of omega-3 polyunsaturated fatty acids, particularly (DHA) is important for the developing fetus and newborn. Since fresh fish is not a staple of most American diets, algeal supplementation in the form of prenatal vitamins, containing DHA is important. Both the March of Dimes and The American College of Obstetricians and Gynecologist concur; recommending 100-200mg supplementation of DHA. Since DHA supplementation as well as other antioxidants, may be contained in prenatal vitamins a comparison of common micronutrient supplements is available are listed on Table 1.

	RDA (FNB 2009)	PreQue 10	OB complete 400	PreNexa[3]	Prenate DHA[4]	Vitafol OB+DHA[5]	Citranata l Assure[6]	Gesticare DHA[7]	OB Complete One[8]	Prenate Essentia[9]	Citranatal Harmony[10]	Prefera OB One[11]	Neevo DHA[12]	Concept DHA[13]
Administration	---	2 tablets once daily or 1 tablet twice daily	Once daily	Once daily	Once daily	2 pills once daily	2 pills once daily	2 pills once daily	Once daily	Once daily	Once daily	Once daily	Once daily	Once daily
Antioxidants														
CoQ10 (co-enzyme Q-10)	0	100 mg	0	0	0	0	0	0	0	0	0	0	0	0
Lycopene	0	10 mg	0	0	0	0	0	0	0	0	0	0	0	0
Vitamins														
Vitamin A (Beta-Carotene)	0.75-0.77 mg	2500 IU	0	0	0	2700 IU	0	0	0	0	0	0	0	0
Vitamin B_1 (Thiamine Monoitrate)	1.4 mg	2 mg	2 mg	0	0	1.6 mg	3 mg	3 mg	2 mg	0	0	0	0	2 mg
Vitamin B_2 (Riboflavin)	1.4 mg	3.4 mg	3.4 mg	0	0	1.8 mg	3.4 mg	3 mg	4 mg	0	0	0	0	3 mg
Vitamin B_6 (Pyridoxine HCl)	1.9 mg	0	25 mg	25 mg	25 mg	2.5 mg	25 mg	50 mg	30 mg	25 mg	25 mg	50 mg	25 mg	25 mg
Vitamin B_{12} (Cyanocobalamin)	26 mcg	2 mcg	26 mcg	0	12 mcg	12 mcg	0	8 mcg	50 mcg	12 mcg	0	12 mcg	50 mcg	12.5 mcg
Folate/fFolic aAcid	0.6 mg	1 mg	1.2 mg	1.2 mg	1.0 mg	1.0 mg	1.0 mg	1.0 mg	1.0 mg	1.0 mg	1.0 mg	1.0 mg	1.0 mg	1.0
Vitamin D_3 (Cholecalciferol)	200 IU	240 IU	800 IU	170 IU	200 IU	400 IU	400 IU	410 IU	1200 IU	200 IU	400 IU	400 IU	400 IU	0
Vitamin C	80-85 mg	60 mg	100 mg (as ascorbic acid with calcium ascorbate and calcium theonate)	25 mg	85 mg	70 mg	120 mg	120 mg	70 mg	85 mg	0	25 mg	40 mg	25 mg
Vitamin E (d-alpha tocopherol)	22.35 IU	30 IU	30 IU (as Hypersorb vitamin E)	30 IU	10 IU	30 IU	30 IU	30 IU	30 IU	10 IU	30 IU	10 IU	30 IU	0
Niacin (Niacinamide)	18 mg	0	10 mg	0	0	18 mg	20 mg	20 mg	10 mg	0	0	17 mg	0	1.8 mg

Minerals														
Copper	1 mg	2 mg	1 mg	0	0	2 mg	2 mg	0	1 mg	0	0	0	0	2 mg
Zinc (Zinc Oxide)	11-12 mg	25 mg	25 mg	0	0	25 mg	25 mg	15 mg	15 mg	0	0	15 mg	0	10 mg
Iron	27 mg	30 mg	40 mg (as Ferronyl and Ferrochel)	30 mg	27 mg	65 mg	35 mg	27 mg	40 mg (ferronyl) 10 mg Sumalate (elemental iron)	28 mg (ferrous fumarate)	27 mg (carbonyl iron)	22 mg Polysaccharide Iron Complex 6 mg as HIP (heme iron polypeptide)	27 mg (ferrous fumarate)	17.5 mg (ferrous fumarate) 17.5 mg Polysaccharide Iron Complex
Calcium	1000-1300 mg	0	0	160 mg	140 mg	100 mg	125 mg	200 mg	25 mg (DimaCal) & 25 mg calcium carbonate	140 mg	100 mg	0	75 mg	0
Magnesium (Magnesium Oxide)	350-400 mg	20 mg	0	0	45 mg	25 mg	0	0	25 mg	45 mg	0	0	0	5 mg
Selenium (as Sodium Selenate)	0	15 mcg	0	0	0	0	0	0	0	0	0	0	0	0
Purified Fish Oil														
Docosahexaenoic Acid (DHA)	NA	100 mg	≥320 mg	265 mg	300 mg	250 mg	300 mg	250 mg	300 mg	300 mg	250 mg	200mg	250 mg	156 mg
Other Omegas									≥40 mg	40 mg				
Other Micronutrients														
Iodine (Potassium Iodide)	0.22 mg	0	0	0	0	0	150 mcg	150 mcg	150 mcg	150 mcg	0	175 mcg	0	0
Choline (Choline Bitartrate)	450 mg	0	0	0	0	0	0	55 mg	0		0	0	0	0

Table 1. Prenatal micronutrient supplements.

3. Oxidative stress in preterm infants

As shown on Fig. 1, antioxidant defenses include the enzymes superoxide dismutase, catalase, and glutathione. Antioxidants cross the placenta, and include vitamins A, C, E, and CoQ_{10} as well as lycopene and DHA. Premature infants are at particular risk from oxidative stress because both endogenous and passively acquired exogenous antioxidant defense systems do not accelerate in maturation until late in the third trimester. (Finer & Leone, 2009; Baba & McGrath, 2008) Oxidative stress is a contributing factor for tissue injury through formation of free radicals and reactive oxygen/nitrogen species leading to inflammatory cytokines which result in premature birth. (Pressman, 2011) The evidence is growing that oxidative stress is the final common endpoint for a complex of events that either are genetically determined or are triggered by an in utero stressor. The newborn infant, especially those delivered prematurely, is very susceptible to free radical-induced oxidative damage. First, the premature infant is frequently exposed to oxygen therapy and hyperoxia which is richer in oxygen than the intrauterine environment exposing the infant to an excess of free radicals. (Maulik et al., 1999) Second, the antioxidant defense mechanism and its ability to be induced by hyperoxia is relatively impaired in preterm infants. (Speer & Silverman, 1998) Third, the preterm infant has an increased susceptibility to infection and inflammation, which increases oxidative stress. (Saugstad, 1988) Finally, free iron is found in the plasma and tissue of premature infants to a greater extent than in the term infants. Oxidative stress is likely a contributing factor in the development and severity of several newborn conditions to the extent that Saugstad (1988, 2005) has suggested the phrase "oxygen radical disease of neonatology". The idea suggests that oxidative stress affects a variety of organs, often simultaneously, causing neonatal diseases such as bronchopulmonary dysplasia (BPD), retinopathy of prematurity (ROP), necrotizing enterocolitis (NEC), intraventricular hemorrhage (IVH), and periventricular leukomalacia (PVL). (Clyman, 1989; Archer et al., 1989; Sanderud, 1993)

3.1 Free radicals, reactive oxygen species, reactive nitrogen species and antioxidant defense

Preterm infants are at risk of unique immaturity-related neonatal diseases and a common factor in the pathogenesis of such diseases is the free radical tissue injury from oxidative stress. (Pressman, 2001) Free radicals may be generated by exposure of preterm infants to high oxygen concentrations during resuscitation and mechanical ventilation as well as by hyperoxia during the reperfusion phase of a hypoxic-ischemic brain insult, primarily in the presence of high concentrations of non-protein bound iron. (Saugstad, 1996) Small amounts of free radicals are generated continuously in living organisms and are important for normal cell reactions and cell growth. Under normal circumstances, there is a critical balance between pro-oxidant and antioxidant forces. Normally, the body's antioxidant defenses will handle free radicals, which are produced. On the other side, excessive production of ROS enhances many diseases associated with deficient antioxidant defenses and produces tissue injury in preterm infants. Many lifesaving procedures in the neonatal intensive care units may produce ROS an possible tissue damage due to the newborn's poorly developed antioxidant systems. The preterm infants are frequently exposed to excessive oxidative stress generated by the high oxygen concentrations used in neonatal resuscitation or mechanical ventilation, by inflammation and infection, and by parenteral nutrition.

As shown on Fig. 1, the antioxidant defense mechanisms are both enzymatic and nonenzymatic. (Shoji & Koletzko, 2007; Thibeault, 2000)

3.2 Enzymatic antioxidant defenses

Antioxidant enzyme activities have been shown to increase in response to oxidative stresses (Fig. 1). Antioxidant enzymes participate in a complex interaction of reducing and oxidizing molecules that defines the cellular milieu necessary for maintaining cellular, placental, fetal, and postnatal growth. (Dennery, 2004) Such enzymes have low activity in preterm infants and cannot balance excessive ROS production. The most important antioxidant enzymes are copper-zinc superoxide dismutases (SOD), which are found in cytoplasm as well as peroxisomes, and manganese SOD from mitochondria. SOD catalyzes the dismutation of superoxide anion to H2O2. Glutathione peroxidase (GPx) in mitochondria and catalase (CAT) in peroxisomes catalyze the reaction of H2O2 to molecular oxygen and water. These enzymes, together with vitamin E, play an important role in the peroxidation of polyunsaturated free fatty acids in cell membranes. (Thibeault, 2000)
In extremely low birth weight (<1500gms) infants, structural immaturity and surfactant deficiency necessitate mechanical ventilation and oxygen administration, both of which contribute to an inflammatory response. Oxidative stress in preterm infants is expressed by lower (reduced) and higher (oxidized) glutathione concentrations in plasma of preterm infants compared with term infants and lower glutathione levels in tracheal aspirates of preterm infants developing BPD. (Smith et al., 1993; Grigg et al., 1993) Glutathione peroxidase is important for removal of intracellular hydrogen peroxide and lipid peroxides, and glutathione is a direct scavenger of oxidants both intracellularly and extracellularly. Its role in lung protection is suggested by the high concentrations of glutathione in the lining fluid of lower airways and alveoli, with a transient postnatal decrease in preterm infants. (Jain et al., 1995) Many trials have incorporated enzymes in the process of prevention of tissue damage by oxygen in preterm neonates to prevent chronic lung disease. The challenge is how to introduce them into the cells or maintain them in the circulation when administered systemically. Effective therapy must be directed to the target organ and to a specific ROS or RNS. (Jankov et al., 2001; Thibeault, 2000)

3.3 Non-enzymatic antioxidant defenses

Other pathways to resist oxidative stress include the non-enzymatic pathways (Fig. 1). Nutrients such selenium, copper, and zinc may have antioxidant functions as components of antioxidant enzymes. Vitamins A, E, and C, ceruloplasmin, transferrin, glutathione (GSH), and bilirubin are considered to have antioxidant properties. Prematurity places the preterm infants at risk of ROS-induced injury because of relatively deficient uteroplacental transfer of these nutrients important to antioxidant defense. (Shah MD & Shah SR, 2009) Selenium is involved in many selenoenzymes, with GPx being the most important. Plasma selenium concentrations and Glutathione peroxidase (GPx) activity are associated with the birth weight of infants. (Trindade, 2007) Although selenium deficiency may participate in preterm diseases, the data is not sufficient to support this concept. (Darlow & Austin, 2003) The role of vitamin A likely is mediated through its action on retinol-binding protein and the retinoic acid receptor, rather than direct antioxidant effects. Serum levels of vitamin A have consistently been shown to be reduced in preterm infants. (Darlow & Graham, 2007) Vitamin C (ascorbic acid) concentrations rise in placenta and fetal liver with increasing

gestational age. A number of recent studies have suggested that supplementation with vitamin C or E may prevent teratogenic effects of maternal diabetes, but have not been consistently found to provide other measurable benefits. (Dheen et al., 2009)
Ceruloplasmin, transferrin and ferroxidase participate in the metabolism of iron, which acts as a potent oxidizing agent, so diminished function or bioavailability would be expected to increase susceptibility to oxidative stress. ROS production is enhanced by the presence of free iron. (Brion et al., 2003) Reductions in the concentrations of these non-enzymatic antioxidants may predispose the preterm infant to difficulties with increased production of ROS. Reduced transferrin and ceruloplasmin concentrations have been observed in asphyxiated preterm infants prior to the development of periventricular-intraventricular brain hemorrhage. (Lindeman et al., 2000) Glutathione depletion or inadequate synthesis has been proposed to explain developmental susceptibility of the preterm newborn to oxidative stress. Low levels in the broncho-alveolar fluid predicts the later development of BPD in intubated premature newborns. (Grigg et al., 1993) In vitro bilirubin has been demonstrated as a potent antioxidant scavenger of peroxyl radicals. In the oxidative process, bilirubin reverts to its precursor biliverdin, a nontoxic product. A direct relationship between the total antioxidant status of the newborn plasma and bilirubin concentrations was found in both preterm and term infants. (Wiedemann et al., 2003)

4. Free radical excess and neonatal organ damage

4.1 Neonatal brain injury

Brain injury in neonate can be precipitated by different mechanisms including hypoxia, hyperoxia, ischemia-reperfusion, and infection with the consequent release of oxygen free radicals and inflammatory mediators (cytokines) by activated neutrophils and macrophages. Immature brains are particularly vulnerable to oxidative stress due to poor antioxidant capabilities, high concentration of free iron and increases in unsaturated fatty acids. (Dugan & Choi, 1994) Furthermore, the inadequate scavenging ability of the immature nervous system, characterized by lower SOD and GPx activity, contributes to the accumulation of H2O2 and subsequent neurotoxicity. As H2O2 accumulates, it is exposed to free iron, resulting in generation of OH, a potent cytotoxic free radical. During brain reperfusion in a preterm infant, overload with ionic iron due to low concentrations of iron-oxidizing and iron-binding proteins may induce iron-catalyzed lipid peroxidation of the cerebral endothelial cells, resulting in vascular injury and intraventricular hemorrhage (IVH). (Lackmann et al., 1996)
The process of hypoxic-ischemic brain injury begins with the insult and extends for several hours into the recovery period (reperfusion phase of injury). With an increase in brain oxygenation in the reperfusion phase, superoxide and hydroxyl radicals are formed. (Volpe, 2001) Free radicals alter Na/K ATPase activity in cortical synaptosomal membranes, resulting in glutamate release, membrane injury, and cell death resulting in edema and seizures after 18-24 hours. (Perlman, 2006) Neonatal hypoxia can also upregulate the expression of nitric oxide (NO) synthases in the cerebral cortex, causing increased production of NO which functions as a free radical and also can trigger several neuronal cell death mechanisms, including NMDA receptor and neuronal nuclear membrane modification and transcription of apoptotic genes. (Mishra et al., 2006) Recent studies indicate that inflammatory mediators also contribute to hypoxic-ischemic brain injury, and although hypoxia-ischemia is recognized as a cause of neonatal brain injury, cytokine

mediated maternal-fetal infection (sepsis or fetal inflammatory response syndrome) also plays an important role in the pathogenesis of fetal/neonatal brain damage including early periventricular leukomalacia (PVL). (Mishra et al., 2006; Hitti et al., 2001)

There are several neuroprotective interventions and experimental models aiming at ameliorating brain injury. However, few of these interventions have been confirmed as sufficiently safe for clinical use. Further studies are necessary, but current approaches that appear safe and effective include free radical inhibitors, free radical scavengers, and mild cerebral hypothermia; the latter being the most promising. The neonatal mortality rates in extremely low birth weight infants have been reduced, but with increasing survival rate, the risk of prenatal and neonatal brain damage has not been eliminated and may be increased. (Louis et al., 2004; Marlow et al., 2005) The dilemma of determining the timing in which the potential damaging factor for the brain has occurred is a challenge for all the perinatal and neonatal specialists. In the past, acquired brain damage was mainly attributed to birth trauma, birth asphyxia, and other pathologies occurring around birth. (ACOG/AAP, 2003) With the advances in neonatal brain neuroimaging, especially MRI and MRS, cord blood nucleated red blood cells, and biomarkers for oxidative stress, it has become possible to determine a time window of the brain damage. Regarding the neonatal brain imaging, cranial ultrasound (US) has been used for many years to determine the type, extent, and evolution of brain lesions like hypoxic-ischemic encephalopathy as cerebral edema is almost always seen during the first day of life (12-18-24hrs. after birth). However, the higher sensitivity of MRI has made this study superior to cranial US in detecting early brain damage. Besides hypoxic-ischemic encephalopathy, brain MRI can also detect other lesions such as cortical-subcortical damage, diffuse cortical lesions, bilateral parasagittal lesions, brain stem lesions, cerebellar and hippocampal lesions. Brain MRI can also provide information on brain development changes such as myelination of white matter, glial cell migration and early PVL. (Childs et al., 2001) Diffusion-based MRI can provide the earliest indicators of brain damage and can be used in detecting the antenatal, perinatal, or postnatal timing of hypoxic insult. The MRI has also been used to detect fetal brain damage. (Girard et al., 2003) Nucleated red blood cell (NRBC) count indicates fetal hypoxia in both term and preterm infants. Correlations between NRBC count and cord blood pH with brain damage have been demonstrated. (ACOG/APP, 2003) For cases of intrapartum HIE cord pH is almost always <7.0. (ACOG/AAP, 2003) Also, correlations between high NRBC counts and poor neurological outcomes have been demonstrated. (Buonocore et al., 1999) Although the exact time elapsing between hypoxia and appearance of NRBC is not known, there is evidence that a period of more than 24 hours is necessary between the onset of fetal hypoxia and appearance of NRBC in blood. (Buonocore et al., 1999)

The role of oxidative stress in brain injury after fetal hypoxia has been extensively studied and demonstrated. During hypoxia, free radicals production increases with a possible decreased antioxidant defense which leads to mitochondrial dysfunction, inhibition of protein synthesis, enhanced mechanisms of apoptosis, and increased oxidative stress. (Delivoria & Misbra, 1998) Oxidative stress during fetal and neonatal hypoxia can therefore be assayed in cord blood as a marker of severe prenatal hypoxia/asphyxia. Assessment of oxidative stress is currently made by measuring advanced glycation end products from oxidation of proteins, carbohydrates, and lipids in cytoplasm, nucleus, and membranes. (Yamamoto et al., 2002) In conclusion, in addition to information provided by the obstetricians, neonatologists can have other tools of determining whether brain damage has occurred in the prenatal, intrapartum, or postnatal period, however, each tool has its limitations.

4.2 Retinopathy of prematurity: (ROP)

Retinopathy of prematurity which is a disease limited almost exclusively to premature infants. It is characterized by abnormal vascularization of the retina, causing a range of vision impairment, and remains a major cause of morbidity for premature neonates. The discovery of the relationship between hyperoxia and the development of ROP represented a breaking point in modern neonatology. (Ashton & Cook, 1954; Campbell, 1951; Patz et al., 1952) The fetus in utero is exposed to arterial oxygen pressure of 22–24 mm Hg. After delivery, the premature infant may be exposed to a relative hyperoxia that may downregulate vascular endothelial growth factor (VEGF) production leading to vaso-obliteration of existing vessels and arrest of the vascularization. As ROP has been related to hyperoxia, reactive oxygen stress may be involved in this disease. (Shweiki et al., 1992)
As the retina develops anterior to the arrested vascularization area, there will be increased oxygen demand, which creates localized physiological hypoxia which will increase the expression of the VEGF in response to hypoxia. With maturation, the non-vascularized retina becomes increasingly metabolically active and consequently hypoxic. Hypoxia leads to more VEGF, which induces neo-vascularization of the retina, which in severe cases may result in retinal fibrosis and retinal detachment. (Darlow & Graham, 2002; Penn et al., 1994; Smith et al., 1999) Present therapy for severe ROP is mainly based on laser retinal ablation of the avascular retina. This therapy reduces the incidence of blindness by 25%. (Good, 2004) A number of antioxidants and nutrients have been or may be tested. Vitamins A and C supplementation do not seem to reduce the rate of severe ROP. (Darlow et al., 2005; Lakatos et al., 1986) D-penicillamine, however, is a powerful antioxidant and vasomodulator and there are some promising data which strongly indicate that this drug may reduce the severity of ROP.

4.3 Chronic lung disease/bronchopulmonary dysplasia: (CLD/BPD)

The development of chronic lung disease in infancy remains a significant health problem, particularly in the premature infant. Hyperoxia is an important factor in the development of bronchopulmonary dysplasia and is associated with growth arrest and impaired alveolar septal development in the neonatal lung. (Jobe, 1999) The etiology of CLD is unknown, but many investigators have suggested that free radicals play a key role in its development. The pathogenesis of chronic lung disease/BPD is multi-factorial, and many pre- and postnatal risk factors have been identified, such as chorioamnionitis, systemic infection, inadequate resuscitation, high-inspired oxygen concentrations, barotrauma, volutrauma, and mechanical ventilation. These factor all can injure tissue through oxygen toxicity and pro-inflammatory mediators acting on immature airways and pulmonary tissue. (Saugstad, 1998)
Chemokines (interleukin [IL]-8) and other pro-inflammatory cytokines such as IL-1, IL-6, and tumor necrosis factor-alpha are produced by alveolar macrophages, airway epithelial cells, fibroblasts, type II pneumocytes, and endothelial cells of preterm infants. Activated neutrophils and macrophages release potent proteases together with many enzymes. However, free oxygen radicals inactivate the protease inhibitors (alpha-1-proteinase inhibitor), leading to an imbalance between protease and antiprotease inhibitor,

contributing to damage and excretion of elastic fiber degradation products. Oxidative stress increases both metalloproteins and their inhibitors, causing disruption of the extracellular matrix and contributing to pulmonary fibrosis. (Speer, 2004, 2006) The main source of free radicals in the lungs seems to be phagocyte activation. The increase in phagocyte number and interleukin concentrations in the broncoalveolar fluid obtained from premature infants with CLD indicates that oxygen toxicity and inflammation are involved in the development of lung injury. (Delacourt et al., 1996; Groneck et al., 1993; Pittet et al., 1997)

Several important factors contribute to augmented oxidative stress in the newborn and especially the preterm infant. First, because of immaturity, the lung of preterm infants is frequently exposed to oxygen therapy and hyperoxia. Second, the antioxidant defense and its ability to be induced during a hyperoxic challenge are impaired. Third, the preterm infant has an increased susceptibility to infection and inflammation, which increases oxidative stress. Fourth, free iron, which catalyzes the production of free oxygen radicals, can be detected in preterm infants. (Asikainen & White, 2004; Welty, 2001; Welty & Smith, 2001) Antioxidant nutrients, including inositol, glutamine, cysteine, and methionine, as well as vitamins and some trace elements have been thought to play a role in protection of lung parenchyma. (Binivale & Ehrenkranz, 2006) A trial of parenteral inositol for preterm infants who had respiratory distress showed that inositol supplementation was associated with increased survival and a lower incidence of BPD. Interventions to prevent lung oxidative injury in preterm infants require more basic clinical studies to solve the intricate oxidative mechanisms in the molecular processes and address the use of specific or groups of antioxidants. (Hallman et al., 1992)

4.4 Necrotizing enterocolitis: (NEC)

Oxidative stress is caused by an imbalance between the production of ROS and the ability to detoxify them with the help of antioxidants. The premature infant is especially susceptible to ROS-induced damage because of inadequate antioxidant stores at birth, as well as impaired up-regulation in response to oxidant stress. Several etiologic factors have been identified in the pathogenesis of NEC: immaturity, hypoxia/ischemia, hyperosmolar feedings, and bacterial colonization as well as oxidative stress. (Hsueh et al., 2002) The preterm infants are more vulnerable to NEC by an interaction of local defense, enteral feeding, bacterial colonization, inflammatory response and genetic susceptibility. The preterm infants have inadequate local nonspecific mucosal defenses, delayed gut colonization, and down-regulation of intracellular signaling that inhibit inflammatory reaction. Failure of the intestinal barrier in the preterm infants may induce an excessive inflammatory response resulting in platelet-activating factor (PAF)-induced bowel injury and high concentrations of pro-inflammatory cytokines that trigger the production of free radicals. (Martin & Walker, 2006)

The final pathway in NEC pathogenesis involves free radical injury. During hypoxia the intestine will accumulate xanthine-oxidase with excessive generation of ROS during the reperfusion period, resulting in oxidative cellular damage. This hypothesis is strongly supported by experimental studies that show protective benefit of pretreatment with antioxidants such as allopurinol, superoxide dismutase (SOD), and vitamin E. (Hsueh et al., 2002) Many strategies to prevent NEC have been investigated, but few are promising. Feeding human milk can reduce the incidence of NEC. Human milk antioxidant components include the enzymes superoxide dismutase for dismutation of superoxide anion, catalases for degradation of hydrogen peroxide (H2O2), glutathione peroxidase for destruction of H2O2 and organic peroxides. Human milk contains other molecules including cysteine, vitamins C and E, which are scavengers of oxygen radicals. (L'Abbe & Friel, 2000; Lindmark-Mansson & Akesson, 2000)

5. Preventive and therapeutic strategies against free radical damage

Human studies have demonstrated that a delicate balance between the production of reactive oxygen species and the antioxidant defense factors is essential to prevent cell damage from the ROS/RNS. The premature infant is especially susceptible to oxidation-induced damage because of: first, inadequate concentrations of antioxidants at birth since developmental increases in antioxidant capacity occur in the latter part of gestation and; second, the ability to increase synthesis of antioxidants in response to hyperoxia or other oxidant challenges is deficient. Relative impairments in the induction of antioxidant enzymes may result in an increased risk for the development of free oxygen radical diseases of the newborn such as periventricular leukomalacia, bronchopulmonary dysplasia, and retinopathy of prematurity. (Auten & Davis, 2009) Accordingly the preventive and therapeutic strategies have focused on avoiding the reactive oxygen species as well as using antioxidants; both enzymatic and non-enzymatic.

5.1 Avoid oxidative stress

Increased production of ROS can occur as a result of many conditions affecting the mother (maternal diabetes, maternal drugs, chorioamnionitis, congenital infections), as well as the newborn infant (hyperoxia, reperfusion, inflammation). Prevention and control of maternal diabetes which if not treated, is associated with an increased production of ROS, can minimize the incidence of ROS-induced fetal structural defects. (Wiznitzer et al., 1999) Epidemiologic data have suggested a strong association between chorioamnionitis and the development of bronchopulmonary dysplasia due to increased concentrations of pro-inflammatory cytokines in human amniotic fluid and fetal cord blood, indicating a systemic inflammatory response during chorioamnionitis. Treatment of maternal chorioamnionitis may minimize the ROS-induced fetal insult. (Buhimschi et al., 2009)

Obviously, avoidance of neonatal conditions such as asphyxia, hyperoxia, and retinal phototherapy light exposure which can cause excessive release of free oxygen radicals are the best strategy in avoiding the oxidative stress in neonates. It is also important to consider the fact that infection, especially sepsis, is a significant source of oxidative stress. Accordingly, early identification and treatment of sepsis and the concept of optimal oxygenation are considered important preventive strategies. Conventional indications suggest that optimal oxygen tension should be maintained between 50-70 mmHg. (Wolkoff & Narula, 2000). A significant decrease in chronic lung disease and retinopathy of prematurity without any difference in mortality were observed in extremely low birth weight infants kept at less than 95% oxygen saturation compared to those kept at more than 95%. (Sun, 2002) Hyperoxia and oxidative stress may occur during neonatal resuscitation with a potential risk is associated with resuscitating those infants, especially preterm infants, with 100% oxygen due to more production of ROS compared to room air. (Ramij et al., 1993) Accordingly, it seems reasonable to suggest avoiding routine neonatal resuscitation with 100% oxygen. To avoid hyperoxia in a very pre-term infants (less than, 32 weeks gestation), use of an oxygen blender and pulse oximeter during resuscitation is recommended.

Another preventive strategy is avoiding or at least minimizing the barotrauma and volutrauma caused by mechanical ventilation in preterm infants with respiratory distress syndrome. Barotrauma, volutrauma and oxygen toxicity, during mechanical ventilation, are important factors in the pathogenesis of CLD with the release of multiple pro-inflammatory cytokines and increased production ROS and RNS that are destructive to lipids, proteins and DNA, within the pulmonary cells. Avoidance of the use of pure oxygen during resuscitation as well as avoidance of mechanical ventilation with the use of early surfactant and nasal continuous positive air pressure (CPAP) may reduce respiratory tissue damage. (Schult et al., 2003)

5.2 Antioxidant therapy

The use of antioxidants to suppress or at least minimize the molecular damage by ROS and or RNS could be considered in situations in which hyperoxia is expected. Antioxidants could be both enzymatic and non-enzymatic factors that scavenge various oxidants.

5.2.1 Antioxidant enzymes

Antioxidant enzymes include copper-zinc superoxide dismutase (CuZnSOD), and manganese SOD can catalyze the dismutation of superoxide anion to H2O2. Supplementation with an aerosol-delivered SOD mimetic improved alveolar development in a baboon model of severe BPD caused by prematurity, hyperoxia, and mechanical ventilation. (Chang et al., 2003) Another antioxidant enzyme is the Glutathione peroxidase (GPx) which is also important for removal of intracellular hydrogen peroxide and lipid peroxides, and glutathione is a direct scavenger of oxidants both intracellularly and extracellularly. Its role in lung protection is suggested by the high concentrations of glutathione in the lining fluid of lower airways and alveoli, with a transient postnatal decrease in preterm infants. (Jain et al., 1995) Many trials have been made to incorporate enzymes in the process of prevention of tissue damage by oxygen in preterm neonates to prevent diseases like chronic lung disease. The challenge is how to introduce them into the cells or maintain them in the circulation when administered systemically. Effective therapy must be directed to the target organ and to a specific ROS or RNS. (Jankov et al., 2001; Thibeault, 2000)

5.2.2 Non-enzymatic antioxidants

Non-enzymatic antioxidants include glutathione, thioredoxin, vitamins A, C, and E, melatonin, polyphenols, certain trace elements, and others. As previously mentioned, vitamins A, C, and E are important factors in normal physiology as well as antioxidant defense. The role of Vitamin A is mediated by acting on retinol-binding protein and the retinoic acid receptor. However, serum levels of vitamin A have consistently been shown to be reduced in preterm infants thus increasing their risk for chronic lung disease. (Darlow & Graham, 2007; Debier & Larondelle, 2005) Although vitamin concentrations can be increased in the serum of preterm animal models, this has not resulted in a significant reduction in ROS-induced injury. (Berger et al., 1998; Brion et al., 2003) Studies has shown that Melatonin can reverse oxidant/antioxidant imbalance in damaged lung tissue in neonatal rats and thus it may have a promising beneficial factor on hyperoxia-induced lung disease in human neonates with chronic lung diseases. (Jan et al., 2007; Mollaoglu et al., 2007; Pignone et al., 2006)

5.2.3 Hypothermia

During hypoxia-ischemia, an overproduction of free radicals has been suggested to cause oxidative stress, with harmful effects on cells and tissues. Recent studies have shown therapeutic systemic cooling or hypothermia therapy may exert protective effects against oxidative stress. Term infants were randomly selected for treatment with moderate whole body hypothermia versus standard supportive care after perinatal asphyxia. Total hydroperoxide as a biomarker of oxidative stress, and C-reactive protein as a marker of inflammation, were monitored. The slower increase and lower peaks of total hydroperoxides and the C-reactive protein in the hypothermic group support the hypothesis that hypothermia may reduce the post-asphyxic oxidative stress. (Perrone et al., 2010)

5.2.4 Breast feeding

Another preventive strategy against ROS is the advocacy of breast feeding for all infants as some studies have suggested that increased ROS could be scavenged by feeding human milk. Human milk is recognized as the optimal form of nutrition during the neonatal period, providing nutrients and a variety of components (minerals, vitamins, and enzymes) that can work as antioxidants. Human milk antioxidant components include the enzymes superoxide dismutase for dismutation of superoxide anion, catalase for degradation of hydrogen peroxide (H2O2), glutathione peroxidase for destruction of H2O2 and organic peroxides. Human milk contains other molecules including cysteine, vitamins C and E, which are scavengers of oxygen radicals. (Ledo et al., 2009; Tsopmo & Friel, 2007) Further work may identify micro supplements which could be added to breast milk or formula to address the need for more antioxidants.

6. Conclusion

A physiologic redox state is essential for normal human development. However, pregnant women, their growing fetus as well as preterm newborns are highly susceptible to oxidative stress because they often are exposed to hyperoxia, infectious/inflammatory conditions, and high concentrations of nonprotein- bound iron, which can contribute to increased production of free radicals. It has been shown unequivocally that during pregnancy and in the preterm newborn, there are lower levels of antioxidant factors, which result in an imbalance between oxidant and antioxidant factors that actually trigger free radical injury. Several studies have shown that in women with such an imbalance, preeclampsia, preterm labor, intrauterine growth restriction, and preterm premature rupture of the membranes, can result. Also, investigations have suggested that oxidative stress is involved in the pathogenesis of neonatal diseases such as periventricular leukomalacia, intraventricular hemorrhage, and bronchopulmonary dysplasia, retinopathy of prematurity and necrotizing enterocolitis. Clinical trials in pregnant women have shown that increasing the amount of lycopene, and CoQ_{10}, as well as DHA, seems to reduce the burden of the maternal fetal disorders listed above. Single supplementations of vitamins A, C, E, have not shown salutary results. However, has shown on Table 1, many of the market leaders in prenatal micronutrients supplementation include many of these antioxidant vitamins, minerals, and trace elements. Also, clinical trials have provided indirect evidence supporting the concept that free radicals play a key role in the pathogenesis of neonatal diseases. Although free radical injury is well recognized in neonatal disease pathogenesis, a clear definition of its degree of participation, the precise mechanisms, and the specific radicals involved in every disease need to be established. While well accepted in obstetric practice, the impact of antioxidant therapy in the neonatal period remains under investigation. Although research is promising, further studies for early identification of infants at risk from oxidative stress and the development of safe and efficient antioxidant strategies to prevent or minimize oxidative damage are required.

7. References

ACOG/AAP, Neonatal Encephalopathy and Cerebral Palsy. 2003 Washington, D.C.

Adam O, et al. Influence of dietary linoleic acid intake with different fat intake on arachidonic acid concentrations in plasma and platelet lips and eicosanoid biosynthesis in female volunteers. Ann Nutr Metab 2003;47:31-36.

Agarwal A, Gupta S, Sharma RK. Role of oxidative stress in female reproduction. Reprod Biol Endocrinol. 2005;3:28.

Apollinaire Tsopmo and James K. Friel. Human Milk has Anti-Oxidant Properties to Protect Premature Infants. Current Pediatric Reviews, 2007;3:45-51

Archer SL, Peterson D, Nelson DP et al. Oxygen radicals and antioxidant enzymes alter pulmonary vascular reactivity in the rat lung. J Appl Physiol 1989;66:102–111.

Arterburn LM, Oken HA, Hall EB, Hamersely J, Kuratko CN, Hoffman JP. Algal oil capsules and cooked salmon: nutritionally equivalent sources of docosahexaenoic acid. J Am Diet Assoc 2008; in press.

Arterburn LM, Oken HA, Hoffman JP Bailey-Hall EB, Chung G, Hamersely J, et al. Bioequivalence of docosahexaenoic acid from different algal oils in capsules and a DHA-fortified food. Lipids 2007;42:1011-1024.

Ashton N, Cook C. Direct observation of the effect of oxygen on developing vessels: preliminary report. Br J Ophthalmol 1954;38:433–440.

Asikainen TM, White CW. Pulmonary antioxidant defenses in the preterm newborn with respiratory distress and bronchopulmonary dysplasia in evolution: implications for antioxidant therapy. Antioxid Redox Signal 2004;6:155-67.

Auten RL, Davis JM. Oxygen toxicity and reactive oxygen species: the devil is in the details. Pediatr Res 2009;66:121e7.

Baba L, McGrath JM. Oxygen free radicals: effects in the newborn period. Adv Neonatal Care 2008;8(5):256-264.

Bell SJ, Bradley D, Forse RA, et al. The new dietary fats in health and disease. J Am Diet Assoc. 1997;97:280-286.

Berger TM, Frei B, Rifai N, et al. Early high dose antioxidant vitamins do not prevent bronchopulmonary dysplasia in premature baboons exposed to prolonged hyperoxia: a pilot study. Pediatr Res 1998;43:719e26.

Binivale MA, Ehrenkranz RA. The role of nutrition in the prevention and management of bronchopulmonary dysplasia. Semin Perinatol. 2006;30:200–208.

Blondi et al. Curr Pharma Des. 2005:11:2075-2089; Suhi et al. Am J Obstet Gynecol 2008;541:e7.

Boutet M, Roland L, Thomas N, Bilodeau JF. Specific systemic antioxidant response to preeclampsia in late pregnancy: the study of intracellular glutathione peroxidases in maternal and fetal blood. Am J Obstet Gynecol 2009;200:530.e1-530.e7.

Bresolin N, Bet L, Binda A, Moggio M, Comi G, Nador F, Ferrante C, Carenzi A, Scarlato G. Clinical and biochemical correlations in mitochondrial myopathies treated with coenzyme Q10. Neurology 1988;38:892-899.

Brion LP, Bell EF, Raghuveer TS. Vitamin E supplementation for prevention of morbidity and mortality in preterm infants. Cochrane Database Syst Rev. 2003. CD003665.

Brion LP, Bell EF, Raghuveer TS. Vitamin E supplementation for prevention of morbidity and mortality in preterm infants. Cochrane Database Syst Rev;2003. CD003665.

Buhimschi CS, Dulay AT, Abdel-Razeq S, Zhao G, Lee S, Hodgson EJ, Bhandari V, Buhimschi IA: Fetal inflammatory response in women with proteomic biomarkers characteristic of intra-amniotic inflammation and preterm birth. Br J Obstet Gynaecol 2009;116:257–267.

Buhimschi IA, Buhimschi CS, Pupkin M, Weiner CP. Beneficial impact of term labor: nonenzymatic antioxidant reserve in the human fetus. Am J Obstet Gynecol. 2003;189:181-188.

Buonocore G, Perrone S, Gioia D, Gatti MG, Massfra C, Agosta R, Bracci R: Nucleated red blood cell count at birth as an index of perinatal brain damage. Am J Obstet Gynecol 1999;181:1500-1505.

Burton GJ, Jauniaux E. Oxidative stress, Best Practice & Research Clinical Obstetrics and Gynaecology. 2010;doi:10.1016/j.bpobgyn.2010.10.016.

Campbell K. Intensive oxygen therapy as a possible cause of retrolental fibroplasias: a clinical approach. Med J Aust 1951;2:48–50.

Chang LY, Subramaniam M, Yoder BA, et al. A catalytic antioxidant attenuates alveolar structural remodeling in bronchopulmonary dysplasia. Am J Respir Crit Care Med 2003;167:57e64.

Childs AM, Cornette L, Ramenghi LA, Tanner SP, Arthur RJ, Martinez D, Levene MI; Magnetic reasonance and cranial ultrasound characteristics of periventricular white matter abnormalities in newborn infants. Clin Radiol 2001;56:647-655.

Clinton SK. Lycopene: chemistry, biology, and implications for human health and disease. Nutr Rev. 1998;56:35-51.

Clyman RI, Saugstad OD, Mauray F. Reactive oxygen metabolites relax the lamb ductus arteriosus by stimulating prostaglandin production. Circ Res 1989;64:1–8.

Crane FL, Navas P. The diversity of coenzyme Q function. Mol Aspects Med. 1997;18(suppl):S1-S6.

Darlow BA, Austin NC. Selenium supplementation to prevent short-term morbidity in preterm neonates. Cochrane Database Syst Rev. 2003;4:CD003312

Darlow BA, Buss H, McGill F, Fletcher L, Graham P, Winterbourn CC.Vitamin C supplementation in very preterm infants: a randomized controlled trial. Arch Dis Child Fetal Neonatal Ed 2005;90: F117–122.

Darlow BA, Graham PJ. Vitamin A supplementation for preventing morbidity and mortality in very low birthweight infants (Review). Cochrane Collaboration Syst Rev 2002;4.

Darlow BA, Graham PJ. Vitamin A supplementation to prevent mortality and short and long-term morbidity in very low birthweight infants. Cochrane Database Syst Rev. 2007. CD000501.

Darlow BA, Graham PJ. Vitamin A supplementation to prevent mortality and short and long-term morbidity in very low birthweight infants. Cochrane Database Syst Rev;2007. CD000501.

Debier C, Larondelle Y. Vitamins A and E: metabolism, roles and transfer to offspring. Br J Nutr 2005;93:153e74.

Delacourt C, D'Ortho M-P, Maquin-Mavier I, et al. Oxidantantioxidant balance in alveolar macrophages from newborn rats. Eur Respir J 1996;9:2517–2524.

Delivoria M, Misbra OP; Mechanisms of cerebral injury, perinatal asphyxia and strategies for prevention. J Pediatr 1998;132:830-834.

Dennery PA. Role of redox in fetal development and neonatal diseases. Antioxid Redox Signal. 2004;6:147–153

Dheen ST, Tay SS, Boran J, et al. Recent studies on neural tube defects in embryos of diabetic pregnancy: an overview. Curr Med Chem 2009;16:2345e54.

Dugan, L.L.; Choi, D.W. Excitotoxicity, free radicals; cell membrane changes. Ann. Neurol., 1994; 35:S17-S21.

Elliott JP, Morrison JC. Uterine Contraction, In Press,

Endermann DH, Schiffrin B. J Am Soc Nephrd. 2004;15:1983-1992.

Finer N, Leone T. Oxygen saturation monitoring for the preterm infant: the evidence basis for current practice. Pediatr Res 2009;65(4):375-380.

Foklers K, Osterborg A, Nylander M, Morita M, Mellstedt H. Activities of vitamin Q10 in animal models and a serious deficiency in patients with cancer. Biochem. Biophys. Res. Commun. 1997;234;296-299.

Gallagher S. Omega 3 oils and pregnancy. Midwifery Today 2004;26-31.

Girard N, Gire C, Sigandy S, Porcu G, Brander GF, Raybaud C, Grouny SC: MR imaging of acquired fetal brain disorders. Child Nerv Syst 2003;19:490-500.

Goldenberg RL, Culhan JF, Iams JD & Romero R (2008). Epidemiology and causes of preterm birth. The Lancet, Vol. 371, No. 9606, pp. 75-84.

Good WW. Early treatment for retinopathy of prematurity cooperative group. Trans Am Opthalmol 2004;102:233–248.

Greenberg JA, Bell SJ, Van Ausdal W. Omega-3 fatty acid supplementation during pregnancy. Rev Obstet Gnecol 2008;1(4):162-169.

Grigg J, Barber A, Silverman M. Bronchoalveolar lavage fluid glutathione in intubated premature infants. Arch Dis Child 1993;69:49-51.

Grigg J, Barber A, Silverman M. Bronchoalveolar lavage fluid glutathione in intubated premature infants. Arch Dis Child 1993;69:49e51.

Groneck P, Reuss D, Gotze-Speer B, et al. Effects of dexamethasone on chemotactic activity and inflammatory mediators in tracheobronchial aspirates of preterm infants at risk for chronic lung disease. J Pediatr 1993;22:938–944.

Hallman M, Bry K, Hoppu K, Lappi M, Pohjavuori M. Inositol supplementation in premature infants with respiratory distress syndrome. N Engl J Med. 1992;326:1233–1239.

Hawthorne et al. Plasma phospholipid levels in children improve with supplementation of DHA to orange juice. J Am Diet Assoc 2007;107(Suppl 3):A56.

Helzlsouer KJ, Constock GW, Morris JS. Selenium, lycopene, α-tocopherol, β-carotene, retinol, and subsequent bladder cancer. Cancer Res 1989;49:6144-6148.

Hitti J, Tarczy-Hornoch P, Murphy J, Hillier SL, Aura J, Eschenbach DA. Amniotic fluid infection, cytokines, and adverse outcome among infants at 34 weeks' gestation or less. Obstet Gynecol 2001;98:1080-8.

Hsueh W, Caplan MS, Qu X-W, Tan X-D, De Plaen IG, Gonzalez-Crussi F. Neonatal necrotizing enterocolitis: clinical considerations and pathogenetic concepts. Pediatr Dev Pathol. 2002;6:6–23.
Hsueh W, Caplan MS, Qu X-W, Tan X-D, De Plaen IG, Gonzalez-Crussi F. Neonatal necrotizing enterocolitis: clinical considerations and pathogenetic concepts. Pediatr Dev Pathol. 2002;6:6–23.
Jain A, Mehta T, Auld PA, Rodrigues J, Ward RF, Schwartz MK, et al.Glutathione metabolism in newborns: evidence for glutathione deficiency in plasma, bronchoalveolar lavage fluid, and lymphocytes in prematures. Pediatr Pulmonol 1995;20:160-6.

Jan JE, Wasdell MB, Freeman RD, Bax M. Evidence supporting the use of melatonin in short gestation infants. J Pineal Res 2007;42:22-27.

Jankov RP, Negus A, Tanswell AK. Antioxidants as therapy in the newborn: some words of caution. Pediatr Res. 2001;50:681–687.

Jobe, A. J. 1999. The new BPD: an arrest of lung development. Pediatr. Res. 46:641–643.

Joshi SR, Mehendale SS, Dangat KD, Kilari AS, Yadav HR, Taralekar VS. High maternal plasma antioxidant concentrations associated with preterm delivery. Ann Nutr Metab. 2008;53:276-82.

Kaiser LL, Allen L; American Diatetic Association. Position of the American Dietetic Association: nutrition and Lifestyle for a healthy pregnancy outcome. J Am Diet Assoc. 2002;102:1479-1490.

Kontic-Vucinic O, Sulovic N, Radunovic N. Micronutrients in women's reproductive health: I. Vitamins. Int J Fertil Womens Med. 2006;51:106-115.

Kramer MS, Kahn SR, Platt RW, et al. Antioxidant vitamins, long-chain fatty acids, and spontaneous preterm birth. Epidemiology. 2009;20:707-13.

L'Abbe M, Friel JK. Glutathione peroxidase and superoxide dismutase concentrations in milk from mothers of premature and full-term infants. J Pediatr Gastr Nutr 2000;31:270-4.

Lackmann GM, Hesse L, To¨llner U. Reduced iron-associated antioxidants in premature newborns suffering intracerebral hemorrhage. Free Rad Biol Med. 1996;20:407–409.

Lakatos L, Hatvani I, Oroszlan G, Balla G, Karmazsin L, Alaka O et al. Controlled trial of D-penicillamine to prevent retinopathy of prematurity. Acta Paediatr Hung 1986;27:47–56.

Landmesser U, Merten R, Spiekermann S, Büttner K, Drexler H, Hornig B. Vascular extracellular superoxide dismutase activity in patients with coronary artery disease: relation to endothelium-dependent vasodilation. Circulation. 2000;101:2264-2270.

Langsjoen P, Langsjoen P, Willis R, Folkers K. Treatment of essential hypertension with coenzyme Q10. Mol. Aspects Med. 1994;15:S265-S272.

Ledo A, Arduini A, Asensi MA, et al. Human milk enhances antioxidant defenses against hydroxyl radical aggression in preterm infants. Am J Clin Nutr 2009;89:210e5.

Lindeman JH, Lentjes EG, van Zoeren-Grobben D, Berger HM. Postnatal changes in plasma ceruloplasmin and transferrin antioxidant activities in preterm babies. Biol Neonate 2000;78:73e6.

Lindmark-Mansson H, Akesson B. Antioxidative factors in milk. Br J Nutr 2000;84(Suppl. 1): S103-10.

Luo ZC, Fraser WD, Julien P, et al. Tracing the origins of "fetal origins" of adult diseases: programming by oxidative stress? Med Hypotheses. 2006;66:38-44.

Louis JM, Ehrenberg HM, Collin MF, Mercer BM. Perinatal intervention and neonatal outcomes near the limit of viability. Am J Obstet Gynecol 2004;191:1398-403.

Makrides M, Gibson RA, McPhee AJ, et al. Effect of DHA supplementation during pregnancy on maternal depression and neurodevelopment of young children. JAMA. 2010;304:1675-1683.

Marlow N, Wolke D, Bracewell MA, Samara M. Neurologic and developmental disability at six years of age after extremely preterm birth. N Engl J Med 2005;352:9-19.

Martin CR, Walker WA. Intestinal immune defences and the inflammatory response in necrotising enterocolitis. Semin Fetal Neonatal Med. 2006;11:369–377.

Masters ET, Jedrychowski W, Schleicher RL, et al. Relation between prenatal lipid-soluble micronutrient status, environmental pollutant exposure, and birth outcomes. Am J Clin Nutr. 2007;86:1139-1145.

Maulik D, Zanelli S, Numagami Y, Ohnishi ST, Mishra OP, Delivoria PM. Oxygen free radical generation during in-utero hypoxia in the fetal guinea pig brain: the effects of maturity and of magnesium sulfate administration. Brain Res. 1999;817:117-22.

Mishra OP, Mishra R, Ashraf QM, Delivoria-Papadopoulous M. Nitric oxide-mediated mechanism of neuronal nitric oxide synthase and inducible nitric oxide synthase expression during hypoxia in the cerebral cortex of newborn piglets. Neuroscience. 2006;140:867–863.

Mollaoglu H, Topal T, Ozler M, Uysal B, Reiter RJ, Korkmaz A, et al. Antioxidant effects of melatonin in rats during chronic exposure to hyperbaric oxygen. J Pineal Res 2007;42:50-54.

Morrison JC, Elliott J, Knuppel RA, Siabi B, Pill MW. Dove Medical Press. Current issues and perspectives in prenatal nutrition. Research and Reports in Neonatology 2011;1:25-38.

O'Donovan DJ, Fernandes CJ. Free radicals and diseases in premature infants. Antioxidants and redox signaling 2004;6(1):169-176.

Oken E, Belfort MB. (Editorial) DHA Supplementation. JAMA 2010;304:1632-33.

Olsen SF, Hansen HS, Secher JN, Jensen B, Sandstrom B. Gestation length and birth weight in relation to intake of marine n-3 fatty acids. Br J Nutr 1995;73:397-404.

Olsen SF, Secher NJ, Tabor A, Weber T, Walker JJ, Gluud C. Randomized clinical trials of fish oil supplementation in high-risk pregnancies. Fish Oil Trials in Pregnancy (FOTIP) Team. Br J Obstet Gynaecol 2000;107:382-95.

Otto SJ, Houwelingen ACv, Hornstra G. The effect of different supplements containing docosahexaenoic acid on plasma and erythrocyte fatty acids of health non-pregnant women. Nutr Res 2000;20:917-927.

Patz A, Hoeck LE, DeLaCruz E. Studies on the effect of high oxygen administration in retrolental fribroplasia. I. Nursery Observations. Am J Ophthalmol 1952;35:1248–1253.

Penn JS, Henry MM, Tolman BL. Exposure to alternating hypoxia and hyperoxia causes severe proliferative retinopathy in the newborn rat. Pediatric Res 1994;36(6):724-731.

Perlman JM. Summary proceedings from the neurology group on hypoxic-ischemic encephalopathy. Pediatrics. 2006;117:S28–S32.

Perrone S, Szabo´ M, Bellieni CV, Longini M, Bango´ M, Kelen D, Treszl A, Negro S, Tataranno ML, Buonocore G. Whole body hypothermia and oxidative stress in babies with hypoxic-ischemic brain injury. Pediatr Neurol 2010;43:236-240.

Pignone AM, Rosso AD, Fiori G, Matucci-Cerinic M, Becucci A, Tempestini A, et al. Melatonin is a safe and effective treatment for chronic pulmonary and extrapulmonary sarcoidosis. J Pineal Res 2006;41:95-100.

Pittet JF, Mackersie RC, Martin TR, et al. Biological markers of acute lung injury: prognostic and pathogenetic significance. Am J Respir Crit Care Med 1997;155:1187–1205.

Poston L, Briley AL, Seed PT, Kelly FJ, Shennan AH. Vitamin C and vitamin E in pregnant women at risk for pre-eclampsia (VIP trial): randomized placebo-controlled trial. Lancet 2006;367:1145-54.

Pressman EK, Thornburg LL, Glantz JC, et al. Inflammatory cytokines and antioxidants in midtrimester amniotic fluid: correlation with pregnancy outcome. Am J Obstet Gynecol 2011;204:155.e1-7.

Ramij S, Abuja S, Thirupuram S, et al. Rususcitation of asphyxiated newborn infants with room air or 100% oxygen. Pediatr Res 1993;34:809-12.

Sanderud J, Bjoro K, Saugstad OD. Oxygen radicals stimulate thromboxane and prostacyclin synthesis and induce vasoconstriction in pig lungs. Scand J Clin Lab Invest 1993; 53:447–455.

Saugstad OD. Bronchopulmonary dysplasia-oxidative stress and antioxidants. Semin Neonatol 2003;8(1):39-49.

Saugstad OD. Chronic lung disease: the role of oxidative stress. Biol Neonate 1998; 74: Suppl. 1, 21–28.

Saugstad OD. Hypoxanthine as an indicator of hypoxia: its role in health and disease through free radical production. Pediatr Res 1988;23:143–150.

Saugstad OD. Mechanism of tissue injury by oxygen radicals: implications for neonatal disease. Acta Paediatr 1996; 85:1-4.

Saugstad OD. Oxidative stress in the newborn – a 30-year perspective. Biol Neonate 2005; 88:228–236.

Scholl TO. Maternal nutrition before and during pregnancy. Nestle Nutr Workshop Ser Pediatr Program. 2008;61:79-89.

Schultz C, Tautz J, Reiss I, et al. Prolonged mechanical ventilation induces pulmonary inflammation in preterm infants. Biol Neonate 2003;84:64–66.

Shah MD, Shah SR. Nutrient deficiencies in the premature infant. Pediatr Clin North Am 2009;56:1069e83.

Sharma JB, Kumar A, Kumar A, Malhotra M, et al. Effect of lycopene on pre-eclampsia and intra-uterine growth retardation in primigravidas. International J Gynecol Obstet 2003;81:257-262.

Shoji H, Koletzko B. Oxidative stress and antioxidant protection in the perinatal period. Curr Opin Clin Nutr Metab Care. 2007;10:324–328

Shweiki D, Itin A, Soffer D, Keshet E. Vascular endothelial growth factor induced by hypoxia may mediate hypoxia-induced angiogenesis. Nature 1992;359:843–845.

Smith CV, Hansen TN, Martin NE, McMicken HW, Elliott SJ. Oxidant stress responses in premature infants during exposure to hyperoxia. Pediatr Res 1993;34:360-5.

Smith LE, Shen W, Perruzzi C, Soker S, Kinose F, Xu X et al. Regulation of vascular endothelial growth factor-dependent retinal neovascularization by insulin-like growth factor-1 receptor. Nat Med 1999;5:1390–1395.

Smuts CM, Huang M, Mundy D, Plasse T, Major S, Carlson SE. A randomized trial of docosahexaenoic acid supplementation during the third trimester of pregnancy. Obstet Gynecol 2003;101:469:79.

Speer CP, Silverman M. Issues relating to children born prematurely. Eur Respir J Suppl. 1998;27:13s-16s.

Speer CP. Inflammation and bronchopulmonary dysplasia: a continuing story. Semin Fetal Neonatal Med. 2006;11:354–362

Speer CP. Pre- and postnatal inflammatory mechanisms in chronic lung disease of preterm infants. Paediatr Respir Rev. 2004;5:S241–S244.

Stein P, Scholl TO, Schluter MD, et al. Oxidative stress early in pregnancy and pregnancy outcome. Free Res. 2088;42:841-8.

Sun SC. Relation of target SpO2 levels and clinical outcome in Extremely Low Birth Weight infants on supplemental oxygen. Pediatr Res 2002;51:350A.

Teran E, Hernandez I, Nieto B, Tavara R, Ocampo JE, Calle A. Coenzyme Q10 supplementation during pregnancy reduces the risk of pre-eclampsia. Int J Gynaecol Obstet. 2009;105:43-45.

Teran E, Racines-Orbe M, Vivero S, Escudero C, Molina G, Calle A. Preeclampsia is associated with a decrease in plasma coenzyme Q10 levels. Free Radic Biol Med. 2003;35(11):1453-1456.

Thibeault DW. The precarious antioxidant defenses of the preterm infant. Am J Perinatol. 2000;4:167–181.

Tiano L, Belardinelli R, Carnevali P, Principi F, Seddaiu G, Llttarru GP. Effect of coenzyme Q10 administration on endothelial function and extracellular superoxide dismutase in patients with ischaemic heart disease: a double-blind, randomized controlled study. Eur Heart J. 2007;28:2249-2255.

Trindade CEP. Microelements and vitamins in the nutrition of very low-birthweight preterm infants: a Brazilian perspective. NeoReviews. 2007;8:e3–e13

Volpe JJ. Perinatal brain injury: from pathogenesis to neuroprotection. Ment Retard Dev Disabil Res Rev. 2001;7:56–64.

Welty SE, Smith CV. Rationale for antioxidant therapy in premature infants to prevent bronchopulmonary dysplasia. Nutr Rev 2001;59:10-7.

Welty SE. Antioxidants and oxidations in bronchopulmonary dysplasia: there are no easy answers. J Pediatr 2003;143:697-8.

Wiedemann M, Kontush A, Finckh B, Wege HH, Kohlschu¨tter A. Neonatal blood plasma is less susceptible to oxidation than adult plasma owing to its higher content of bilirubin and lower content of oxidizable fatty acids. Pediatr Res. 2003;53:843–849.

Wiznitzer A, Furman B, Mazor M, Reece EA. The role of prostanoids in the development of diabetic emberyopathy. Semin Reprod Endocrinol 1999;17:175-81.

Wolkoff LI, Narula P. Issue in neonatal and pediatric oxygen therapy. Respir Care Clin N AM 2000;6:675-91.

Xu H, Perez-Cuevas R, Xiong X, et al. An international trial of antioxidants in the prevention of preeclampsia (INTAPP). Am J Obstet Gynecol 2010;202:239.e1-10.

Yamamoto T, Shibata N, Maramatsu F, Sakayori N, Kobayashi M; Oxidative stress in the human fetal brain; an immunohistochemical study. Pediatr Neurol 2002;26:116-122.

6

Weakening and Rupture of Human Fetal Membranes – Biochemistry and Biomechanics

N. Rangaswamy[1], D. Kumar[1], R.M. Moore[1], B.M. Mercer[2], J.M. Mansour[3], R. Redline [4] and J.J. Moore[1,2]

[1]*Department of Pediatrics,*
[2]*Department of Reproductive Biology,*
[3]*Department of Mechanical and Aerospace Engineering,*
[4]*Department of Pathology, Case Western Reserve University, Cleveland, OH, USA*

1. Introduction

In spite of advances in the quality of prenatal care, management of high-risk pregnancies and treatment strategies targeting prevention of preterm births, the rate of preterm births in the US has continued to rise over the last two decades and is associated with high mortality and morbidity. Care of preterm infants also poses a significant financial burden on limited health care resources. Infants born at less than 37 weeks gestation account for 69% of all US infant deaths and their care has been modestly estimated at 26 billion dollars per year (Behrman et al., 2006; MacDorman et al., 2008). Preterm Premature Rupture of Membranes (PPROM) causes 30 - 40% of all preterm births and is disproportionately distributed such that African Americans suffer twice the rate of PPROM than Caucasians (Goldenberg et al., 1996a). Although some limited success has been achieved in the treatment of iatrogenic fetal membrane (FM) rupture resulting from amniocentesis or fetal surgery (Quintero et al., 1999; Young et al., 2000; O'Brien et al., 2001; Bilic et al., 2010), there has been no success in the repair of spontaneously ruptured FM, as occurs with PPROM (Quintero et al., 1998; Sciscione et al., 2001; Young et al., 2004b; Devlieger et al., 2006). Recent progress in the understanding of the biochemically-mediated processes which lead to FM weakening and rupture suggests that inhibition of these processes may be possible. This generates hope that many cases of PPROM may ultimately be preventable (R.M. Moore et al., 2009b, 2010; Kumar et al., 2011).

2. New techniques used in the studies on FM rupture

2.1 Mapping procedure

We have developed and utilized a systematic procedure to map the rupture strength of FM over its entire topographic surface, thereby identifying relatively weak areas for further biochemical, proteomic, and sophisticated biomechanical testing.

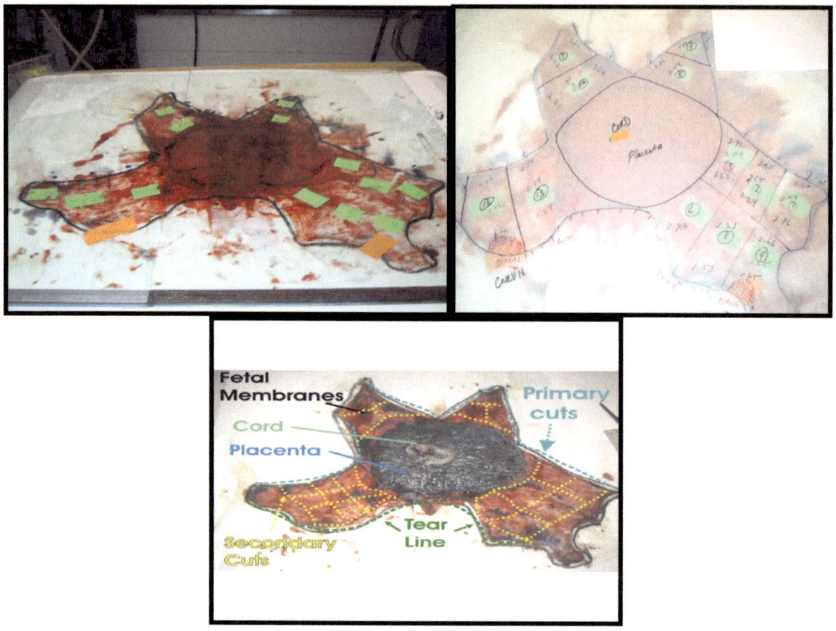

Fig. 1. Fetal Membrane cutting procedure. (Top Left) Marked membranes showing location of primary cuts required to lay the membranes flat. (Top Right) Membrane fragments removed with outlines of pieces on lab table paper. (Bottom) Paper tracing reproduction showing cuts, orientation and location of all pieces, and strength results. (Reproduced with permission from El-Khwad et al. Biol Reprod 72:720-726, 2005.)

Although animal data document homogeneous weakening of the FM over the entire surface with increasing gestation (Lei et al., 1995, 1997; Paavola et al., 1995; Parry et al., 1998), attempts to demonstrate similar gestational changes in human FM were unsuccessful (Manabe et al., 1991). Studies in which whole FM or randomly selected pieces were sampled showed high variability and no definite pattern of remodeling and apoptosis. In response to the challenge of interpreting variable data, we developed a systematic method of cutting the membranes (El-Khwad et al., 2005; Fig. 1.). Fetal membranes to be tested were cut along specific grids. We identified the region of the membranes overlying the cervix by marking it in utero with Gentian Violet. As a result, the exact location and orientation of each piece cut from the membranes relative to both the placental disc and to the region that formerly overlay the cervix was determined. A paper model (tracing) mapping the location and the rupture strength data of each piece is ultimately constructed. This two dimensional map can be folded to show the original three-dimensional physical configuration of the amniotic sac with superimposed Rupture Strength results. This approach confirmed an inherent inhomogeneity in the biomechanics of the gestational sac and clearly demonstrated the para-cervical weak zone. These features had been camouflaged in many previous studies where parts of weak and strong regions were tested together with the assumption of FM homogeneity over its entire surface.

2.2 Rupture test equipment

Specialized equipment is necessary to determine FM physical properties. Our testing apparatus, developed in collaboration with Com-Ten industries (a national supplier of tensile testing equipment) (Moore et al., 2006), has a number of advantages over that used in previous biomechanical studies of FM: 1. It applies a bi-axial (two dimensional) stretch on the membranes similar to normal physiology; 2. It uses the puncture mode with any size probe and tissue clamp - it is thus possible to perform a detailed survey of physical properties over the entire fetal membrane surface in a reasonable time period; 3. It will hold preset displacements or forces for viscoelastic studies; 4. Probes may be fit with ultrasound sensors for simultaneous measurement of membrane thickness; 5. High precision - calibrated accuracy is 0.05 Newton force and 0.01 cm displacement over appropriate intervals; 6. Tissue specimens are kept moist at all times. 7. Data is captured in digital form, displayed graphically, and analyzed by the software. A force-displacement curve (Fig. 2.) is computer generated during each experiment and the strength characteristics (membrane Rupture Strength, Work to Rupture, Stiffness and other physical properties) are derived and calculated from the data. Data is also exportable for independent analysis.

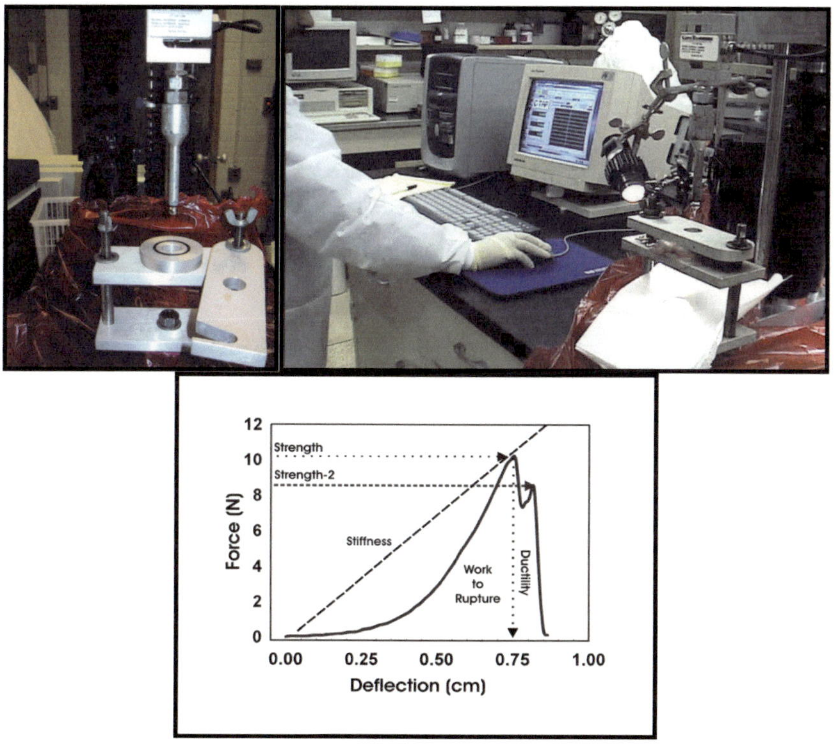

Fig. 2. Strength testing equipment. (Top Left) Close-up view of fetal membrane holding apparatus (from top to bottom - load cell force sensor, rupture probe with spherical tip, membrane holding assembly). (Top Right) Com-Ten Ball-Burst Compression Testing Equipment (from left to right - computer controller, analog-digital converter, membrane rupture assembly). (Bottom) Typical force displacement curve. (Reproduced with permission from El-Khwad et al. Biol Reprod 72:720-726, 2005.)

Development of rupture test equipment and use of this mapping methodology helped us establish the following:

2.2.1. Both term and preterm FM are biomechanically and biochemically heterogeneous over their surfaces. Only by use of this mapping procedure and equipment have we been able to identify and topologically map weak areas so that characterization can lead to direct investigation of the mechanism of weakening (El-Khwad et al., 2005, 2006; Rangaswamy et al., 2011).

2.2.2. Sequence of FM rupture - amnion and choriodecidua first stretch together followed by their separation, then choriodecidua ruptures prior to reaching its elastic limit and amnion stretches further in a non-elastic fashion, then ruptures (Arikat et al., 2006).

2.2.3. FM strain hardens with acute cyclical stretch. Like metal pulled into wire it becomes stronger and less elastic. It does not weaken (Pandey et al., 2007).

2.2.4. Determine which physiological agents or processes cause sufficient FM weakening to precipitate rupture, and under what conditions (dose, duration, etc.) this occurs.

2.3 Equipment to measure adhesion of amnion to choriodecidua

Discovery that FM (amnion and choriodecidua) separate during the process of rupture led to development of equipment to measure their adherence and allowed us demonstrate that FM peel apart and become less adherent with increasing gestation (Kumar et al., 2009; Strohl et al., 2010). Commercial industrial tensile testing equipment (Com-Ten) was adapted to perform a standard engineering T-peel test to measure the adhesive force of FM (Fig. 3.). Use of this equipment allowed us to determine that FM components become less adherent and separate with increasing gestational age (Strohl et al., 2010).

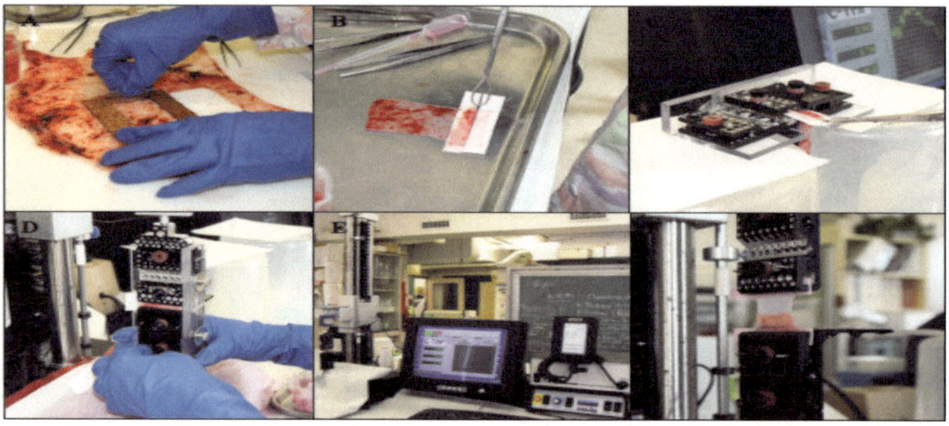

Fig. 3. Peel testing procedures. Tissue samples are cut out from FM kept moist and laid flat and kept moist (A). Stiff filter paper stints assist in holding and mounting the partially manually peeled amnion and choriodecidua by maintaining shape (B). Membrane piece mounted on custom clamps which are maintained in fixed position by a plexiglass mount support to assist sample loading (C). Sample loaded clamps with supporting Plexiglas mount as a single unit attached to the peel testing device (D). The peel tester with the FM piece loaded and the plexiglass mount support removed before beginning the test (E). FM components, amnion and choriodecidua, being peeled apart between the clamp jaws (F).

3. Para-cervical weak zone in FM – A result of programmed biochemical weakening processes

Rupture of FM (ROM) is an integral event in the onset and development of labor. Even though ROM usually follows uterine contractions, it precedes the onset of contractions in at least 10% of term labor and 40% of premature labor. This implies that the stretch force alone is not the cause of FM weakening.

3.1 Term FM develops a para-cervical "weak zone" where rupture initiates

Rat model studies suggest that amnion, the strongest component of FM undergoes collagen remodelling as gestation progresses (Paavola et al., 1995; Lockwood et al., 1999). As a result of these phenomena, FM is postulated to weaken and become more susceptible to rupture near the end of gestation. Apoptosis has also been suggested to occur near term in human amnion and chorion (McLaren et al., 2000a). Malak and Bell first identified an area of so-called "high morphological change" in the zone of FM overlying the cervix (Malak & Bell, 1994). This distinct para-cervical region has been demonstrated in the FM from both term vaginal and caesarean section deliveries without labor and comprises approximately 2-10% of the total FM surface area (McLaren et al., 1999a; McParland et al., 2003). Bell's group further characterized this area of FM as having increased matrix metalloproteinase (MMP) -9, increased trophoblast apoptosis, differences in the thickness of membrane sub layers, and increased myofibroblasts in this area (McLaren et al., 1999b, 2000a, 2000b; McParland et al., 2003). Lappas and colleagues have confirmed an increase in apoptotic markers, and have reported increased NF-kB activity and acetylated-forkhead box O1 protein expression in the para-cervical FM region (Reti et al., 2007; Lappas et al., 2009). All these studies have presumed that remodelling in this para-cervical zone leads to FM weakening and subsequent rupture.

We have identified a focal "weak zone" with biochemical characteristics equivalent to the previously described "zone of high morphological change" in the para-cervical region of FM. Using FM from repeat cesarean section performed prior to any labor, we showed that this region ruptures with only 20 - 50% of the force required to rupture other areas of the FM (Fig. 4.), and that it exhibits a biochemical signature of increased collagen remodeling and apoptosis (El-Khwad et al., 2005). Western Blot analysis indicated increases in matrix metalloproteinase 9 (MMP-9) and cleaved PARP, and decreases in fibulins 1, 3, 5 and TIMP-3 in the Weak Zone. MMP-2 did not show differences. TIMP-1 was barely detectable; TIMP-2 and TIMP-4 protein were detectable in all specimens but did not change with Strength. Other groups have also confirmed the increase in markers of collagen remodeling and apoptosis (Malak & Bell et al., 1994; El-Khwad et al., 2005, 2006; Meinert et al., 2007, Reti et al., 2007; Han et al., 2008; Lappas et al, 2008, 2009, 2010a, 2010b).

Using FM from patients with AROM (artificial rupture of membranes) and SROM (spontaneous rupture of membranes), we have further demonstrated that the para-cervical weak zone persists with the same biochemical signature as that identified in pre-labor cesarean section membranes. As the rupture tear line usually extends through the weak zone, we have postulated that it contains the site of initiation of FM rupture (El-Khwad et al., 2005, 2006). We have also demonstrated that acute, repetitive stretch does not weaken, but paradoxically strengthens FM (Pandey V et al., 2007). Our studies, those of the Bell group, and now those of four other groups (as indicated above) thus strongly support the concept of regional differences in FM properties, most specifically, that the area over the cervix is significantly weaker than the rest of the FM with concomitant differences in biochemical and histological properties. Taken together, the data indicate that term FM normally weakens in late gestation as a result of programmed biochemically mediated processes. Presumably, spontaneous FM rupture at term usually results from the mechanical stresses of labor upon biochemically pre-weakened membranes.

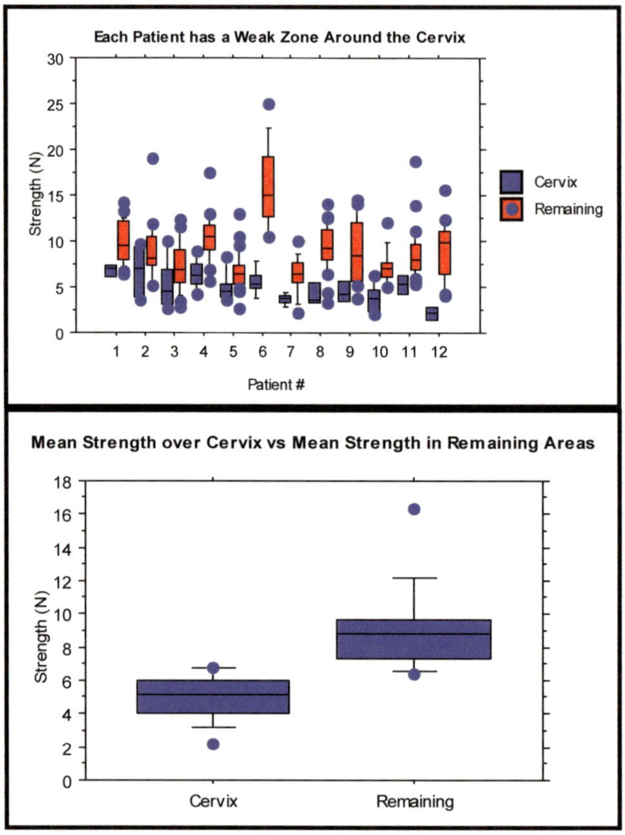

Fig. 4. Fetal membrane strength. [Bottom] Mean strength of cervical zones for each patient is less than the mean strength of the remaining areas ($P < 0.001$). [Top] Individual patient data showing a weaker cervical zone for each of the 12 patients relative to the remaining areas. (Reproduced with permission from El-Khwad et al. Biol Reprod 72:720-726, 2005.)

3.2 Role of MMP activation and apoptosis in the weak zone formation

Fortunato and Menon (2004) have extensively reviewed the roles played by MMPs and apoptosis in FM rupture. The strength of amnion and chorion is largely due to collagen. Collagens I, III, IV, V and VI have been described in various layers of amniochorion. The major strength in amnion is derived from collagen I (seen extensively in the compact layer and adjacent mesoderm) and collagen IV (a major component of the basement membrane and of the bundles connecting the mesenchymal layer and the epithelium) (Bachmaier et al., 1999). Degradation of collagen is controlled by specific MMPs as modulated by tissue inhibitors of matrix metalloproteinases (TIMPs). Thus, the ratio of MMPs and TIMPs is a good indicator of collagen degradation, which along with the deposition rate of new collagen by fibroblasts, determines the ultimate tissue strength. Although MMP types 1, 2, 3, 8 and 9 have been well described in amniochorion; major investigative work in FM has been done with MMP types 2 and 9. MMP-1 predominates prior to the onset of contractions as described by Bryant-Greenwood and Yamamoto. FM MMP-2 is constitutive and reportedly does not respond to cytokines or change with PPROM or labor (term or preterm) [Fortunato et al., 1999; Maymon et al., 2001; Xu et al., 2002]. In contrast, both active and latent forms of

MMP-9 have been shown to increase in human amniotic fluid with PPROM and in amniotic fluid of rhesus monkeys after inducing labor with cytokines (Bryant-Greenwood et al., 1995; Osmers et al., 1995; Athayde et al., 1999; Vadillo-Ortega et al., 2002). MMP-9 can also be induced in FM tissue with PGE_2, $PGF_{2\alpha}$, TNF_α and ROS (Buhimschi et al., 2000; Sciscione et al., 2001; Ulug et al., 2001; Arechavaleta-Velasco et al., 2002; Zaga et al., 2004). TIMP-1, which controls the activity of MMP-9, has been extensively studied in FM and found to decrease with PROM and labor (Ulug et al., 2001; Arechavaleta-Velasco et al., 2002; Buhimschi et al., 2000; Zaga et al., 2004; McLaren et al., 2000b). Thus we conclude that MMP-9 plays a major role in FM remodeling, weakening and rupture. Our work also demonstrates that MMP-9 levels are an excellent marker for FM strength (El-Khwad et al., 2005, 2006; Kumar et al., 2006; R.M. Moore et al., 2009b) [Fig. 5, 7, 8, 10]. TIMP-3 has a direct correlation with FM rupture strength (unlike TIMP types 1 and 2) and was significantly decreased in the weak zone (El-Khwad et al., 2005, 2006). Unlike other TIMPs, TIMP-3 inhibits all the gelatinases, TNF-α, and also is stored within ECM (Mannello et al., 2001).

MMP activation and apoptosis are often interrelated. The ECM acts a major stabilizing factor in many tissue systems. This stability is compromised when MMP activation leads to the breakdown of ECM leading to apoptosis (Boudreau et al., 1995; Chintala e al., 2002). MMPs may also induce apoptosis by cleaving membrane bound cytokines, including TNFα and FasL (Gearing et al., 1994; Kayagaki et al., 1995). Apoptosis can also induce activation of MMPs. In addition, the same agents which have been reported to cause apoptosis in FM tissue also activate and increase transcription of MMPs, specifically, MMP-1, MMP-9 (So et al., 1992; Fortunato et al., 2002). We have reported a parallel increase in prostaglandins with induction of apoptosis in amnion epithelial, mesenchymal and WISH cells with several non-physiological (actinomycin D, cycloheximide, staurosporin) and physiological (ceramide, lactosylceramide, PGJ2 metabolites) apoptotic agents (Moore et al., 1988, 1993).

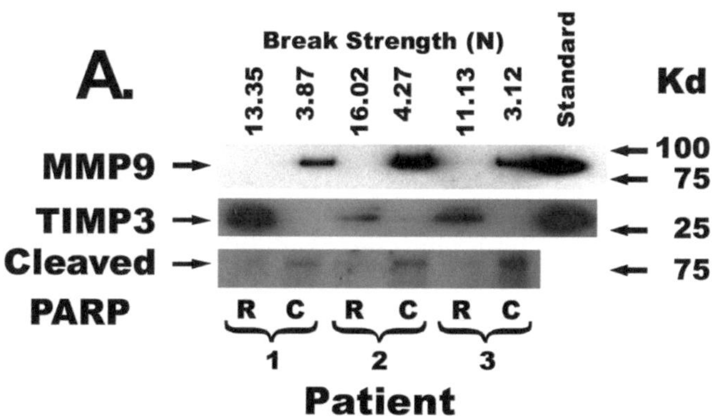

Fig. 5. Biochemical characteristics of fetal membrane regions: Western blot showing differences in MMP-9, TIMP-3 and PARP cleavage between weak, paracervical regions (C) and relatively strong remaining areas (R). Typical Western blot showing parallel strength differences in cervical (C) and remaining (R) areas of the fetal membranes from three patients. (Reproduced with permission from El-Khwad et al. Biol Reprod 72:720-726, 2005.)

Prostaglandins also induce transcription and activate MMPs in most tissues (Lyons et al., 2002; Yoshida et al., 2002). The apoptotic process, thus, potentially weakens FM by eliminating fibroblastic cells, which lay down new collagen, and simultaneously activates

enzyme systems, which break down existing collagen. Activation of MMPs feeds forward to increase apoptosis, which subsequently feeds back to further increase MMP activation.
The physiological mechanisms that initiate MMP activation and apoptosis in FM are not understood. Many constituents of amniotic fluid whose concentrations increase with gestation, with infection, or even with rupture of membranes (TNFα, IL-1β, lactosylceramide, etc) have been shown to cause apoptosis in cells derived from FM and intact membranes (Moore et al., 1988, 1993). Most of these "apoptotic" agents also increase transcription or activation of MMPs, especially MMP-9 (Kumar et al., 2006; R.M. Moore et al., 2009b; Menon et al., 2004; Zaga et al., 2004). Several groups have proposed the synergistic effects of MMP activation and apoptosis leading to rupture of the FM (McLaren et al., 2000a; Fortunato et al., 2000; Bowen et al., 2002; Lei et al., 1996). The promoter polymorphisms in some cytokines (TNFα and IL-1β) and MMPs (-1,-8,-9) have been identified to be associated with PPROM (Ferrand et al., 2002; Fujimoto et al., 2002; Hernandez-Guerrero et al., 2003; Roberts et al., 1999). Patients with these polymorphisms may have earlier initiation of the programmed weakening process resulting in premature rupture of FM and earlier deliveries.

3.3 Structural protein changes in the extracellular matrix of the "weak zone" in FM

As part of the remodeling processes in the weak zone, there must be changes in the structural proteins that could contribute to the weakening of FM. Changes in MMPs and TIMPs on their own do not result in weakening and rupture of FM. The collagen structural units or other components of extracellular matrix (ECM) may undergo degradation resulting in weakening of FM. At least half of the published reports found no decrease in fibrillar collagen in the area of the rupture site in human FM, however (Manabe et al., 1991; Al-Zaid et al., 1980; Evaldson et al., 1987; Halaburt et al., 1989). This is in contrast to animal studies in which collagen degradation is the major factor in remodeling of FM (Lei et al., 1996). There is some evidence that other processes play a crucial role in human FM weakening: 1. Collagen fiber bundles are more dispersed and less well organized in the area of FM rupture site as demonstrated through X-ray diffraction and microscopy (Connon et al., 2007). This disorganization is also supported by evidence that decorin and biglycan are decreased and increased respectively at the site of FM rupture (Meinert et al., 2001 & 2007). Decorin is a protein that promotes protein fiber organization and biglycan has the opposite effect. 2. FM mesenchymal cells undergo "phenotypic switching" from strength promoting myofibroblasts to macrophages that are capable of producing cytokines which weaken the FM (Kim et al., 2008). 3. Numerous studies have demonstrated increased apoptotic activity near the site of SROM (Runic et al., 1998; Yuan et al., 2009; Sagol et al., 2002). 4. We have reported that three members of the fibulin protein family are decreased in the para-cervical weak zone (R.M. Moore et al., 2009a). These proteins are involved in making bridges in the microfibrillar component of the ECM, thus this protein family is clearly of potential interest in the remodeling process that weakens FM prior to rupture. There have been no previous reports describing fibulin family proteins in amnion. We also demonstrated that amnion epithelial and mesenchymal cells produced all three fibulins and their abundance was inhibited by TNF-α, a cytokine involved in weakening of FM (Ossovskaya et al., 2004). We speculate that the amnion microfibrillar layer undergoes significant remodeling with the development of FM weak zone.

3.4 Stretch forces increase rupture strength of the FM rather than decreasing it

It was previously thought that during labor, the FM weakens progressively as a result of repetitive stretching due to contractions. Toppozada (Toppozada et al., 1970) showed that the specific contraction causing rupture of membranes was rarely the most forceful contraction that had been experienced up to that time. They reasoned that prior contractions weakened the membrane so that it subsequently gave way with less force. Lavery described stress relaxation, creep and thinning in FM as part of their study of viscoelastic properties (Lavery et al., 1977, 1982). They assumed, but did not demonstrate, that membranes were weaker (had a lower Rupture Strength) after experiencing viscoelastic, non-recoverable deformation. To test this hypothesis, we collected term vaginally delivered, FM, which were strength tested after being cyclically stretched (Pandey et al., 2007). Rupture Strength and Work to rupture were determined for intact unstretched FM (control) and compared with topographically adjacent FM pieces which were stretched to 75 % of the Rupture Strength of controls, for 5, 10 or more cycles of 10 seconds each. Repeated stretching caused non-elastic deformation of the FM as reported by Lavery et al but the Rupture Strength after repeated stretching paradoxically increased rather than decreased. Stretched FM Rupture Strength increased 20-40% with respect to controls after 5 or 10 cycles. In contrast, Work to Rupture decreased. After a large number of cycles (20-30), Rupture Strength ultimately decreased. The number of cycles of stretch required to promote weakening of the FM was highly variable and may be related to the cycles that the membrane had gone through prior to delivery. When separated FM components were tested, amnion alone showed the same altered pattern of Rupture Strength and Work to Rupture after stretch cycling as the intact tissue - Rupture Strength initially increased while Work to Rupture decreased. Choriodecidua did not exhibit properties of stretch induced deformation. FM thus undergo deformation with stretch cycling. The initial cycles of high force stretching causes an increase in FM Rupture Strength, but decreased Work to Rupture (likely due to the amnion component alone). With continued cycling, Rupture Strength also ultimately decreased. We speculate that collagen fibers in FM may realign during initial stretch cycles as they do in stretched skin and cartilage. This may effectively strain harden the FM, increasing Rupture Strength and thus protecting the FM from precipitous rupture. This protective mechanism may fail after many cycles of stretch allowing FM to rupture at lower Rupture Strength and lower Work to Rupture.

4. Preterm Premature Rupture of FM

The precipitant causes of preterm FM weakening leading to PPROM remain uncertain. Limited data is available on FM physical properties in preterm patients. The studies in our laboratory utilizing our methodology confirm that premature FM are stronger than term with a significant drop-off after 37 to 38 weeks gestation (Rangaswamy et al., 2011; fig. 6.). Other researchers (Pressman et al., 2002; Lavery et al., 1979; Chua et al., 2009) have studied the effects of gestational age on FM strength and noted a statistically significant decrease in FM tensile strength after 39 weeks gestation which is consistent with our findings. Our study is the first to demonstrate heterogeneity in biomechanical properties across preterm FM as we have previously shown in term FM (El-Khwad et al., 2005). This mandates that a greater degree of remodeling and/or degradation would be necessary for preterm FM to rupture than occurs in term FM. Although a definitive para-cervical Weak Zone cannot usually be located in PPROM FM because the para-cervical region cannot be marked prior to delivery, a relative weak zone along the rupture tear line is generally present.

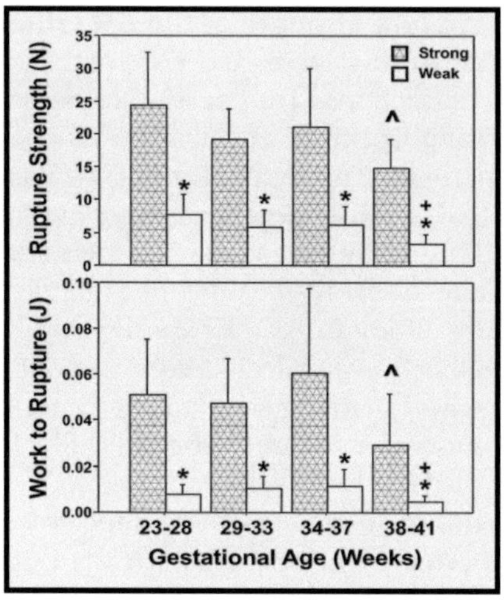

Fig. 6. FM rupture strength (upper panel) and work to rupture (lower panel) comparing the weak zone vs. strong areas across gestational groups: A decreasing trend in both rupture strength and work to rupture is shown from preterm to term gestation (Data are presented as the mean ± SD, +^* indicate $p < 0.001$). Reproduced with permission from Gynecol Obstet Fertil. 2011 ; 39(6):373-377 (Rangaswamy et.al., 2011).

Although the mechanism of FM rupture at term or with PPROM is not well understood, we believe that PPROM occurs due to an abnormal early activation of the processes that weaken FM at term. Supportive findings of this theory are the marked upregulation of MMPs, pro-inflammatory cytokines and chemokines in amniotic fluid and FM in PPROM and chorioamnionitis (Cox et al., 1997; Maymon et al., 1999; Thomakos et al., 2010; Bryant-Greenwood et al., 1995; Fortunato et al., 2003; Riley et al., 1999; Locksmith et al., 2001; Xu et al., 2002). TNF and IL-1β specifically have been shown to induce apoptosis, induce MMP 9 and increase PGE_2 production in chorioamnion and cultured primary amnion cells (R.M. Moore et al., 2009b; Runic et al., 1998; Fortunato et al., 2001; Furuta et al., 2000; Lundin-Schiller et al., 1991; Garcia-Lloret et al., 1996; Lockwood et al., 2008). We previously reported that several physiological agents and reactive oxygen species (hydrogen peroxide) induce apoptosis with concomitant PGE_2 release in amnion derived WISH cells, primary amnion cells and intact amnion (Kumar et al., 2004 a, 2004 b).

Inflammation due to an ascending bacterial infection from the female genital tract remains the most widely speculated cause as up to 55 percent of patients with PPROM had culture or PCR evidence of infection (Jones et al., 2009). Inflammatory processes at sites remote from the female genital tract (e.g.: periodontal infections) may also increase the levels of proinflammatory cytokines at the materno-fetal, interface (Offenbacher et al., 2006; Carta et al., 2004). Decidual hemorrhage/abruption is also highly associated with PPROM (Harger et al., 1990; Salafia et al., 1995). Additional risk factors include advanced maternal age, primiparity, (Ladfors et al., 2000) smoking, (Burguet et al., 2004) short cervical length (Iams et al., 1996) structural abnormality of chorioamniotic membranes (Stuart et al., 2005), and PPROM with preterm birth in a previous pregnancy (Ladfors et al., 2000; Lee et al., 2003; Shen et al., 2008). African American women are at higher risk of PPROM than Caucasian women (Goldenberg et al., 1996a), which might be due to racial differences in the regulation of promoter activity of pro-inflammatory cytokines and MMPs (Simhan et al., 2003; Ferrand et al., 2002).

Two major processes that have been associated with PPROM are inflammation (due to infection and other etiologies) and decidual hemorrhage/abruption. We have developed and utilized a unique model system to investigate FM weakening due to each of these etiologies and identified a pharmacological agent with potential role in preventing this weakening process, which will be discussed in the next two sections.

5. Investigations to understand mechanism(s) of FM weakening and rupture

5.1 Development of an in vitro model system to study the mechanisms of FM rupture

There are no animal models for the study of human FM weakening and rupture. We have used FM strength testing equipment and methods that allow us to systematically measure and map human FM biomechanical properties over the entire FM surface and correlate these with local biochemical properties (as discussed above) in conjunction with an adaptation of the explant culture system developed by Fortunato and Menon (Fortunato et al., 1994) to produce a model system to study the process of human FM weakening (R.M. Moore et al., 2006, 2009b, 2010; Kumar et al., 2011; Mercer et al., 2010). Full thickness FM explants are cut from regions of the FM distant from the Weak Zone of FM from unlabored Cesarean deliveries. The explants are then incubated for 2 to 4 days with agents postulated to affect the weakening process. Biomechanical testing is then performed and correlated with local induced biochemical changes in the immediately adjacent tissue. This model system is novel and unique in its ability to quantitatively measure FM weakening, the major parameter of clinical interest, as well as the associated biochemical changes. We are using this model system to explore the mechanisms by which FM weakening occurs as the result of two processes, *inflammation/infection and decidual hemorrhage/abruption,* which are both highly associated with preterm birth due to PPROM.

5.2 Inflammation/Infection induced FM weakening

Under normal circumstances, pregnancy is regulated by a balanced activity of anti-inflammatory and pro-inflammatory cytokines/chemokines (Ugwumadu et al., 2002; Diehl et al., 2002). They play an important role in placental growth and development (Croy et al., 2002). Progesterone may play an important role in continuation of pregnancy by promoting anti-inflammatory cytokines over pro-inflammatory cytokines. During the end of pregnancy at term, the activity of pro-inflammatory cytokines dominates resulting in the weakening and rupture of FM. At term, the amniotic fluid contains anti-inflammatory cytokines IL-10, IL-4, IL-1 receptor antagonist (Il-1RA) and transforming growth factor -β (TGF-β) [Jones et al., 1997; Dudley et al., 1996; Baergen et al., 1994; Romero et al., 1992b; A.G. Moore et al., 2000; Heikkinen et al., 2001]. The functions of these cytokines include suppressing pro-inflammatory cytokines (by IL-4), modulation of IL-1 mediated inflammatory effects (by IL-1RA) and inhibition of production of pro-inflammatory cytokines and suppression of the activity of antigen presenting cells (by IL-10).

The role of cytokines is not just limited to normal childbirth but also occurs in births (including preterm births) associated with infection. However, there are likely some differences (Bryant-Greenwood et al., 2007; Osman et al., 2006; Haddad et al., 2006; Beutler et al., 2004). The severity of inflammatory response that occurs in normal labor is relatively less compared to that seen in infections (Rusterholz et al., 2007). Relaxins, nuclear factor (NF)-kB and toll-like receptor (TLR)-2 are all part of the inflammatory cascade that result in term/preterm labor or weakening and rupture of FM (Bryant-Greenwood et al., 2009; Millar et al., 1998; Werner et al., 2005; Hoebe et al., 2004). The amniotic fluid in normal uncomplicated pregnancy shows elevated pro-inflammatory cytokines (IL-1β, IL-6 and TNF-α) with increasing gestation (Opsjln et al., 1993; Romero et al., 1990b; Laham et al., 1994 & 1996), which is further increased during labor at term (Opsjln et al., 1993; Romero et al., 1990b; Laham et al., 1994; Cox et al., 1997; Maymon et al., 1999; Gunn et al., 1996; Romero et al., 1990a & 1992a). Infection during pregnancy further elevates the levels of these cytokines in amniotic fluid, FM and decidua (Goldenberg et al., 2000). This fact holds well even in preterm deliveries (compared to term) especially with infection and PPROM (Cox et al., 1997; Maymon et al., 1999; Romero et al., 1988 & 1993). The source of these cytokines is the infiltrating leucocytes as demonstrated by immunolocalization studies of gestational tissues (Young et al., 2002). Both amniotic fluid IL-16 and IL-18 are increased with infection. IL-18 is a pleiotropic cytokine that plays a role in host defense against infection whereas IL-16 is unique, functioning as a chemoattractant, modulator of lymphocytes, monocytes, eosinophils and dendritic cells, and in cell cycle control (Jones et al., 2009). On the other hand, the anti-inflammatory cytokines also increase with term and preterm labor, the most marked elevation occurring in preterm delivery with infection.

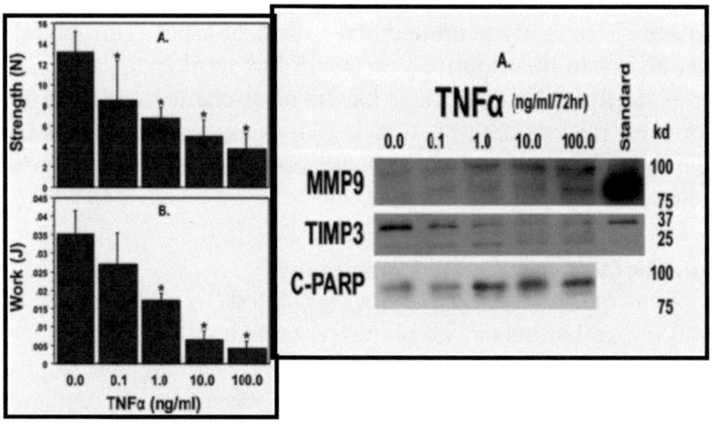

Fig. 7. TNF weakens full thickness FM. [Left] TNF-induced dose-dependent decreases in FM strength (A) and work to rupture (B). Incubations were for 72 h. [Right] TNF (0–100 ng/ml for 72 h) induced increases in MMP9 protein (upper panel) and decreased TIMP3 protein (middle panel) in FM explants in a dose-dependent manner. TNF also induced apoptosis in FM explants as evidenced by cleavage of PARP1 (113 kD) into 85 kD fragments (lower panel). Reproduced with permission from Biol Reprod 74:29-34, 2006 (Kumar D et al., 2006).

The tissue and cellular pathways involved in cytokine induced FM weakening are not fully understood. Although it has been generally assumed that collagen remodeling and apoptosis lead to FM weakening and rupture, this had not been directly demonstrated prior to our recent studies. Using our *in vitro* model system we have shown that inflammatory cytokines (TNF and IL-1β) weaken full thickness FM explants in a dose dependent manner concomitant with biochemical changes that mimic the signature of the natural Weak Zone (Fig. 7.) Cytokines act on FM in a complex manner. As the amnion is the strongest component of the FM, it must be significantly weakened in any mechanistic schema leading to rupture (Arikat et al., 2006). Our published data show that cytokines do not weaken the isolated amnion, but readily weaken amnion when it is adherent to the choriodecidua as part of the full thickness FM (Kumar et al., 2011) [Fig. 8.]. In contrast, conditioned media produced by incubating isolated choriodecidua with cytokines readily weaken the amnion. It is thus clear that a critical cytokine target for FM weakening is in the choriodecidua, where one or more soluble products are produced which are necessary for TNF or IL-1β induced weakening of the amnion.

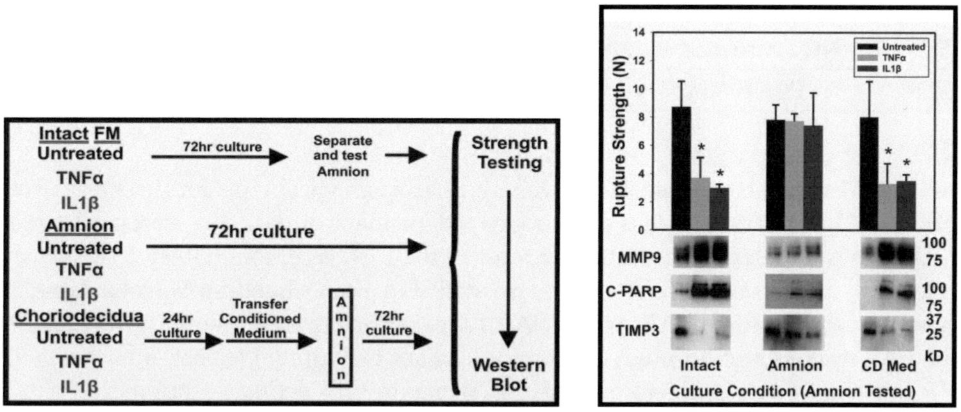

Fig. 8. TNF and IL-1β cannot weaken isolated amnion directly: Experiment description [left] and results [right]. Isolated amnion when incubated with cytokines (center group of results) showed no decrease in strength and minimal changes in MMP9, TIMP3 and cleaved PARP. Amnion exposed to conditioned media from choriodecidua incubated with cytokines showed weakening and biochemical changes (right group of results). Control study results show amnion weakening with intact FM stimulation (left group of results). Reproduced with permission from Placenta 32(3):206-213, 2011 (Kumar D et al., 2011).

5.3 Decidual hemorrhage/abruption induced FM weakening

Thrombin may be produced in FM by decidual hemorrhage/abruption and activation of the extrinsic coagulation cascade. Decidual cells have been shown to have abundant tissue factor thus facilitating the production of Thrombin after hemorrhage (Lockwood et al., 1993 & 2001). PPROM patients have increased tissue factor (Erez et al., 2008). Thrombin is known to have many actions not related to coagulation. Thrombin can act directly on the extracellular matrix (ECM) by converting MMPs 1, 2, 3 and 9 from zymogen to active forms (Fang et al., 2006; Lafleur et al., 2001). Alternatively, it can act indirectly, through cells, by activating Protease Activated Receptors (PAR) (Hollenberg et al., 2005; Ossovskaya et al., 2004) and thereby inducing MMPs and other proteins, which may remodel the ECM. Thrombin has been shown to induce MMP9 in monocytes (Chi-Jen Chang et al., 2009), oral squamous cell carcinoma (Liu et al., 2001), human dermal fibroblast (Wang et al., 2007) and mesangial cells (Liu et al., 2000), microvascular endothelial cells from human brain (Kolev et al., 2003) and rabbit aortic smooth muscle cells (Fabunmi et al., 1996). Four PARs (1 - 4) have been described but none have yet been reported in FM. PARs are activated by the proteolytic activity of thrombin and other serine proteases (thrombin acts on PARs 1, 3 and 4 and trypsin acts upon PAR 2). These enzymes cleave the N-terminus of the receptor, which thereafter permanently acts as a tethered ligand causing a physiological response. Synthetic PAR activating peptides (PAR-AP) composed of the initial amino acid string of the new N-terminus generated when thrombin cleaves PAR, can activate their specific PAR independent of thrombin or receptor cleavage (Refer table below).

Receptor	Activating Peptide	Control Peptide
PAR 1	TFLLR-NH2	FTLLR-NH2
PAR 2	SLIGRL-NH2; 2furoyl-LIGRLO-NH2	LSIGRL-NH2; 2furoyl-OLRGIL-NH2
PAR 3	NOT activated by PAR-APs	---------
PAR 4	AYPGKF-NH2	YAPGKF-NH2

Table 1.

These PAR-APs have been used extensively as pharmacological tools for probing the effects of specific PAR activation in cells and tissues independent of the other effects of thrombin. PAR-APs are commercially available for most of the PAR receptors (table). Inactive control peptides with a reversal of two AA's are also available (Ramachandran & Hollenberg, 2008). We have evidence that the PAR-AP for PAR 1 weakens isolated amnion (fig 10 – sub figure 2). The PAR receptors act through G-proteins families including: I (cAMP inhibitory), 12/13 (Raf/Ras activation) or q (calcium signaling) which in turn activate a number of signaling cascades including MAP kinases, Akt/PKB, P13 kinase and NFkB (101).
Our recent report demonstrates that Thrombin weakens full thickness FM in a dose dependent fashion in our model system (Moore et al., 2010, fig. 9). We have also reported that Thrombin increases both the zymogen and active forms of MMP-9 and MMP-3 in the amnion (Furuta et al., 2000). The latter is particularly interesting as MMP-3 can activate other MMPs, especially MMP-2, which is prevalent in the amnion but is not further induced by either cytokines or Thrombin.

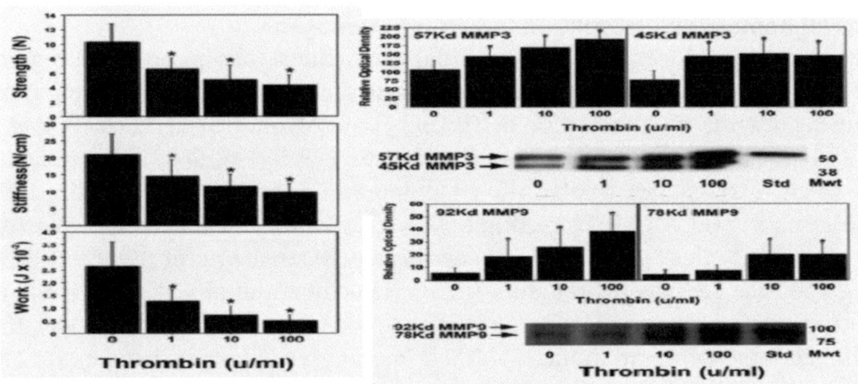

Fig. 9. Thrombin weakens full thickness FM. [Left] Thrombin-induced dose-dependent decreases in FM strength, stiffness and work to rupture. All incubations were for 48 h. (* P < 0.01). [Right] Thrombin induced increases in MMP3 protein (upper panel) and MMP9 protein (lower panel) in FM explants in a dose-dependent manner. (Reproduced with permission from Moore et al. Placenta 2010.)

In further work we have found that, unlike cytokines, thrombin can directly weaken the isolated amnion. The critical targets for thrombin are thus in amnion rather than the choriodecidua. [Fig. 10 – subfigures 1, 3 & 4]

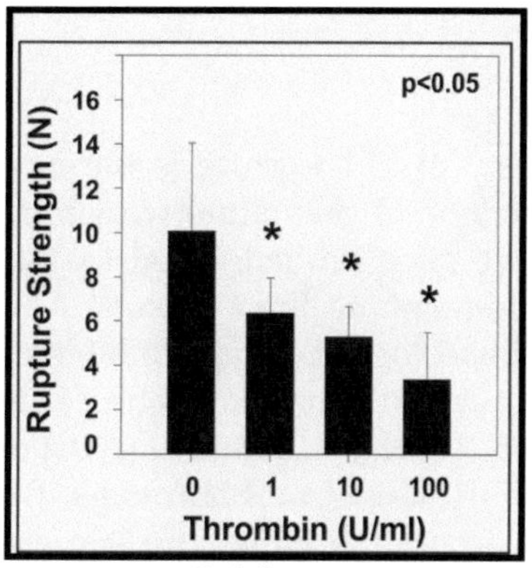

Subfigure 1

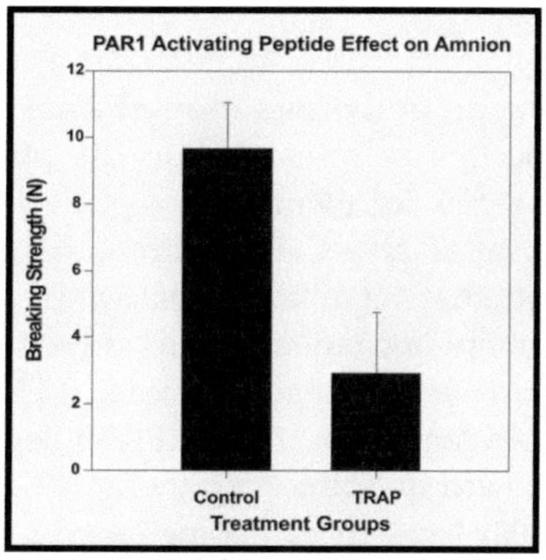

Subfigure 2

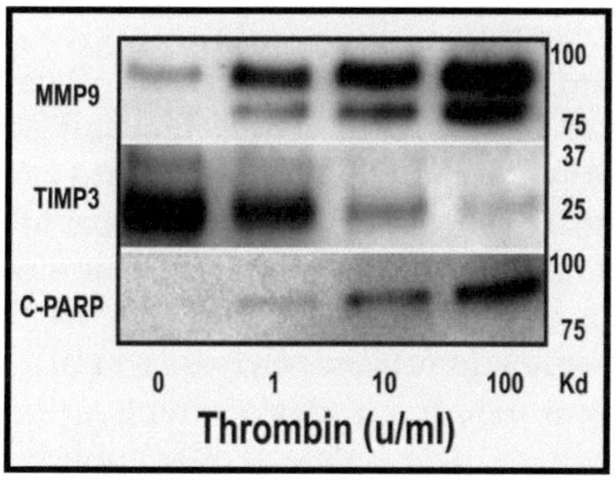

Subfigure 3

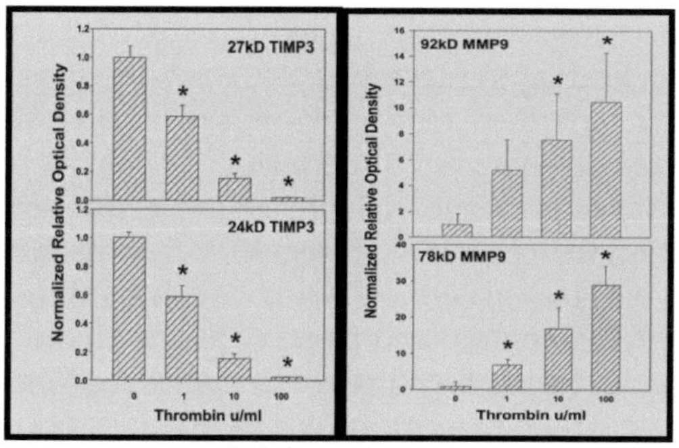

Subfigure 4

Fig. 10. [Top Left] Thrombin weakens isolated amnion. (* p < .01 vs. control),
[Top Right] PAR 1 (1 uM) activating peptide (TRAP) weakens isolated amnion (p<.001),
[Below] Thrombin increases MMP9, decreases TIMP3 and increases PARP cleavage in isolated amnion (all *p<.001). . (Reproduced with permission from Kumar et al. Placenta 2011.)

5.4 Inflammatory cytokines and thrombin have different mechanisms of FM weakening

As the amnion is the strongest component of the FM, it must be significantly weakened in any mechanistic schema leading to rupture. For this reason agents that weaken FM were tested for their effect upon isolated amnion membranes. Cytokines (TNF or IL-1β) do not weaken the isolated amnion, but readily weaken amnion when it is adherent to the choriodecidua as part of the full thickness FM. In contrast, conditioned media produced by incubating isolated choriodecidua with these cytokines readily weaken the amnion. It is thus clear that a critical cytokine target for FM weakening is in the choriodecidua, where one or more soluble products are produced which are necessary for TNF or IL-1β induced weakening of the amnion (Kumar et al., 2011). On the other hand Thrombin can directly weaken the isolated amnion. The critical targets for Thrombin induced FM weakening are thus in amnion rather than the choriodecidua (Kumar et al., 2011).

6. Investigations targeting the potential prevention of FM weakening and rupture

6.1 Tissue repair and prevention of weakness

A major objective of research into the physiology of FM rupture is the development of possible strategies for membrane repair or prevention of premature weakening. Studies of tissue repair after physically induced injury have been limited. Artal (Artal et al., 1976) demonstrated that membranes placed in pseudo-amniotic fluid become weaker over 24 hours but remain unchanged if a mixture of pharmacological enzyme inhibitors is included. The tissue surrounding a stab wound in FM has been shown to be viable for up to 12 days but the wound remained unhealed (Devlieger et al., 2000a). Millar et al (2003) demonstrated increased growth of amnion epithelium with IGF-II. Using a rabbit model, Devlieger et al (2000b & 2003) have shown some success in incorporating plugs into iatrogenic ruptured sites. Growth factors, TGFβ and FGFβ, which normally accelerate repair in other tissues, were shown by the same group to improve the rate of FM repair, although the concomitant increased inflammatory response was of concern because of its possible exacerbation of events leading to premature delivery (Devlieger et al., 2003). FM injured *in vitro,* thus seem to have minimal tendency for self-repair. Clinical studies of FM sealants and sealing techniques have been undertaken in hopes of restoring amniotic fluid volume and averting the risks of prolonged oligohydramnios after extremely early PPROM. An *in vitro* study has revealed that platelets aggregate with exposure to amnion, but not to chorion or amniotic fluid, and that platelet adhesion and activation occur with exposure to the connective tissues underlying amnion and chorion but not amniotic epithelium (Louis-Sylvestre et al., 1998). Similarly, Harmali et al have demonstrated improved membrane tensile strength (Rupture Tension, Strain to Rupture, and Work to Rupture) with iatrogenic defects after application of a fibrin sealant, but that the membrane strength remains less than that of unruptured membrane segments (Harmanli et al., 1998). Fibrin/thrombin based sealants, but not platelet infusions, have been shown to cause temporary cessation of leakage (Reddy et al., 2001). Regarding non-biologic barriers, O'Brien et al (2001) evaluated gelatin sponge (Gelfoam, TM) applied over larger defects and found it to effectively dam linear defects of up to 7 mm in length, but not complex defects. The ability to fuse ("weld") FM with Nd: YAG Laser applied to polytetrafluoroethylene has also been demonstrated *in-vitro,* though the ability of such intervention to seal a membrane defect has not (Mendoza et al., 1999).

There has been some success in the treatment of iatrogenic membrane rupture. In 1999, Quintero and co-workers (Quintero et al., 1998 & 1999) demonstrated successful membrane sealing for persistent oligohydramnios after amniocentesis and fetoscopy, using intra-amniotic injection of platelets and cryoprecipitate ("amniopatch") through a 22-gauge needle. Successful membrane sealing has been achieved with intrauterine injection of gelatin sponge (O'Brien et al., 2002). Sciscione and co-workers (2001) were able to achieve cessation of leakage and restoration of normal amniotic fluid volume in some women with intracervical instillation of fibrin sealants. However, the need for concurrent cervical cerclage placement to decrease fluid leakage has been described (Baumgarten & Moser, 1986). Young and colleagues (Young et al., 2000, 2004a) demonstrated successful endoscopically guided sealing of an iatrogenic membrane defect using maternal platelets and fibrinogen/thrombin and subsequently demonstrated success with fibrin glue and powdered collagen slurry applied to puncture sites. While these studies, and other small case series, have raised the potential that membrane sealing can be performed effectively when the defect occurs in otherwise normal FM, further study regarding the optimal timing and method of intervention after iatrogenic PROM is needed.

Ultimately, because of the presence of antecedent membrane degradation and sub-clinical inflammation in the fetal membranes, membrane sealing may not be appropriate for those with spontaneous membrane rupture. It is not surprising that membranes that have ruptured as the result of having undergone extensive extracellular remodeling and cellular apoptosis may not readily reverse their physiological direction and repair themselves. Further study regarding the maternal/fetal risks and fetal benefits of invasive interventions for membrane rupture remote from term are warranted before such practices are incorporated into clinical practice. A detailed understanding of the process of physiological and pathological fetal membrane weakening may allow appropriate early intervention. Our models of in vitro tissue weakening with biochemical agents and stretch may prove useful in evaluating potential repair strategies.

6.2 Prevention of weakening and rupture – Identification of at risk pregnancies

If the potential for FM repair after rupture is limited, perhaps premature weakening of the fetal membranes can be prevented. To be medically and ethically acceptable, any procedure done on pregnant women to prevent possible FM weakening must be either totally innocuous or highly targeted toward women at significant risk for PPROM. In order to target women at risk they must first be reliably identified.

Spontaneous preterm birth due to preterm labor and PROM is associated with a variety of clinical characteristics and also with abnormal ancillary test findings (e.g. short cervix on transvaginal ultrasound, a positive cervicovaginal fetal-fibronectin screen) (Rangaswamy et al., 2011; Iams et al., 1996; Mercer et al., 1996; Goldenberg et al., 1996b). However, such evaluations are neither sensitive nor specific when applied to asymptomatic women, and there is significant overlap in the characteristics of women who ultimately deliver due to preterm labor and PROM (Mercer et al., 2000). As such, it remains difficult to identify those who will develop PROM before the fact. Recently, several groups have demonstrated that African Americans, a group with a high incidence of PPROM with early delivery, have a higher incidence of certain more active polymorphisms of MMPs and pro-inflammatory cytokines (Ferrand et al., 2002; Fujimoto et al., 2002; Hernandez-Guerrero et al., 2003; Roberts et al., 1999). It is possible that a combination of genes and historical factors could eventually lead to prediction of risk of PPROM with adequate certainty that procedures designed to prevent FM rupture that carry some inherent risk would be justifiable.

In the presence of minimal or no identified risk, administration of vitamin C alone or in combination with vitamin E has been suggested for the prevention of PPROM, mainly for their antioxidant effect (Siega-Riz et al., 2003). However, there are concerns regarding the use of vitamin C as it can increase or decrease apoptosis (Orzechowski et al., 2002) depending on the cell system, dose, and co-effectors present. We have shown that vitamin C does not inhibit, and may exacerbate H_2O_2 induced apoptosis in amnion-derived WISH cells, amnion cell cultures, and amnion membrane explants (Kumar et al., 2004a, 2004b). In vivo studies have also shown mixed results with use of vitamin C. Although a single clinical trial of oral vitamin C demonstrated a decrease in PROM but not premature delivery, three much larger studies showed increased PROM and PPROM in the vitamin-supplemented groups (Spinnato et al., 2008; Hauth et al., 2010; Xu et al., 2010). Warnings were issued in these publications about use of vitamins C/E, at least at the doses utilized. Using our *in vitro* model of TNF-α-induced FM weakening, we have demonstrated that vitamin C preincubation does not prevent TNF-α induced FM weakness. In fact, high doses of vitamin C actually increase MMP-9 activity and weaken the FM.

6.3 Alpha-Lipoic Acid (LA) inhibits cytokine and thrombin induced weakening

In contrast, we have shown that Lipoic acid, a naturally occurring dietary supplement [routinely used as part of prophylaxis for diabetic neuropathy (Ziegler et al., 2009)], with anti-oxidant and NFkB inhibitory properties prevented TNF-α induced FM weakening and also prevented concomitant TNF-α induced increases in MMP-9 and PGE2 (Fig. 11.) [R.M. Moore et al, 2009]. The mechanism of Lipoic acid action is unclear but this effect on FM is not isolated. It has been shown to inhibit TNF- α induced NF-κB transcriptional activity and MMP-9 expression in vascular smooth muscle cells, and attenuate LPS-induced NF-κB: DNA-binding in monocytes by activating the PI3K/AKT pathway (Kim et al., 2007; Zhang et al., 2007). It also metabolically regenerates glutathione and other antioxidants (Bilska & Wlodek et al., 2005). We have also demonstrated that LA inhibits FM weakening by Thrombin and inhibits Thrombin induced weakening of the isolated amnion (Kumar et al., 2011). As Lipoic acid inhibits both cytokine and thrombin induced FM weakening and remodeling, it is a promising candidate for possible clinical use to prevent PPROM. LA has been investigated in dozens of clinical trials (41 trials are now listed on clinicaltrials.gov) with no adverse effects reported. Unfortunately, all of the trials excluded pregnant women (Clinicaltrials.gov). There have also been promising toxicity studies in pregnant rats (Shirpoor A et al., 2008). A trial of LA in pregnant women at risk for PPROM awaits more definitive information of its mechanism of action in the prevention of FM weakening in addition to safety data.

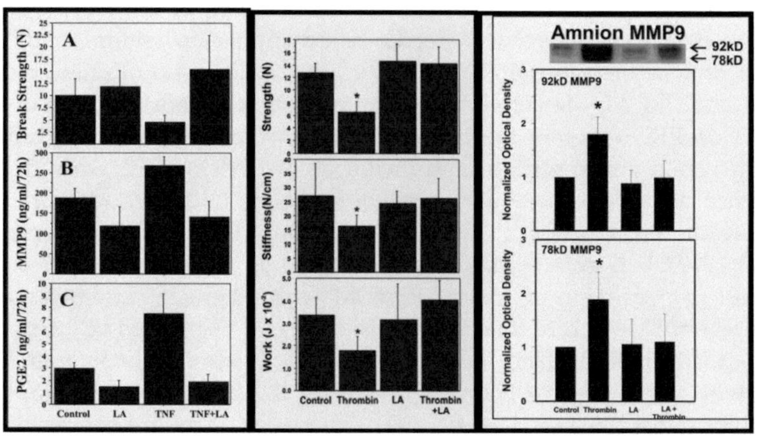

Fig. 11. Lipoic Acid inhibits TNF and Thrombin induced weakening and biochemical changes: [Left] TNF (50 ng/ml) induced weakening, increases in MMP9 and increases in PGE2 are inhibited by Lipoic Acid (0.5 mM); [Middle] Thrombin (10 U/ml) induced changes in biomechanics are inhibited by lipoic acid (.25 mM); [Right] Thrombin (10 U/ml) induced increases in MMP9 zymogen and active forms are inhibited by Lipoic Acid (.25 mM). Reproduced from Moore et al. Biol Reprod 80:781-87, 2009 and Placenta 31:886-892, 2010 with permission.

7. Conclusions

It had been previously thought that the mechanical force due to uterine contraction during labor weakens the FM. This theory has been negated by the clinical fact that the FM rupture prior to the onset of contractions and by our finding that the force required to rupture the membranes is increased rather than decreased by cyclical mechanical stretching of FM *in vitro*. We have demonstrated that a weak zone develops in the FM overlying the cervix at the end of gestation. This weak zone is associated with collagen remodeling and apoptosis as evidenced by elevated MMP-9, decreased TIMP-3 and elevated PARP cleavage. Even though the process of weakening in term FM has been described, detailed molecular mechanisms and the initiating signals have yet to be unraveled. Our in vitro model system has facilitated demonstration that the weakening effect of cytokines (TNF-α and IL-1β) and thrombin on FM results in collagen remodeling and apoptosis, similar to that observed in term FM delivered by unlabored cesarean and labored vaginal deliveries. Lipoic acid has been shown to inhibit the weakening effect of both these agents *in vitro,* suggesting that it could be a promising drug in the prevention of PPROM. However, studies are required to demonstrate its safety and efficacy in pregnant women.

8. References

Al-Zaid, N.S., Bou-Resli, M.N. & Goldspink, G. (1980). Bursting pressure and collagen content of fetal membranes and their relation to premature rupture of the membranes, *Br J Obstet Gynaecol* 87(3):227-229.

Arechavaleta-Velasco, F., Ogando, D., Parry, S. & Vadillo-Ortega, F. (2002). Production of matrix metalloproteinase-9 in lipopolysaccharide-stimulated human amnion occurs through an autocrine and paracrine proinflammatory cytokine-dependent system, *Biol Reprod* 67(6):1952-1958.

Arikat, S., Novince, R., Kumar, D., Fox, J., Mercer, B., Mansour, J.M. & Moore J.J. (2006). Separation of amnion from Choriodecidua is an integral event to the rupture of normal term fetal membranes and constitutes a significant proportion of the work required, *Am J OB Gynecol.* 194 (1):211-217.

Artal, R., Sokol, R.J., Neuman, M., Burstein, A.H. & Stojkov, J. (1976). The mechanical properties of prematurely and non--prematurely ruptured membranes. Methods and preliminary results, *Am J Obstet Gynecol.* 125(5):655-659.

Athayde, N., Romero, R., Gomez, R., Maymon, E., Pacora, P., Mazor, M., Yoon, B.H., Fortunato, S., Menon, R., Ghezzi, F & Edwin, S.S. (1999). Matrix metalloproteinases-9 in preterm and term human parturition, *J Matern Fetal Med.* 8(5):213-219.

Athayde, N., Romero, R., Maymon, E., Gomez, R., Pacora, P., Yoon, B.H. & Edwin, S.S. (2000). Interleukin 16 in pregnancy, parturition, rupture of fetal membranes, and microbial invasion of the amniotic cavity, *Am J Obstet Gynecol.* 182(1 Pt 1):135-141.

Bachmaier, N. & Graf, R. (1999). The anchoring zone in the human placental amnion: bunches of oxytalan and collagen connect mesoderm and epithelium, *Anat Embryol (Berl).* 200(1):81-90.

Baergen, R., Benirschke, K. & Ulich, T.R. (1994). Cytokine expression in the placenta. The role of interleukin 1 and interleukin 1 receptor antagonist expression in chorioamnionitis and parturition, *Arch Pathol Lab Med.* 118(1):52-55.

Baumgarten, K. & Moser, S. (1986). The technique of fibrin adhesion for premature rupture of the membranes during pregnancy, *J Perinat Med.* 14(1):43-49.

Behrman, R.E., Adashi, E.Y., Allen, M.C., Carouso, R.L et al. (2006). Preterm Birth: Causes, Consequences, Prevention, *Report of the Institute of Medicine.*

Beutler, B. (2004). Inferences, questions and possibilities in Toll-like receptor signaling, *Nature.* 430(6996):257-263.

Bilic, G., Brubaker, C., Messersmith, P.B., Mallik, A.S., Quinn, T.M., Haller, C., Done, E., Gucciardo, L., Zeisberger, S.M., Zimmermann, R., Deprest, J. & Zisch, A.H. (2010). Injectable candidate sealants for fetal membrane repair: bonding and toxicity in vitro, *Am J Obstet Gynecol.* 202(1):85.e1-9

Bilska, A. & Włodek, L. (2005). Lipoic acid - the drug of the future? *Pharmacol Rep.* 57(5):570-7.

Boudreau, N., Sympson, C.J., Werb, Z. & Bissell, M.J. (1995). Suppression of ICE and apoptosis in mammary epithelial cells by extracellular matrix, *Science.* 267(5199):891-893.

Bowen, J.M., Chamley, L., Keelan, J.A. & Mitchell, M.D. (2002). Cytokines of the placenta and extra-placental membranes: roles and regulation during human pregnancy and parturition, *Placenta.* 23(4):257-273.

Bryant-Greenwood, G.D. & Yamamoto, S.Y. (1995). Control of peripartal collagenolysis in the human chorion-decidua, *Am J Obstet Gynecol.* 172(1 Pt 1):63-70.

Bryant-Greenwood G.D., Kern, A., Yamamoto, S.Y., Sadowsky, D.W. & Novy, M.J. (2007). Relaxin and the human fetal membranes, *Reprod Sci.* 14(8 Suppl):42-45.

Bryant-Greenwood, G.D., Yamamoto, S.Y., Sadowsky, D.W., Gravett, M.G. & Novy, M.J. (2009). Relaxin stimulates interleukin-6 and interleukin-8 secretion from the extraplacental chorionic cytotrophoblast, *Placenta.* 30(7):599-606.

Buhimschi, I.A., Kramer, W.B., Buhimschi, C.S., Thompson, L.P. & Weiner, C.P. (2000). Reduction-oxidation (redox) state regulation of matrix metalloproteinase activity in human fetal membranes, *Am J Obstet Gynecol.* 182(2):458-464.

Burguet, A., Kaminski, M., Abraham-Lerat, L., Schaal, J.P., Cambonie, G., Fresson, J., Grandjean, H., Truffert, P., Marpeau, L., Voyer, M., Rozé, J.C., Treisser, A. & Larroque, B; EPIPAGE Study Group. (2004). The complex relationship between smoking in pregnancy and very preterm delivery, *BJOG.* 111(3):258-265.

Carta, G., Persia, G., Falciglia, K. & Iovenitti, P. (2004). Periodontal disease and poor obstetrical outcome, *Clin Exp Obstet Gynecol.* 31(1):47-49.

Chang, C.J., Hsu, L.A., Ko, Y.H., Chen, P.L., Chuang, Y.T., Lin, C.Y., Liao, C.H. & Pang, J.H. (2009). Thrombin regulates matrix metalloproteinase-9 expression in human monocytes, *Biochemical and Biophysical Research Communications.* 385(2):241–246.

Chintala, S.K., Zhang, X., Austin, J.S. & Fini, M.E. (2002). Deficiency in matrix metalloproteinase gelatinase B (MMP-9) protects against retinal ganglion cell death after optic nerve ligation, *J Biol Chem.* 277(49):47461-47468.

Chua, W.K. & Oyen, M.L. (2009). Do we know the strength of the chorioamnion? A critical review and analysis, *Eur J Obstet Gynecol Reprod Biol.* 144 Suppl 1:S128-33.

Connon, C.J., Nakamura, T., Hopkinson, A., Quantock, A., Yagi, N., Doutch, J. & Meek, K.M. (2007). The biomechanics of amnion rupture: an X-ray diffraction study, *PLoS One.* 2(11):e1147.

Cox, S.M., Casey, M.L. & MacDonald, P.C. (1997). Accumulation of interleukin-1beta and interleukin-6 in amniotic fluid: a sequela of labour at term and preterm, *Hum Reprod Update.* 3(5):517-527.

Croy, B.A., Chantakru, S., Esadeg, S., Ashkar, A.A. & Wei, Q. (2002). Decidual natural killer cells: key regulators of placental development (a review), *J Reprod Immunol.* 57(1-2):151-168.

Devlieger, R., Gratacos, E., Wu, J., Verbist, L., Pijnenborg, R. & Deprest, J.A. (2000a). An organ-culture for in vitro fetal membrane healing capacity, *Eur J Obstet Gynecol Reprod Biol.* 92(1):145-150.

Devlieger, R., Deprest, J.A., Gratacós, E., Pijnenborg, R., Leask, R. & Riley, S.C. (2000b). Matrix metalloproteinases -2 and -9 and their endogenous tissue inhibitors in fetal membrane repair following fetoscopy in a rabbit model, M*ol Hum Reprod.* 6(5):479-485.

Devlieger, R., Ardon, H., Verbist, L., Gratacós, E., Pijnenborg, R. & Deprest, J.A. (2003). Increased polymorphonuclear infiltration and iatrogenic amniotic band after closure of fetoscopic access sites with a bioactive membrane in the rabbit at midgestation, *Am J Obstet Gynecol.* 188(3):844-848.

Devlieger, R., Millar, L.K., Bryant-Greenwood, G., Lewi, L. & Deprest, J.A. (2006). Fetal membrane healing after spontaneous and iatrogenic membrane rupture: a review of current evidence, *Am J Obstet Gynecol.* 195(6):1512-1520.

Diehl, S. & Rincón, M. (2002). The two faces of IL-6 on Th1/Th2 differentiation, *Mol Immunol.* 39(9):531-536.

Dudley, D.J., Hunter, C., Varner, M.W & Mitchell, M.D. (1996). Elevation of amniotic fluid interleukin-4 concentrations in women with preterm labor and chorioamnionitis, *Am J Perinatol.* 13(7):443-447.

El-Khwad, M., Stetzer, B., Moore, R.M., Kumar, D., Mercer, B., Arikat, S., Redline, R.W., Mansour, J.M. & Moore, J.J. (2005). Pre-labor fetal membranes have a weak zone overlying the lower uterine pole and cervix, *Biol Reprod.* 72(3):720-726.

El-Khwad, M., Stetzer, B., Moore, R.M., Kumar, D., Arikat, S., Redline, R.W., Mansour, J.M. & Moore, J.J. (2006). A circumscribed area along the tear line in human fetal membranes of vaginal deliveries demonstrates marked physical weakness and coincident evidence of apoptosis and remodeling, *JSGI.* 13(3):191-195.

Erez, O., Espinoza, J., Chaiworapongsa, T., Gotsch, F., Kusanovic, J.P., Than, N.G., Mazaki-Tovi, S., Vaisbuch, E., Papp, Z., Yoon, B.H., Han, Y.M., Hoppensteadt, D., Fareed, J., Hassan, S.S. & Romero, R. (2008). A link between a hemostatic disorder and preterm PROM: a role for tissue factor and tissue factor pathway inhibitor, *J Matern Fetal Neonatal Med.* 21(10):732-744.

Evaldson, G.R., Larsson, B. & Jiborn, H. (1987). Is the collagen content reduced when the fetal membranes rupture? A clinical study of term and prematurely ruptured membranes, *Gynecol Obstet Invest.* 24(2):92-94.

Fabunmi, R.P., Baker, A.H., Murray, E.J., Booth, R.F. & Newby, A.C. (1996). Divergent regulation by growth factors and cytokines of 95 and 72 kDa gelatinases and tissue inhibitors or metalloproteinases-1, -2, and -3 in rabbit aortic smooth muscle cells, *Biochem. J.* 315(Pt 1)335–342.

Fang, Q., Liu, X., Al-Mugotir, M., Kobayashi, T., Abe, S., Kohyama, T. & Rennard, S.I. (2006). Thrombin and TNF-alpha/IL-1beta synergistically Induce Fibroblast-Mediated Collagen Gel Degradation, *Am J Respir Cell Mol Biol.* 35(6):714–721.

Ferrand, P.E., Parry, S., Sammel, M., Macones, G.A., Kuivaniemi, H., Romero, R. & Strauss III, J.F. (2002). A polymorphism in the matrix metalloproteinase- 9 promoter is associated with increased risk of preterm premature rupture of membranes in African Americans, *Mol Hum Reprod.* 8(5):494-501.

Fortunato, S.J., Menon, R., Swan, K.F. & Lyden, T.W. (1994). Organ culture of amniochorionic membrane in vitro, *Am J Reprod Immunol.* 32(3):184-187.

Fortunato, S.J., Menon, R. & Lombardi, S.J. (1999). MMP/TIMP imbalance in amniotic fluid during PROM: An indirect support for endogenous pathway to membrane rupture, *J Perinat Med.* 27(5):362-368.

Fortunato, S.J., Menon, R., Bryant, C. & Lombardi, S.J. (2000). Programmed cell death (apoptosis) as a possible pathway to metalloproteinase activation and fetal membrane degradation in premature rupture of membranes, *Am J Obstet Gynecol.* 182(6):1468-1476.

Fortunato, S.J. & Menon, R. (2001). Distinct molecular events suggest different pathways for preterm labor and premature rupture of membranes, *Am J Obstet Gynecol.* 184(7):1399-1405.

Fortunato, S.J., Menon, R. & Lombardi, S.J. (2002). Role of tumor necrosis factor-alpha in the premature rupture of membranes and preterm labor pathways, *Am J Obstet Gynecol.* 187(5):1159-1162.

Fortunato, S.J. & Menon, R. (2003). IL-1 beta is a better inducer of apoptosis in human fetal membranes than IL-6. *Placenta.* 24(10): 922-928.

Fujimoto, T., Parry, S., Urbanek, M., Sammel, M., Macones, G., Kuivaniemi, H., Romero, R. & Strauss, J.F. 3rd. (2002). A single nucleotide polymorphism in the matrix metalloproteinase-1 (MMP-1) promoter influences amnion cell MMP-1 expression and risk for preterm premature rupture of the fetal membranes, *J Biol Chem.* 277(8):6296-6302.

Furuta, I., Yamada, H., Sagawa, T. & Fujimoto, S. (2000). Effects of inflammatory cytokines on prostaglandin E(2) production from human amnion cells cultured in serum-free condition, *Gynecol Obstet Invest.* 49(2):93-97.

Garcia-Lloret, M.I., Yui, J., Winkler-Lowen, B. & Guilbert, L.J. (1996). Epidermal growth factor inhibits cytokine-induced apoptosis of primary human trophoblasts, *J Cell Physiol.* 167(2):324-332.

Gearing, A.J., Beckett, P., Christodoulou, M., Churchill, M., Clements, J., Davidson, A.H,, Drummond, A.H,, Galloway, W.A., Gilbert, R., Gordon, J.L., et al. (1994). Processing of tumour necrosis factor-alpha precursor by metalloproteinases, *Nature.* 370(6490):555-557.

Goldenberg, R.L., Mercer, B.M., Meis, P.J., Copper, R.L., Das, A. & McNellis D. (1996b). The preterm prediction study: fetal fibronectin testing and spontaneous preterm birth. NICHD Maternal Fetal Medicine Units Network, *Obstet Gynecol.* 87(5 Pt 1):643-648.

Goldenberg, R.L., Cliver, S.P., Mulvihill FX, Hickey, C.A., Hoffman, H.J., Klerman, L.V. & Johnson, M.J. (1996a). Medical, psychosocial, and behavioral risk factors do not explain the increased risk for low birth weight among black women, *Am J Obstet Gynecol.* 175(5):1317-1324.

Goldenberg, R.L., Hauth, J.C. & Andrews, W.W. (2000). Intrauterine infection and preterm delivery, *N Engl J Med.* 342(20):1500-1507.

Gunn, L., Hardiman, P., Tharmaratnam, S., Lowe, D. & Chard, T. (1996). Measurement of interleukin-1 alpha and interleukin-6 in pregnancy-associated tissues, *Reprod Fertil Dev.* 8(7):1069-1073.

Haddad, R., Tromp, G., Kuivaniemi, H., Chaiworapongsa, T., Kim, Y.M., Mazor, M. & Romero, R. (2006). Human spontaneous labor without histologic chorioamnionitis is characterized by an acute inflammation gene expression signature, *Am J Obstet Gynecol.* 195(2):394.e1-24.

Halaburt, J.T., Uldbjerg, N., Helmig, R. & Ohlsson, K. (1989). The concentration of collagen and the collagenolytic activity in the amnion and the chorion, *Eur J Obstet Gynecol Reprod Biol.* 31(1):75-82.

Han YM, Romero R, Kim JS, Tarca AL, Kim SK, Draghici S, Kusanovic JP, Gotsch F, Mittal P, Hassan SS, Kim CJ. (2008). Region-specific gene expression profiling: novel evidence for biological heterogeneity of the human amnion. *Biol Reprod.* 79(5):954-61.

Harger, J.H., Hsing, A.W., Tuomala, R.E., Gibbs, R.S., Mead, P.B. & Eschenbach, D.A. (1990). Risk factors for preterm rupture of fetal membranes: a multicenter case-control study, *Am J Obstet Gynecol.* 163 (1 Pt 1):130–137.

Harmanli, O.H., Wapner, R.J. & Lontz, J.F. (1998). Efficacy of fibrin glue for in vitro sealing of human chorioamniotic membranes, *J Reprod Med.* 43(11):986-990.

Hauth, J.C., Clifton, R.G., Roberts, J.M., Spong, C.Y., Myatt, L., Kenneth, J., et al for the Eunice Kennedy Shriver National Institute of Child Health and Human Development (NICHD) Maternal-Fetal Medicine Units Network (MFMU). Vitamin C and E Supplementation to Prevent Spontaneous Preterm Birth: A Randomized Controlled Trial, *Obstet Gynecol.* 2010; 116(3):653-658.

Heikkinen, J., Möttönen, M., Pulkki, K., Lassila, O. & Alanen, A. (2001). Cytokine levels in midtrimester amniotic fluid in normal pregnancy and in the prediction of pre-eclampsia, *Scand J Immunol.* 53(3):310-314.

Hernandez-Guerrero, C., Monzon-Bordonaba, F., Jimenez-Zamudio, L., Ahued-Ahued, R., Arechavaleta-Velasco, F., Strauss, J.F. 3rd. &Vadillo-Ortega, F. (2003). In-vitro secretion of proinflammatory cytokines by human amniochorion carrying hyper-responsive gene polymorphisms of tumour necrosis factor-alpha and interleukin-1beta, *Mol Hum Reprod.* 9(10):625-629.

Hoebe, K., Janssen, E. & Beutler, B. (2004). The interface between innate and adaptive immunity, *Nat Immunol.* 5(10):971-974.

Hollenberg, M.D. (2005). Physiology and Pathophysiology of Proteinase-Activated Receptors (PARs): Proteinases as Hormone-Like Signal Messengers: PARs and More, *J Pharmacol Sci.* 97(1):8-13.

Iams, J.D., Goldenberg, R.L., Meis, P.J., et al. (1996). The length of the cervix and the risk of spontaneous premature delivery: National Institute of Child Health and Human Development Maternal Fetal Medicine Unit Network, *N Engl J Med.* 334(9):567-572.

Jones, C.A., Finlay-Jones, J.J. & Hart, P.H. (1997). Type-1 and type-2 cytokines in human late-gestation decidual tissue, *Biol Reprod.* 57(2):303-311.

Jones, H.E., Harris, K.A., Azizia, M., Bank, L., Carpenter, B., et al. (2009). Differing Prevalence and Diversity of Bacterial Species in Fetal Membranes from Very Preterm and Term Labor, *PLoS One.* 4(12): e8205.

Kayagaki, N., Kawasaki, A., Ebata, T., Ohmoto, H., Ikeda, S., Inoue, S., Yoshino, K., Okumura, K., Yagita, H. (1995). Metalloproteinase-mediated release of human Fas ligand, *J Exp Med.* 182(6):1777-1783.

Kim, H.S., Kim, H.J., Park, K.G., Kim, Y.N., Kwon, T.K., Park, J.Y., Lee, K.U., Kim, J.G., Lee, I.K. (2007). Alpha-lipoic acid inhibits matrix metalloproteinase-9 expression by inhibiting NF-kappaB transcriptional activity, *Exp Mol Med.* 39(1):106-113.

Kim, S.S., Romero, R., Kim, J.S., Abbas, A., Espinoza, J., Kusanovic, J.P., Hassan, S., Yoon, B.H. & Kim, C.J. (2008). Coexpression of myofibroblast and macrophage markers: novel evidence for an in vivo plasticity of chorioamniotic mesodermal cells of the human placenta, *Lab Invest.* 88(4):365-374.

Kolev, K., Skopal, J., Simon, L., Csonka, E., Machovich, R. & Nagy, Z. (2003). Matrix metalloproteinase-9 expression in post-hypoxic human brain capillary endothelial cells: H2O2 as a trigger and NF-kappaB as a signal transducer, *Thromb. Haemost.* 90(3)528–537.

Kumar, D., Lundgren, D.W., Moore, R.M., Silver, R.J. & Moore, J.J. (2004a). Hydrogen peroxide induced apoptosis in amnion-derived WISH cells is not inhibited by Vitamin C, *Placenta.* 25(4):266-272.

Kumar, D., Moore, R.M., El-khwad, M., Silver, R.J. & Moore, J.J. (2004b). Vitamin C exacerbates hydrogen peroxide induced apoptosis and concomitant PGE2 release in amnion epithelial and mesenchymal cells and in intact amnion, *Placenta.* 25(6):573-579.

Kumar, D., Fung, W., Moore, R.M., Pandey, V., Fox, J., Stetzer, B., Mansour, J.M., Mercer, B.M., Redline, R.W. & Moore, J.J. (2006). Inflammatory mediators found in amniotic fluid induce collagen remodeling, apoptosis, and biophysical weakening of cultured fetal membranes, *Biol Reprod.* 74(1):29-34.

Kumar, D., Novince, R., Strohl, A., Mercer, B.M., Mansour, J.M., Moore, R.M. & Moore, J.J. (2009). A new methodology to measure strength of adherence of the fetal membrane components, amnion and the choriodecidua, *Placenta.* 30(6):560-563.

Kumar, D., Schatz, F., Moore, R.M., Mercer, B.M., Rangaswamy, N., Mansour, J.M., Lockwood, C.J. & Moore, J.J. (2011). The effects of Thrombin and Cytokines upon the Biomechanics and Remodeling of Isolated Amnion, *In Vitro, Placenta.* 2011. 32(3):206-213.

Ladfors, L., Mattsson, L.A., Eriksson, M. & Milsom, I. (2000). Prevalence and risk factors for prelabor rupture of the membranes (PROM) at or nearterm in an urban Swedish population, J *Perinat Med.* 28(6):491-496.

Lafleur, M.A., Hollenberg, M.D., Atkinson, S.J., Knauper,.V., Murphy, G. & Edwards, D.R. (2001). Activation of pro-(matrix metalloproteinase-2) (pro-MMP-2) by thrombin is membrane-type-MMP-dependent in human umbilical vein endothelial cells and generates a distinct 63 kDa active species, *Biochem. J.* 357(Pt 1):107-115.

Laham, N., Brennecke, S.P., Bendtzen, K. & Rice, G.E. (1994). Tumour necrosis factor alpha during human pregnancy and labour: maternal plasma and amniotic fluid concentrations and release from intrauterine tissues, *Eur J Endocrinol.* 131(6):607-614.

Laham, N., Brennecke, S.P., Bendtzen, K. & Rice GE. (1996). Differential release of interleukin-6 from human gestational tissues in association with labour and in vitro endotoxin treatment, *J Endocrinol.* 149(3):431-439.

Lappas M, Odumetse TL, Riley C, Reti NG, Holdsworth-Carson SJ, Rice GE, Permezel M. (2008). Pre-labour fetal membranes overlying the cervix display alterations in inflammation and NF-kappaB signalling pathways. *Placenta.* 29(12):995-1002.

Lappas, M., Riley, C., Rice, G.E. & Permezel M. (2009). Increased Expression of ac-FoxO1 Protein in Prelabor Fetal Membranes Overlying the Cervix: Possible Role in Human Fetal Membrane Rupture, *Reprod Sci.* 16(7):635-641. 1.

Lappas M, Mitton A, Lim R, Barker G, Riley C, Permezel M. (2010a). SIRT1 is a novel regulator of key pathways of human labor. *Biol Reprod.* 84(1):167-178.

Lappas M, Lim R, Riley C, Menon R, Permezel M. (2010b). Expression and Localisation of FoxO3 and FoxO4 in Human Placenta and Fetal Membranes. Placenta 31:1043-1050.

Lavery, J.P. & Miller, C.E. (1977). The viscoelastic nature of chorioamniotic membranes, *Obstet Gynecol.* 50(4):467-472.

Lavery, J.P. & Miller, C.E. (1979). Deformation and creep in the human chorioamniotic sac. *Am J Obstet Gynecol.* 134(4):366-375.

Lavery, J.P., Miller, C.E. & Knight, R.D. (1982). The effect of labor on the rheologic response of chorioamniotic membranes, *Obstet Gynecol.* 60(1):87-92.

Lee, T., Carpenter, M.W., Heber, W.W. & Silver, H.M. (2003). Preterm premature rupture of membranes: risks of recurrent complications in the next pregnancy among a population-based sample of gravid women, *Am J Obstet Gynecol.* 188(1):209-213.

Lei, H., Vadillo-Ortega,,F., Paavola, L.G. & Strauss, J.F. (1995). 92-kDa gelatinase (matrix metalloproteinase-9) is induced in rat amnion immediately prior to parturition, *Biol Reprod.* 53(2); 339-344.

Lei, H., Furth, E.E., Kalluri, R., Chiou, T., Tilly, K.I., Tilly, J.L., Elkon, K.B., Jeffrey, J.J. & Strauss, J.F. 3rd. (1996). A program of cell death and extracellular matrix degradation is activated in the amnion before the onset of labor, *J Clin Invest.* 98(9):1971–1978.

Liu, W.H., Chen, X.M. & Fu, B. (2000). Thrombin stimulates MMP-9 mRNA expression through AP-1 pathway in human mesangial cells, *Acta Pharmacol. Sin.* 21(7)641-645.

Liu, Y., Gilcrease, M.Z., Henderson, Y., Yuan, X.H., Clayman, G.L. & Chen, Z. (2001). Expression of protease-activated receptor 1 in oral squamous cell carcinoma, *Cancer Lett.* 169(2)173–180.

Locksmith, G.J., Clark, P., Duff, P., Saade, G.R. & Schultz, G.S. (2001). Amniotic fluid concentrations of matrix metalloproteinase 9 and tissue inhibitor of metalloproteinase 1 during pregnancy and labor, *Am J Obstet Gynecol.* 184(2):159-164.

Lockwood, C.J., Nemerson, Y., Guller, S., Krikun, G., Alvarez, M., Hausknecht, V., Gurpide, E. & Schatz, F. (1993). Progestational regulation of human endometrial stromal cell tissue factor expression during decidualization, *J Clin Endocrinol Metab.* 76(1):231–236.

Lockwood, C.J. & Kuczynski, E. (1999). Markers of risk for preterm delivery, *J Perinat Med.* 27(1):5-20.

Lockwood, C.J., Krikun, G., Schatz, F. (2001). Decidual cell-expressed tissue factor maintains hemostasis in human endometrium, *Ann NY Acad Sci*. 943:77–88

Lockwood, C.J., Oner, C., Uz, Y.H., Kayisli, U.A., Huang, S.J., Buchwalder, L.F., Murk, W., Funai, E.F. & Schatz, F. (2008). Matrix metalloproteinase 9 (MMP9) expression in preeclamptic deciduas and MMP9 induction by tumor necrosis factor alpha and interleukin 1 beta in human first trimester decidual cells, *Biol Reprod*. 78(6):1064-1072.

Louis-Sylvestre, C., Rand, J.H., Gordon, R.E., Salafia, C.M. & Berkowitz, R.L. (1998). In vitro studies of the interactions between platelets and amniotic membranes: a potential treatment for preterm premature rupture of the membranes, *Am J Obstet Gynecol*. 178(2):287-293.

Lundin-Schiller, S. & Mitchell, M.D. (1991). Prostaglandin production by human chorion laeve cells in response to inflammatory mediators, *Placenta*. 12(4):353-363.

Lyons, C.A., Beharry, K.D., Nishihara, K.C., Akmal, Y., Ren, Z.Y., Chang, E., Nageotte, M.P. (2002). Regulation of matrix metalloproteinases (type IV collagenases) and their inhibitors in the virgin, timed pregnant, and postpartum rat uterus and cervix by prostaglandin E(2)-cyclic adenosine monophosphate, *Am J Obstet Gynecol*. 187(1):202-208.

MacDorman, M.F. & Mathews, T.J. (2008). Recent Trends in Infant Mortality in the United States, NCHS Data Brief. (9):1-8.

Malak, T.M. & Bell, S.C. (1994). Structural characteristic of term human fetal membranes: a novel zone of extreme morphological alteration within the rupture site, *Br J Obstet Gynecol*. 101(5):375-386.

Manabe, Y., Himeno, N. & Fukumoto, M. (1991). Tensile strength and collagen content of amniotic membrane do not change after the second trimester or during delivery, *Obstet Gynecol*. 78(1):24-27.

Mannello, F. & Gazzanelli, G. (2001). Tissue inhibitors of metalloproteinases and programmed cell death: conundrums, controversies and potential implications, *Apoptosis*. 6(6):479-482.

Maymon, E., Ghezzi, F., Edwin, S.S., Mazor, M., Yoon, B.H., Gomez, R. & Romero, R. (1999). The tumor necrosis factor alpha and its soluble receptor profile in term and preterm parturition, *Am J Obstet Gynecol*. 181(5 Pt 1):1142-1148.

Maymon, E., Romero, R., Pacora, P., Gomez, R., Mazor, M., Edwin, S., Chaiworapongsa, T., Kim, J.C., Yoon, B.H., Menon, R., Fortunato, S. & Berry, S.M. (2001). A role for the 72 kDa gelatinase (MMP-2) and its inhibitor (TIMP-2) in human parturition, premature rupture of membranes and intraamniotic infection, *J Perinat Med*. 29(4):308-316.

McLaren, J., Malak, T.M. & Bell, S.C. (1999a). Structural characteristics of term human fetal membranes prior to labour: identification of an area of altered morphology overlying the cervix, *Hum Reprod*. 14(1):237-241.

McLaren, J., Taylor, D.J. & Bell, S.C. (1999b). Increased incidence of apoptosis in non-labour -affected cytotrophoblast cells in term fetal membranes overlying the cervix, *Human Reprod*. 14(1):2895-2900.

McLaren, J., Taylor, D.J. & Bell, S.C. (2000a). Increased concentration of pro-matrix metalloproteinase 9 in term fetal membranes overlying the cervix before labor: implications for membrane remodeling and rupture, *Am J Obstet Gynecol*. 182(2):409-416.

McLaren, J., Taylor, D.J. & Bell, S.C. (2000b). Prostaglandin E(2)-dependent production of latent matrix metalloproteinase-9 in cultures of human fetal membranes, *Mol Hum Reprod.* 6(11):1033-1040.
McParland, P.C., Taylor, D.J. & Bell, S.C. (2003). Mapping of zones of altered morphology and chorionic connective tissue cellular phenotype in human fetal membranes (amniochorion and decidua) overlying the lower uterine pole and cervix before labor at term, *Am J Obstet Gynecol.* 189(5):1481-1488.
Meinert, M., Eriksen, G.V., Petersen, A.C., Helmig, R.B., Laurent, C., Uldbjerg, N. & Malmström, A. (2001). Proteoglycans and hyaluronan in human fetal membranes, *Am J Obstet Gynecol.* 184(4):679-685.
Meinert, M., Malmström, A., Tufvesson, E., Westergren-Thorsson, G., Petersen, A.C., Laurent, C., Uldbjerg, N., Eriksen, G.V. (2007). Labour induces increased concentrations of biglycan and hyaluronan in fetal membranes, *Placenta.* 28(5-6):482-486.
Mendoza, G.A., Acuña, E., Allen, M., Arroyo, J. & Quintero, R.A. (1999). In vitro laser welding of amniotic membranes, *Lasers Surg Med.* 24(5):315-318.
Menon, R. & Fortunato, S.J. (2004). The role of matrix degrading enzymes and apoptosis in rupture of membranes, *J Soc Gynecol Investig.* 11(7):427-437.
Mercer, B.M., Goldenberg, R.L., Das, A., Moawad, A.H., Iams, J.D., Meis, P.J., Copper, R.L., Johnson, F., Thom, E., McNellis, D., Miodovnik, M., Menard, M.K., Caritis, S.N., Thurnau, G.R., Bottoms, S.F. & Roberts, J. (1996). The preterm prediction study: a clinical risk assessment system, *Am J Obstet Gynecol.* 174(6):1885-1893; discussion 1893-1895.
Mercer, B.M., Goldenberg, R.L., Moawad, A.H., Meis, P.J., Iams, J.D., Das, A.F., Caritis, S.N., Miodovnik, M., Menard, M.K., Thurnau, G.R., Dombrowski, M.P., Roberts, J.M. & McNellis, D. (1999). The preterm prediction study: effect of gestational age and cause of preterm birth on subsequent obstetric outcome. National Institute of Child Health and Human Development Maternal-Fetal Medicine Units Network, *Am J Obstet Gynecol.* 181(5 Pt 1):1216-1221.
Mercer, B.M., Goldenberg, R.L., Meis, P.J., Moawad, A.H., Shellhaas, C., Das, A., Menard, M.K., Caritis, S.N., Thurnau, G.R., Dombrowski, M.P., Miodovnik, M., Roberts, J.M., McNellis, D. (2000). The Preterm Prediction Study: prediction of preterm premature rupture of membranes through clinical findings and ancillary testing. The National Institute of Child Health and Human Development Maternal-Fetal Medicine Units Network, *Am J Obstet Gynecol.* 183(3):738-745.
Mercer, B.M., Abdelrahim, A., Moore, R.M., Novak, J., Kumar, D., Mansour, J.M., Perez-Fournier, M., Milluzzi, C. & Moore, J.J. (2010). The impact of Vitamin C supplementation in pregnancy and in-vitro upon fetal membrane strength and remodeling, *Reprod Sciences.* 17(7):685-695.
Millar, L.K., Boesche, M.H., Yamamoto, S.Y., Killeen, J., DeBuque, L., Chen, R. & Bryant-Greenwood, G.D. (1998). A relaxin-mediated pathway to preterm premature rupture of the fetal membranes that is independent of infection, *Am J Obstet Gynecol.* 179(1):126-134.
Millar, L.K., Reiny, R., Yamamoto, S.Y., Okazaki, K., Webster, L. & Bryant-Greenwood, G.D. (2003). Relaxin causes proliferation of human amniotic epithelium by stimulation of insulin-like growth factor-II, *Am J Obstet Gynecol.* 188(1):234-241.

Moore, A.G., Brown, D.A., Fairlie, W.D., Bauskin, A.R., Brown, P.K., Munier, M.L., Russell, P.K., Salamonsen, L.A., Wallace, E.M. & Breit, S.N. (2000). The transforming growth factor-ss superfamily cytokine macrophage inhibitory cytokine-1 is present in high concentrations in the serum of pregnant women, *J Clin Endocrinol Metab.* 85(12):4781-4788.

Moore, J.J., Dubyak, G., Moore, R. & Vander Kooy D. (1988). Oxytocin activates the inostisol-phospholipid - protein kinase C system and stimulates prostaglandin production in human amnion cells, *Endocrinology.* 123(4):1771-1777.

Moore, J.J., Moore, R.M., Collins, P.L. (1993). Protein kinase A activators inhibit agonist induced prostaglandin production in human amnion cells, *Prostaglandins Leukotrienes and Essential Fatty Acids.* 48(5):355-361.

Moore, R.M., Mansour, J.M., Redline, R., Mercer, B.M. & Moore, J.J. (2006). The physiology of fetal membrane rupture: insight gained from the determination of physical properties, *Placenta.* 27(11-12):1037-1051.

Moore, R.M., Redline, R.W., Kumar, D., Mercer, B.M., Mansour, J.M., Yohannes, E., Novak, J.B., Chance, M.R., Moore, J.J. (2009a). Differential expression of fibulin family proteins in the para-cervical weak zone and other areas of human fetal membranes, *Placenta.* 30(4):335-341.

Moore, R.M., Novak, J.B., Kumar, D., Mansour, J.M., Mercer, B.M. & Moore, J.J. (2009b). Alpha-lipoic acid inhibits Tumor Necrosis Factor-induced remodeling and weakening of human fetal membranes, *Biol Reprod.* 80(4):781-787.

Moore, R.M., Schatz, F., Kumar, D., Mercer, B.M., Rangaswamy, N., Abdelrahim, A., Bartel, C., Mansour, J.M., Lockwood, C.J. & Moore JJ. (2010). Alpha-Lipoic Acid Inhibits Thrombin-Induced Fetal Membrane Weakening *In Vitro, Placenta.* 31(10):886-892.

O'Brien, J.M., Mercer, B.M., Barton, J.R. & Milligan, D.A. (2001). An in vitro model and case report that used gelatin sponge to restore amniotic fluid volume after spontaneous premature rupture of the membranes, *Am J Obstet Gynecol.* 185(5):1094-1097.

O'Brien, J.M., Barton, J.R. & Milligan, D.A. (2002). An aggressive interventional protocol for early midtrimester premature rupture of the membranes using gelatin sponge for cervical plugging, *Am J Obstet Gynecol.* 187(5):1143-1146.

Offenbacher, S., Boggess, K.A., Murtha AP, et al. (2006). Progressive periodontal disease and risk of very preterm delivery, *Obstet Gynecol.* 107(1):29-36.

Opsjłn, S.L., Wathen, N.C., Tingulstad, S., Wiedswang, G., Sundan, A., Waage, A. & Austgulen, R. (1993). Tumor necrosis factor, interleukin-1, and interleukin-6 in normal human pregnancy. *Am J Obstet Gynecol.* 169(2 Pt 1):397-404.

Orzechowski, A., Łokociejewska, M., Muras, P. & Hocquette, J.F. (2002). Preconditioning with millimolar concentrations of vitamin C or N-acetylcysteine protects L6 muscle cells insulin-stimulated viability and DNA synthesis under oxidative stress, *Life Sci.* 71(15):1793-1808.

Osman, I., Young, A., Jordan, F., Greer, I.A. & Norman, J.E. (2006). Leukocyte density and proinflammatory mediator expression in regional human fetal membranes and decidua before and during labor at term, *J Soc Gynecol Investig.* 13(2):97-103.

Osmers, R.G.W., Blaser, J., Kuhn, W. & Tschesche, H. (1995). Interleukin-8 synthesis and the onset of labor, *Obstet. Gynecol.* 86(2):223-229.

Ossovskaya, V.S. & Bunnett, N.W. (2004). Protease-Activated Receptors: Contribution to Physiology and Disease, *Physiol Rev.* 84(2): 579–621.

Paavola, L.G., Furth, E.E., Delgado, V., Boyd, C.O., Jacobs, C.C., Lei, H., Strauss, J.F.3rd. (1995). Striking changes in the structure and organization of rat fetal membranes precede parturition, *Biol Reprod.* 53(2):321-338.

Pandey, V., Jaremko, K., Moore, R.M., Mercer, B., Stetzer, B., Kumar, D., Fox, J., Mansour, J., Moore, J.J. (2007). The force required to rupture fetal membranes paradoxically increases with acute in vitro repeated stretching, *Am J OB Gynecol.* 196(2):165.e1-7.

Parry, S. & Strauss, J.F. (1998). Premature rupture of the fetal membranes, *N Engl J Med.* 338(10):663-670.

Pressman, E.K., Cavanaugh, J.L. & Woods, J.R. (2002). Physical properties of the chorioamnion throughout gestation, *Am J Obstet Gynecol.* 187(3):672-675.

Quintero, R.A., Morales, W.J., Kalter, C.S., Allen, M., Mendoza, G., Angel, J.L. & Romero, R. (1998). Transabdominal intra-amniotic endoscopic assessment of previable premature rupture of membranes, *Am J Obstet Gynecol.* 179(3):71-76.

Quintero, R.A., Morales, W.J., Allen, M., Bornick, P.W., Arroyo, J. & LeParc, G. (1999). Treatment of iatrogenic previable premature rupture of membranes with intra-amniotic injection of platelets and cryoprecipitate (amniopatch): preliminary experience, *Am J Obstet Gynecol.* 181(3):744-749.

Ramachandran, R. and Hollenberg, M.D. (2008). Proteinases and signaling: pathophysiological and therapeutic implications via PARs and more, *British Journal of Pharmacology.* 153, S263–S282

Rangaswamy, N., Abdelrahim, A., Moore, R.M., Uyen, L., Mercer, B.M., Mansour, J.M., Kumar, D., Sawady, J. & Moore, J.J. (2011). Biomechanical characteristics of human fetal membranes. Preterm fetal membranes are stronger than term fetal membranes. *Gynecol Obstet Fertil.* 39(6):373-377.

Reddy, U.M., Shah, S.S., Nemiroff, R.L., Ballas, S.K., Hyslop, T., Chen, J., Wapner, R.J., Sciscione, A.C. (2001). In vitro sealing of punctured fetal membranes: potential treatment for midtrimester premature rupture of membranes, *Am J Obstet Gynecol.* 185(5):1090-1093.

Reti, N.G., Lappas, M., Riley, C., Wlodek, M.E., Permezel,.M., Walker, S. & Rice, G.E. (2007). Why do membranes rupture at term? Evidence of increased cellular apoptosis in the supracervical fetal membranes, *Am J Obstet Gynecol.* 196(5):484.e1-10.

Riley, S.C., Leask, R., Chard, T., Wathen, N.C., Calder, A.A. & Howe, D.C. (1999). Secretion of matrix metalloproteinase-2, matrix metalloproteinase-9 and tissue inhibitor of matrix metalloproteinases into the intrauterine compartments during early pregnancy, *Mol Hum Reprod.* 5(4):376-381.

Roberts, A.K., Monzon-Bordonaba, F., Van Deerlin, P.G., Holder, J., Macones, G.A., Morgan, M.A., Strauss, J.F. 3rd. & Parry, S. (1999). Association of polymorphism within the promoter of the tumor necrosis factor alpha gene with increased risk of preterm premature rupture of the fetal membranes, *Am J Obstet Gynecol.* 180(5):1297-1302.

Romero, R., Mazor, M., Wu, Y.K., Sirtori, M., Oyarzun, E., Mitchell, M.D. & Hobbins, J.C. (1988). Infection in the pathogenesis of preterm labor. *Semin Perinatol.* 12(4):262-279.

Romero, R., Parvizi, S.T., Oyarzun, E., Mazor, M., Wu, Y.K., Avila, C., Athanassiadis, A.P. & Mitchell, M.D. (1990a). Amniotic fluid interleukin-1 in spontaneous labor at term, *J Reprod Med.* 35(3):235-238.

Romero, R., Avila, C., Santhanam, U. & Sehgal, P.B. (1990b). Amniotic fluid interleukin 6 in preterm labor. Association with infection, *J Clin Invest.* 85(5):1392-1400.

Romero, R., Mazor, M., Sepulveda, W., Avila, C., Copeland, D. & Williams, J. (1992a). Tumor necrosis factor in preterm and term labor, *Am J Obstet Gynecol.* 166(5):1576-1587.

Romero, R., Sepulveda, W., Mazor, M., Brandt, F., Cotton, D.B., Dinarello, C.A. & Mitchell, M.D. (1992b). The natural interleukin-1 receptor antagonist in term and preterm parturition, *Am J Obstet Gynecol.* 167(4 Pt 1):863-872.

Romero, R., Baumann, P., Gomez, R., Salafia, C., Rittenhouse, L., Barberio, D., Behnke, E., Cotton, D.B. & Mitchell, M.D. (1993). The relationship between spontaneous rupture of membranes, labor, and microbial invasion of the amniotic cavity and amniotic fluid concentrations of prostaglandins and thromboxane B2 in term pregnancy, *Am J Obstet Gynecol.* 168(6 Pt 1):1654-1664.

Runić, R., Lockwood, C.J., LaChapelle, L., Dipasquale, B., Demopoulos, R.I., Kumar, A. & Guller, S. (1998). Apoptosis and Fas expression in human fetal membranes, *J Clin Endocrinol Metab.* 83(2):660-666.

Rusterholz, C., Hahn, S. & Holzgreve, W. (2007). Role of placentally produced inflammatory and regulatory cytokines in pregnancy and the etiology of preeclampsia, *Semin Immunopathol.* 29(2):151-162.

Sağol, S., Sağol, O., Ozkal, S. & Asena, U. 2002. Role of apoptosis, bcl-2 and bax protein expression in premature rupture of fetal membranes, *J Reprod Med.* 47(10):809-815.

Salafia CM, Lopez-Zeno JA, Sherer DM, Whittington SS, Minior VK, Vintzileos AM et al. Histologic evidence of old intrauterine bleeding is more frequent in prematurity. *Am J Obstet Gynecol.* 1995; 173:1065–1070.

Sciscione, A.C., Manley, J.S., Pollock, M., Maas, B., Shlossman, P.A., Mulla, W., Lankiewicz, M. & Colmorgen, G.H. (2001). Intracervical fibrin sealants: A potential treatment for early preterm premature rupture of the membranes, *Am J Obstet Gynecol.* 184(3):368-373.

Shen, T.T., DeFranco, E.A., Stamilio, D.M., Chang, J.J. & Muglia, L.J. (2008). A population-based study of race-specific risk for preterm premature rupture of membranes, *Am J Obstet Gynecol.* 199:373.e1-7.

Shirpoor, A., Minassian, S., Salami, S., Khadem-Ansari, M.H. & Yeghiazaryan, M. (2008). Alpha--lipoic acid decreases DNA damage and oxidative stress induced by alcohol in the developing hippocampus and cerebellum of rat, *Cell Physiol Biochem.* 22(5-6):769-776.

Siega-Riz, A.M., Promislow, J.H., Savitz, D.A., Thorp, J.M. Jr. & McDonald, T. (2003). Vitamin C intake and the risk of preterm delivery, *Am J Obstet Gynecol.* 189(2):519-525.

Simhan, H.N., Krohn, M.A., Roberts, J.M., Zeevi, A. & Caritis, S.N. (2003). Interleukin-6 promoter -174 polymorphism and spontaneous preterm birth, *Am J Obstet Gynecol.* 189(4):915-918.

So, T., Ito, A., Sato, T., Mori, Y., Hirakawa, S. (1992). Tumor necrosis factor-alpha stimulates the biosynthesis of matrix metalloproteinases and plasminogen activator in cultured human chorionic cells, *Biol Reprod.* 46(5):772-778.

Spinnato, J.A. II., Freire, S., Pinto e Silva, J.L., et al. Antioxidant supplementation and premature rupture of the membranes: a planned secondary analysis, *Am J Obstet Gynecol.* 2008; 199(4):433.e1-8.

Strohl, A., Kumar, D., Novince, R., Shaniuk, P., Smith, J., Bryant, K., Moore, R.M., Novak, J., Stetzer, B., Mercer, B.M., Mansour, J.M. & Moore, J.J. (2010). Decreased Adherence and Spontaneous Separation of Fetal Membrane Layers--Amnion and Choriodecidua—a Possible Part of the Normal Weakening Process, *Placenta.* 31(1): 18–24.

Stuart, E.L., Evans, G.S., Lin, Y.S. & Powers, H.J. (2005). Reduced collagen and ascorbic acid concentrations and increased proteolytic susceptibility with prelabor fetal membrane rupture in women, *Biol Reprod.* 72(1):230-235.

Thomakos, N., Daskalakis, G., Papapanagiotou, A., Papantoniou, N., Mesogitis, S. & Antsaklis, A. (2010). Amniotic fluid interleukin-6 and tumor necrosis factor-a at mid-trimester genetic amniocentesis: Relationship to intra-amniotic microbial invasion and preterm delivery, *European Journal of Obstetrics & Gynecology and Reproductive Biology.* 148(2):147-151.

Toppozada, M.K., Sallam, N.A., Gaafar, A.A., el-Kashlan, K.M. (1970). Role of repeated stretching in the mechanism of timely rupture of the membranes, *Am J Obstet Gynecol.* 108(2):243-249.

Ugwumadu, A.H. (2002). Bacterial vaginosis in pregnancy, *Curr Opin Obstet Gynecol.* 14(2):115-118.

Ulug, U., Goldman, S., Ben-Shlomo, I., Shalev, E. (2001). Matrix metalloproteinase (MMP)-2 and MMP-9 and their inhibitor, TIMP-1, in human term decidua and fetal membranes: the effect of prostaglandin F(2alpha) and indomethacin, *Mol Hum Reprod.* 7(12):1187-1193.

Vadillo-Ortega, F., Sadowsky, D.W., Haluska, G.J., Hernandez-Guerrero, C., Guevara-Silva, R., Gravett, M.G. & Novy, M.J. (2002). Identification of matrix metalloproteinase-9 in amniotic fluid and amniochorion in spontaneous labor and after experimental intrauterine infection or interleukin-1b infusion in pregnant rhesus monkeys, *Am J Obstet Gynecol* 186(1):128-138.

Wang, L., Luo, J. & He, S. (2007). Induction of MMP-9 release from human dermal fibroblasts by thrombin: involvement of JAK/STAT3 signaling pathway in MMP-9 release, *BMC Cell Biol* 8:14.

Werner, S.L., Barken, D. & Hoffmann, A. (2005). Stimulus specificity of gene expression programs determined by temporal control of IKK activity, *Science* 309(5742):1857-1861.

Xu, P., Alfaidy, N. & Challis, J.R. (2002). Expression of matrix metalloproteinase (MMP)-2 and MMP-9 in human placenta and fetal membranes in relation to preterm and term labor, *J Clin Endocrinol Metab* 87(3):1353-1361.

Xu, H., Perez-Cuevas, R., Xiong X, et al. (2010). An international trial of antioxidants in the prevention of preeclampsia (INTAPP). *Am J Obstet Gynecol* 202(3):239.e1-10.

Yoshida, M., Sagawa, N., Itoh, H., Yura, S., Takemura, M., Wada, Y., Sato, T., Ito, A. & Fujii, S. (2002). Prostaglandin F (2alpha), cytokines and cyclic mechanical stretch augment matrix metalloproteinase-1 secretion from cultured human uterine cervical fibroblast cells, *Mol Hum Reprod* 8(7):681-7.

Young, A., Thomson, A.J., Ledingham, M., Jordan, F., Greer, I.A. & Norman, J.E. (2002). Immunolocalization of proinflammatory cytokines in myometrium, cervix, and fetal membranes during human parturition at term, *Biol Reprod* 66(2):445-449.

Young, B.K., Roque, H., Abdelhak, Y.E., Poiolek, D., Demopulos, R. & Lockwood, C.J. (2000). Minimally invasive endoscopy in the treatment of preterm premature rupture of membranes by application of fibrin sealant, *J Perinat Med* 28(4):326-330.

Young, B.K., Roman, A.S., MacKenzie, A.P., Stephenson, C.D., Minior, V., Rebarber, A. & Timor-Tritsch, I. (2004a). The closure of iatrogenic membrane defects after amniocentesis and endoscopic intrauterine procedures, *Fetal Diagn Ther* 19(3):296-300.

Young, B.K., MacKenzie, A.P., Roman, A.S., Stephenson, C.D., Minior, V., Rebarber, A. & Timor-Tritsch, I. (2004b). Endoscopic closure of fetal membrane defects: comparing iatrogenic versus spontaneous rupture cases, *J Matern Fetal Neonatal Med* 16(4):235-240.

Yuan, B., Ohyama, K., Takeichi, M. & Toyoda, H. (2009). Direct contribution of inducible nitric oxide synthase expression to apoptosis induction in primary smooth chorion trophoblast cells of human fetal membrane tissues, *Int J Biochem Cell Biol* 41(5):1062-1069.

Zaga, V., Estrada-Gutierrez, G., Beltran-Montoya, J., Maida-Claros, R., Lopez-Vancell, R. & Vadillo-Ortega, F. (2004). Secretions of interleukin-1beta and tumor necrosis factor alpha by whole fetal membranes depend on initial interactions of amnion or choriodecidua with lipopolysaccharides or group B streptococci, *Biol Reprod* 71(4):1296-1302.

Zhang, W.J., Wei, H., Hagen, T. & Frei, B. (2007). Alpha-lipoic acid attenuates LPS-induced inflammatory responses by activating the phosphoinositide 3-kinase/Akt signaling pathway, *Proc Natl Acad Sci U S A* 104(10):4077-4082.

Ziegler, D. (2009). Painful diabetic neuropathy: Advantage of novel drugs over old drugs, *Diabetes Care* 32:S414-419.

7

The Effect of Inflammation on Preterm Birth

Grazzia Rey, Silvana Pereyra, Tatiana Velazquez, Daniel Grasso, Justo Alonso, Bernardo Bertoni and Rossana Sapiro
School of Medicine, University of the Republic
Uruguay

1. Introduction

1.1 General considerations

The World Health Organization defines preterm birth as the delivery of an infant between 20 and 37 weeks of gestation (Martin et al., 2005, Beck et al., 2010). Preterm birth (PTB) is a worldwide health problem and remains the leading cause of perinatal morbidity and mortality. PTB rates have been reported as 11% in the United States, and approximately 5 to 7% in Europe (Goldenberg, 2002). In industrialized countries, preterm delivery is responsible for 70% of mortality and 75% of morbidity in the neonatal period, contributing to significant long-term neurodevelopmental problems, pulmonary dysfunction, and visual impairment (Challis et al., 2001; Wen et al., 2004; Iacovidou et al., 2010). In South America, more than 10% of newborns are preterm, and the incidence is between 8% and 10% in Uruguay (Rey et al., 2008; Sosa et al., 2011). Unfortunately, the rate of PTB continues to rise according to recent incidence reports, and is currently 12–13% in the USA (Ananth et al., 2006).

1.2 Etiology

Over the last decade, it has become increasingly apparent that the cause of PTB and preterm premature rupture of membranes (PPROM) is multifactorial and involves both genetic and environmental factors (Romero et al., 1994; Romero et al., 2000; Crider et al., 2005; Romero et al., 2006; Goldenberg et al., 2008). Similar observations have been made in other complex diseases such as coronary heart disease (Talmud & Humphries, 2004), hypertension (Hamet et al., 1998; Zhu, 2005) and psychiatric conditions (Lau & Eley, 2004). Consequently, researchers focused on the search for a genetic background that predispose to complex diseases when unfavorable environmental conditions are present. Preterm labor is considered the final common pathway of different complications of pregnancy such as infection, placental abruption, smoking, poor nutrition, alcoholism, multiple gestation, endocrine and coagulation disorders and fetal or maternal genetic susceptibility (Goldenberg, 2002; Wen et al., 2004; Goldenberg et al., 2008; Iacovidou et al., 2010). Regarding genetic susceptibility the single best predictor of PTB among multiparous pregnant women is past history of preterm delivery: women with one prior PTB have a recurrence risk of PTB of 15% and those with two or more prior PTBs have a recurrence risk of 32% (Pennell et al., 2007). The risk of PTB tends to remain with the mother through multiple pregnancies, even with increased levels of prenatal surveillance and preventive interventions (Carr-Hill & Hall, 1985). Twin studies have suggested that heritability for PTB ranges from 17% to 36% (Clausson et al., 2000). Women who themselves were born preterm have an increased risk of PTB. The risk of PTB increases as the gestational age of the mother's birth decreases, with mothers born at less than 30 weeks having a 2.4-fold (95% CI 1.4 - 4.2) increase in risk of PTB (Porter et al., 1997). Furthermore, there is a well-described ethnic difference in the rate of PTB (even when controlling for mother contributing etiologic factors). In 2005, the incidence of preterm delivery among African Americans and European Americans in the U.S. was 18.4% and 11.7%, respectively (Anum et al., 2009). This ethnic disparity in PTB between African Americans and European Americans has been present for decades. The inequity is likely the consequence of multiple factors, including socioeconomic status, access to care, environment, and differences in genetic background (Anum et al., 2009).

1.3 Inflammatory pathways and preterm birth

Preterm labor is considered a syndrome because there are many causes that lead to different pathological processes. Most of them involve an inflammatory cytokine-mediated response. The fetus loses some of its immunological defense in their presence and becomes vulnerable to destruction by the immune system (Vrachnis et al., 2010). Infection has been regarded as one of the most heralded causes of preterm birth due to the drastic link between underlying infectious agents and their ability to promote inflammatory responses (Goldenberg et al., 2000; Thaxton et al., 2010). Infections like chorioamnionitis may initiate preterm labor. Bacterial vaginosis is associated with increased PTB risk even without infection of the fetal membranes (Slattery & Morrison, 2002). Increased inflammation occurs in normal parturition, and inflammatory cytokines are higher in women who deliver preterm (Keelan et al., 2003). Infection, stress, and obesity promote inflammation, suggesting that these environmental exposures may promote an inflammation-mediated mechanism resulting in early parturition (Crider et al., 2005). Inflammation and immune response are universal mechanisms of host defense against infection. They function on the basis of special receptors called pattern-recognition receptors which recognize conserved microbial structures called pathogen-associated molecular patterns. Due to pattern-recognition receptors, the human organism is able to discriminate between self- and non-self-antigens (Li et al., 2010).

1.4 The role of toll-like receptors

A strong explanation for initiation of distinct immune pathways could be the activation of toll-like receptors (TLRs). TLRs are a diverse set of innate immune sentinel receptors of pathogens highly conserved throughout evolution (Bauer et al., 2009). TLRs are a group of pattern-recognition receptors that play a crucial role in 'danger' recognition and the induction of immune response. The human TLR family comprises at least 13 distinctive proteins (TLR1 - TLR13) that are able to recognize typical microbial agents and subsequently facilitate an early immune response via downstream different signaling pathways (Medzhitov et al., 1997; O'Neill, 2008). The human TLR member best characterized to date is toll-like receptor 4 (TLR4), as this signaling molecule is essential for the recognition of bacterial lipopolysaccharides (LPS) among other microbial agents (Krishnan et al., 2007). LPS represent a key element of gram-negative bacteria and contain fatty acids in their lipid-A domain anchoring LPS into the bacterial cell wall (Raetz & Whitfield, 2002). LPS are thought to play a key role in eliciting an inflammatory response including the activation of the immune cells and the release of enzymes involved in the remodeling of the extracellular matrix leading to preterm delivery. TLRs are highly expressed at the maternal-fetal interface on trophoblasts and uterine immune cells (Patni et al., 2007). It is likely that differential uterine immune responses occur due to the diversity of pathogens that ensues activation of any one of the TLRs, ultimately leading to deleterious inflammation and preterm birth (Li et al., 2010; Thaxton et al., 2010). In particular, TLR4 is widely expressed in different cell types of the placenta compared to others members of the TLR family (Ma et al., 2007). Human TLR4 gene is polymorphic. Combination of distinct alleles of polymorphic genes could account for individual and ethnic differences in the rate and extent of production of individual proteins as well as variations in the acquisition and/or severity of a particular disorder. Sequencing of the human TLR4 revealed that most of the variation in non-synonymous polymorphisms is located in the third exon (Smirnova et al., 2001). The non-synonymous polymorphism localized on position 896 (rs4986790) is an A/G transition causing an aspartic acid/glycine substitution at amino acid location Asp299Gly. Arbour *et al.* were the first to report that individuals with Asp299Gly polymorphism had a blunted response toward inhaled LPS (Arbour et al., 2000; Ferwerda et al., 2008). Individuals carrying the variant alleles are at increased risk of Gram-negative infections (Agnese et al., 2002) and premature birth (Lorenz et al., 2002a) but not for preterm premature rupture of membranes (PPROM) in African Americans (Ferrand et al., 2002). Animal models seem to confirm the critical role of TLR4 in induced preterm delivery by inflammation (Li et al., 2010).

1.5 Our goal

More evidences support the complexity of preterm birth (Plunkett & Muglia, 2008). Modeling procedures used by twin studies suggest that additive genetic factors and environmental risk factors that are not shared among siblings both influence preterm birth (Clausson et al., 2000). Additionally, interactions between genes (Kalish et al., 2006; Menon et al., 2006) have been associated with preterm birth risk. Several studies suggest that gene-environment interactions, such as interactions between inflammatory gene risk alleles and bacterial infections (Macones et al., 2004b; Engel et al., 2005) also influence the disorder. Together, these studies imply that the etiology of preterm birth likely involves genetic as well as environmental factors in complex interactions. However the physiological and molecular bases of these interactions are not well understood. Our goal is to advance on the knowledge of how genetic and environmental factors combine to affect the risk of PTB and, more specifically, how the variations in the human genome (polymorphisms) can modify the effects of demographic conditions and exposures to environmental health hazards. We focused on TLR4 pathway. TLR4 genetic variations of our population have been looked closely trying to associate single nucleotide polymorphisms (SNP) to the commonly demographic, social, and ethnic accepted factors that contribute or cause PTB. Since PTB likely depends on a number of interacting risk factors, our genetic studies try to identify markers or pathways involved in the disorder. The goal is to find risk factors in the context of particular populations that might predict preterm birth more accurately than those currently identified.

2. Materials and methods

2.1 Subjects

A case-control study was conducted. Subjects were offspring of women receiving obstetrical care at the Pereira Rossell Hospital, Montevideo, Uruguay. Cases (n = 276) were neonates from pregnancies complicated by spontaneous PTB. Preterm birth was considered the delivery of an infant between 20 and 37 weeks of gestation (Martin et al., 2005). Two subgroups were distinguished; neonates born between 33 and 36 weeks were catalogued as moderate PTB (n = 169) and neonates of gestational age (GA) less than 33 weeks were included in a group of severe PTB (n = 117). Control subjects (n = 295) were neonates delivered at term (≥ 37 weeks of gestation) but not after 42 weeks of GA. The study protocol was approved by the School of Medicine Ethics Committee of the University of the Republic, Uruguay.

Sociodemographic characteristics, obstetric history, risk factors for PTB and data from the new born were collected from the perinatal informatics system. Perinatal informatics system registers all pregnancies in Uruguay since 1990 (Díaz A. et al., 1990). Confidentiality was assured by assigning numbers to the samples and deleting names and other information of patients in data collection forms. Informed consent was obtained from the mothers in all cases.

2.2 DNA extraction and Asp299Gly TLR4 genotyping

DNA was extracted either from umbilical cords or from newborn cheek swabs by conventional methods (Rey et al., 2008). To detect Asp299Gly polymorphism, we used the Polymerase Chain Reaction-Restriction Fragment Length Polymorphism (PCR-RFLP) strategy previously described by Lorenz et al. (2001) (Figure 1a) and a High Resolution-Melting Analysis (HRM) developed in our laboratory (Figure 1b).

2.3 Real time PCR and high-resolution -melting analysis

HRM analysis was performed on the Rotor-Gene 6000™ real-time instrument (Corbett Life Science) with Eva Green, a saturating dye technology (Type-it HRM PCR Kit, Qiagen). PCRs were performed in 10µl reaction volumes, containing 1X Qiagen HRM-typing buffer. The primers used were forward 5´ATTTGACCATTGAAGAATTCCG3´ and reverse 5′TGTTGCCATCCGAAATTATAAG3′. PCR reaction was carried out with an initial hold at 95°C for 5 min, followed by 35 cycles of 95°C for 15 s and 60°C for 1 min, and then HRM ramps were generated by acquiring florescence data at a temperature ramp from 72 to 80°C. Individuals with homozygous and heterozygous genotypes were included as controls in all experiments. HRM curves were normalized and genotype was assigned according to HRM curve shape by the Rotor-Gene software and visual inspection (Figure 1b).

2.4 Immunohistochemistry

A total of 6 chorioamniotic membranes were collected immediately after either preterm or term labor and processed for immunochemistry by standard methods. Briefly, all samples were formalin-fixed, paraffin-embedded, and 10 µm sections of the tissues were obtained. Blocking was performed by application of 5% goat blocking serum, followed by incubation with 2 µg/ml polyclonal goat anti-human TLR4 antibody (sc-8694, Santa Cruz Biotechnology, Santa Cruz, CA) with demonstrated specificity in placenta (Holmlund et al., 2002). Sections were incubated overnight at 4°C. A streptavidin-conjugated secondary antibody-mediated peroxidase development system (Elite Universal Vectastain ABC kit Vector Laboratories, Burlingame, CA) was used and antibody complexes visualized using DAB (BioFX Labs, Owing Mills, Maryland, USA). Tissues were counterstained with Mayer's hematoxylin and imaged by light microscopy (Nikon Eclipse E200). Images were imported into Adobe Photoshop Elements (Adobe, San Jose, California).

2.5 Statistics

Comparisons of allele frequencies were performed using the χ^2 test or Fisher's exact test. Means between groups were compared using Student's *t*-Test. The association between TLR4 genotypes and PROM related to GA was examined by logistic regression analysis. The presence of differential effects of TLR4 genotypes on the risk of PROM was explored by the inclusion of interaction or conditional terms. The analysis was performed with the Epi Info 2000 software (Center for Disease Control and Prevention, Atlanta, GA, USA). Probability values of 0.05 or less were considered significant.

3. Results

A total of 571 women were included in the study. Main characteristics of our study population are shown in the Table 1. No differences were detected in both groups regarding mother's age mean (25.8 ±0.9 mother's age who delivered at term vs. 25.0 ±0.9 at preterm), parity (26% mothers delivering at term were nuliparous vs. 29% of mothers who delivered preterm their first child) and poor obstetric history (8% of mothers delivering at term vs. 16% of mothers who delivered preterm). Poor obstetric history includes previous preterm birth, low birth weight, or recurrent miscarriage. No differences were found when the three causes of poor obstetric history were discriminated. In contrast with other studies, no statistical differences were found between mothers that delivered at term and preterm regarding their history of previous PTB (7% of mothers delivering at term had at least one previous PTB vs. 17% of mothers who delivered preterm). Teenage mothers tend to have more preterm children than older ones. Also, pregnant women that do not attend medical visits have an elevated frequency of preterm delivery. However, education level does not affect the incidence of PTB. Smoking strongly associates to PTB. Hypertension, pregnancy bleeding, premature rupture of membranes (PROM) and intra uterine growth restriction (IUGR) are conditions statistically significant associated to preterm birth. Anemia and previous mother pathologies are not (Table 1). Maternal infections during pregnancy do not associate to PTB. Infections included here were urinary tract infections, low genital infections and syphilis but not HIV that was excluded of the study. We did not find statistically significance neither when infections were considered together nor when they were analyzed individually (Table 1).

Genotyping was assigned by RFLP (Figure 1b) in most of the sample. HRM analysis was applied in 100 newborns with the procedure designed in our laboratory. In a blinded study, fifty random samples from our previous data assigned by RFLP were used and re genotyped by real time followed by HRM (Figure 1b). Consistency was one hundred percent, indicating an excellent accuracy. Hardy-Weinberg (H-W) disequilibrium exact test indicates that TLR4 Asp299Gly variation is in Hardy-Weinberg equilibrium ($p > 0.05$), even when case and control groups are discerned, or the data are stratified by medical conditions (data not shown). Only the wild type (wt) and the Asp299Gly allele were present in our sample. No individual carrying the homozygous variant was found. Association tests indicate none significant value with respect to preterm birth and the SNP, with OR's yielding non-significant values ($p > 0.05$) (Table 2). Logistic regression analysis (Table 3) included only most powerful variables that determine PTB in our model, based on data from Table 1. Under this consideration, TLR4 SNP is not significantly associated to PTB (data not shown). However, a significant association is found when TLR4 Asp299Gly is conditionally by PROM between severe preterm newborns and babies born at term (table 4). Immunolocalization of TLR4 performed in fetal membranes demonstrated the presence of the protein in the epithelium of both, preterm and term amnios (Figure 2).

	Term (%) N= 271	Preterm (%) N=261	OR (CI 95%)	p-value
Maternal Age (<19)	10.6	19.3	2.01 (1.23 - 3.27)	0.003
Education Level *	47.0	48.1	0.96 (0.68 - 1.34)	0.432
Prenatal visits (< 5)	5.2	9.4	1.88 (0.90 - 3.92)	0.063
Smoking	46.1	63.9	2.07 (1.46 - 2.93)	0.0000039
Hypertension	2.9	10.5	3.89 (1.74 - 8.67)	0.0000021
Pregnacy bleeding	1.8	5.1	2.87 (1.02 - 8.09)	0.031
Infections	30.1	34.7	1.23 (0.86 - 1.77)	0.149
IUGR	3.0	6.8	2.41 (1.03 - 5.63)	0.029
PPROM	15.9	36.0	2.98 (1.98 - 4.51)	0.0000004
Anemia	2.6	3.0	1.73 (0.42 - 3.28)	0.482

* at least one year of high school
PROM, premature rupture of membranes
IUGR, intra uterine growth restriction

Table 1. Sociodemographic and medical characteristics of mothers and their newborns. Odds ratios and p-values between term and preterm births.

TLR4*	Term	Preterm
Asp299Gly/wt	10.6 (7.2 - 14.8)	11.2 (7.7 - 15.5)
wt/wt	89.4 (85.2 - 92.8)	88.8 (84.5 - 92.3)

Table 2. Asp299Gly TLR4 Genotype frequencies. * Fisher Test, p value=0.463

Trait	OR (CI 95%)	P-value
Hypertension	4.978 (2.068 - 11.985)	0.0003
Smoking	2.182 (1.512 - 3.149)	0.000002
PROM	3.185 (2.078 - 4.881)	0.0000003
TLR4	0.834 (0.445 - 1.561)	0.5694

Table 3. Logistic Regression model built using main socio-demographic and medical mother's characteristics. P-value: preterm vs. term.

Gestational Age (GA)	**Without PROM** **n = 415**	**With PROM** **n = 159**
> 37 weeks	0.0438	0.067
33-36 weeks	0.038	0.040
< 33 weeks	0.043	0.109*

Table 4. Minor Allele Frequency (MAF) of Asp299Gly according to GA. *Fisher test p value: 0.007 severe preterm vs. term.

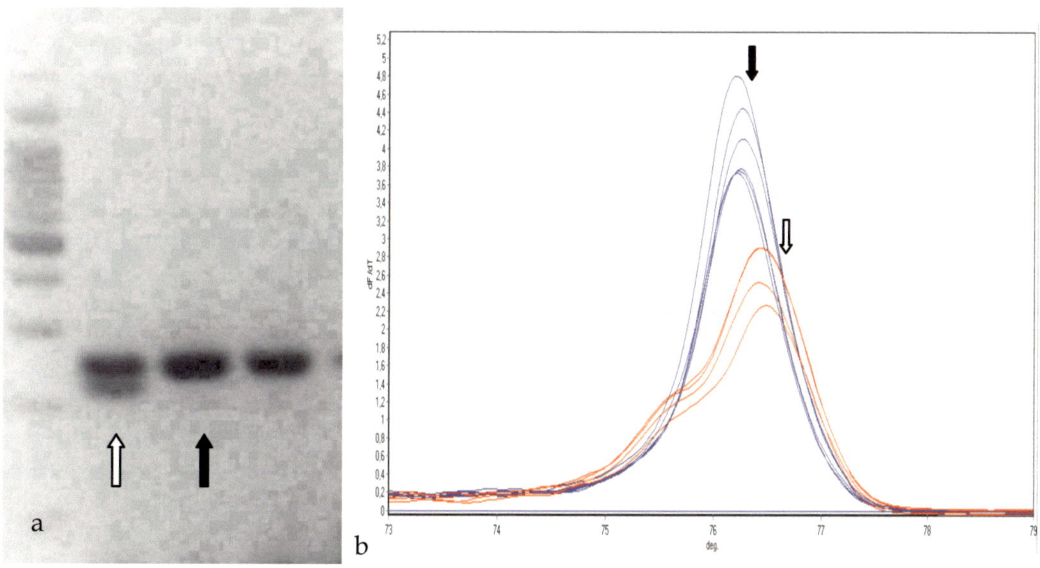

Fig. 1. a: Genotype patterns after PCR-RFLP. b: representative HRM melting curve. Black arrows: homozygous AA, White arrows: heterozygous GA.

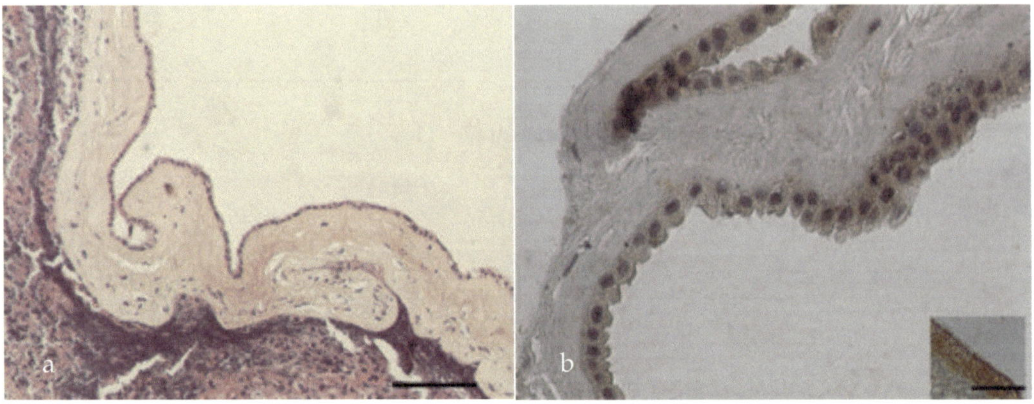

Fig. 2. Section of fetal membranes. a: 36 weeks gestation: HE (bar 100 μm).
b: Immunolocalization of TLR4 human protein at 36 weeks gestation.
Inset: term membranes (bar20μm).

4. Discussion

For the last eight years our group has been analyzing clinical, obstetric and environmental characteristics in association to genetic background of mothers and their offspring who have delivered at a public hospital in Montevideo, Uruguay. A case control study was conducted with the intention of advancing a research agenda to understand and diminish the population health burden embodied by PTB.

In view of the fact that PTB is considered a complex condition, it was not surprising the finding of strong association of the syndrome to several binomial mother-fetus socio-economical and clinical factors. Linkage of PTB to hypertension, PROM, bleedings, IUGR, and smoking suggested the possibility of vasoconstriction and/or an altered liberation of cytokines as a common basis of the process that leads to preterm labor. In addition, recent studies demonstrated associations between elevated levels of circulating proinflammatory cytokines, particularly interleukin (IL) 6, IL-1beta, and tumor necrosis factor alpha (TNF-alpha) and preterm birth (Lyon et al., 2010). These inflammatory cytokines might link the pathology of uterine contraction, uterine cervical ripening, and preterm premature rupture of membranes (Noguchi et al., 2010). Stimulation of TLRs with their ligands has been shown to induce proinflammatory cytokine release in uterine epithelial cells, fetal membranes and placenta (Schaefer et al., 2004; Noguchi et al., 2010). Moreover, the presence of TLR4 detected by immunohistochemistry in the amnios of women at labor suggested the possibility that stimulation of TLRs with their ligands induce proinflammatory cytokine release, conducting to labor (Schaefer et al., 2004; Noguchi et al., 2010). We were able to localize TLR4 in term and preterm membranes. It is probable that TLR4 pathway is playing a role in normal delivery but at the same time, some environmental conditions should also be present in order to produce PTB. Namely, when some environmental factors are present, interaction between unfavorable external conditions (e.g., infections) and TLR4 could be the ultimate cause of PTB.

Since TLRs play a key role in those pathways and the Asp299Gly variation has been associated to a blunted response toward pathogens (Arbour et al., 2000; Ferwerda et al., 2008), an association of the SNP and PTB was expected. The biological relevance of this

TLR4 SNPs has been widely investigated; individuals carrying the variant alleles are at increased risk of Gram-negative infections (Arbour et al., 2000; Agnese et al., 2002; Lorenz et al., 2002b). An association between the presence of TLR4 Asp299Gly polymorphisms and the occurrence of serious infections in HIV-1 infected patients was also reported (Papadopoulos et al., 2010). The same variant protects individuals from atherosclerosis (Kiechl et al., 2002; Ameziane et al., 2003). As we mentioned earlier, regarding preterm birth, results vary according to different studies. Lorenz et al. (2002a) in a Finish population found that fetuses carrying the Asp299Gly variation had an increased risk for preterm birth. On the other hand, there is no association between the rare variant and the risk for PPROM in African Americans (Ferrand et al., 2002). However, in our study PTB was not linked directly to the presence of TLR4 variation. We did find an association between severe PTB (less than 34 weeks of gestation), PROM and the presence of the Asp299Gly variation (see also previous work; Rey et al., 2008), suggesting possible differences between the pathogenesis of severe and moderate preterm birth. Is it possible that genetic component plays a key role in severe preterm but not in moderate preterm? Is PTB in accordance with other complex diseases where younger affected individuals show a greater genetic component? While prematurity is a continuum, with the whole population of births before 37 weeks' gestation experiencing some increased risk compared with term birth, it is the extreme of the distribution, very preterm birth, that accounts for a third of all infant deaths, 67% of neonatal mortality (Callaghan et al., 2006), and a significant prevalence of acquired developmental disabilities and severe cognitive disability in USA (Kramer & Hogue, 2009). Several issues should be considered in order to explain the differences found between studies that associates genetics and PTB.

4.1 Ethnic disparities

As far as our knowledge concerns, there is not enough evidence in South American populations that could conclusively indicate that there is Hispanic disparity in PTB. Although the utility of considering genetics at all in understanding ethnic disparities in health is being vigorously debated (Ioannidis et al., 2004; Kaufman & Cooper, 2008), the goal of gene-environment studies in specific populations is to advance in the knowledge of how genetic and environmental factors combine to affect the risk of the disease (Kelada et al., 2003) for a specific group of people. The studies of the impact of different polymorphism on inflammatory diseases in South American population have only recently started and sufficient data have yet to be collected and reported (Santos et al., 2006; Garza-Gonzalez et al., 2007; Jorge et al., 2010; Pontillo et al., 2010). Regarding PTB Romero et al. (2010) conducted a large, candidate gene association study of women and their offspring who experienced birth after preterm labor with intact membranes, in a Hispanic population from Chile. They identified sequence variants in genes involved in inflammation and extracellular matrix biology that were associated with preterm birth. TLR4 SNPs were included in their study but no differences were reported between cases and controls. Moura et al. (2009) in a study that included more than 400 Brazilian women did not find any association between spontaneous PTB and any of six gene variations of cytokines included in their studies. They did find a significant association between PTB and a combination of variants by a multi-locus analysis. TLR SNPs were not included (Moura et al., 2009).

Uruguayan population has been described fundamentally as of European origin. However, more recently, genetic admixture analysis demonstrated a Native American and African contribution to the Uruguayan population of 10.4% and 5.6%, respectively (Hidalgo et al., 2005; Sans et al., 2006). The Uruguayan Asp299Gly observed frequency is lower than that of Europeans or Africans and equal to the admixed Chilean population (Rey et al., 2008), which suggests the effect of admixture on this gene. We published the first report concerning association between TLR4 and PTB or PPROM on a South American country and the data presented here confirm this link. The body of literature that mentions genetics as an explanation for the racial disparity in preterm birth is large, but notable for rarely measuring genes; most studies suggest that residual racial variation in preterm birth risk is genetic after statistical control for measured socioeconomic and behavioral risk factors (Kramer & Hogue, 2009). Our data combine severe PTB, PROM and the association of the SNPs which is not considered in those previous studies. Specifically, severe PTB birth could be linked stronger to genetic factors than moderate PTB. Interestingly, while severe preterm birth is a poor outcome for any pregnancy, African-American women experience nearly 3 times the risk of severe PTB birth when compared with non-Hispanic white women (Kramer & Hogue, 2009), meaning that probably genetic component is stronger when birth is produced before 33 weeks of gestational age.

4.2 Interactions with environmental factors

Again, it is possible that the aforementioned SNP could influence the PTB only when some environmental conditions are present. Indeed, some of these genetic variations require the presence of certain environmental stimuli to have any clinical significance. To date, however, only relatively few studies on the association of gene-environment interactions with preterm birth have been published (e.g. Wang et al., 2002; Genc et al., 2004; Macones et al., 2004; Nukui et al., 2004; Genc & Schantz-Dunn, 2007; Gracie et al., 2010; Menon et al., 2010; Genc & Onderdonk, 2011). Macones et al. (2004) described a gene–environment interaction between the tumor necrosing factor (TNF) alpha polymorphism and bacterial vaginosis. Women found to have both the TNF alpha polymorphism and bacterial vaginosis were at synergistically increased risk of PTB when compared with women with only the TNF alpha polymorphism or bacterial vaginosis alone (Macones et al., 2004). In our study neither environmental nor clinical conditions were found to have association to TLR4 Asp299Gly variation when preterm labor is considered as a whole. Interestingly, infection was not always present at detectable levels. Probably this is not surprising. The characteristics of intrauterine inflammation are histologic chorioamnionitis and elevated amniotic fluid concentrations of cytokines or metalloproteases. The major cause of PTB prior to 32 weeks of gestation is intrauterine infection and/or inflammation (Romero et al., 2007; Goldenberg et al., 2008; Keelan, 2011) but only a minor proportion of such pregnancies exhibit clinical signs of chorioamnionitis (Romero et al., 2007; Keelan, 2011). Intrauterine infection most commonly arises from the ascending route (associated with abnormal vaginal flora), with colonization first of the decidual membrane, followed by chorion, amnion, amniotic fluid and fetus. Chorioamnionitis can be present at all stages of the colonization process (Grigsby et al., 2010). Intrauterine infection arising from a haematogenous route is an alternative cause of PTB, although considered less common (Keelan, 2011). Various findings suggest that in some pregnancies, the infective organism may be present in placental tissues from mid-gestation. In fact, it has been suggested that intrauterine infections may originate pre-conceptually, possibly arising from organisms residing in the endometrium prior to implantation which subsequently activate the maternal innate immune system as a result of a change in growth or immune surveillance (Oh et al., 2010). It is possible that an altered cytokine expression can cause *per se* preterm labor, namely an overproduction of cytokines can be harmful to the fetus because of the activation of the cytokine flow (Vrachnis et al., 2010). Since inflammation-driven preterm labor can happen in the absence of overt amniotic infection, it is assumed that this cascade of events can also occur as a consequence of exposure to blood organisms or endotoxins, or possibly via exposure to non-microbial triggers of the innate immune system (Romero et al., 2007; Keelan, 2011).

4.3 Genetic background, interaction between SNPs

Inflammatory signaling is highly complex and subject to modulation by numerous factors responding to multiple external and internal signals (Keelan, 2011). TLR signaling employs the NF-κB signal transduction pathway, a key regulator of inflammatory gene expression (Medvedev et al., 2000; Lu et al., 2008; Vallabhapurapu & Karin, 2009). Key steps in the TLR4 signal pathway include recruitment of adapter proteins (MyD88, IRAK1/4 and TRAF6), activation of intermediate kinases (RIP1, TAB2/3, TAK1 and IKKα/β) and phosphorylation/degradation of the chaperone protein IκB (Martinon & Tschopp, 2007). In theory, variations in any of the genes that codify for the proteins involved may affect inflammatory pathway and labor. That means that few candidate gene studies could be an endless trade with the danger of leading to an imperfect understanding of the biological pathways that end in PTB. It was also shown that the associations found are difficult to replicate (Todd, 2006; Manolio et al., 2009). Genome-wide association studies (GWAS), in which several hundred thousand to more than a million SNPs are assayed in thousands of individuals, represent a powerful new tool for investigating the genetic architecture of complex diseases (Hardy & Singleton, 2009; Manolio, 2010). The GWAS represent an important advance compared to 'candidate gene' studies, in which sample sizes are generally smaller and the variants assayed are limited to a selected few. However, most common variants individually or in combination confer relatively small increments in risk (1.1 to 1.5-fold) and explain only a small proportion of heritability (Hindorff et al., 2009). According to Dolan et al. (2010) genetic associations with preterm birth reveals a paucity of research in the area, compared with more mature genetic association fields like schizophrenia and Alzheimer's disease (Allen et al., 2008; Sun et al., 2008; Dolan et al., 2010). So far, no robustly replicated genetic variants contributing to this complex disease have been identified (Dolan et al., 2010).

GWAS research focusing on known pathways of PTB like inflammatory pathways, involved in host defense mechanisms, innate immunity activation and infection, could narrow the list of SNPs to study and produce more reliable data. Web-based reference databases that link the genome to biologic systems (e.g. Kyoto Encyclopedia of Genes and Genomes, www.genome.jp/kegg/pathway.html) are excellent tools to manage this information. The data collected so far in our group could be the first step to conduct a GWAS that associates wide amount genetic variations to a well studied population of preterm and term newborns. Uruguay has 3.5 million people (July 2010) and shares population characteristics with both developed countries and Latin American underdeveloped regions. Example of the foremost is the low birth rate (13.91 births/1,000 population; https://www.cia.gov/library/publications/the-world-factbook/). In Uruguay, nearly 10% of total newborns are preterm. The demographic characteristic of Uruguay, namely the comparatively low population and the lack of natural hazards, will make it easy to increase the number of cases and analyze not only the newborns but also their family in order to link genetic studies to social, environmental or pathological conditions where the newborns are raised. Finally genetic profiles will help to develop treatments according different susceptibilities. Because preterm labor is a final common pathway for multiple etiologies, it is reasonable to think that it will not be a single therapy that will work optimally for all binomial mother-fetus. As patient-specific pharmacogenomic profiles are developed, it will be possible to create patient-specific treatment regimens. It may become possible to identify those women and their fetuses who are predisposed to preterm labor and to institute patient-specific preventive measures (Esplin & Varner, 2005).

5. Conclusions

Understanding causes of PTB is especially important in underdeveloped countries. Complications of PTB are associated with increase of medical expenses, representing billions of dollars of direct costs and unrealized potential each year, sometimes unaffordable for poor countries. On another hand individual and ethnic differences exist both in the prevalence of infection related preterm birth and in the extent of immune responses to infection. Diversity of immune responses may influence the levels of susceptibility in women to preterm labor. Given individual genetic variations and differential environmental exposures, stratification of study subjects by genotype may allow the detection of risk of preterm birth among individuals exposed to different environmental effects. Furthermore, enhanced understanding of pathologic mechanisms may allow the development of drugs or interventions that can be used to prevent or treat preterm birth. On the basis of our current understanding of the role of intrauterine inflammation in the etiology of preterm birth, therapeutics should be directed to the well known pathways that conduct to inflammation.
Finally, preterm birth research will likely benefit greatly from GWAS findings and PTB Gene will incorporate data from such studies. Large scale multi-center collaborations using common standards and high throughput platforms that accounts for ethnic and environmental local conditions are needed to improve newborn health. They will direct progress in deciphering the genetic factors underlying preterm birth and consecutively help to bring basic research discoveries to the bedside.

6. Acknowledgments

Funding for this work was provided by Fogarty International Center 'National Institutes of Health' grant RO1TW006223 and and Comision Sectorial de Investigacion Cientifica (Uruguay). We acknowledge Mrs. Souza, from Dickens Institute, for her careful review of the manuscript language. We would to like to specially thank all the mothers that agreed to participate in this study.

7. References

Agnese DM, Calvano JE, Hahm SJ, Coyle SM, Corbett SA, Calvano SE & Lowry SF. 2002. Human toll-like receptor 4 mutations but not CD14 polymorphisms are associated with an increased risk of gram-negative infections. J Infect Dis 186:1522-1525.

Ameziane N, Beillat T, Verpillat P, Chollet-Martin S, Aumont MC, Seknadji P, Lamotte M, Lebret D, Ollivier V & de Prost D. 2003. Association of the Toll-like receptor 4 gene Asp299Gly polymorphism with acute coronary events. Arterioscler Thromb Vasc Biol 23:e61-64.

Allen NC, Bagade S, McQueen MB, Ioannidis JP, Kavvoura FK, Khoury MJ, Tanzi RE & Bertram L. 2008. Systematic meta-analyses and field synopsis of genetic association studies in schizophrenia: the SzGene database. Nat Genet 40:827-834.

Ananth CV, Getahun D, Peltier MR, Salihu HM & Vintzileos AM. 2006. Recurrence of spontaneous versus medically indicated preterm birth. Am J Obstet Gynecol 195:643-650.

Anum EA, Springel EH, Shriver MD & Strauss JF, 3rd. 2009. Genetic contributions to disparities in preterm birth. Pediatr Res 65:1-9.

Arbour NC, Lorenz E, Schutte BC, Zabner J, Kline JN, Jones M, Frees K, Watt JL & Schwartz DA. 2000. TLR4 mutations are associated with endotoxin hyporesponsiveness in humans. Nat Genet 25:187-191.

Bauer S, Muller T & Hamm S. 2009. Pattern recognition by Toll-like receptors. Adv Exp Med Biol 653:15-34.

Beck S, Wojdyla D, Say L, Betran AP, Merialdi M, Requejo JH, Rubens C, Menon R & Van Look PFA. 2010. The worldwide incidence of preterm birth: a systematic review of maternal mortality and morbidity. Bulletin of the World Health Organization 88:31-38.

Díaz A, Schwarcz R,. Díaz Rossello JL, Símini F, Giacomini H, López R, Martell M, Fescina R, De Mucio B, Martínez G 1990. Sistema informático perinatal. Rev Med Uruguay; 6: 75-83

Callaghan WM, MacDorman MF, Rasmussen SA, Qin C & Lackritz EM. 2006. The Contribution of Preterm Birth to Infant Mortality Rates in the United States. Pediatrics 118:1566-1573.

Carr-Hill RA & Hall MH. 1985. The repetition of spontaneous preterm labour. Br J Obstet Gynaecol 92:921-928.

Clausson B, Lichtenstein P & Cnattingius S. 2000. Genetic influence on birthweight and gestational length determined by studies in offspring of twins. Bjog 107:375-381.

Crider KS, Whitehead N & Buus RM. 2005. Genetic variation associated with preterm birth: a HuGE review. Genet Med 7:593-604.

Challis JR, Lye SJ, Gibb W, Whittle W, Patel F & Alfaidy N. 2001. Understanding preterm labor. Ann N Y Acad Sci 943:225-234.

Dolan SM, Hollegaard MV, Merialdi M, Betran AP, Allen T, Abelow C, Nace J, Lin BK, Khoury MJ, Ioannidis JP, Bagade S, Zheng X, Dubin RA, Bertram L, Velez Edwards DR & Menon R. 2010 . Synopsis of Preterm Birth Genetic Association Studies: The Preterm Birth Genetics Knowledge Base (PTBGene). Public Health Genomics13:514 - 523.

Engel SA, Erichsen HC, Savitz DA, Thorp J, Chanock SJ & Olshan AF. 2005. Risk of spontaneous preterm birth is associated with common proinflammatory cytokine polymorphisms. Epidemiology 16:469-477.

Esplin MS & Varner MW. 2005. Genetic factors in preterm birth--the future. Bjog 112 Suppl 1:97-102.

Ferrand PE, Fujimoto T, Chennathukuzhi V, Parry S, Macones GA, Sammel M, Kuivaniemi H, Romero R & Strauss JF, 3rd. 2002. The CARD15 2936insC mutation and TLR4 896 A>G polymorphism in African Americans and risk of preterm premature rupture of membranes (PPROM). Mol Hum Reprod 8:1031-1034.

Ferwerda B, McCall MB, Verheijen K, Kullberg BJ, van der Ven AJ, Van der Meer JW & Netea MG. 2008. Functional consequences of toll-like receptor 4 polymorphisms. Mol Med 14:346-352.

Garza-Gonzalez E, Bosques-Padilla FJ, Mendoza-Ibarra SI, Flores-Gutierrez JP, Maldonado-Garza HJ & Perez-Perez GI. 2007. Assessment of the toll-like receptor 4 Asp299Gly, Thr399Ile and interleukin-8 -251 polymorphisms in the risk for the development of distal gastric cancer. BMC Cancer 7:70.

Genc MR & Onderdonk A. 2011. Endogenous bacterial flora in pregnant women and the influence of maternal genetic variation. BJOG: An International Journal of Obstetrics & Gynaecology 118:154-163.

Genc MR & Schantz-Dunn J. 2007. The role of gene-environment interaction in predicting adverse pregnancy outcome. Best Pract Res Clin Obstet Gynaecol.

Genc MR, Vardhana S, Delaney ML, Onderdonk A, Tuomala R, Norwitz E & Witkin SS. 2004. Relationship between a toll-like receptor-4 gene polymorphism, bacterial vaginosis-related flora and vaginal cytokine responses in pregnant women. European Journal of Obstetrics & Gynecology and Reproductive Biology 116:152-156.

Goldenberg RL, Culhane JF, Iams JD & Romero R. 2008. Epidemiology and causes of preterm birth. Lancet 371:75-84.

Goldenberg RL, Hauth JC & Andrews WW. 2000. Intrauterine infection and preterm delivery. N Engl J Med 342:1500-1507.

Goldenberg RL. 2002. The management of preterm labor. Obstet Gynecol 100:1020-1037.

Gracie S, Lyon A, Kehler H, Pennell C, Dolan S, McNeil D, Siever J, McDonald S, Bocking A, Lye S, Hegadoren K, Olson D & Tough S. 2010. All Our Babies Cohort Study: recruitment of a cohort to predict women at risk of preterm birth through the examination of gene expression profiles and the environment. BMC Pregnancy and Childbirth 10:87.

Grigsby PL, Novy MJ, Waldorf KMA, Sadowsky DW & Gravett MG. 2010. Choriodecidual Inflammation: A Harbinger of the Preterm Labor Syndrome. Reproductive Sciences 17:85-94.

Hamet P, Pausova Z, Adarichev V, Adaricheva K & Tremblay J. 1998. Hypertension: genes and environment. J Hypertens 16:397-418.

Hardy J & Singleton A. 2009. Genomewide association studies and human disease. N Engl J Med 360:1759-1768.

Hidalgo PC, Bengochea M, Abilleira D, Cabrera A, Alvarez I. 2005. Genetic Admixture Estimate in the Uruguayan Population Based on the Loci LDLR, GYPA, HBGG, GC and D7S8. Int J Hum Genet 5: 217-22.

Hindorff LA, Sethupathy P, Junkins HA, Ramos EM, Mehta JP, Collins FS & Manolio TA. 2009. Potential etiologic and functional implications of genome-wide association loci for human diseases and traits. Proc Natl Acad Sci U S A 106:9362-9367.

Holmlund U, Cebers G, Dahlfors AR, Sandstedt B, Bremme K, Ekstrom ES & Scheynius A. 2002. Expression and regulation of the pattern recognition receptors Toll-like receptor-2 and Toll-like receptor-4 in the human placenta. Immunology 107:145-151.

Iacovidou N, Varsami M & Syggellou A. 2010. Neonatal outcome of preterm delivery. Ann N Y Acad Sci 1205:130-134.

Ioannidis JPA, Ntzani EE & Trikalinos TA. 2004. 'Racial' differences in genetic effects for complex diseases. Nat Genet 36:1312-1318.

Jorge Y, Duarte M & Silva A. 2010. Gastric cancer is associated with NOS2 -954G/C polymorphism and environmental factors in a Brazilian population. BMC Gastroenterology 10:64.

Kalish RB, Vardhana S, Normand NJ, Gupta M & Witkin SS. 2006. Association of a maternal CD14 -159 gene polymorphism with preterm premature rupture of membranes and spontaneous preterm birth in multi-fetal pregnancies. J Reprod Immunol 70:109-117.

Kaufman JS & Cooper RS. 2008. Race in epidemiology: new tools, old problems. Ann Epidemiol 18:119-123.

Keelan JA. 2011. Pharmacological inhibition of inflammatory pathways for the prevention of preterm birth. J Reprod Immunol 88:176-184.

Keelan JA, Blumenstein M, Helliwell RJ, Sato TA, Marvin KW & Mitchell MD. 2003. Cytokines, prostaglandins and parturition--a review. Placenta 24 Suppl A:S33-46.

Kelada SN, Eaton DL, Wang SS, Rothman NR & Khoury MJ. 2003. The role of genetic polymorphisms in environmental health. Environ Health Perspect 111:1055-1064.

Kiechl S, Lorenz E, Reindl M, Wiedermann CJ, Oberhollenzer F, Bonora E, Willeit J & Schwartz DA. 2002. Toll-like receptor 4 polymorphisms and atherogenesis. N Engl J Med 347:185-192.

Kramer MR & Hogue CR. 2009. What Causes Racial Disparities in Very Preterm Birth? A Biosocial Perspective. Epidemiologic Reviews 31:84-98.

Krishnan J, Selvarajoo K, Tsuchiya M, Lee G & Choi S. 2007. Toll-like receptor signal transduction. Exp Mol Med 39:421-438.

Lau JY & Eley TC. 2004. Gene-environment interactions and correlations in psychiatric disorders. Curr Psychiatry Rep 6:119-124.

Li L, Kang J & Lei W. 2010. Role of Toll-like receptor 4 in inflammation-induced preterm delivery. Mol Hum Reprod 16:267-272.

Lorenz E, Hallman M, Marttila R, Haataja R & Schwartz DA. 2002a. Association between the Asp299Gly polymorphisms in the Toll-like receptor 4 and premature births in the Finnish population. Pediatr Res 52:373-376.

Lorenz E, Jones M, Wohlford-Lenane C, Meyer N, Frees KL, Arbour NC & Schwartz DA. 2001. Genes other than TLR4 are involved in the response to inhaled LPS. Am J Physiol Lung Cell Mol Physiol 281:L1106-1114.

Lorenz E, Mira JP, Frees KL & Schwartz DA. 2002b. Relevance of mutations in the TLR4 receptor in patients with gram-negative septic shock. Arch Intern Med 162:1028-1032.

Lu YC, Yeh WC & Ohashi PS. 2008. LPS/TLR4 signal transduction pathway. Cytokine 42:145-151.

Lyon D, Cheng CY, Howland L, Rattican D, Jallo N, Pickler R, Brown L & McGrath J. 2010. Integrated review of cytokines in maternal, cord, and newborn blood: part I--associations with preterm birth. Biol Res Nurs 11:371-376.

Ma Y, Krikun G, Abrahams VM, Mor G & Guller S. 2007. Cell type-specific expression and function of toll-like receptors 2 and 4 in human placenta: implications in fetal infection. Placenta 28:1024-1031.

Macones G, Parry S, Elkousy M, Clothier B, Ural S & Strauss J. 2004a. A polymorphism in the promoter region of TNF and bacterial vaginosis: preliminary evidence of gene-environment interaction in the etiology of spontaneous preterm birth. Am J Obstet Gynecol 190:1504 - 1508.

Macones GA, Parry S, Elkousy M, Clothier B, Ural SH & Strauss JF, 3rd. 2004b. A polymorphism in the promoter region of TNF and bacterial vaginosis: preliminary evidence of gene-environment interaction in the etiology of spontaneous preterm birth. Am J Obstet Gynecol 190:1504-1508; discussion 1503A.

Manolio TA. 2010. Genomewide association studies and assessment of the risk of disease. N Engl J Med 363:166-176.

Manolio TA, Collins FS, Cox NJ, Goldstein DB, Hindorff LA, Hunter DJ, McCarthy MI, Ramos EM, Cardon LR, Chakravarti A, Cho JH, Guttmacher AE, Kong A, Kruglyak L, Mardis E, Rotimi CN, Slatkin M, Valle D, Whittemore AS, Boehnke M, Clark AG, Eichler EE, Gibson G, Haines JL, Mackay TF, McCarroll SA & Visscher PM. 2009. Finding the missing heritability of complex diseases. Nature 461:747-753.

Martin JA, Hamilton BE, Menacker F, Sutton PD & Mathews TJ. 2005. Preliminary Births for 2004: Infant and Maternal Health. In: *Centers for Disease Control and Prevention*, 05.07.2011, Available from: http://www.cdc.gov/nchs/products/pubs/pubd/hestats/prelimbirths04/prelimbirths/04health.htm

Martinon F & Tschopp J. 2007. Inflammatory caspases and inflammasomes: master switches of inflammation. Cell Death Differ 14:10-22.

Medvedev AE, Kopydlowski KM & Vogel SN. 2000. Inhibition of lipopolysaccharide-induced signal transduction in endotoxin-tolerized mouse macrophages: dysregulation of cytokine, chemokine, and toll-like receptor 2 and 4 gene expression. J Immunol 164:5564-5574.

Medzhitov R, Preston-Hurlburt P & Janeway CA, Jr. 1997. A human homologue of the Drosophila Toll protein signals activation of adaptive immunity. Nature 388:394-397.

Menon R, Velez DR, Simhan H, Ryckman K, Jiang L, Thorsen P, Vogel I, Jacobsson B, Merialdi M, Williams SM & Fortunato SJ. 2006. Multilocus interactions at maternal tumor necrosis factor-alpha, tumor necrosis factor receptors, interleukin-6 and interleukin-6 receptor genes predict spontaneous preterm labor in European-American women. Am J Obstet Gynecol 194:1616-1624.

Menon R, Fortunato SJ, Edwards DR & Williams SM. 2010. Association of genetic variants, ethnicity and preterm birth with amniotic fluid cytokine concentrations. Ann Hum Genet 74:165-183.

Moura E, Mattar R, de Souza E, Torloni MR, Goncalves-Primo A & Daher S. 2009. Inflammatory cytokine gene polymorphisms and spontaneous preterm birth. J Reprod Immunol 80:115-121.

Noguchi T, Sado T, Naruse K, Shigetomi H, Onogi A, Haruta S, Kawaguchi R, Nagai A, Tanase Y, Yoshida S, Kitanaka T, Oi H & Kobayashi H. 2010. Evidence for activation of Toll-like receptor and receptor for advanced glycation end products in preterm birth. Mediators Inflamm 2010:490-406.

Nukui T, Day RD, Sims CS, Ness RB & Romkes M. 2004. Maternal/newborn GSTT1 null genotype contributes to risk of preterm, low birthweight infants. Pharmacogenetics 14:569-576.

O'Neill LA. 2008. The interleukin-1 receptor/Toll-like receptor superfamily: 10 years of progress. Immunol Rev 226:10-18.

Oh KJ, Lee SE, Jung H, Kim G, Romero R & Yoon BH. 2010. Detection of ureaplasmas by the polymerase chain reaction in the amniotic fluid of patients with cervical insufficiency. Journal of Perinatal Medicine 38:261-268.

Papadopoulos AI, Ferwerda B, Antoniadou A, Sakka V, Galani L, Kavatha D, Panagopoulos P, Poulakou G, Kanellakopoulou K, van der Meer JW, Giamarellos-Bourboulis EJ & Netea MG. 2010. Association of toll-like receptor 4 Asp299Gly and Thr399Ile polymorphisms with increased infection risk in patients with advanced HIV-1 infection. Clin Infect Dis 51:242-247.

Patni S, Flynn P, Wynen LP, Seager AL, Morgan G, White JO & Thornton CA. 2007. An introduction to Toll-like receptors and their possible role in the initiation of labour. Bjog 114:1326-1334.

Pennell CE, Jacobsson B, Williams SM, Buus RM, Muglia LJ, Dolan SM, Morken NH, Ozcelik H, Lye SJ & Relton C. 2007. Genetic epidemiologic studies of preterm birth: guidelines for research. Am J Obstet Gynecol 196:107-118.

Plunkett J & Muglia LJ. 2008. Genetic contributions to preterm birth: implications from epidemiological and genetic association studies. Ann Med 40:167-195.

Pontillo A, Brandao L, Guimaraes R, Segat L, Araujo J & Crovella S. 2010. Two SNPs in NLRP3 gene are involved in the predisposition to type-1 diabetes and celiac disease in a pediatric population from northeast Brazil. Autoimmunity 43:583-589.

Porter TF, Fraser AM, Hunter CY, Ward RH & Varner MW. 1997. The risk of preterm birth across generations. Obstet Gynecol 90:63-67.

Raetz CR & Whitfield C. 2002. Lipopolysaccharide endotoxins. Annu Rev Biochem 71:635-700.

Rey G, Skowronek F, Alciaturi J, Alonso J, Bertoni B & Sapiro R. 2008. Toll receptor 4 Asp299Gly polymorphism and its association with preterm birth and premature rupture of membranes in a South American population. Mol Hum Reprod 14:555-559.

Romero R, Espinoza J, Goncalves LF, Kusanovic JP, Friel L & Hassan S. 2007. The role of inflammation and infection in preterm birth. Semin Reprod Med 25:21-39.

Romero R, Espinoza J, Kusanovic JP, Gotsch F, Hassan S, Erez O, Chaiworapongsa T & Mazor M. 2006. The preterm parturition syndrome. Bjog 113 Suppl 3:17-42.

Romero R, Maymon E, Pacora P, Gomez R, Mazor M, Yoon BH & Berry SM. 2000. Further observations on the fetal inflammatory response syndrome: a potential homeostatic role for the soluble receptors of tumor necrosis factor alpha. Am J Obstet Gynecol 183:1070-1077.

Romero R, Mazor M, Munoz H, Gomez R, Galasso M & Sherer DM. 1994. The preterm labor syndrome. Ann N Y Acad Sci 734:414-429.

Romero R, Velez Edwards DR, Kusanovic JP, Hassan SS, Mazaki-Tovi S, Vaisbuch E, Kim CJ, Chaiworapongsa T, Pearce BD, Friel LA, Bartlett J, Anant MK, Salisbury BA, Vovis GF, Lee MS, Gomez R, Behnke E, Oyarzun E, Tromp G, Williams SM & Menon R. 2010. Identification of fetal and maternal single nucleotide polymorphisms in candidate genes that predispose to spontaneous preterm labor with intact membranes. Am J Obstet Gynecol 202:431 e431-434.

Sans M, Merriwether DA, Hidalgo PC, Bentancor N, Weimer TA, Franco MH, Alvarez I, Kemp BM & Salzano FM. 2006. Population structure and admixture in Cerro Largo, Uruguay, based on blood markers and mitochondrial DNA polymorphisms. Am J Hum Biol 18:513-524.

Santos JL, Lera L, Perez-Bravo F & Albala C. 2006. Adiposity and bone mineral density of Chilean elderly women in relation to toll-like receptor 4 gene polymorphisms. Ann Hum Biol 33:585-592.

Schaefer TM, Desouza K, Fahey JV, Beagley KW & Wira CR. 2004. Toll-like receptor (TLR) expression and TLR-mediated cytokine/chemokine production by human uterine epithelial cells. Immunology 112:428-436.

Slattery MM & Morrison JJ. 2002. Preterm delivery. Lancet 360:1489-1497.

Smirnova I, Hamblin MT, McBride C, Beutler B & Di Rienzo A. 2001. Excess of rare amino acid polymorphisms in the Toll-like receptor 4 in humans. Genetics 158:1657-1664.

Sosa CG, Althabe F, Belizan JM & Buekens P. 2011. Use of oxytocin during early stages of labor and its effect on active management of third stage of labor. Am J Obstet Gynecol. 204(3):238.e1-5.

Sun J, Kuo PH, Riley BP, Kendler KS & Zhao Z. 2008. Candidate genes for schizophrenia: a survey of association studies and gene ranking. Am J Med Genet B Neuropsychiatr Genet 147B:1173-1181.

Talmud PJ & Humphries SE. 2004. Gene: environment interactions and coronary heart disease risk. World Rev Nutr Diet 93:29-40.

Thaxton JE, Nevers TA & Sharma S. 2010. TLR-mediated preterm birth in response to pathogenic agents. Infect Dis Obstet Gynecol 2010.

Todd JA. 2006. Statistical false positive or true disease pathway? Nat Genet 38:731-733.

Vallabhapurapu S & Karin M. 2009. Regulation and function of NF-kappaB transcription factors in the immune system. Annu Rev Immunol 27:693-733.

Vrachnis N, Vitoratos N, Iliodromiti Z, Sifakis S, Deligeoroglou E & Creatsas G. 2010. Intrauterine inflammation and preterm delivery. Ann N Y Acad Sci 1205:118-122.

Wang X, Zuckerman B, Pearson C, Kaufman G, Chen C, Wang G, Niu T, Wise PH, Bauchner H & Xu X. 2002. Maternal cigarette smoking, metabolic gene polymorphism, and infant birth weight. JAMA 287:195-202.

Wen SW, Smith G, Yang Q & Walker M. 2004. Epidemiology of preterm birth and neonatal outcome. Semin Fetal Neonatal Med 9:429-435.

Zhu X. 2005. Admixture mapping for hypertension loci with genome-scan markers. 37:177-181.

8

Uterine Contraction Monitoring, Maintenance Tocolysis, and Preterm Birth

John C. Morrison[1], John P. Elliott[2] and Stephen Jones[3]
[1]*Departments of Obstetrics and Gynecology, University of Mississippi Medical Center, Jackson, Mississippi,*
[2]*Magella Medical Group, an affiliation of Obstetrix Medical Group, Laguna Hill, California,*
[3]*Christus Schumpert Hospital, Shreveport, Louisianna, USA*

1. Introduction

Uterine contractions occur in runs of 1-3/hr throughout pregnancy from early in the second trimester until full term usually without consequence. Regular uterine contractions are essential in every case of preterm labor (PTL) resulting in preterm delivery at <37 weeks. It has been demonstrated that women are unable to accurately perceive the contractions associated with preterm labor while uterine contraction monitoring can frequently detect these contractions at an early enough time that acute tocolysis can stop preterm labor in most cases and significantly prolong the pregnancy. In women who have cervical shortening, those who have preterm labor symptomatology with multifetal gestations, or patients who have already had an episode of preterm labor, uterine contraction monitoring has been helpful in prolonging the pregnancy by early detection. As an example, women, after receiving tocolysis for true preterm labor, are monitored (tertiary prevention) in the home (whether or not they are receiving maintenance tocolytics) and when a second episode of PTL occurs, the majority reach the hospital for appropriate treatment before excessive cervical dilatation has occurred. Alternatively, following successful acute tocolysis in the hospital, patients may receive maintenance tocolysis with a subcutaneous terbutaline infusion pump and are also managed at home with continued contraction assessment. This chapter will review the available literature regarding the use of contraction monitoring for tertiary prevention as well as subcutaneous terbutaline maintenance therapy for treatment of contractions.

2. Background

2.1 General

The incidence of preterm birth (PTB), or delivery at <37 weeks, continues to increase and accounts for 75% of all neonatal mortality and morbidity.(Hamilton *et al.*, 2006) All physicians agree that preterm delivery (PTD) following preterm labor (PTL) involves frequent uterine contractions which dilate the cervix. In fact, the definition of preterm labor involves uterine contractions $\leq$5 minutes apart and cervical change (usually $\geq$1cm dilatation or cervical shortening (or thinning) by ultrasound). Contractions that do not meet that frequency or contractions without cervical change several hours after uterine activity starts are called uterine irritability, irregular contractions, Braxton Hicks contractions, or false labor, but have no effect on the cervix are never called preterm labor. In order to delay or prevent PTD, true uterine contractions should be detected sufficiently early (cervical dilatation <4 cm), to allow reasonable success of tocolytic drugs to result in meaningful pregnancy prolongation.(ACOG Practice Bulletin, 2007) Unfortunately, painful, irregular uterine contractions can also be associated with false labor or uterine irritability and even when they are strong, much less than 50% are perceived by patients.(Beckmann *et al.*, 1996; Faustin *et al.*, 1997) PTL can be acute (abruptly going from normal contraction frequency of 1-2/hr on average to $\geq$8 ctx/hr) or gradual (over days). Basal uterine activity is important clinically, since the goal is to detect an increase in contractions in a timely fashion.

2.2 Uterine contraction monitoring

The detection of contractions in asymptomatic patients to rule out true preterm labor for some identified risk factor by uterine activity assessment or palpation alone has meet with variable success.(Faustin *et al.*, 1997; Martin *et al.*, 1990; Dyson *et al.*, 1998) The use of uterine contraction monitoring and patient recorded signs and symptoms is more successful (secondary prevention) but does not yield high enough positive predictive value to be useful as a assessment tool for those with high risk factors.(Dyson *et al.*, 1998) Some patients are at extremely high risk for preterm delivery such as those who have already experienced an episode of true preterm labor with cervical dilatation or women with multi-fetal gestations (MFG), or those with a significantly shortened cervix. These patients have all been shown to benefit from uterine activity monitoring (tertiary prevention).(Morrison *et al.*, 2001; Katz *et al.*, 1986; Watson *et al.*, 1990; Kosasa *et al.*, 1990) Contraction assessment is particularly important in MFG as the contraction pattern is different from that in singletons. Newman *et al., (1986)* demonstrated that twins have statistically more contractions/hr than singletons averaging 2/hr at 29 weeks, 3/h at 33 weeks, and 4/h at 36 weeks. Garite *et al.*, (1990) demonstrated a crescendo of contractions in twins, triplets and quads starting approximately 48 hrs prior to PTL (3.5 ctx/hr $\pm$ 1.4) and at 24 hrs prior to PTL (5.3 ctx / hr $\pm$ 1.3) Hernandez *et al.*, (2008) demonstrated that twins who developed PTL with or without early delivery had significantly more baseline contractions compared to twins who never developed PTL. Contractions exceeded 3.5/hr at 29-1/2 weeks in those developing PTL. Newman *et al.*, (2006) could not identify a threshold number of uterine contractions that would predict PTL but confirmed that twins have more UC at each gestational age (GA) than singletons and that UC increase with advancing GA and also time of day (1600-0359 hours). Rust *et al.*, (1997) compared twins who developed PTL <24 weeks. In this study, 31 patients had been placed on contraction monitoring prior to PTL and 32 were prescribed home contraction monitoring after PTL was arrested. The GA at diagnosis of PTL was similar, but cervical dilation was significantly different, with the twins already on a monitor being less dilated (1.1 $\pm$ 0.5 cm vs 2.3 $\pm$ 0.8 cm p .0001). The twin pregnancies already undergoing contraction monitoring delivered at a mean GA 34.7± 2.8 wks compared to 27.6 ± 2.5 wks for those placed on monitoring after PTL was arrested at <24 wks ($p < .001$).

2.3 Higher order multiples

Triplets and quadruplets are referred to as high order multiple (HOM) pregnancies. Preterm labor is confirmed in 80% of triplet pregnancies and 98% of quads, occurs at an earlier gestational age, and the mothers are almost always unaware of the contractions due to increased fetal movement.(Elliott *et al.*, 1995) Elliott *et al.*, (1995) utilized HUAM to determine a weekly average of contractions/hour for patients with HOM gestation. With two, one-hour monitoring sessions per day the total number of observed contractions were divided by 14 and utilized as an average number (eg 3.9 ctx /hr) that week. In support, Garite *et al.*, (1990) reported that patients with singleton pregnancies increased their contractions to 3.5/hr 48 hours prior to PTL developing, while (Elliott *et al.*, 1995) found that HOM gestations who were given betamethasone developed increasing contractions and true PTL/delivery statistically more frequently if the baseline number of UC was greater than 3.5/hr compared to those with a baseline contraction frequency that was less than 3.5/hr. Based on this arbitrary number of contractions/hr (3.5 UC/hr) (Elliott *et al.*, 1997) started tocolysis prophylactically, utilizing terbutaline pump therapy to attempt to prevent PTL that can result in PTD. The results of this report showed that in 15 sets of triplets and 6 sets of quads only 14% delivered due to PTL; much less than the reported incidence in other series. This underscores the importance of determining uterine contraction frequency and then potentially initiating preventative therapy. Therefore, the rationale of using contraction monitoring for tertiary prevention as well as treatment using subcutaneous terbutaline is supported by various studies but what are the clinical results of such investigations?

2.4 Contraction monitoring with maintenance tocolysis

In general, tertiary assessment results in an earlier diagnosis of recurrent preterm labor at less cervical dilatation, which improves the success of tocolysis and results in greater pregnancy prolongation when compared with standard care even when both groups used maintenance tocolysis.(Morrison *et al.*, 2001; Katz *et al.*, 1986; Watson *et al.*, 1990; Kosasa *et al.*, 1990; Smith *et al.*, 1994) Furthermore, after tocolysis of the second PTL episode or in pregnancies with advanced cervical dilation (>3-4cm), the combination of continued uterine contraction monitoring along with subcutaneous terbutaline infusion using a programmable pump have resulted in significantly prolonged gestation compared to no treatment or oral maintenance therapy.(Elliott *et al.*, 2001; Morrison *et al.*, 2003; Lam *et al.*, 2001) Both contraction monitoring and terbutaline administration by subcutaneous pump, when used in appropriate patients, significantly increased the length of pregnancy, resulted in fewer low birth weight infants, and reduced neonatal stay as well as neonatal cost.(Martin *et al.*, 1990; Smith *et al.*, 1994; Morrison *et al.*, 2003; Lam *et al.*, 2001)

2.5 Purpose

The purpose of this chapter is to review the literature regarding uterine contraction monitoring, when used for tertiary prevention, and to assess studies using subcutaneous terbutaline infusion (when employed in conjunction with uterine contraction monitoring) in women who had previously had an episode of confirmed preterm labor, and those with twins or higher order multiples demonstrating cervical change.

3. Tertiary uterine contraction monitoring

3.1 Method of contraction monitoring

Regarding contraction monitoring for tertiary prevention, only randomized clinical trials (RCT) or cohort studies with appropriate matched controls were considered. A review of the literature revealed seven acceptable trials from 1985 to 2005, using uterine contraction monitoring for tertiary care. There were three additional studies that were eliminated because the HUAM group was not compared to a standard of care control group or because women with current preterm labor as a subgroup were never reported separately. Women using contraction assessment in the home monitored uterine activity for two hours per day (usually once in the morning and once in the afternoon) using a sensitive guard-ring principal monitoring. On a daily basis a nurse initiated a phone call and transmitted the two hours of monitoring to assess the number and quality of the contractions present. During this daily phone call the nurse asked about symptoms of preterm labor, such as pelvic heaviness, uterine contractions, tightening increase in cervical discharge, etc. If signs and symptoms of preterm labor where present or if there were >4 contractions per hour, the patient was asked to hydrate and re-monitor. If these repeat data were not satisfactory, the patient was sent to the hospital. In addition, during the daily phone call, the education regarding signs or symptoms of PTL and patient's specific educational objectives were reinforced. Finally, these women had access to a 24/7 availability toll free calls to a nurse other than the person who made the daily phone call. All women attended a special preterm birth prevention clinic, where cervical assessment digitally or by ultrasound was carried out along with an assessment of preterm labor signs and symptoms and other testing such as, cultures, fetal fibronectin, and a variety of educational techniques at the discretion of the physician. Women in the various cohort or control groups frequently attended the same clinics with the same education, but were taught palpation for uterine activity, which they recorded daily.

3.2 Results of tertiary contraction monitoring

As shown in Table I, the study by Katz revealed an average of 68% reduction in preterm birth when patients using uterine contraction monitoring in the home were compared to the standard care control group.(Katz *et al.*, 1986) In the prospective controlled study by Kosasa, preterm delivery rates were not reported, but in women prescribed contraction monitoring after preterm labor was arrested, there was a pregnancy prolongation of 4.6 weeks and an average gestational age of delivery at 36.7 weeks.(Kosasa *et al.*, 1990) In addition, there was a cost savings of $21,200.00 in the contraction monitoring group versus the standard care group for such high risk patients. Katz *et al.*, (1988) studied 120 women after an episode of confirmed preterm labor. Half of the patients received contraction monitoring compared to self-palpation. Preterm births among monitored patients were significantly less than the control group (15 versus 34%, $p<.05$) and more importantly time gained *in utero* was 7.4 ± 3.0 weeks in the monitored group versus 4.0 ± 1.2 weeks in controls.(Katz *et al.*, 1988) Morrison *et al.*, (2001) found similar results in a Medicaid population where pregnancy prolongation was extended, there were fewer preterm births, and the cost saving was significantly more ($14,459.00) among monitored patients when compared to controls. Morrison *et al.*, (2001) Watson *et al.*, (1990) in a randomized clinical trial among women discharged on monitoring versus control patients, found that there were 44% fewer preterm births compared to control women ($p<.05$) with a higher incidence of failed tocolysis also among control women resulting in a longer mean time gained *in utero* for monitored women.

STUDIES INVOLVING CURRENT PRETERM LABOR PATIENTS AND COMMERCIALLY AVAILABLE HUAM SERVICE COMPARED TO THE STANDARD OF CARE							
STUDY	RESEARCH DESIGN	QUALITY OF EVIDENCE	N	PTD RATE REDUCTIONS IN MONITORED GROUP		$ SAVINGS / PREGNANCY	COMMENTS
				<35 WKS	<37 WKS		
Katz et al., 1986	Matched Trial	II-2	120	*	56%	*	Pregnancy prolongation was 7.4 weeks for HUAM group compared to 4.0 weeks
Watson et al., 1990	RCT	I	67	*	44%	*	Greater than 2 weeks improvement in gestational age at birth with HUAM
Kosasa et al 1990	Prospective Cost Effectiveness Study	II-1	43	*	*	$21,200	$24,000 Savings/CPTL Patient - $2,800 cost of HUAM/PT = $21,200. Greater than 4 weeks prolongation of pregnancy. Savings from lower NICU days and reduction in antenatal days
Nagey et al., 1993	RCT	I	56			*	HUAM group had 43% dropout rate which made final sample size too small to detect differences
Smith et al., 1994	Matched Trial	II-2	58	*	39%	*	47% delivered <37 weeks in the control group compared to 8% in the HUAM group
Brown et al., 1999	RCT	I	186	27%	19%	*	11% lower NICU admits, 25% lower NICU days/1000 births, and 37% less respiratory ventilation in the HUAM group
Morrison et al., 2001	Cohort Trial	II-2	100	95%	80%	$14,459	Actual claims data shows a significant savings in the HUAM group
* Not reported in study							

Table 1. Utilization of huam for tertiary care evidence table.

Nagey *et al.*, (1993) studied 28 women who were discharged from the hospital after tocolysis and received HUAM versus 29 women who received routine care. Since there was no daily perinatal contact or 24/7 availability of calling the nurse, there was considerably more non-compliance (26/28) in the monitored group and accordingly there was no difference in pregnancy prolongation or preterm deliveries. Additionally, 4 patients out of the 28 in the monitoring group were never discharged and did not receive monitoring at all. Finally, the authors did not meet their power calculation, as 45 in each group were needed to show a detectable difference for contraction monitoring. Pregnancy prolongation and neonatal morbidity statistics were not reported in this study. Smith *et al.*, (1994) studied women discharged after preterm labor using contraction monitoring versus a like number who served as matched controls. Among monitoring women, pregnancy prolongation, gestational age at birth, and number delivering <37 weeks compared to control patients were significantly improved (p<.011). Brown *et al.*, (1999) studied 86 women who were assigned to monitoring compared to 80 in an unmonitored group following effective acute tocolysis. Unfortunately, the number needed to show a significant difference in preterm delivery was 438 and only 162 were enrolled over a 7-year period. Therefore, no differences in preterm delivery or pregnancy prolongation were noted but since daily contact with a nurse was allowed, the number of NICU admissions was reduced in both groups (24%, 27%) compared to other studies.

3.3 Contraction monitoring: Pooled results

When these studies are pooled, the preterm delivery rate (<37 weeks) in the monitored group was 30.6% versus 48.9% among control patients. In the 2 studies reporting data for <35 week deliveries, the monitored group was favored (7.7% versus 22.9%).(Morrison *et al.*, 2001; Brown *et al.*, 1999) This translated into a pregnancy prolongation of 7.8 weeks in the monitored group versus 4.4 weeks in the control group. Two studies reported NICU rates of admission (Smith *et al.*, 1994; Brown *et al.*, 1999) and the pooled data reveals a 7.2% NICU admission rate for monitored patients versus 36.2% among the infants of control women.

Pregnancy prolongation resulted in a total cost savings amongst the studies who collected financial data (Morrison *et al.*, 2001; Kosasa *et al.*, 1990) of $413,153 or $13,153/per pregnancy compared to control group women. Among secondary prevention studies including patients who had preterm labor in the current gestation, Floyd and Morrison also revealed benefit for these monitored patients versus control subjects with respect to pregnancy prolongation and preterm deliveries.(Floyd *et al.*, 1993; Morrison *et al.*, 1990) In sum, when patients use contraction monitoring for tertiary care (after discharge from an episode of acute preterm labor in the current pregnancy), there is a significant prolongation of pregnancy and fewer preterm deliveries, which results in fewer NICU admissions and less neonatal morbidity as well as cost among monitored patients compared to controls.

4. Maintenance tocolysis

4.1 Tocolytic choices

The data presented in Table I supports monitoring contractions, particularly to detect recurrent preterm labor after successful treatment of the initial episode of early labor. The therapeutic strategies for such women, however is disparate. Although there is not reliable data because such women are rarely studied, a large number of patients each year who have been successfully treated for preterm labor remain in the hospital until delivery, rather than being sent home. To be sure this appropriately includes some patients with advanced cervical dilatation (≥4cm), others with concominant medical/obstetric problems or women who have geographic difficulties with transportation or patients who are considered to be unreliable. In our clinical experience however, these are the minority and most women remaining in hospital simply do so to reduce medical/legal risks or assuage maternal/physician anxiety. Clearly this is not cost or health effective. Many of these patients would qualify for discharge and monitoring with terbutaline subcutaneous therapy or oral tocolytic treatment in the home. Secondly, many physicians do not prescribe tocolytic maintenance therapy to women who are sent home because studies have shown that oral therapy does not extend pregnancy compare to placebo.(Rust *et al.*, 1996) Calcium channel blockers such as nifedipine are also utilized for maintenance tocolysis. There have been two placebo controlled trials with nifedipine and neither have shown any difference in gestational age at delivery, time gained *in utero*, deliveries at term, or composite neonatal morbidity when compared to placebo patients.(Carr *et al.*, 1999; Lyell *et al.*, 2008) In addition, maternal myocardial infarction, hepatic toxicity, and hypotension with fetal distress, as well as a reduction in uterine artery pulsatility index with fetal death have all been reported with the oral use of nifedipine for preterm labor particularly when the dose is increased.(Abbasi *et al.*, 2003; van Geijn *et al.*, 2005) Therefore, the choice of oral nifedipine for maintenance tocolysis, similar to oral terbutaline or oral magnesium, does not appear to be solid as its efficacy is questionable and there are significant maternal and fetal side effects. Regardless, women who are discharged after acute preterm labor is stopped, need uterine contraction monitoring whether they use oral tocolytics, the terbutaline pump, or no medication.

4.2 Do oral tocolytics work

It is clear that many patients in the treatment arm of these studies whether it be, oral terbutaline, oral magnesium or nifedipine simply did not receive an adequate dose of the drug due to maternal side effects. For example, there are several studies which show that when maintenance tocolysis is discontinued, between 30% and 50% of patients deliver within 24 to 72 hours.(Jones *et al.*, 2006; Rebarber *et al.*, 2009) Teleologically, it seems unlikely that patients who have been on tocolysis for several weeks or months would deliver within 1-3 days (and 70-80% within 1 week) if the tocolytic agent did not cause cessation of uterine contractions. Therefore, it may not be that oral tocolytics don't work when given in a maintenance form, it may just be, that the effective dosage of medications have side effects resulting in poor compliance or discontinuation of treatment. In summary, the issue of maintenance tocolysis is not clear-cut. While it is not cogent to leave all patients in the hospital after an episode of acute preterm labor, if one is not going to use maintenance tocolysis on an ambulatory basis, at the very least, home contraction monitoring with daily nursing calls should be utilized in our opinion to detect recurrent preterm labor at the earliest time.

5. Subcutaneous terbutaline pump usage

5.1 Requirements for terbutaline pump

Another area in which contraction monitoring is essential is during maintenance tocolysis therapy employing a subcutaneous terbutaline infusion pump. When the subcutaneous terbutaline pump was used versus or maintenance drugs (or no oral tocolysis) 46 peer review studies were noted. In each study involving the terbutaline pump, it was required that uterine contraction monitoring was utilized since this end organ response (uterine contraction) was necessary to guide bolus terbutaline dosing. Additionally, it was required that such investigations utilize pharmacy consultation to calculate the volume of distribution in order to give an appropriate basal dose of terbutaline parenterally. Daily nursing contact (usually by phone) was carried out to detect patient reported signs and symptoms as well as two, one hour monitoring periods (usually one in the morning and one in the evening). Of all the terbutaline studies, there were three randomized clinical trials (Level I), 26 observational case control/cohort studies (Level II), and 17 descriptive case series (Level III). Two studies (Wenstrom *et al.*, 1997; Guinn *et al.*, 1998) were eliminated because they did not allow proper usage of terbutaline treatment (pharmacy consultation to adjust basal dosage, contraction monitoring to adjust bolus terbutaline therapy, daily nursing contact, or emergency patient contact) and in addition both were vastly underpowered (94 enrolled, 320 required by power calculations). In the other studies, the outcomes of interest in both groups under study (tertiary prevention, terbutaline pump treatment), included pregnancy prolongation, preterm delivery rate (<37 weeks/<35 weeks), gestational age at delivery, also NICU admission rate, as well as, the length of stay were noted, and if available, the cost savings per pregnancy. These were compared between the treatment and control group.

In this therapy a basal rate of subcutaneous terbutaline is determined (.045-.075mg/hr) in consultation with a pharmacist so that the patient's volume of distribution is calculated verifying that the constant level of terbutaline is optimized for that patient. Importantly, the basal rate is supplemented by intermittent boluses (usually .25mg terbutaline each) programmed by the patient during the daily nursing call timed to address increased uterine activity detected by contraction monitoring. These bolus doses are critical as each patient's contraction pattern is different. The advantage of the small subcutaneous dosage per day, combining the basal rate and bolus rate (usually 2.5-3.5mg), is that there is less down regulation of beta-agonist receptors and a reduction in maternal side effects when compared to oral maintenance therapy with terbutaline (20-40mg per day).

5.2 Results of terbutaline pump maintenance tocolysis

As shown in Table II, the data for continuous subcutaneous terbutaline infusion is voluminous. There are 46 peer review publications over a 20-year period (1988-2008) involving over 30,000 patients. Of these 46 there are only 2 studies which did not find increased pregnancy prolongation, less NICU admissions and lowered cost.(Wenstrom *et al.*, 1997; Guinn *et al.*, 1998) Both of these studies had critical flaws. First they were small, only involving 94 total patients of which 39 received the terbutaline pump, but also importantly a fixed basal dosage of terbutaline was used without volume of distribution calculations so that a 150-pound woman received the same dosage as a 350-pound woman. Also, there was no measurement of end organ response as contraction monitoring to determine if changes in bolus dosage were needed, was not allowed. Finally, neither study had enough patients (94 enrolled, 320 in each group required to meet a power calculation) to demonstrate efficacy. Of the other 44 studies, all were positive; demonstrating fewer preterm deliveries, greater pregnancy prolongation, less NICU admission and/or enhanced cost savings.

- Lam et al, 1987
- Lam et al, 1988
- Lam et al, 1988
- McGettigan et al, 1991
- Gianopoulos et al, 1991
- Jones et al, 1991
- Fischer et al, 1991
- Wolfsen et al, 1992
- Allbert et al, 1992
- Moise et al, 1992
- Weinbaum et al, 1992
- Elliott et al, 1992
- Lindenbaum et al, 1992
- Regenstein et al, 1993
- Adkins et al, 1993
- Allbert et al, 1994
- Perry et al, 1995
- Wenstrom et al, 1997
- Elliott et al, 1997
- Lam et al, 1998
- Guinn et al, 1998
- Berkus et al, 1999
- Hamersley et al, 1999
- Lam et al, 2000
- Elliott et al, 2001
- Elliott et al, 2001
- Lam et al, 2001
- Viscarello et al, 2002
- Viscarello et al, 2002
- Elliott et al, 2002
- Hamersley et al, 2002
- Morrison et al, 2003
- Lam et al, 2003
- Fleming et al, 2004
- Ambrose et al, 2004
- Roman et al, 2004
- Rebarber et al, 2004
- Gaziano et al, 2004
- Gaziano et al, 2004
- Brown et al, 2005
- Rittenberg et al, 2006
- Jones et al, 2006
- Mcweeney, 2006
- de la Torre, 2008
- Flick, 2008
- Rebarber, 2008

Table 2. Evidence - Continuous SQ Terbutaline. 46 Peer Review Studies 1988-2008.

Table III, shows the pregnancy prolongation amongst all studies where it was reported. In these 20 studies, pregnancy prolongation ranges from 2.4 to 11 weeks averaging 4.6 weeks in the treatment group. Finally, in a meta-analysis Lam *et al.*, analyzed 6 studies with 858 patients using subcutaneous terbutaline and contraction monitoring versus 897 patients who were not treated or received oral terbutaline/nifedipine.(Lam *et al.*, 2009) It was noted that in the monitored group there was a 73% reduction in preterm birth <32 weeks and the NICU admission rate was 28.8% versus 40.7%. Overall, there was a $7,100 - $10,500 cost saving amongst studies who reported financial data.

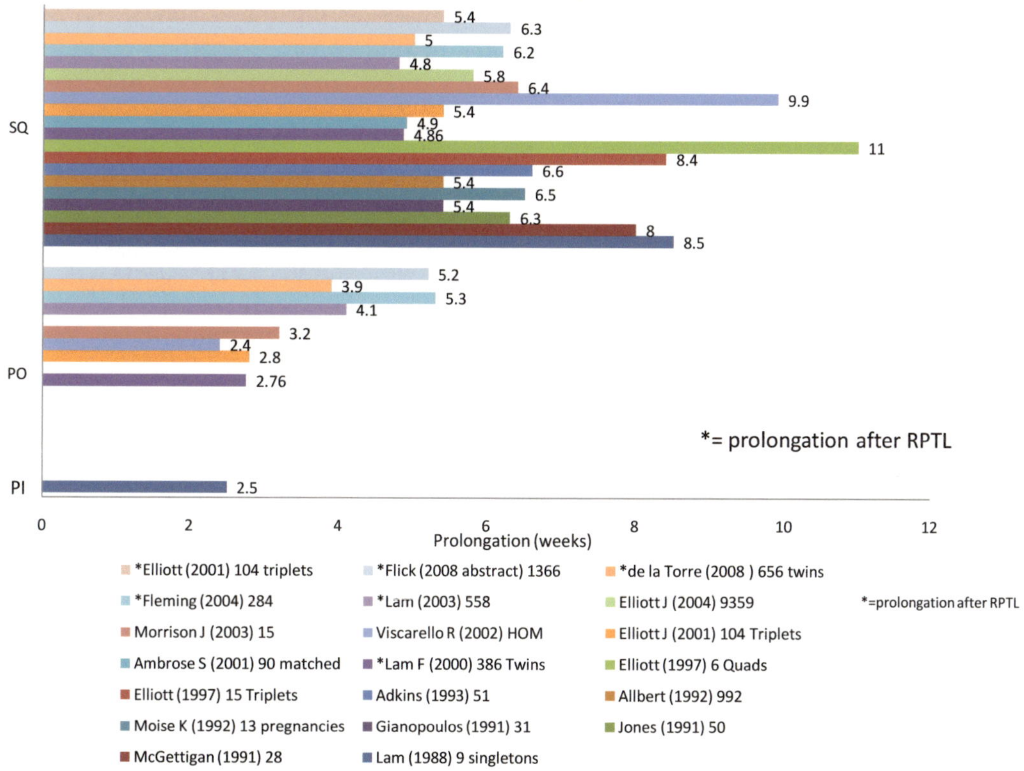

Table 3. Clinical Experience - Pregnancy Prolongation.

6. Summary

Following tocolysis of acute preterm labor, women discharged on maintenance therapy or on no tocolytic agent at all, appear to benefit from tertiary contraction assessment and daily nursing contact. Critical to the contraction-monitoring program, whether subcutaneous terbutaline is used or not, is the daily nursing assessment for signs and symptoms of preterm labor and monitoring of uterine activity. If the program is used correctly as indicated above, patients will experience a greater pregnancy prolongation resulting in fewer preterm births which translates into less NICU admissions and reduced neonatal morbidity and greater cost savings. When uterine contraction monitoring without tocolytics are used in these very high-risk patients the goal is to identify recurrent preterm labor at the earliest possible time so that advanced cervical dilatation does not occur before tocolysis can be initiated. Among women using the subcutaneous terbutaline pump the goal is to maintain uterine quiescence by giving the appropriate basal dose (calculated on volume of distribution) while using uterine contraction assessment to adjust bolus therapy to extend the gestation as long as possible. Should recurrent preterm labor occur with either of these therapies, then primary or acute treatment with magnesium sulfate is indicated. Since several studies have noted that there is an advantage, if preterm delivery does occur, in treating with magnesium sulfate (decreased cerebral palsy) this should be the drug of choice for acute treatment of any episode of preterm labor. (Elliott et al., 2009)

In summary, it would appear that in appropriate cases (as illustrated above) the use of contraction monitoring in the home is extremely helpful in early detection of recurrent preterm labor and extending the gestation as far as possible. This would seem to benefit the patient, the neonate, and society in general.

7. References

Abbasi, S, Gerdes JS, Sehdev HM, Samini SS, Ludmir J. "Neonatal outcome after exposure to indomethacin in utero: A retrospective case cohort study." Am J Obstet Gyne 2003; 189: 782-5.

ACOG Practice Bulletin. "Management of Preterm Labor." Compendium of selected publications 2007;Volume 2:688-695.

Beckmann CA, Beckmann CRB, Stanziano GJ, Bergauer NK, Martin CB. Accuracy of maternal perception of preterm uterine activity. Am J Obstet Gynecol 1996;174:672-5.

Brown HL, Britton KA, Brizendino EJ, Hiett AK, Ingram D, Turnquca MA et al. A randomized comparison of home uterine activity monitoring in the out-patient management of women treated for preterm labor. Am J Obstet Gynecol 1999;180:798-805.

Carr DB, Clark AL, Kernek K, Spinnato, JA. "Maintenance oral nifedipine for preterm labor: A randomized clinical trail." Am J Obstet Gynecol 1999; 181: 822-7.

Dyson DC, Danbe KH, Bamber JA, Crites YM, Field DR, Maier JA, et al. Monitoring women at risk for preterm labor. N Engl J Med 1998;338:15-9.

Elliott et al. "Pregnancy prolongation in triplet pregnancies oral vs continuous subcutaneous terbutaline." J Reprod Med 2001;46:975-82.

Elliott JP and Radin TG. The effect of corticosteroid administration on uterine activity and preterm labor in high-order multiple gestation. Obstet Gynecol 1995;85:250-254.

Elliott JP, Lewis DF, Morrison JC, Garite TJ. In Defense of Magnesium Sulfate. Obstet Gynecol 2009; 113:1341-8

Elliott JP, Flynn M, Kaemmerer EL, et al. Terbutaline pump tocolysis in high order multiples. J Reprod Med 1997;42:687-693.

Faustin D, Klein S, Spector IJ, Nelson J. Maternal perception of preterm labor: is it reliable? J Matern Fetal Med 1997;6:184-6.

Floyd RC, Martin RW, McLaughlin BN, Roberts WE, Morrison JC. Preterm birth prevention in a large Medicaid population. Am J Gynecol Health 1993;7:65-70S.

Garite TJ, Bentley DL, Hamer CA and Porto ML. Uterine activity characteristics in multiple gestations. Obstet & Gynecol 1990;76:565-595.

Guinn D, Goepfert A, Owen J. Terbutaline pump maintenance therapy for prevention of preterm delivery; a double-blind trial. Am J Obstet Gynecol 1998;179:874-8.

Hamilton BE, Martin JA, Ventura SJ. Births; preliminary data for 2005. Natl Vital Stat Rep 2006;55(11):1-18.

Hernandez AR, Gonzalez-Quintero VH, Istwan N, Rhea D, Vazquez-Vera E, Flick AA, Stanziano G. Antepartum uterine contraction patterns in twin pregnancies with and without preterm labor and delivering before or after 36 weeks. *Am J Obstet Gynecol* 2008;198(5):328-9.

Jones JS, Morrison JC, Istwan N, Rhea B, Collins, A, Stanziano G. "The interval to spontaneous delivery following discontinuation of maintenance tocolysis." J Mater Fetal Neon Med 2006; 19(6) 331-335.

Katz M, Gill PJ, Newman RB. Detection of preterm labor by ambulatory monitoring of uterine activity for the management of oral tocolysis. Am J Obstet Gynecol 1988;154:1253-6.

Katz M. Newman RB, Gill PH. Assessment of uterine activity in ambulatory patients at high risk of preterm labor and delivery. Am J Obstet Gynecol 1986;154:44-7.

Kosasa TS, Abou-Sayf FK, Li-Ma G, Hale RW. Evaluation of the cost-effectiveness of home monitoring of uterine contractions. Obstet Gynecol 1990;76:71-5.

Lam et al. "Clinical and cost effectiveness of continuous subcutaneous terbutaline versus oral tocolytics for treatment of recurrent preterm labor in twin gestations. J Perinatol 2001;21:444-450.

Lam F, Rhea D, Stanziano G. Using meta-analysis methodology to evaluate treatment of preterm labor. *Obstet Gynecol 2009;113:875*

Lyell DJ, Pullen KM, Mannan J, *et al.* Maintenance nifedipine tocolysis compared with placebo. Obstet Gynecol 2008;112:1221-6.

Martin RW, Gookin KS, Hill WC, Fleming AD, Knuppel RA, Lake MF, et al. Uterine activity compared with symptomatology in the detection of preterm labor. Obstet Gynecol 1990;76:19-23S.

Morrison JC, Bergauer NK, Jaques D, Coleman SK, Stanziano GJ. Telemedicine: cost-effective management of high risk pregnancy. Manag Care 2001;10:42-9.

Morrison JC, Chauhan SP, Carroll CS, Bofill JA, Magann EF. "Continuous subcutaneous terbutaline administration prolongs pregnancy after recurrent preterm labor." Am J Obstet Gynecol 2003;188:1460-7.

Morrison JC, Pittman KP, Martin RW, McLaughlin BN. Cost/health effectiveness of home uterine activity monitoring in a Medicaid population. Obstet Gynecol 1990;76:76-81.

Nagey DA, Bailey-Jones C, Herman AA. Randomized comparison of home uterine activity monitoring and routine care in patients discharged after treatment for preterm labor. Obstet Gynecol 1993;82(3):19-23.

Newman RB, Gill PJ, Katz M. Uterine activity during pregnancy in ambulatory patients: Comparison of singleton and twin gestations. Am J Obstet Gynecol 1986;154:530-531.

Newman RB, Iams JD, Das A, Goldenberg RL et al. A prospective masked observational study of uterine contraction frequency in twins. Am J Obstet Gynecol 2006;195:1564-1570.

Rebarber A, Cleary-Goldman J, Istwan N, Rhea D, Stanziano G, Saltzman D. "The association of elective cessation of tocolysis and preterm birth in singleton gestations." Am J Perinatol 2009; 26: 351-55.

Rust OA, Bofill JA, Arriola RM, Andrew ME, Morrison JC. "The clinical efficacy of oral tocolytic therapy." Am J Obstet Gynecol 1996; 175: 838-842.

Rust OA, Perry KG, Andrew ME, Roberts WE et al. Twins and preterm labor. J Reprod Med1997;42:229-234.

Smith JC, Floyd RC, Pittman KP, et al. Reduction of preterm births in a low-income population utilizing home uterine activity monitoring. J Matern Fetal Invest 1994;4:87-92.

van Geijn HP, Lenglet JE, Bolte AC. "Nifedipine trails: effectiveness and safety aspects." BJOG: an internal J of Obstet Gynecol 2005; 112: Supplement 1, 79-83.

Watson DL, Welch RA, Marlona FG, Lake MF, Knuppel RA, Martin RW, et al. Management of preterm labor patients at home: does daily uterine activity monitoring and nursing support make a difference? Obstet Gynecol 1990;76:3 2S-5S.

Wenstrom K, Weiner C, Merrill D. A placebo-controlled randomized trial of the terbutaline pump for prevention of preterm delivery. Am J Perinatol 1997;14:87-91.

9

Progestins and Preterm Birth

Helen Y. How[1] and Baha M. Sibai[2]
[1]*Norton Healthcare System, Louisville, Ky,*
[2]*Department of Obstetrics and Gynecology,*
University of Texas Health Sciences, Houston, Texas,
USA

1. Introduction

Premature delivery (PTD), defined as birth prior to 37 weeks' gestation, remains one of the major problems that lead to perinatal morbidity and mortality in the developed countries (Goldenberg et al., 2008). It affects approximately 12.7% of all deliveries in the United States and 4.4 - 8.2% in many other developed countries such as Australia, New Zealand, Sweden, Canada and Japan (Hamilton et al., 2006; Jenkins et al., 2006; Morken et al., 2005; Health Canada 2003). One third of these occur before 34 weeks' gestation (Amon, 1999; Behrman & Butler et al., 2007). In the United States, the preterm birth (PTB) rate has increased more than 30% since 1984 and equates to nearly 500,000 PTBs each year (March of Dimes, 2007). This prematurity rate has been increasing probably as a result of delayed child bearing, increased frequency of multifetal pregnancies from assisted reproductive technology (Tough et al., 2002; Reynolds et al.,2003), general non-interventional approach at or beyond 34 weeks' gestation and the increase in labor inductions and cesarean deliveries including those medically indicated (Damus et al., 2008).

Prematurity causes an estimated 60-80% of all neonatal deaths of non-anomalous infants in developed countries (Guyer et al., 1997). Neonatal mortality is directly correlated with gestational age (GA) at delivery. For example, the mortality rate for infants born at less than 32 weeks' gestation is almost 70 times the rate of a term infant, and for infants born less than 37 weeks' gestation it is 15 times the term infant rate (2.6/1000 live births)(March of Dimes Birth Defects Foundation, 2005). Reported neonatal morbidity is also a major concern, especially for infants born at less than 32 weeks' gestation. Neonatal complications include intraventricular hemorrhage (IVH), necrotizing enterocolitis (NEC), respiratory distress syndrome (RDS), bronchopulmonary dysplasia (BPD), jaundice and anemia (Behrman and Butler et al., 2007). Economically, care for these infants is responsible for an estimated $51,600 investment per child in neonatal care, contributing more than $26 billion to annual healthcare costs in the US (Behrman and Butler et al., 2007). Among the infants who survive, 10% -15% are burdened with significant handicaps, such as cerebral palsy, mental retardation, retinopathy, or hearing impairment (Gluckman & Hanson, 2004). More importantly, low birth weight (LBW) infants who are spared significant neonatal morbidity are at higher risk for cardiovascular disease (myocardial infarction, stroke, and hypertension) and diabetes as adults (Gluckman & Hanson, 2004). Therefore, greater attention should be focused on very PTBs < 32 weeks' gestation, because, although this group represents only 1-2% of all deliveries, it accounts for about 60% of perinatal mortality

and nearly 50% of all long term neurological morbidity (Hack & Fanaroff, 1999). Judgment on the success of any preventative treatment should focus on deliveries occurring before 33 completed weeks of gestation, when the morbidity and mortality rates are high (Campbell, 2011). Preterm delivery is due to either spontaneous preterm labor (PTL) (40%-50%), spontaneous preterm premature rupture of membranes (PPROM)(25%-40%), or obstetrically indicated PTD (20%-25%) as a result of maternal, placental or fetal complications (preeclampsia, renal disease, diabetes mellitus with vasculopathy, placenta previa or abruption, and fetal growth restriction). (Tucker et al., 1991).
Although secondary and tertiary interventions such as antenatal corticosteroids, postnatal surfactant, and improved neonatal care have led to reduced morbidity and mortality caused by PTB, effective primary preventive interventions have remained elusive. Encouragingly, accumulating data suggest that progestins may be effective in preventing PTB. The exact **mechanism of progesterone** in prevention of PTB is not known. Previous studies have demonstrated a number of actions which support gestation (Henderson & Wilson, 2001; Karalis et al., 1996) and inhibit uterine activity, including actions that relax smooth muscle in the pregnant uterus (Lye & Porter et al., 1978), prevents formation of myometrium gap junction (Garfield et al., 1982) and oxytocin receptors (Fuchs et al., 1983), blockade of the effects of oxytocin on the myometrium (Grazzini et al., 1998), as well as having immunosuppressive activity against activation of T lymphocytes (Siiteri & Seron-Ferre , 1981; Garfield et al., 1980). Studies have suggested that a significant portion of spontaneous PTB < 34 weeks' gestation has an infectious or inflammatory etiology. In many patients with infection, elevated levels of lipoxygenase and cyclooxygenase pathway products can be demonstrated (Romero et al., 1989). There are also increased concentrations of cytokines in the amniotic fluid of such women. It is possible that progesterone's anti-inflammatory or immunosuppressive activity may underlie the improvement seen in women with a previous spontaneous PTB < 34 weeks' gestation; however, this remains speculative.

2. Pharmacokinetics of progestins

Progestins are available in natural or synthetic formulations for oral, intramuscular (IM) or vaginal administration in the form of suppository or gel. Natural (micronized) progesterone is an exact duplicate of the progesterone produced in the corpus luteum and placenta. It is therefore more readily metabolized by the body and is associated with minimal side effects. The two naturally occurring products include progesterone and 17-hydroxyprogesterone. The plasma concentration will depend on the dose and route of administration, eg, oral (3-6 ng/ml @100 mg and 30 ng/ml @ 200 mg), transdermal(3 ng/ml @ 45 mg), vaginal cream (19 ng/ml @ 300 mg) or gel (3.9 ng/ml @ 90 mg), vaginal (10-19 ng/ml @ 100 mg, 17-34 ng/ml @ 400 mg) or rectal (15-52 ng/ml @ 100 mg) suppository, IM (40-50 ng/ml @ 100 mg) and sublingual (5 ng/ml @10 mg dose). The time to peak plasma concentration is longest with 90 mg vaginal gel @ 7 hours and shortest with 200 mg oral micronized progesterone @ 0.8 hour. The vaginal suppository (100mg and 400 mg) and 100 mg rectal suppository is about 4 hours and the IM route (100 mg) takes about 2-8 hours (Murray, 1998).
Synthetic progestins are progesterone derivatives and 19 nortestosterone derivatives; their chemical structure is very similar to that of the natural progesterone. 17 alpha hydroxyprogesterone caproate (17OHP-C) is a 17- hydroxyprogesterone derivative; it is the most commonly used synthetic progestin given intramuscularly to prevent PTB. It has been isolated from both adrenal glands and corpora lutea. The synthetic caproate ester is inactive

when given by mouth but works as a long-acting progestin when administered intramuscularly. Pharmacokinetic studies have shown that once-weekly IM administration of 17OHP-C would provide continuous systemic serum levels of 17OHP-C. The half-life of 17OHP-C was estimated to be approximately 7.8 days, compared with approximately 35-55 hours for progesterone (Onsrud et al., 1985). The route of administration plays an important role in the drug's safety and efficacy profile. Oral progesterone has not been used for prevention of PTB because of its first-pass hepatic metabolism, lack of efficacy data, high side-effect profile, and extreme variability in plasma concentrations. Transvaginal administration of progesterone avoids first-pass hepatic metabolism and is associated with rapid absorption, high bioavailability, and local endometrial effects (von Eye et al., 2004). It has been shown to provide higher and more sustained progesterone concentrations and is the preferred route of administration in many cases. Although this route offers no local pain and few side effects, it is associated with variable blood concentrations and patient compliance issues, therefore many favor the intramuscular route (Di Renzo et al., 2005; Penzias & Alper et al., 2003; Posaci et al., 2005).

3. Trials on the use of progestins and PTB

The majority or randomized trials evaluated the prophylactic supplementation of progestins in asymptomatic women at high risk for PTB. Women are considered to be at high risk for several reasons, including past history of spontaneous PTB or miscarriages, multiple gestation, short cervical length (CL), cerclage in place and uterine anomalies. Earlier small trials using 17OHP-C showed mixed results; 4 trials reported benefit (LeVine, 1964; Papiernik, 1970; Johnson et al., 1975; Yemini et al., 1985), whereas 2 trials (Hartikainen-Sorri et al., 1980; Hauth et al., 1983) reported no benefit in reducing the risk of PTB. A meta-analysis over two decade ago (Kierse, 1990) showed that progesterone was beneficial in reducing PTL: odds ratio 0.43 (95% CI, 0.20- 0.89); PTB: odds ratio 0.50 (95% CI, 0.30- 0.85) and LBW (<2500g): odds ratio 0.50 (95% CI, 0.27- 0.80). This meta-analysis concluded that progesterone was the only product that had been proven to be of benefit if used prophylactically to reduce the incidence of PTB. Despite this robust evidence-based conclusion, the information remained dormant for more than two decade.

3.1 Progestins and history of prior PTB

In 2003, two trials rekindled the interest in progestins to prevent PTB. The MFM Network trial (Meis et al., 2003) was conducted by the National Institute for Child Health and Development (NICHD); it is a prospective double blind randomized placebo-controlled trial on 463-singleton gestation with history of spontaneous PTB. Women were treated with weekly intramuscular injections of 250 mg 17OHP-C or placebo from 16 to 20 weeks' gestation until 36 weeks' gestation or birth. The primary outcome of the study was birth before 37 weeks' gestation. Treatment with 17OHP-C reduced the incidence of delivery before 37 weeks (36.3% in the 17OHP-C group vs. 54.9% in the placebo group). In addition, there was a reduction in delivery less than 35 weeks' gestation (20.6% in the 17OHP-C group vs. 30.7% in the control group) and at less than 32 weeks' gestation (11.4% in the 17 OHP-C group vs. 19.6% in the control group). Also, there was a significant reduction in the incidence of LBW (RR 0.66; 95% CI, 0.51-0.87) and rates of IVH (RR 0.25; 95% CI, 0.8-0.82) and need for supplemental oxygen (RR 0.62; CI, 0.42-0.92) in infants of women treated with 17OHP-C. The trial of da Fonseca et al. (da Fonseca et al., 2003) was carried out in Sao Paolo,

Brazil, comprising 142 women considered to be at high risk of PTB due to previous PTB, cervical cerclage and uterine anomalies. These women were randomized to treatment with either vaginal micronized progesterone suppositories 100 mg daily or placebo between 24 and 34 weeks' gestation. Treatment with vaginal progesterone suppositories reduced the rate of PTB before 37 weeks' gestation (13.8% in the progesterone group vs. 28.5% in the placebo group) and before 34 weeks' gestation (2.8% in the progesterone group vs. 18.6% in the placebo group). Both studies found a significant reduction in the incidence of PTB (OR 0.47; 95% CI, 0.31-0.69) (Meis et al., 2003); OR 0.4; 95% CI, 0.4–0.94 (da Fonseca et al., 2003). Neither study found a reduction in the incidence of spontaneous PTL.
Since the publication of these two double blind placebo controlled studies. The National Institute of Child Health and Development (NICHD), the American College of Obstetricians and Gynecologist (ACOG) and the March of Dimes endorsed the prophylactic use of 17OHP-C in women with history of preterm deliveries, although both studies had several limitations. For example: in the da Fonseca et al (da Fonseca et al., 2003) study, the women were not started on non-bioadhesive progesterone vaginal suppository until late gestation, the mean GA at enrollment was 25.2 weeks in the placebo group and 26.5 weeks in the progesterone vaginal suppositories group. In addition, women who delivered preterm following PPROM were excluded. If these women were included in the analysis, the difference in PTB is no longer statistically significant. In the MFM Network (Meis et al., 2003) study, the women enrolled had high rates of PTB, with 54.9 % of the women who received the placebo injections delivering before 37 weeks' gestation. There are some concerns regarding the vehicle, castor oil, used in IM 17OHP-C. The castor oil is thought to induce labor by stimulating the release of prostaglandins, which might negate the potential beneficial effect of IM 17-OHP-C (Brancazio et al., 1988 and O'Sullivan 2010) but this has not been substantiated. However, this high rate of PTD was most likely related to the history of previous preterm deliveries. The earlier in a pregnancy a PTB occurs, the greater the chance of PTD in a subsequent pregnancy. It should also be noted that the mean duration of gestation at the time of the qualifying delivery was 31 weeks' gestation, and a third of the women enrolled had more than one previous PTB. These women were very high risk, strongly motivated and compliant. Iams (Iams, 2010) feels the reasons are primarily based on the demographics of the patient population as well as the obstetric history and feels that the recurrence rate of 55% is about one would expect from patients enrolled in the placebo arm. On the other hand, 17OHP-C may not be effective in women with a lower risk of PTB, and most preterm deliveries occur in women with no previous PTB. Therefore, the result of this (Meis et al., 2003) study should be interpreted with caution and may not be generalizable to women with a lower risk of PTB. In addition, although 17-OHP-C significantly reduced the rate of PTB among the women who received it, the rate of PTB in this group remained very high at 36.3 %. Thus, the identification of other causes of PTB and other methods of preventing it remains a pressing need. Another noteworthy point is that although the study (Meis et al., 2003) demonstrated a statistically significant reduction in the primary endpoint of PTB prior to 37 weeks' gestation, the reduction in PTBs prior to 35 weeks and prior to 32 weeks' gestation which are better surrogates for significant neonatal morbidity and mortality, were not statistically persuasive. Meis and colleagues (Meis et al., 2003) indicated that based on their study results, it would be necessary to treat five to six women with a previous spontaneous PTD to prevent one birth at < 37 weeks' gestation, and to treat 12 women to prevent one birth at < 32 weeks' gestation. In addition, the primary clinical trial did not demonstrate a significant reduction in another secondary endpoint, a composite assessment of infant mortality and morbidity.

In a subsequent data analysis of the NICHD trial evaluating the benefit of 17OHP-C according to the GA of previous delivery, Spong et al (Spong et al., 2005) reported that progesterone did not significantly improve the GA at delivery in women whose earliest previous delivery was at 34 to 35.9 weeks' gestation. However, the recurrence of PTB was significantly less for women treated with 17OHP-C with GA at the earliest previous spontaneous PTB 20 to 27.9 weeks (42% vs. 63%) and 28 to 33.9 weeks (34% vs. 56%). From their data, the authors concluded that for the women with earliest previous spontaneous PTB at 20 to 27.9 weeks and 28 to 33.9 weeks, 4.7 and 4.6 women (respectively for each group) would need to be treated with 17OHP-C to prevent one PTB. In 2007, a multinational double blind placebo controlled trial (O'brien et al., 2007) of 659 women with singleton pregnancies and history of spontaneous PTB demonstrated that daily treatment with 90 mg bioadhesive progesterone vaginal gel (8% Prochieve or Crinone) did not decrease the rate of PTB at < 35 weeks' gestation. This is in contrast to the previously mentioned trial by da Fonseca et al. (da Fonseca et al., 2003). The treatment was initiated between 18 and 22 weeks' gestation and continued until 37 weeks' gestation. The dose of 90 mg progesterone as a bioadhesive gel used in this trial is the therapeutic equivalent of 600 mg progesterone as vaginal suppositories, much higher than the dose used in the Brazilian trial of da Fonseca et al (da Fonseca et al., 2003).

Five good quality meta-analysis and systematic review (Keirse, 1990; Sanchez-Ramos et al., 2005; Coomarasamy et al., 2006; Mackenzie et al., 2006; Dodd et al., 2008) of randomized controlled trials showed that women who received progestational agents had lower rates of LBW and PTB before 37, 35, 34 and 32 completed weeks' gestation. The dose of the 17OHP-C varied between 100 mg and 1000 mg daily for 3-7 days. The timing of initiation ranged between 8 and < 35 weeks' gestation. The timing at which it was discontinued ranged between 34 and 37 weeks' gestation or after eight doses of 17OHP-C or delivery. The progestational agents other than 17OHP-C were medroxyprogesterone, allyslestrenol and progesterone. However, there was no reduction in perinatal morbidity and mortality (Keirse, 1990, Sanchez- Ramos et al., 2005; Mackenzie et al., 2006).

3.2 Progestins and short cervix

Recently, ultrasound assessment of CL has emerged as another effective prognosticator for PTB. Fonseca et al. (Fonseca et al., 2007) published a randomized, double blind placebo-controlled trial of 250 women between 22 and 25 weeks' gestation with a short cervix (≤ 15 mm by transvaginal ultrasound). These women were randomized to receive 200 mg micronized progesterone vaginal capsules or placebo every night from 24 to 34 weeks' gestation. There was a significant 40% reduction in spontaneous PTB at < 34 weeks in the progesterone group (19%) compared with placebo group (34%) (RR 0.56; 95% CI, 0.36-0.86). The effect was limited to singleton pregnancies, as no significant effect was demonstrable in 24 twin pregnancies with a short cervix included in the study. The study was underpowered to show significant effect on perinatal morbidity and mortality. Similarly, in 2011, an international multi-center prospective randomized, placebo-controlled trial (Hassan et al., 2011) showed a reduction in PTD of 50% at < 28 (5.1% vs. 10.3%); of 45% at < 33 (8.9% vs. 13.1%), and of 38% at < 35 (14.5% vs. 23.3%) weeks' gestation with progesterone treatment (90 mg of progesterone in bioadhesive gel daily) in patients between 19 and 24 weeks' gestation whose CL was 10-20 mm. There was also a 53% reduction in very LBW infants (6.4% vs. 13.6%) as well as a significant reduction in the composite neonatal morbidities indices in the progesterone treated group. Hassan et al. excluded CL < 10 mm on the

premise that these patients were less likely to respond to progesterone treatment. This may explain the 50% higher incidence of PTBs in the placebo group in Fonseca study (Fonseca et al., 2007) as the highest incidence of early PTD occurs with CLs of 0-10 mm.
Vaisbuch et al. (Vaisbuch et al., 2010) had previously demonstrated a high incidence of pro-inflammatory cytokines in the amniotic fluid of such cases. A combination of antibiotics and increased vaginal dose of progesterone may result in prolongation of pregnancy in women with CL of < 10 mm. A sub-analysis of O'Brien study (DeFranco et al., 2007), found that in women with a CL < 28 mm, the rate of PTB </= 32 weeks' gestation was significantly lower in the progesterone group, with a significant reduction in RDS in the treated group. This study highlights the problem of all the previous therapeutic intervention studies where randomization is based on a history of PTB, as this is likely to have a small impact on the overall rate of spontaneous PTB because fewer than 10% of spontaneous early PTB occur in women with a previous history. The problem with the DeFranco sub-analysis was that the results of only 46 patients were analyzed (19 in the progesterone group, 27 in the placebo group) and that randomization was based on obstetric history and not on CL. The selection of the 28 mm cut-off for inclusion in the analysis was generated post-hoc for the simple reason that there were only four women available in the study subgroup with a baseline CL of less than 25 mm. These trials suggest that determination of CL is a powerful method for PTB risk assessment. However, until further trials, routine screening of low risk pregnant women by transvaginal ultrasound of CL is still not recommended at least here in the U.S., because only 1.7% (413/24,620) - 2.3% (733/32,091) (Fonseca et al., 2007; Hassan et al., 2011) of the patients screened have short cervix in the mid trimester. It is true that an extension of a routine mid trimester ultrasound examination to include a 5 minute transvaginal scan to measure CL would not involve a significant increase in expenditure in UK and European countries (Campbell, 2011); it may not be the case in the U.S. Routine cervical screening is not recommended by the ACOG Committee Opinion (ACOG #419, 2008). Using statistics from Fonseca et al (Fonseca et al., 2007) trial, the number of women need to be treated to prevent one early birth is only 6.6 (95% CI, 3.8- 22.8). However because of the low prevalence of a short cervix (approx. 1.5%) among low-risk women, the number needed to scan is 650 (95% CI, 379-2248) (Chandiramani, 2007). Nevertheless, many clinicians use vaginal or intramuscular progesterone in women with a true short cervix (CL <25mm) or women with a short cervix who have a cervical cerclage.
A meta-analysis of five randomized control trials (Berghella et al., 2011) including 504 women with previous preterm birth and single gestation with a CL less than 25 mm at randomization before 24 weeks revealed a 30% reduction in recurrent PTB at less than 35 weeks' gestation (28% in the cerclage group and 41% in the non-cerclage group) and a significant and clinically important 36% decrease in perinatal mortality and morbidity. It would take approximately 20 cerclage procedures to prevent one perinatal death. Cerclage has not been shown to be beneficial in other populations including women with only previous PTBs, short CL, multiple gestations or other risk factors for PTB. The authors' explanation is that women with previous PTB with painless CL shortening to less than 25 mm in the subsequent pregnancy before 24 weeks' gestation do have a clinically significant component of cervical insufficiency, and that is why cerclage is beneficial. Base on this data, women with previous spontaneous PTB, between 16 and 34 weeks' gestation, and singleton gestation should be screened for short cervix starting at approximately 16 weeks' gestation and continue every 2 weeks until 23 6/7 weeks' gestation, unless the CL is 25-29 mm, in which case weekly screening is performed. Rafael et al. (Rafael et al., 2011), in a

retrospective cohort study of 58 women with CL of < 25 mm at < 23 6/7 weeks' gestation, found that there was no significant differences in the incidences of spontaneous PTB < 35, < 32, or < 28 weeks' among women with a ultrasound indicated cerclage, regardless of whether or not they received 17OHP-C (15 in the 17OHP-C group vs. 43 in the no 17OHP-C group) during the current pregnancy. Their findings are similar to the results of two other studies concerning 17OHP-C in women with a cerclage in place (Berghella et al., 2010 and Rebarber et al., 2008).

3.3 Progestins and multiple gestations

Twin gestation carries one of the highest risks of PTD. An older study prior to the use of cervical ultrasound was performed in twins with 170HP-C (Hartikainen-Sorri et al., 1980). In this study 77 women with twin gestation were treated only during the last trimester up until 37 weeks with injections of 17OHP-C or placebo. In this randomized clinical trial there were no differences in outcomes such as RDS or perinatal mortality. Likewise, there was no difference in progesterone level (nmoles/liter) between the two groups. In singleton pregnancies, the rate of spontaneous PTB before 34 weeks' gestation is about 1%, while in twins it is 13% (To et al., 2006). These investigators carried out a study of CL measurement at 22 - 24 weeks' gestation in 1163 twin gestations. They found that the rate of PTB before 32 weeks' gestation was strongly associated with CL. Using cut-offs of < 25 mm, <20 mm and <15 mm, the respective detection rates of spontaneous PTB before 32 weeks' gestation were 35%, 49% and 67%. Another small randomized clinical trial (Briery et al., 2009) administered 250mg of 17α-Hydroxyprogesterone IM weekly versus placebo to women with twin gestations. The gestational age at delivery and the incidence of preterm birth at <35 weeks were similar between the two groups as was infant weight, Apgar score and composite neonatal morbidity.

Rouse et al. (Rouse et al., 2003) presented the NICHD network data on the use of 17OHP-C in the prevention of PTB in 655 women with twin gestation; the results showed that treatment with 17OHP-C starting between 16 and 20 weeks and continued until 35 weeks' gestation did not reduce the rate of PTB in twins. Preterm delivery before 35 weeks' gestation occurred in 41.5% of the progestin group vs. 37.3% in the control group. Potential limitations of Rouse trial are: 1) less than 10% of enrolled women had a history of prior PTB; and, 2) they use the same 17OHP-C dose (250 mg) in women with twin gestation, when their plasma volume is known to be 20% greater than that in singleton gestation. A secondary analysis of the NICHD trial (Durnwald et al., 2010) reported that women with twin gestations and a cervical length below the 25th percentile (32 mm) at 16-20 weeks (52/221) had higher rates of PTB. In this subgroup of women, 17OHP-C did not prevent preterm births (56%) before 35 weeks' gestation. A CL above the 75th percentile (44 mm) at 16-20 weeks (53/221) did not significantly reduce the risk of preterm birth (37%) in this high-risk population. The authors attributed this to combination of risk factors, such as multiple gestation and short cervix which may be additive and confer an increased risk for PTB that cannot be overcome by administration of 17OHP-C. Another possible explanation is that cervical shortening in multiple gestations is related to uterine over distension and that this distention is not progesterone sensitive. They concluded that long cervix (44 mm) at 16-20 weeks' gestation may not provide useful clinical information to the obstetrician regarding risk of preterm delivery in twin gestations. Furthermore, a long cervix is likely only reassuring if it is maintained beyond 24 weeks' gestation as demonstrated by Imseis et al. (Imseis et al., 1997).

Norman et al. (Norman et al., 2009), randomized 500 women with twin pregnancy to 90 mg vaginal progesterone or placebo daily from 24-34 weeks' gestation. Again, no effect was seen on the primary outcome of delivery or intrauterine death before 34 weeks' gestation (OR 1.36; 95% CI, 0.89-2.09). In both trials (Rouse et al and Normal et al), a non-significant increase in intrauterine death was seen in the treatment group. Similarly, Caritis et al. (Caritis et al., 2009) demonstrated no reduction in PTB in women with triplet pregnancies treated with 17OHP-C. Healthy women (n= 134) with triplets were randomly assigned to weekly intramuscular injections of either 250 mg of 17OHP-C or placebo, starting at 16 to 20 weeks' gestation and ending at delivery or 35 weeks' gestation. Eighty-three percent of women in the treatment group vs. 84% in the placebo group delivered before 35 weeks' gestation. Another double-blind, randomized (2:1) trial by Combs et al (Combs et al., 2010) on triplets showed no statistically significant difference with regard to primary outcome i.e. composite neonatal morbidity in 17OHP-C (n= 56) and placebo (n=25) groups (38% vs. 41%).

4. Timing and duration of the administration of progestin in women with risk factors

There are 2 published observational data regarding the use of 17 OHP-C in the prevention of recurrent PTB. Rebarber et al. (Rebarber et al., 2007), in a retrospective analysis of data from 481 women who were enrolled for outpatient weekly IM 17OHP-C administrations. They found that women with elective early cessation of weekly 17OHP-C at < 32 weeks' gestation were significantly more likely to have spontaneous recurrent PTD at < 37 weeks, < 35 weeks and < 32 weeks' gestation when compared to the women who received weekly 17OHP-C injections until PTD or 36.9 weeks. Discontinuation of 17OHP-C was defined as being elective when it occurred for any reason other than hospitalization for eminent delivery or an acute condition that led to delivery within 10 days. In this study, whether the elective discontinuation was patient or physician driven is not available from the database. A letter to the AJOG editor, Bernstein (Bernstein, 2008) provided an alternative explanation stating that the 17OHP-C is maybe of no benefit but that the sudden withdrawal of 17OHP-C may be involved in triggering spontaneous PTL. However, most clinicians continue treatment until 37 weeks, with the last injection at 36 weeks, and while the majority begin treatment at 16 weeks, it appears that later initiation of treatment up to 28-30 weeks' gestation may be helpful (Rebarber 2007).
How et al. (How et al., 2007), performed a retrospectively analysis of database of women enrolled for outpatient 17OHP-C prophylaxis for prevention of spontaneous PTB. The data were divided into three groups according to the number of PTB (1, 2, > 2) and stratified to initiation of 17OHP-C at 16-20.9 weeks' and 21-26.9 weeks' gestation. The authors found that the rates of spontaneous PTB were significantly higher in those with ≥ 2 PTB (n=159, 51% vs. 27% at < 37 weeks and 21% vs. 9% at < 35 weeks in the 17OHP-C start at 16-20.9 weeks' gestation group; 18% vs. 2% at < 32 weeks in the 17OHP-C start at 21-26.9 weeks' gestation group) as compared to those with one PTB (n=440). There were no significant differences in spontaneous PTB rates according to the time of initiation of 17OHP-C at 16-20.9 weeks' gestation vs. 21-26.9 weeks' gestation. The authors concluded that women with history of ≥ 2 PTD have a high risk of recurrent spontaneous PTB at < 37 and < 35 weeks despite 17OHP-C prophylaxis. Later second trimester initiation of 17OHP-C prophylaxis is as effective as initiation in the early second trimester. However, these conclusions should be

interpreted with caution because data such as baseline CL, the GA or circumstances of the prior PTB, maternal race, and complete neonatal outcomes were not available.

5. Progestins and threatened or established PTL

Facchinetti et al. (Facchinetti et al., 2007) reported a randomized clinical trial in which symptomatic women with PTL and intact membranes at 25-34 weeks' gestation were allocated to either observation or intramuscular administration of 341 mg of 17OHP-C twice a week until 36 weeks' gestation or delivery. The rationale for using a higher dose in this trial was the onset of PTL requiring tocolysis. In these patients, cervical ripening and the cascade of PTL was already initiated. In this study, 60 women presenting in PTL, treated with atosiban and not delivering within 48 hours were randomly assigned to either treatment with 17OHP-C (n= 30, including 16 with CL </= 25 mm) or expectant management (n=30, including 17 with </= 25 mm). Treatment with 17OHP-C was associated with a reduction in the risk of PTD (OR 0.15; 95% CI, 0.04-0.58). Cervical shortening, as measured by ultrasound performed 7 and 21 days post randomization, was significantly less in the 17OHP-C treated group as compared with placebo.
Another study on progesterone use in patients presenting in PTL was published in 2008 by Borna et al. (Borna & Sahabi et al. 2008). Women between 24 and 34 weeks' gestation with intact membranes were randomized to receive 400 mg of progesterone vaginal suppository (n=37) vs. no treatment (n=33) within 48 hours of arrest of labor with intravenous magnesium sulfate. Progesterone group demonstrated a longer mean latency until delivery (36 +/- 18 days vs. 24 +/- 27) days. However, it failed to reduce the incidence of readmission for PTL. A Cochrane meta-analysis done in 2010 (Su et al., 2010), suggests that progestational agents may be use in the treatment of threatened and preterm labor. However the number of participants in each included study ranged from 35 and 60. Further larger studies are needed.

6. Progestins and preterm premature rupture of membranes

Preterm premature rupture of membranes complicates nearly 3% of all pregnancies and is responsible for one third of all PTB (Mercer et al., 2003). Overall 75% deliver within one week after rupture, but approximately 15% may extend gestation for several weeks (ACOG #1, 1998; Lieman et al., 2005). Briery et al (Briery et al., 2011) randomized women with PPROM at 20-30 weeks' gestation with fetus in cephalic presentation to receive weekly 17OHP-C (n=33) or placebo (n=36) in an attempt to prolong the pregnancy. The report showed that there was no difference in GA at the time of delivery or the interval between randomization and delivery between the 2 groups. The neonatal outcome statistics of morbidity and mortality were similar between the two groups. The authors concluded that in patient with PPROM, 17OHP-C did not extend gestation vs. placebo and cannot be recommended for treatment in such women.

7. Safety and tolerability

Synthetic progestins, including 17OHP-C have been associated with a less desirable side-effect profile than that of natural progesterone, including mood swings, headaches, bloating, abdominal pain, perineal pain, constipation, diarrhea, nausea, vomiting, joint pain, depression, decreased sex drive, difficult or painful intercourse, nervousness, sleepiness, breast enlargement, breast pain, nucturia, dysuria, polyuria, urinary tract infection, allergy, tiredness, dizziness, genital itching, yeast infection, vaginal discharge, fever, flu-like symptoms, back pain, leg pain, sleep disorder, inflammation of a sinus, upper respiratory infection, asthma, acne and pruritus. Although these side effects have been reported with any form of progesterone (for example contraceptive), they rarely are severe and do not usually necessate discontinuing the drug at this dose when given to prevent preterm birth. A case in point, would be the MFM Network trial (Meis et al., 2003), the most common undesirable side effect was injection site pain (35%), injection site swelling (17%), urticaria (12%), pruritus (8%), injection site pruritus (6%), nausea (6%), contusion (6%), injection site nodule (4%), and vomiting (3%) (FDA, 2006). Meis (Meis et al., 2003) and Heinonen (Heinonen et al., 1977) reported a small, statistically non-significant increased in miscarriage and stillbirths in women receiving progesterone. Data from animal studies, suggest that increased plasma levels of progesterone may influence fetal behavior and induce fetal arousal states (Crossley et al., 1997; Nicol et al., 1997). There were no human data regarding long term outcome of women and infants who were exposed to progesterone in-utero until the published NICHD trial (Northen et al., 2007) reported a comprehensive 4 year follow up of children exposed to 17OHP-C in-utero. The children were 30-64 months of age at the time of the follow-up assessments. Of the 348 eligible surviving children, 278 (80%) were available for evaluation (194 17OHP-C, 84 placebo). No significant differences were seen in health status and conditions, or physical exam, including genital anomalies between 17OHP-C and placebo children. The developmental screen including communication, gross motor, fine motor, problem solving, and personal-social issues was not significantly different between 17OHP-C and placebo group. Therefore, it appears that at least with 17OHP-C there are no long term adverse effects in the offspring when used at 250mg per week.

Retrospective data indicate that 17OHP-C exposure may be associated with an increased risk of gestational diabetes (Rebarber et al., 2007; Waters et al., 2009). Hepatic dysfunctions, including cholestasis of pregnancy, have also been reported at a higher rate in women treated with oral micronized progesterone in France (Benifla et al., 1997; Bacq et al., 1997). Weekly IM injections of 17 OHP-C may be undesirable to a portion of the population at risk for PTB. Progesterone administered intramuscularly has been associated with several systemic and local skin complications. Some women may find transvaginal delivery to be more acceptable than injection, but others may not agree. Suppositories can be difficult to place high in the vagina and may liquefy, potentially leads to vaginal discharge, irritation, and infection. Vaginal cream and gel, which do not liquefy and are easier to apply, may alleviate some of the problems associated with transvaginal suppositories. Comparative data on the various methods of administration are thus needed to determine pharmacokinetic or tolerability differences, however, before one method can be recommended over the others.

8. Cost

Treatment with 17OHP-C or progesterone provides a significant reduction in the risk of recurrent PTB. In addition, there is a reduction in direct and indirect costs associated with PTD. For women with a prior PTD treated with 17OHP-C, the projected discounted lifetime medical costs of their offspring could be reduced by more than 2 billion dollars annually

(Bailit &Votruba, 2007). Three U.S. cost-effective analysis studies using decision analysis have been published (Odibo et al., 2006; Cahill et al., 2010; Werner et al., 2011). Odibo et al. (Odibo et al., 2006) compared the cost-effectiveness of using 17OHP-C for the prevention of PTD in cost-savings in women with prior PTD results in cost-savings in women with prior PTD less than 32 weeks and 32 to 37 weeks' gestation. (Cahill et al., 2010) compared the cost effectiveness of universal cervical screening/vaginal progesterone vs. no screening/no treatment on an estimated annual delivery rate of 4 million. The calculated annual cost, based on spontaneous PTBs < 34 weeks' gestation and severe morbidity prevented, fell from $46.2 billion to $33.3 billion annually, an annual saving of $12.9 billion, which was greater than calculated savings from 17OHP-C treatment on the basis of maternal history ($7.9 billion) or cervical-length screening in high risk pregnancies ($3.9 billion). Using a mean estimate of $70 for the second trimester CL scan and $206 for vaginal progesterone treatment, Werner et al. (Werner, 2011) analyze their model using data of Fonseca et al. (Fonseca et al., 2007), the cost saving was $12.1 million for every 100,000 women in the universal screened/vaginal progesterone group. Whereas, using data of Hassan et al (Hassan et al., 2011), the cost saving was $19.6 million per every 100,000 women.

In 2006, a New Drug Approval application was submitted to the FDA for 17 OHP-C, and the rights to produce the drug eventually were bought by KV Pharmaceutical. FDA recommended that the pharmaceutical company perform a confirmatory randomized controlled trial with a larger sample size than the Meis study. Once that confirmatory study was underway and 10% of the total sample size had been recruited from U.S. sites, the FDA approved Makena under the agency's accelerated approval regulations in February 2011. On February 15, 2011, KV Pharmaceutical announced the price of Makena at $1500 per injections, 75-150 times more than what formerly was being charged for the same medication that previously was available through locally regulated compounding pharmacies. The cost of the 17OHP-C was $10 to $20 per injection or $200 or $300 per pregnancy and about $150 per week when home care agencies were used to provide the necessary services. On April 1, 2011, the ACOG and SMFM state that there is no evidence that Makena is more effective or safer than the currently used compounded version. On the same day, KV pharmaceutical reduced the price of Makena from $1500 to $690 per injection or $14,000 to $16,000 per pregnancy. ACOG, SMFM, March of Dimes, American Academy of Family physicians all have responded that this reduction in price is insufficient (Cohen et al., 2011). On May 11, 2011 the pharmacy compounding accreditation board sent a letter to SMFM stating that "unlike most other new FDA approved drugs, the makers of Makena do not have a patent on this preparation. The commercial preparation Makena was approved under the FDA's orphan drug program using an older medication with a formula in the public domain and supported by research conducted by the National Institute of Health. Under the orphan drug program, manufacturers are granted seven years of market exclusivity meaning that they and only they have the ability to promote market and advertise that product for the particular use. While a compounding pharmacy cannot market and promote a commercial competitor to Makena, it can legally compound 17OHP-C on the basis of a prescriber's valid prescription". For comparison, the cost of progesterone USP suppositories is $1-2 per suppository or $ 5-10 per week or $200 per pregnancy, whereas the cost of crinone gel 8% is $15 per week or $100 per week or $2500 per pregnancy (Silver & Cunningham, 2011).

9. Future of progestins and PTB

Data has shown that there is a place for progesterone in the prevention of PTB. However, the optimal dosage, route and timely delivery of the drug remain controversial. It is encouraging that there are multiple ongoing trials that should further clarify the role of progesterone in PTB prevention (www.clincialtrials.gov/ct/show and; www.charttrials.abdn.ac.uk/). To et al (To et al., 2006) , from the fetal Medicine Foundation (FMF), developed a model combining maternal risk factors with CL and found that the inclusion of maternal age and previous history of PTB improved the prediction. The detection rate of screening for PTD before 32 weeks at a fixed false-positive rate of 10% was 38% for maternal factors, 55% for CL and 69% for combined testing. This concept is important when considering which patients to include in spontaneous PTB prevention programs.

10. Conclusions

In summary, the exact mechanism of progestins on reducing preterm birth is speculative at this point. The absence of effect in multiple gestation together with a positive results in women with historical risk, short cervix and the recent cerclage data, suggests that progesterone's effect on preterm birth rates may be related to reducing inflammation rather than acting as a tocolytic agent (Elovitz & Gonzalez et al., 2008). More information is needed not only regarding the mechanism of action, but also in regard to maternal outcomes following antenatal therapy, preference by patient in terms of mode of delivery, satisfaction of care, optimal dose, optimal route of administration and optimal gestational age at which to begin therapy (ACOG #419, 2008).

Although no specific regimen is cited as superior or preferable (ACOG #419, 2008), evidence at this time supports prophylactic administration of progesterone be offered to women with a singleton pregnancy and a previous spontaneous PTB and to pregnant women with a short cervix of </= 25 mm at mid-gestation scan for prevention of PTB (250 mg of weekly IM 17OHP-C or progesterone 100 mg daily vaginally). Current evidence does not support the routine use of progesterone in women with multiple gestations and PPROM nor as a treatment for threatened or established PTL.

11. References

ACOG Committee Opinion. (2008). Use of progesterone to reduce preterm birth. *Obstet Gynecol. 419,963-5.*

ACOG practice bulletin. (1998). Clinical management of preterm premature rupture of membranes. *Obstet Gynecol. 1, 848-57.*

Amon E. (1999) Preterm labor. In: *Medicine of the fetus and mothers*. Reece EA, Hobbins JC, eds. pp. 529-579. Philadelphia, PA.

Bacq Y, Sapey T, Brechot MC, et al. (1997) Intrahepatic cholestasis of pregnancy. *Hepatology* 26,358-64.

Bailit JL, Votruba ME. (2007) Medical cost savings associated with 17 alpha-hydroxyprogesterone caproate. *Am J Obstet Gynecol* 196(3),219. e1-7.

Behrman RE, Butler AS (eds) (2007). Committee on Understanding Premature Birth and Assuring Healthy Outcomes, Board on Health Sciences Policy. *Preterm Birth Causes, Consequences, and Prevention*, Institute of Medicine of the National Academies. The National Academies Press: Washington D.C.

Benifla JL, Dumont M, Levardon M, et al. (1997) Effects of micronized natural progesterone on the liver during the third trimester of pregnancy. *Contracep Fertil Sex*. 25,165-9.

Berghella V, Figueroa D, Szychowski JM, et al. (2010) Vaginal Ultrasound Trial Consortium. 17-alpha-hydroxyprogesterone caproate for the prevention of preterm birth in women with prior preterm bith and a short cervical length. *Am J Obstet Gynecol* 202,351;e1-36.

Berghella V, Rafael TJ, Szychowski JM, et al. (2011) Cerclage for short cervix on ultrasonography in women with singleton gestations and previous preterm birth: a meta-analysis. *Obstet Gynecol*. 117,663-71.

Bernstein PS. (2008). Withdrawal of 17 alpha-hydroxyprosgesterone: a possible trigger for preterm labor? *Am J Obstet Gynecol, 198(2),244;author reply 244-5.*

Bonesca EB, Celik E, Parra M. et al. (2007) Progesterone and the risk of preterm birth among women with a short cervix. *N Engl J Med*. 357,462-9.

Borna S, Sahabi N. (2007) Progesterone for maintenance tocolytic therapy after threatened preterm labour: A randomized controlled trial. *Aust N Z J Obstet and Gynaecol*. 48(1),58-63.

Brancazio LR, Murtha AP, Heine RP. (2003) Prevention of recurrent preterm delivery by 17 alpha-hydroxyprogesterone caproate. *N Engl J Med*. 349,1987-8.

Briery CM, Veillon EW, Klauser CK et al. (2009) Progesterone does not prevent preterm births in women with twins. Southern Med J. 2009;102(9):900-904.

Briery CM, Ve*llon EW, Klauser CK. et al. (2011)* Women with preterm premature rupture of the membranes do not benefit from weekly progesterone. *Am J Obstet Gynecol*. 204,54.31-5.

Cahill AG, Odibo AO, Caughey AB et al. (2010). Universal cervical length screening and treatment with vaginal progesterone to prevent preterm birth: a decision and economic analysis. *Am J Obstet Gynecol. 202,:548.e1-8.*

Campbell S. (2011). Universal cervical-length screening and vaginal progesterone prevents early preterm births, reduces neonatal morbidity and is cost saving: doing nothing is no longer an option. *Ultrasound Obstet Gynecol. 38, 1-9.*

Caritis SN, Rouse DJ, Peaceman AM, et al. (2009) Prevention of preterm birth in triplets using 17 alpha-hydroxyprogesterone caproate: a randomized controlled trial. *Obstet Gynecol* . 113 (2 Pt 1), 285-92.

Chandiramani M. (2007). Progesterone and preterm birth. *N Engl J Med. 357(22); correspondence 2306-7.*

Cohen AW, Copel JA, Macones GA et al. (2011). Unjustified increase in cost of care resulting from U.S. Food and Drug Administration approval of makena (17 alpha hydroprogesterone caproate). *Obstet Gynecol. 117(6), 1408-12.*

Combs CA, Garite T, Maurel K, et al. (2010) Failure of 17-hydroxyprogesterone to reduce neonatal morbidity or prolong triplet pregnancy: a double-blind, randomized clinical trial. *Am J Obstet Gynecol*. 203,248.e1-9.

Coomarasamy A, Thangaratinam S, Gee H, et al. (2006) Progesterone for the prevention of preterm birth: a critical evaluation of evidence. *Eur J Obstet Gynecol Reprod Biol. 129,111-18.*

Crossley KJ, Nicol MB, Hirst JJ, et al. (1997) Suppression of arousal by progesterone in fetal sheep. *Reprod Fertil Dev.* 9,767-73.

da Fonseca E, Bittar RE, Carvalho MHB, et al. (2003). Prophylactic administration of progesterone by vaginal suppository to reduce the incidence of spontaneous preterm birth in women at increased risk: A randomized placebo-controlled, double-blind study. *Am J Obstet Gynecol.* 188, 419-24.

Damus K. (2008). Prevention of preterm birth: a renewed national priority. *Curr Opin Obstet Gynecol.* 20, 590-6.

DeFranco EA, O'Brien JM, Adair CD, et al. (2007) Progesterone vaginal gel for the reduction of recurrent preterm birth: primary results from a randomized, double-blind, placebo-controlled trial. *Ultrasound Obstet Gynecol.* 30:687-96.

Di Renzo GC, Mattei A, Gojnic M, et al. (2005). Progesterone and pregnancy. *Curr Opin Obstet Gynecol.* 17, 598-600.

Durnwald CP, Momirova V, Rouse DJ, et al., for the Eunice Kennediy Shriver National Institute of Child Health and Human Development Maternal-Feal Medicine Units Network. (2010) Second trimester cervical length and risk of preterm birth in women with twin gestations treated with 17-□ hydroxyprogesterone caproate. *The Journal of Maternal-Fetal and Neonatal Medicine.* 23(12),1360-4.

Elovitz M, Gonzalez J. (2008). Medroxyprogesterone acetate modulates the immune response in the uterus, cervix, and placenta in a mouse model of preterm birth. *J. Matern. Fetal Neonatal Me. 21(4), 223-30.*

Facchinetti F, Paganelli S, Comitini G, et al. (2007) Cervical length changes during preterm cervical ripening: effects of 17-alpha-hydroxyprogesterone caproate. *Am J Obstet Gynecol.* 196,453-4.

FDA issues NDA 21-945. Proposed Indication. "Gestiva is indicted for the prevention of preterm birth in...www.fda.gov/ohms/dockets/ac/06/briefing/2006-422B1-02-FDA-background.pdf.

Fonseca EB, Celik E, Parra M. et al. (2007). Progesterone and the risk of preterm birth among women with a short cervix. *N Engl J Med. 357,462-9.*

Fuchs AR, Peryasamy S, Alexandrova M, et al. (1985). Correlation between oxytocin receptor concentration and responsiveness to oxytocin in pregnant rat myometrium: effects of ovarian steroids. *Endocrinology.* 113, 742-9.

Garfield RE, Dannan MS, Daniel EE. (1980). Gap junction formation in myometrium: control by estogens, progesterone, and prostaglandins. *Am J Physiol.* 238, C81-9.

Garfield RE, Puri CP, Csapo AI. (1982). Endocrine, structural, and functional changes in the uterus during premature labor. *Am J Obstet Gynecol.* 142, 21-7.

Gluckman PD, Hanson MA. (2004). Living with the past: evolution, development and patterns of disease. *Science.* 305, 1733-6.

Goldenberg RL, Culhane JF, Iams J, et al. (2008). The epidemiology and etiology of preterm birth. *Lancet* 371, 75-84.

Grazzini E, Guillon G, Mouillac B, et al. (1998). Inhibition of oxytocin receptor function by direct binding of progesterone. *Nature.* 392, 509-12.

Guyer B, Martin JA, MacDorman MF, et al. (1997). Annual summary of vital statistics-1996. *Pediatrics*. 100, 905-18.

Hack M, Fanaroff AA. (1999). Outcomes of children of extremely low birth weight and gestational age in the 1990s. *Early Hum Dev.* 53, 193-218.

Hamilton, BE, Martin JA, Ventura SJ. (2005). Births: preliminary data for 2005. *Natl Vital Stat Rep.* 55, 1-18.

Hartikainen-Sorri A-L, Kauppila A, Tuimala R. (1980). Inefficacy of 17 □-hydroxyprogesterone caproate in the prevention of prematurity in twin pregnancy. *Obstet Gynecol.* 56, 692-5.

Hassan SS, Romero R, Vidyadhari D, et al., for the PREGNANT Trial. (2011). Vaginal progesterone reduces the rate of preterm birth in women with a sonographic short cervix: a multicenter, randomized, double-blind, placebo-controlled trial. *Ultrasound Obstet Gynecol.* 38, 18-31.

Hauth JC, Gilstrap LC III, Brekken AL, et al. (1983). The effect of 17 alpha-hydroxyprogesterone caproate on pregnancy outcome in an active-duty military population. *Am J Obstet Gynecol.* 146, 187-90.

Health Canada. Canadian Perinatal Surveillance System. Canadian Perinatal Health Report 2003. Chapter 4;73-6. Available at: http://www.hc.sc.gc.ca/pphb-dgspsp/rhs-ssg/index.html. Accessed July 10, 2005.

Heinonen PP, Slone D., Shapiro S. (1977). *Birth defects and Drugs in Pregnancy.* Littleton, Mass. PSG Publishing.

Henderson D, Wilson T. (2001). Reduced binding of progesterone receptor to its nuclear response element after human labor onset. *Am J Obstet Gynecol.* 194, 579-85.

How HY, Barton J, Istwan N, et al. (2007). Prophylaxis with 17 Alpha-hdroxyprogesterone caproate for prevention of recurrent preterm delivery: Does gestational age at initiation of treatment matter? *Am J Obstet Gynecol.* 197,260.e1-260.e4.

Iams JD. (2010) Was the preterm birth rate in the placebo group too high in the Meis MFMU Network trial of 17-OHPC? Am J Obstet Gynecol 409-410.

Imseis H, Albert T, Iams J. (1997). Identifying twin gestations at low risk for preterm birth with a transvaginal ultrasonographic cervical measurement at 24 to 26 weeks'; gestation. *Am J Obstet Gynecol.* 177,1149-55.

Institute of Medicine of the National Academies. Preterm Birth: Causes, Consequences, and Prevention, Washington DC; National Academies Press; 2006. Accessed September 1, 2006. Available at: http://www.iom.edu/CMS/3740/25471/35813.aspx.

Jenkins-Manning, Flenady V. Dodd J, et al. (2006). Care of women at risk of preterm birth: a survey of reported practice in Australia and New Zealand. *Aust. NZ J.* 46(6), 546-8.

Johnson JWC, Austin KL, Jones CS, et al. (1975). Efficacy of 17□-hydroxyprogesterone caproate in the prevention of premature labor. *N Engl J Med.* 293, 675-80.

Karalis K, Goodwin G, Majzoub JA. (1996). Cortisol blockade of progesterone: a possible molecular mechanism involved in the initiation of human labor. *Nature Medicine.* 2(5), 556-60.

Keirse MJNC. (1990). Progesterone administration in pregnancy may prevent preterm delivery. *Br J Obstet Gynecol.* 96,275-80.

LeVine L. (1964). Habitual abortion: a controlled clinical study of Progestational therapy. *West J Surg Obstet Gynecol.* 72, 3036.

Lieman JM, Brumfield CG, Carlo W et al. (2005). Preterm premature rupture of the membranes: is there an optimal gestational age for delivery? *Obstet Gynecol. 105, 12-7.*

Lye SJ, Porte DG. (1978). Demonstration that progesterone blocks uterine activity in the ewe in vivo by a direct action on the myometrium. *Journal of Reproduction and Fertility.* 52, 87-94.

Mackenzie R, Walker M, Armson A, et al. (2006). Progesterone for the prevention of preterm birth among women at increased risk: a systematic review and meta-analysis of randomized controlled trials. *Am J Obstet Gynecol. 194, 1234-42.*

March of Dimes Birth Defects Foundation. (2005). Accessed July 11. Available at: http://www.marchofdimes.com.

March of Dimes (2007).: United States infant mortality overview. http://www.marchofdimes.com/peristats/tlanding.aspx?reg=99&lev=0&top=6&slev=1&tlv=qf,

Accessed May 26, 2007.

Meis PJ, Klebanoff M, Thom E, et al. NICHD MFMU Network. (2003). Prevention of recurrent preterm delivery by 17 alpha-hydroxyprogesterone caproate. *N Engl J Med.* 348(24), 2379-85.

Mercer BM. (2003). Preterm premature rupture of the membranes. *Obstet Gynecol. 101,178-93.*

Morken N, Killen K, Hagberg H, et al. (2005). Preterm birth in Sweden 1973-2001: rate, subgroups, and effect of changing patterns in multiple births, maternal age, and smoking: preterm delivery. *Acta Obstet Gynecol Scand.* 84(6), 558-65.

Murray JL (1998). Natural Progesterone: what role in women's health care? *Health Primary Care.* 1,671-87.

Nicol MB, Hirst JJ, Walker D, et al. (1997) Effect of alteration of maternal plasma progesterone concentration on fetal behavioral state during late gestation. *J Endocrinol.* 152,379-86.

Norman JE, Mackenzie F, Owen P, et al. (2009) Progesterone for the prevention of preterm birth in twin pregnancy (STOPPIT): a randomized, double-blind, placebo-controlled study and meta-analysis. *Lancet.* 373:2034-40.

Northen AT, Norman, GS, Anderson K, et al. for NICHD MFMU Network. (2007). Follow-up of children exposed to 17 Alpha-hydroxyprogesterone caproate compared with placebo. *Obstet Gynecol* 110,865-72.

O'Brien JM, Adair CD, Lewis DF, e t al. (2007). Progesterone vaginal gel for the reduction of recurrent preterm birth: Impact of gestational age at pevious delivery. *Ultrasound Obstet Gynecol.* 30,687-96.

Odibo AO, Stamilio DM, Macones GA, et al. (2006). 17 alpha-hydroxyprogesterone caproate for the prevention of preterm delivery: a cost-effectiveness analysis. *Obstet Gynecol* 108(3 Pt 1):492-9.

Onsrud M, Paus E, Haug E, et al. (1985). Intramuscular administration of hydroxyprogesterone caproate in patients with endometrial carcinoma. Pharmacokinetics and effects on adrenal function. *Acta Obstet Gynecol Scand.* 64, 519-23.

O'Sullivan MD, Hehir MP, O'Brien YM, Morrison JC. 17 alpha-hydroxprogesterone caproate vehicle, castor oil, enhances the contractile effect of oxytocin in human myometrium in pregnancy. Am J Obstet Gynecol 2010;202:453.e1-4.

Papiernik E. (1970). Double-blind study of an agent to prevent pre-term delivery among women at increased risk. Schering ed. Series 4. P. 65-68.

Penzias AS & Alper MM. (2003). Luteal support with vaginal micronized progesterone gel in assisted reproduction. *Reprod Biomed Online.* 6, 287-95.

Posaci C, Smitz J, Camus M, et al. (2000). Progesterone for the luteal support of reproductive technologies: clinical options. *Human Reprod.* 15 (suppl I), 129-48.

Progesterone therapy. Progesterone…what is it? (2006). Available at: http://progesteronetherapy.com/.

Rafael TJ, Dhanya Mackeen A, Berghella V. (2011). The Effect of 17α-Hydroxyprogesterone Caproate on Preterm Birth in Women with an Ultrasound-Indicated Cerclage. *Am J Perinatol* 28:389-94.

Rebarber A, Cleary-Goldman J, Istwan NB, et al. (2008). The use of 17 alpha-hydroxyprogesterone caproate (17p) in women with cervical cerclage. *Am J Perinatol* 25:271-5.

Rebarber A, Ferrara, LA, Hanley ML, et al. (2007). Increased recurrence of preterm delivery with early cessation of 17-alpha-hydroxyprogesterone caproate. *Am J Obstet Gynecol.* 196,224.e1-224.e4.

Rebarber A, Istwan N, Russo-Stieglitz K et al. (2007). Increased incidence of gestational diabetes in women receiving prophylactic 17 alpha-hydroxyprogesterone caproate for prevention of recurrent preterm delivery. *Diabetes Care. 30,2277-80.*

Reynolds MM, Schieve LA, Martin JA, et al. (2003). Trends in multiple births conceived using assisted reproductive technology, United States, 1997-2000. *Pediatrics.* 111(5), 1159-62.

Romero R, Wu YK, Mazor M. (1989). Amniotic fluid arachidonate lipoxygenase metabolites in preterm labor. *Prostaglandins Leukot Essent fatty acids. 36, 69-75.*

Rouse DJ, Caritis SN, Peaceman AM, et al.(2007). National Institute of Child Health and Human Developmetn Maternal-Fetal Medicine Units Nretwork. A trial of 17 alpha-hydroxyprogeterone caproate to prevent prematurity in twins. *N Engl J Med* 357, 454-61.

Sanchez-Ramos L, Kaunitz AM, Delke I. (2005). Progestational agents to prevent preterm birth: a meta-analysis of randomized controlled trials. *Obstet Gynecol.* 105,273-9.

Siiteri PK, Seron-Ferre M. (1981). Some new thoughts on the feto-placental unit and parturition in primates. IN: *Fetal endocrinology.* Novy JM, Reskko AJ, editors. P.1. Academic Press. New York.

Silver RM & Cunningham FG. (2011). Deus ex Makena? *Obstet Gynecol. 117(6), 1263-65.*

Spong CY, Meis PJ, Thom EA, et al. (2005). Progesterone for prevention of recurrent birth: Impact of gestational age at previous delivery. *Am J Obstet Gynecol.* 193,1127-31.

Su LL, Samuel M, Chong YS. (2010). Progestational agents for treating threatened or established preterm labour. (Review) *The Cochrane Collaboration.* Published by John Wiley & Sons, Ltd.

To MS, Fonseca EB, Molina FS, et al. (2006). Maternal characteristics and cervical length in the prediction of early spontaneous preterm delivery in twins. *Am J Obstet Gynecol.* 194:1360-5.

To MS, Skentou CA, Royston P, et al. (2006). Prediction of patient-specific risk of early preterm delivery using maternal history and sonographic measurement of cervical length: a population-based prospective study. *Ultrasound Obstet Gynecol* 27,362-7.

Tough SC, Newburn-Cook C, Johnston DW. (2002). Delayed childbearing and its impact on population rate changes in lower birth weight, multiple birth, and preterm delivery. *Pediatrics.* 109(3), 399-403.

Tucker JM, Goldenberg RI, Davis RO, et al. (1991). Etiologies of preterm birth in an indigent population: Is prevention a logical expectation? *Obstet Gynecol.* 77, 343-7.

Vaisbuch E, Hassan SS, Mazaki-Tovi S, et al. (2010). Patients with an asymptomatic short cervix (< or = 15 mm) have a high rate of subclinical intraamniotic inflammation: implications for patient counseling. *Am J Obstet Gynecol* 202,433.e1-8.

von Eye Corleta H, Capp E, Ferreira MBC. (2004). Pharmacokinetic of natural progesterone vaginal suppository. *Gynecol Obstet Invest.* 58, 105-8.

Waters TP, Schultz BAH, Mercer BM. et al. (2009). Effect of 17 alpha- hydroxyprogesterone caproate on glucose intolerance in pregnancy. *Obstet Gynecol. 114:45-9.*

Werner EF, Han CS, Pettker CM et al. (2011). Universal cervical-length screening to prevent preterm birth:a cost-effective analysis. *Ultrasound Obstet Gynecol 38:32-7*

Yemini M, Borenstein R, Dreazen E, et al. (1985). Prevention of premature labor by 17 alphahydroxyprogesterone caproate. *Am J Obstet Gynecol.* 293,675-80.

10

Management of Abnormal Vaginal Flora as a Risk Factor for Preterm Birth

Gilbert G.G. Donders[1,2] and Gert Bellen[2]
[1]*Department of Obstetrics and Gynaecology of the Regional Hospital, Heilig Hart Tienen and University Hospital Gasthuisberg Leuven,*
[2]*Femicare vzw, Clinical Research for Women, Tienen, Belgium*

1. Introduction

Prevention of preterm birth remains a major challenge in obstetrics. While over the years a lot of attention has been given to the structural deficiencies, like uterine abnormalities, or 'weak' or 'insufficient' cervix, during the last decades the importance of ascending infection as a possible cause of preterm birth, preterm rupture of the membranes and intrauterine infection has become increasingly evident (Martius & Eschenbach, 1990). The earlier the preterm labor starts, the higher the likelihood an underlying chorio-amnionitis will be found. While for term deliveries the risk of chorio-amnionitis is around 1%,it is more than 45% in preterm deliveries (Scherman et al., 1997). The damage intrauterine infection causes to the fetus is not limited to the complications and sequels of being born preterm, but also is due to brain damage, like intra- or peri-ventricular hemorrhages and cerebral palsy, caused by the inflammatory reaction due to infection (Romero et al., 2007). Furthermore, such gestational ascending infections may cause maternal complications like sepsis, septic arthritis, maternal respiratory distress (Garland et al., 2002).

Bacterial vaginosis (BV) in pregnancy has an acknowledged increased risk of preterm delivery, but treatment with metronidazole is not beneficial, and if anything, harmful for the pregnancy. Use of broader spectrum antibiotics like clindamycin, or combination antibiotherapy, have shown better results, but still not all studies are in agreement with this. Therefore, critical reappraisal of the prevailing data are crucial, and new studies may need to incorporate new findings and insights. For one, the diagnostic accuracy needs to be refined, as it became increasingly clear that aerobic pathogens and the inflammation caused by aerobic vaginitis (AV), may play a more important role than previously thought. In recent studies meticulously discriminating these differences between BV, AV and mixed AV-BV flora by phase contrast microscopy, it became evident that not only BV may be primarily associated to intrauterine growth restriction and preterm birth, but also the aerobic component may lead to inflammatory reactions in placenta, amniotic fluid and fetus, preterm rupture of the membranes and preterm birth. In this review, emphasis is placed on the most crucial differential diagnostic characteristics, and the treatment adjustments these findings require. Part of this review has been published in the British Journal of Gynecology (Donders et al, 2011).

2. Definition of AV

Diagnosis of AV is based on wet mount microscopy. Normal and abnormal lactobacillary flora are divided into 3 to 4 flora types, also depicted as lactobacillary grades (LBG's). LBG 1 corresponds to a 'healthy' microflora, and has predominant lactobacillary morphotypes of variable size. Lactobacillary grade III is a condition wherein the lactobacillary morphotypes are completely replaced by other bacterial morphotypes. Lactobacillary grade II is an intermediate group, with partial replacement of the lactobacilli by other bacteria. Due to their specific link to pathology, we refined the three grades, and divided grade 2 (LBGII) in a less severe (LBGIIa) and a more severe (LBGIIb) variety (Donders, 1999). As LBG 3, and to a lesser extent LBG IIb are more likely to be linked with pathological conditions, they are entitled 'abnormal vaginal flora'. LBG's are the basis for a composite score to which the following four variables were added: 1) proportional number of leukocytes, 2) presence of toxic leukocytes, 3) presence of parabasal epithelial cells and 4) type of background flora (Donders, 2002). This condition is a screening tool that should not be confused with bacterial vaginosis. Bacterial vaginosis is a condition with abnormal vaginal flora, but abnormal vaginal flora is not always bacterial vaginosis. Some studies demonstrate that the absence of lactobacilli is a more powerful predictor of preterm birth than the presence of bacterial vaginosis (Donders et al., 2008a; Hay et al., 1994). In order to diagnose such abnormal lactobacillary grades, the use of wet mount is preferred above the use of Gram stains due to superior accuracy (Donders et al., 2000c; Donders et al 1996) and better correlation with lactate in the vaginal content (Donders et al., 1998), a functional test for lactobacillary defence function.

Therefore, in this classification, the immune reaction of the host is also taken into account for the diagnosis. Parabasal cells are considered a sign of severe epithelial inflammation usually not seen in uncomplicated BV. They are encountered only in moderate or severe forms of aerobic vaginitis (AV), such as in desquamative inflammatory vaginitis (Newbern et al., 2002; Sobel, 1994). Background flora was allocated score 0 if the background flora was unremarkable or showed debris and bare nuclei from lysed epithelial cells (cytolysis), score 1 if the lactobacillary morphotypes were very coarse or resembled small bacilli (rather than lactobacilli), and 2 if there were prominent cocci, or chained cocci visible. Leukocytes were scored according to their proportional number when compared with epitheliocytes. More than 10 leukocytes per epithelial cell is assigned 2 points, while less than 10 per epithelial cell, but more than 10 per high power field corresponds to 1 point. Adding these points together comprises a composite score, the 'AV'-score. A composite score of 1 to 4 represents normal flora. A score of 5 to 6 to moderate AV, and a score above 6 (to max. 10) to severe AV. In practice, a score of 8 to 10 matches the definition of 'desquamative inflammatory vaginitis'.

The use of this AV criterion enables us to divide the flora in a more detailed and comprehensive way, avoiding undefined and unclear categories. Bacterial flora is lactobacillary type predominant (normal), or it is abnormal. If abnormal the flora can be disturbed by anaerobic overgrowth (BV) or by aerobic micro-organisms, such as E coli, group B streptococci, enterococci etc (AV), or can be a mixture of both (mixed AV-BV). Therefore one has to be continuously aware that concomitant infections may occur, and also concurrent infections with *Candida sp.*, *Trichomonas vaginalis*, mycoplasmata or cervicitis (*Chlamydia trachomatis*, *Neisseria gonorrhoeae* and other) (Donders et al., 1993b).

One of the disadvantages of the Nugent score system that is used on Gram stained specimens to diagnose BV (Nugent et al., 1991), is that one does not realize more than one condition may co-occur. In studying wet mounts and applying the BV and AV criteria at the same time, pure BV can be clearly distinguished from pure AV, but at the same time combined forms can be discovered where wherein anaerobic BV flora and AV flora coincide. This mixed AV-BV flora may well be a transient condition between BV and AV, but most likely a prolonged co-infection of both may also occur.

3. Abnormal vaginal flora subtypes in pregnancy

For a few genital infections with severe impact on the outcome of the pregnancy, such as syphilis and gonorrhoea, a 'screen and treat' policy is almost always cost-effective (Donders et al., 1993a; Elliot et al., 1990), while for other infectious conditions, like vaginal overgrowth with mycoplasmata, the jury is still out there to define its precise role in the pathogenesis of infection related preterm birth and fetal injury (Lee et al., 2009; Harada et al., 2008; Carey et al., 1991; Gravett & Eschenbach, 1986).

From the early 90ies it became evident that not only typical pathogens like *C. trachomatis*, *T. vaginalis* and *N. gonorrhoeae* could harm the pregnancy, but also merely aberrations from the normal lactobacilli dominant vaginal flora could endanger the fetus. Although all in the same line, these aberrations were all studied form a different perspective. Most studies used Nugent's or Spiegel's score on Gram stains to detect an association between bacterial vaginosis (BV) and intermediate flora with adverse pregnancy outcome (Hay et al., 1994; Elliot et al., 1990; Lee et al., 2009; Thorp et al., 2008; Cauci et al., 2002c; Hauth et al., 2003; Kekki et al., 2001; Kiss et al., Klebanoff et al., 2005; McDonald et al., 1997; Oakeshott et al., 2004; Verstraelen et al., 2007), but similar findings could be obtained with clinical Amsel criteria to diagnose BV (Honest et al., 2004; Rouse et al., 2009), abnormal lactobacillary grades on both Pap smears, gram stains, and wet mount preparations (Hay et al., 1994; Donders et al., 1993b; Mass et al., 1999; Donders et al., 2009) and with other abnormalities of the bacterial flora than full BV (Donders et al., 2002; Donders et al., E pub ahead of print 2010; Donders et al., 2009).

As is generally acknowledged, Nugent score above 7 on Gram stained specimens corresponds well with BV, and is nowadays accepted as golden standard for the diagnosis of BV in most clinical trials. Compared to this method, wet mount is said to be less sensitive. However, some constraints have to be taken into consideration. First of all, on a continuous scale of 1 to 10, there is no consensus on what the intermediate group with a score of 4 to 6 stands for. If Nugent were an ideal scoring system for bacterial vaginosis, with score 1 to 3 being normal and 7 or above being full blown BV, score 4 to 6 should be transitional, partial or intermediate BV, but in reality it is not. Ideally this intermediate flora state represents a turning point from a normal state into BV, or on the opposite, from BV to normal. However, most of these women with so-called intermediate BV according to Nugent will neither have BV, nor will they become normal. In fact, as they are not having normal flora, nor BV, they rather resemble a sort of 'garbage bin', but this does not mean that they do not represent important pathology. Most intriguing, in almost all studies addressing the importance of BV and the intermediate group as a separate category, it was clear that the intermediate group was linked to a different, and usually more serious scope of complications (e.g. mid trimester pregnancy loss) than the 'classic', full-blown BV (Hay et al., 1994; McDonald et al., 1994).

4. Pathogenesis, immunology and genetics

As AV only rather recently became recognized as an entity that differs in several aspects from BV, lot of its ethiology and pathogenesis remains unraveled. It is not known why the vagina harbours 2 to 3 predominant lactobacillary species (e.g. L. gasseri, L. cripatus, L. iners or L.) in normal women (Verstraelen et al., 2009) while in others anaerobes or aerobic commensals overgrow the vagina. It may well be that AV and BV are both ends of the same spectrum of bacterial abnormalities in the vagina, explaining the frequent occurrence of both conditions combined, also in pregnancy (Zodzika et al, 2011). Although it is not clear how the one condition can evolve into the other, it is certainly evident that both conditions express a completely different immunology pattern. Pro-inflammatory cytokines IL1b, IL6 and IL 8 are clearly linked to LBG's in pregnant women, cytokines going up with decreasing numbers of lactobacilli (Donders et al., 2003; Donders et al., 2000a). As was also shown by Cauci et al, BV does express an elevated pro-inflammatory cytokine IL1 b as well, but not the promoter cytokines of the prostaglandin cascade, IL-6 and IL-8 (Cauci et al., 2003), whereas in AV not only IL1b but also dramatic concentrations of IL6 and IL 8 are formed in the vagina (Donders, 2002). As the pro-inflammatory cytokine producers, especially IL-8, in BV women have a different pathogenesis than the (more common) non-producers, and are linked to several risk factors in pregnancy (Cauci et al., 2008; Cauci et al. 2002a, 2002b), likewise the enormous production of prostaglandin provoking cytokines IL 6 and IL 8 in AV patients make them likely candidates for causing preterm labor and delivery (Donders, 2002; Donders, 2007). The links between the presence of vaginal infections, increased levels of IL 6 and IL 8 in both vagina and amniotic fluid and chorio-amnionitis, PPROM and preterm birth are confirmed in several studies (Massaro et al., 2009; Hitti et al., 2001; Rizzo et al., 1996).

5. Prevalence

Prevalence of BV in pregnancy is very variable according to the geographical and socio-demographic area of sampling and ranges from as low as 9% (Larsson et al., 2007) to as high as 48% (Tann et al., 2006). Longitudinal studies show invariably a decrease of BV during pregnancy and a lower likelihood to acquire I with the weeks the gestation progresses (Waters et al., 2008). The prevalence of abnormal aerobic flora or aerobic vaginitis is much more difficult to determine. Besides the prevalence studies on GBS colonization, which ranges between 7 and 25% between 35 and 37 weeks, until recently only sporadic papers have been published on the frequency of AV. Due to the high concentrations of circulating estrogens, severe AV, typically with increased numbers of parabasal cells, is infrequent in pregnancy. However, the prevalence of less extensive types , mild to moderate AV, may range from 8 to 10% according to sporadic studies done during pregnancy (Donders et al., 2009; Zodzika et al., 2011; Rezeberga et al., 2008). Also, it has to be acknowledged that many BV patients have AV to a certain extent as well, - only, the score obtained by Nugent's method will never tell you. Therefore we plea to look for both AV and BV in pregnancy as both conditions are present, need different management approaches and are both linked to adverse pregnancy outcome.

6. Diagnostic techniques and screening

Some authors used aspecific substitute markers instead of Nugent Score for BV detection for exploring risk factors in the vaginal flora during pregnancy. Being one of the crucial criteria of the Amsel diagnosis of BV, pH is often used as such a surrogate point of care test for BV (Madhivanan et al., 2009). However, in a study where pH was used as a screening tool in pregnancy, only 40% of women with increased vaginal pH had BV (Zodzika et al., 2011). When screening random women in Uganda, we discovered BV in only 27% of women with pH above 4.4 and 39% of women with pH above 4.7 had BV, while another 11% and 25% had coccoid AV respectively (unpublished results). The study demonstrated that AV and mixed AV-BV flora is also a frequent cause of abnormal pH in pregnancy. Hoyme et al. installed a screening in a German state by self measurements of the vaginal pH followed by treatment and found a dramatic reduction of preterm births (<37 gestational weeks at delivery) and early preterm births (<32 weeks) (Hoyme & Saling, 2004). As no specific search for BV was done, the proportion of women treated for other conditions than BV in this study in unkown.

On several occasions, our group could demonstrate that the finding of decreased lactobacilllary morphotypes in the beginning of pregnancy is a marker which is strongly linked to preterm birth, even more convincingly so than full BV on its own (Donders et al., 2008a; Donders et al., 1993b; Donders et al., 2009; Madhivanan et al., 2009; Donders et al., 2008b). As is the case with increased pH, also deficient lactobacillary grades are part of the clinical diagnosis of BV, without implying that all abnormal cases necessarily have BV.

7. Outcome

7.1 Miscarriage

Although BV is linked to the increased incidence of spontaneous first and second trimester miscarriage (Hay et al., 1994; Donders et al., 2000b; Larsson et al., 2006; Oakeshott et al., 2002) and reduced baby-take-home-rates in pregnancies obtained through assisted fertility procedures like in vitro fertilization, these data are less clear for AV. In in vitro fertilization procedures, a relation was found between BV and implantation failures (Ralph et al., 1999), but this relation was not confirmed in another observation (Liversedge et al., 1999). Furthermore, amongst these patients a clear relation of BV with tubal infertility was present, (Liversedge et al., 1999; Wilson et al., 2002) indicating indirectly BV is a risk factor for ascending infection and tubal damage. Interestingly, in one study, not BV, but decreased lactobacilli (AVF) was found to be the risk factor of implantation failure at IVF (Eckert et al., 2003). In animals, experiments have shown that *E. coli* derived lipopolysaccharides (LPS) cause implantation failure associated with increased anti-inflammatory cytokines (Deb et al., 2004a, 2004b). No data are available yet about the chances to conceive and keep the pregnancy in women with clinical AV or AV flora, but in sporadic cases pathogenic *E. coli* serotypes were involved in recurrent abortion cases (Blum-Oehler et al., 1997).

7.2 Midtrimester chorioamnionitis

The problem of amniotic fluid infection is that most of the time regular culture techniques are insufficiently sensitive to detect bacterial infection. Therefore, if PCR is used, frequent infection with E coli could be detected amongst these cases even when cultures were negative (Daoud et al., 2008). Also GBS and gram negative rods (Sherman et al., 1997) are frequent causes of intrauterine infections and histologic chorioamnionitis, often leading to midtrimester abortion, and even recurrences in two thirds of the women who have experienced it before.

7.3 Preterm birth

In one study H Mc Donald et al. found an association between midtrimester vaginal colonization with *U urealyticum* and bacterial vaginosis (culture of *G vaginalis*) and preterm birth, but not with enteropathogens such as E coli and enterococci (McDonald et al., 1992), but in another study the same authors found such enteropathogens and *S. aureus* to be predictive for preterm birth before 37 and 34 weeks (McDonald et al., 1991). Others have consistently linked colonization of *U urealyticum* of *M hominis* with preterm labor, short cervix, intrauterine infection and preterm birth (Donders et al., E pub ahead of print 2010; Donati et al., 2010; Holst et al., 2006; Hassan et al., 2006). In studies addressing the different subtypes of abnormal vaginal flora, aerobic vaginitis, mixed flora, and partial bacterial vaginosis show a significant relation with preterm birth alongside bacterial vaginosis (Donders et al., E pub ahead of print 2010; Donders et al., 2009; Donati et al., 2010), the latter being more related to growth restriction. After analyzing their studies, Carey and Klebanoff came to the conclusion that rather than just anaerobic BV, overgrowth with *S. aureus* and *E. coli* were the only vaginal bacterial flora linked to preterm birth (Carey et al., 2005). By looking at the microscopic flora patterns as possible risk factors early in pregnancy, we and others came to exactly the same conclusions, namely that aerobic abnormal flora early in pregnancy constitutes a significant risk of preterm labor, chorioamnionitis and funisitis of the newborn (Donders et al., 2008a; Donders et al., 2009; Rezeberga et al., 2008). Our hypothesis is that this link of preterm birth risk with the presence of vaginal flora disturbances associated with overgrowth of aerobic commensal bacteria may be the main reason why treatment with the broader spectrum antibitiotic clindamycin is a better approach to reduce preterm birth and preterm rupture of the membranes than metronidazole, which eliminates only the anaerobes (Donders et al., 2009; Larsson et al., 2006; Lamont et al., 2003).

7.4 Intrauterine infection

This would also explain why the pro-inflammatory cytokines that are most closely linked to intrauterine infection and preterm labor, IL 6 and IL 8 are not produced in uncomplicated full BV, but are found in dramatic concentrations in AV (Donders, 2002) and explain the closer association with these cytokines with lactobacillary grades than with anaerobic BV (Donders et al., 2003). In a comprehensive review Roberto Romero and coworkers summarized their voluminous work showing the importance of intrauterine inflammation induced by ascending infection and causing periventricular leucomalacia and cerebral palsy (Romero et al., 2004). Furthermore he and others emphasized the role of genetic variations in polymorphisms creating different responses amongst women to intrauterine infectious challenges (Holst & Garnier, 2008). While it was known since a long time that anaerobic BV associated bacteria can frequently recovered from the uterine cavity in amniocentesis specimens of women with preterm labor (Martius & Eschenbach, 1990; Hitti et al., 2001; Rizzo et al., 1996; Newton et al., 1997; Krohn et al., 1995; Hillier et al., 1995; Newton, 1993; Gibbs, 1993), most cases of neonatal sepsis are not caused by these BV associated bacteria, but by aerobic bacteria, mainly group B streptococcus, *E. coli* and *S. aureus*. Only recently, for the first time, Rezeberga et al could demonstrate that AV at the first prenatal visit before 12 weeks, detected both clinically as on cultures, was related to an increased risk of chorioamnionitis and funisitis (Rezeberga et al., 2008). Neonatal sepsis, most with *S. aureus* , was also a frequent finding in growth restricted fetuses (Vedmedovska et al., 2010a).

7.5 Intrauterine growth restriction

While women with AV and inflammatory reaction are more likely to develop intrauterine infection, chorioamnionitis, funisitis (Rezeberga et al., 2008) and preterm delivery, the merely non-inflammatory bacterial vaginosis may rather cause growth restriction and preterm delivery of small for date fetuses (Rezeberga et al., 2008). Also in the work of Vedmedovska et al., it was found that genital infections, primarily bacterial vaginosis, was linked to fetal growth restriction (Vedmedovska et al., 2010b).

8. Treatment

8.1 Antibiotics

It is not yet clear which should be the best approach to treat for AV in non-pregnant women, let alone during pregnancy. The inflammatory component of most patients with AV makes one think that antibiotics may not be the best, or not the only approach. But IF is chosen to give antibiotics in pregnancy to reduce preterm birth and intrauterine infection, it became clear after a placebo controlled studies that metronidazole is not the answer as it does not decrease the preterm birth rate in women with bacterial vaginosis (McDonald et al., 1997; McDonald et al., 2007; Carey et al., 2000; Odendaal et al., 2002). Even worse, Klebanoff's (Klebanoff et al., 2001) and Odendael's study (Odendaal et al., 2002) on the treatment of trichomoniasis and BV, respectively, rather demonstrated an increased risk of preterm birth after treatment with metronidazole, leading several authors to the compelling conclusion that metronidazole should not be used in pregnancy with the purpose to reduce the risk of preterm birth (Donders et al., 2009; Odendaal et al., 2002; Carey et al., 2003; Morency & Bujold, 2007). Investigators using broader spectrum antibiotics, also covering gram positive cocci and E coli, on the other hand, were successful in the reduction of preterm birth in several placebo controlled studies (Larsson et al., 2006; Lamont et al., 2003; Ugwumadu et al., 2003), although not all (Kekki et al., 2001; Kurkinen-Raty et al., 2000; Rosenstein et al., 2000). As most studies used a single treatment course of 5 to 7 days, and test of cure was not always done, one can ask whether a more intensive and repetitive treatment regimen would not be indicated, but studies are lacking.

Use of other antibiotics, aiming at *U urealyticum* and *C trachomatis*, like amoxicillin and erythromycin, have not been successful in the reduction of preterm birth or other infection-related complications in pregnancy (Andrews et al., 2003; Goldenberg et al., 2006; McGregor et al., 1990). Tempera et al tested local kanamycin for paitents with AV and performed a detailed analysis of the culture results, proving this may be a successful approach (Tempera et al., 2004). However, even though this antibiotic is not absorbed, tests in pregnancy with this and other similar products have not yet been done yet. Some local, non absorbable with antibiotics, like rifaximin, may have a special promise, due to favorable anti- inflammatory action reducing pro-inflammatory cytokine production as a surplus (Brown et al., 2010). As this has lead to high cure rates in inflammatory bowel diseases such as Crohn's disease, diverticulitis and colitis ulcerosa (Guslandi, 2010; Shafran & Burgunder, 2010; Latella & Scarpignato, 2009), and given the non-absorbable nature, studies exploring the potential of this antibiotic in the treatment of vaginal flora disturbances could be interesting, also in pregnancy.

Finally, also the level of preterm threat may play a crucial role in the efficiency of the BV treatment. Women with BV who have contractions and other symptoms of preterm labor extend their gestation longer when treated for BV than when untreated, whereas asymptomatic women show no difference between treatment versus placebo (Stevens et al, 2004; Briery et al, 2011).

8.2 Antiseptics

Only sporadic and older studies addressed the topic of using antiseptic medication with chlorhexidin, povidine iodine or chloramine as a preventive measure to prevent perinatal and maternal infectious complications in pregnancy, usually without any success (Watanabe et al., 1998; Rouse et al., 1997; Broe et al., 1992). Hence the therapy has been largely abandoned during pregnancy. A recent study shows a beneficial effect of dequalinium chloride vaginal tablets on BV that is comparable to treatment with intravaginal clindamycin, but the effect of this new disinfectant on AV is not known, and studies in pregnancy were not yet performed (Weisenbacher et al., 2011).

8.3 Probiotics

Acidifying or probiotic therapy has also sporadically been tested for women with AVF or BV in pregnancy, but not specifically for AV. In 1990, Holst et al reported a clear benefit of using acidifying cream for BV in a small group of women during pregnancy (Holst & Brandberg, 1990), but this paper was never followed by larger series. A Cochrane review of all randomized trial using probiotics indicated a clear reduction of vaginal infection after the use of oral or vaginal lactobacillus acidophilus containing milk products or yogurt, but data on the outcome of pregnancy were lacking (Othman et al., 2007).

9. References

Andrews WW, Sibai BM, Thom EA, Dudley D, Ernest JM, McNellis D et al. Randomized clinical trial of metronidazole plus erythromycin to prevent spontaneous preterm delivery in fetal fibronectin-positive women. Obstet Gynecol 2003; 101(5 Pt 1):847-855.

Blum-Oehler G, Heesemann J, Kranzfelder D, Scheutz F, Hacker J. Characterization of Escherichia coli serotype O12:K1:H7 isolates from an immunocompetent carrier with a history of spontaneous abortion and septicemia. Eur J Clin Microbiol Infect Dis 1997; 16(2):153-155.

Briery CM, Chauhan SP, Magann EF, Martin RW, Bofill JA, Cushmanh JL, Morrison JC. Treatment of bacterial vaginosis does not reduce preterm birth among high-risk asymptomatic women. J of MSMA 2011; 52:72-75.

Broe D, Van DJ, Cowley D, Vacca A, Voreteliac V, Maquire D et al. Detection of premature rupture of membranes by measuring diamine oxidase in vaginal fluid: false-negative results caused by obstetric antiseptic creams. Clin Chem 1992; 38(5):784.

Brown EL, Xue Q, Jiang ZD, Xu Y, Dupont HL. Pretreatment of epithelial cells with rifaximin alters bacterial attachment and internalization profiles. Antimicrob Agents Chemother 2010; 54(1):388-396.

Carey JC, Blackwelder WC, Nugent RP, Matteson MA, Rao AV, Eschenbach DA et al. Antepartum cultures for Ureaplasma urealyticum are not useful in predicting pregnancy outcome. The Vaginal Infections and Prematurity Study Group. Am J Obstet Gynecol 1991; 164(3):728-733.

Carey JC, Klebanoff MA, Hauth JC, Hillier SL, Thom EA, Ernest JM et al. Metronidazole to prevent preterm delivery in pregnant women with asymptomatic bacterial vaginosis. National Institute of Child Health and Human Development Network of Maternal-Fetal Medicine Units. N Engl J Med 2000; 342(8):534-540.

Carey JC, Klebanoff MA. What have we learned about vaginal infections and preterm birth? Semin Perinatol 2003; 27(3):212-216.

Carey JC, Klebanoff MA. Is a change in the vaginal flora associated with an increased risk of preterm birth? Am J Obstet Gynecol 2005; 192(4):1341-1346.

Cauci S, Driussi S, Guaschino S, Isola M, Quadrifoglio F. Correlation of local interleukin-1beta levels with specific IgA response against Gardnerella vaginalis cytolysin in women with bacterial vaginosis. Am J Reprod Immunol 2002; 47(5):257-264.

Cauci S, Guaschino S, Driussi S, De SD, Lanzafame P, Quadrifoglio F. Correlation of local interleukin-8 with immunoglobulin A against Gardnerella vaginalis hemolysin and with prolidase and sialidase levels in women with bacterial vaginosis. J Infect Dis 2002; 185(11):1614-1620.

Cauci S, Hitti J, Noonan C, Agnew K, Quadrifoglio F, Hillier SL et al. Vaginal hydrolytic enzymes, immunoglobulin A against Gardnerella vaginalis toxin, and risk of early preterm birth among women in preterm labor with bacterial vaginosis or intermediate flora. Am J Obstet Gynecol 2002; 187(4):877-881.

Cauci S, Guaschino S, De AD, Driussi S, De SD, Penacchioni P et al. Interrelationships of interleukin-8 with interleukin-1beta and neutrophils in vaginal fluid of healthy and bacterial vaginosis positive women. Mol Hum Reprod 2003; 9(1):53-58.

Cauci S, Culhane JF, Di SM, McCollum K. Among pregnant women with bacterial vaginosis, the hydrolytic enzymes sialidase and prolidase are positively associated with interleukin-1beta. Am J Obstet Gynecol 2008; 198(1):132-137.

Daoud GA, Suzuki Y, Yamamoto T, Suzuki T, Suzumori N, Tanemura M. Establishment of a polymerase chain reaction method for detection of Escherichia coli in amniotic fluid in patients with chorioamnionitis. Fetal Diagn Ther 2008; 24(2):132-139.

Deb K, Chaturvedi MM, Jaiswal YK. Comprehending the role of LPS in Gram-negative bacterial vaginosis: ogling into the causes of unfulfilled child-wish. Arch Gynecol Obstet 2004; 270(3):133-146.

Deb K, Chatturvedi MM, Jaiswal YK. Gram-negative bacterial endotoxin- induced infertility: a birds eye view. Gynecol Obstet Invest 2004; 57(4):224-232.

Donati L, Di VA, Nucci M, Quagliozzi L, Spagnuolo T, Labianca A et al. Vaginal microbial flora and outcome of pregnancy. Arch Gynecol Obstet 2010; 281(4):589-600.

Donders GG, Desmyter J, De Wet DH, Van Assche FA. The association of gonorrhoea and syphilis with premature birth and low birthweight. Genitourin Med 1993; 69(2):98-101.

Donders G, De Wet HG, Hooft P, Desmyter J. Lactobacilli in Papanicolaou smears, genital infections, and pregnancy. Am J Perinatol 1993; 10(5):358-361.

Donders GG, Vereecken A, Salembier G, Van BB, Spitz B. Assessment of Vaginal Lactobacillary Flora in Wet Mount and Fresh or Delayed Gram's Stain. Infect Dis Obstet Gynecol 1996; 4(1):2-6.

Donders GG, Desmyter J, Vereecken A. Vaginitis. N Engl J Med 1998; 338(21):1548.

Donders GG. Microscopy of the bacterial flora on fresh vaginal smears. Infect Dis Obstet Gynecol 1999; 7(3):126-127.

Donders GG, Bosmans E, Dekeersmaecker A, Vereecken A, Van BB, Spitz B. Pathogenesis of abnormal vaginal bacterial flora. Am J Obstet Gynecol 2000; 182(4):872-878.

Donders GG, Van BB, Caudron J, Londers L, Vereecken A, Spitz B. Relationship of bacterial vaginosis and mycoplasmas to the risk of spontaneous abortion. Am J Obstet Gynecol 2000; 183(2):431-437.

Donders GG, Vereecken A, Dekeersmaecker A, Van BB, Spitz B. Wet mount microscopy reflects functional vaginal lactobacillary flora better than Gram stain. J Clin Pathol 2000; 53(4):308-313.

Donders GG. Definition of a type of abnormal vaginal flora that is distinct from bacterial vaginosis: aerobic vaginitis. Br J Obstet Gynecol. 2002; 109: 1-10.

Donders GG, Vereecken A, Bosmans E, Dekeersmaecker A, Salembier G, Spitz B. Definition of a type of abnormal vaginal flora that is distinct from bacterial vaginosis: aerobic vaginitis. BJOG 2002; 109(1):34-43.

Donders GG, Vereecken A, Bosmans E, Spitz B. Vaginal cytokines in normal pregnancy. Am J Obstet Gynecol 2003; 189(5):1433-1438.

Donders GG. Definition and classification of abnormal vaginal flora. Best Pract Res Clin Obstet Gynaecol 2007; 21(3):355-373.

Donders GGG, Odds A, Vereecken A, Van Bulck B, Caudron J, Londers L, Salembier G and Spitz B. Abnormal vaginal flora in the first trimester, but not full blown bacterial vaginosis is associated with preterm birth. Prenat Neonat Med 2008;(3):588-593.

Donders GGG, Spitz B, Vereecken A, Van Bulck B, Cornelis A, Dekeersmaeker A, Klerckx P, Londers L and Caudron J. The Ecology of the Vaginal Flora at First Prenatal Visit is Associated with Preterm Delivery and Low Birth Weight. The Open Inf Dis J 2008; 2:45-51.

Donders GG, Van Calsteren K, Bellen G, Reybrouck R, Van den Bosch T, Riphagen I et al. Predictive value for preterm birth of abnormal vaginal flora, bacterial vaginosis and aerobic vaginitis during the first trimester of pregnancy. BJOG 2009; 116(10):1315-24.

Donders GG, Van Calsteren C, Bellen G, Reybrouck R, Van den Bosch T, Riphagen I et al. Association between abnormal vaginal flora and cervical length as risk factors for preterm birth. Ultrasound Obstet Gynecol, E pub ahead of print 26 Jan 2010.

Donders GG, Bellen G, Rezeberga D. Aerobic vaginitis in pregnancy. BJOG, 2011;118:1163-70.

Eckert LO, Moore DE, Patton DL, Agnew KJ, Eschenbach DA. Relationship of vaginal bacteria and inflammation with conception and early pregnancy loss following in-vitro fertilization. Infect Dis Obstet Gynecol 2003; 11(1):11-17.

Elliott B, Brunham RC, Laga M, Piot P, Ndinya-Achola JO, Maitha G et al. Maternal gonococcal infection as a preventable risk factor for low birth weight. J Infect Dis 1990; 161(3):531-536.

Garland SM, Ni CF, Satzke C, Robins-Browne R. Mechanisms, organisms and markers of infection in pregnancy. J Reprod Immunol 2002; 57(1-2):169-183.

Gravett MG, Eschenbach DA. Possible role of Ureaplasma urealyticum in preterm premature rupture of the fetal membranes. Pediatr Infect Dis 1986; 5(6 Suppl):S253-S257.

Gibbs RS. Chorioamnionitis and bacterial vaginosis. Am J Obstet Gynecol 1993; 169(2 Pt 2):460-462.

Goldenberg RL, Mwatha A, Read JS, Adeniyi-Jones S, Sinkala M, Msmanga G et al. The HPTN 024 Study: the efficacy of antibiotics to prevent chorioamnionitis and preterm birth. Am J Obstet Gynecol 2006; 194(3):650-661.

Guslandi M. Rifaximin for Inflammatory Bowel Disease. Dig Dis Sci 2010.

Hassan S, Romero R, Hendler I, Gomez R, Khalek N, Espinoza J et al. A sonographic short cervix as the only clinical manifestation of intra-amniotic infection. J Perinat Med 2006; 34(1):13-19.

Harada K, Tanaka H, Komori S, Tsuji Y, Nagata K, Tsutsui H et al. Vaginal infection with Ureaplasma urealyticum accounts for preterm delivery via induction of inflammatory responses. Microbiol Immunol 2008; 52(6):297-304.

Hauth JC, Macpherson C, Carey JC, Klebanoff MA, Hillier SL, Ernest JM et al. Early pregnancy threshold vaginal pH and Gram stain scores predictive of subsequent preterm birth in asymptomatic women. Am J Obstet Gynecol 2003; 188(3):831-835.

Hay PE, Lamont RF, Taylor-Robinson D, Morgan DJ, Ison C, Pearson J. Abnormal bacterial colonisation of the genital tract and subsequent preterm delivery and late miscarriage. BMJ 1994; 308(6924):295-298.

Hillier SL, Krohn MA, Cassen E, Easterling TR, Rabe LK, Eschenbach DA. The role of bacterial vaginosis and vaginal bacteria in amniotic fluid infection in women in preterm labor with intact fetal membranes. Clin Infect Dis 1995; 20 Suppl 2:S276-S278.

Hitti J, Hillier SL, Agnew KJ, Krohn MA, Reisner DP, Eschenbach DA. Vaginal indicators of amniotic fluid infection in preterm labor. Obstet Gynecol 2001; 97(2):211-219.

Holst E, Brandberg A. Treatment of bacterial vaginosis in pregnancy with a lactate gel. Scand J Infect Dis 1990; 22(5):625-626.

Holst RM, Jacobsson B, Hagberg H, Wennerholm UB. Cervical length in women in preterm labor with intact membranes: relationship to intra-amniotic inflammation/microbial invasion, cervical inflammation and preterm delivery. Ultrasound Obstet Gynecol 2006; 28(6):768-774.

Holst D, Garnier Y. Preterm birth and inflammation-The role of genetic polymorphisms. Eur J Obstet Gynecol Reprod Biol 2008; 141(1):3-9.

Honest H, Bachmann LM, Knox EM, Gupta JK, Kleijnen J, Khan KS. The accuracy of various tests for bacterial vaginosis in predicting preterm birth: a systematic review. BJOG 2004; 111(5):409-422.

Hoyme UB, Saling E. Efficient prematurity prevention is possible by pH-self measurement and immediate therapy of threatening ascending infection. Eur J Obstet Gynecol Reprod Biol 2004; 115(2):148-153.

Kekki M, Kurki T, Pelkonen J, Kurkinen-Raty M, Cacciatore B, Paavonen J. Vaginal clindamycin in preventing preterm birth and peripartal infections in asymptomatic women with bacterial vaginosis: a randomized, controlled trial. Obstet Gynecol 2001; 97(5 Pt 1):643-648.

Kiss H, Petricevic L, Husslein P. Prospective randomised controlled trial of an infection screening programme to reduce the rate of preterm delivery. BMJ 2004; 329(7462):371.

Klebanoff MA, Carey JC, Hauth JC, Hillier SL, Nugent RP, Thom EA et al. Failure of metronidazole to prevent preterm delivery among pregnant women with asymptomatic Trichomonas vaginalis infection. N Engl J Med 2001; 345(7):487-493.

Klebanoff MA, Hillier SL, Nugent RP, Macpherson CA, Hauth JC, Carey JC et al. Is bacterial vaginosis a stronger risk factor for preterm birth when it is diagnosed earlier in gestation? Am J Obstet Gynecol 2005; 192(2):470-477.

Krohn MA, Hillier SL, Nugent RP, Cotch MF, Carey JC, Gibbs RS et al. The genital flora of women with intraamniotic infection. Vaginal Infection and Prematurity Study Group. J Infect Dis 1995; 171(6):1475-1480.

Lamont RF, Duncan SL, Mandal D, Bassett P. Intravaginal clindamycin to reduce preterm birth in women with abnormal genital tract flora. Obstet Gynecol 2003; 101(3):516-522.

Larsson PG, Fahraeus L, Carlsson B, Jakobsson T, Forsum U. Late miscarriage and preterm birth after treatment with clindamycin: a randomised consent design study according to Zelen. BJOG 2006; 113(6):629-637.

Larsson PG, Fahraeus L, Carlsson B, Jakobsson T, Forsum U. Predisposing factors for bacterial vaginosis, treatment efficacy and pregnancy outcome among term deliveries; results from a preterm delivery study. BMC Womens Health 2007; 7:20.

Latella G, Scarpignato C. Rifaximin in the management of colonic diverticular disease. Expert Rev Gastroenterol Hepatol 2009; 3(6):585-598.

Lee SE, Romero R, Kim EC, Yoon BH. A high Nugent score but not a positive culture for genital mycoplasmas is a risk factor for spontaneous preterm birth. J Matern Fetal Neonatal Med 2009; 22(3):212-217.

Liversedge NH, Turner A, Horner PJ, Keay SD, Jenkins JM, Hull MG. The influence of bacterial vaginosis on in-vitro fertilization and embryo implantation during assisted reproduction treatment. Hum Reprod 1999; 14(9):2411-2415.

Kurkinen-Raty M, Vuopala S, Koskela M, Kekki M, Kurki T, Paavonen J et al. A randomised controlled trial of vaginal clindamycin for early pregnancy bacterial vaginosis. BJOG 2000; 107(11):1427-1432.

Madhivanan P, Krupp K, Hardin J, Karat C, Klausner JD, Reingold AL. Simple and inexpensive point-of-care tests improve diagnosis of vaginal infections in resource constrained settings. Trop Med Int Health 2009; 14(6):703-708.

Martius J, Eschenbach DA. The role of bacterial vaginosis as a cause of amniotic fluid infection, chorioamnionitis and prematurity--a review. Arch Gynecol Obstet 1990; 247(1):1-13.

Mass SB, Brennan JP, Silverman N, van Hoeven KH. Association between a shift in vaginal flora on Papanicolaou smear and acute chorioamnionitis and preterm delivery. Diagn Cytopathol 1999; 21(1):7-9.

Massaro G, Scaravilli G, Simeone S, Capuano S, Pastore E, Forte A et al. Interleukin-6 and Mycoplasma hominis as markers of preterm birth and related brain damage: our experience. J Matern Fetal Neonatal Med 2009; 22(11):1063-1067.

McDonald HM, O'Loughlin JA, Jolley P, Vigneswaran R, McDonald PJ. Vaginal infection and preterm labour. Br J Obstet Gynaecol 1991; 98(5):427-435.

McDonald HM, O'Loughlin JA, Jolley P, Vigneswaran R, McDonald PJ. Prenatal microbiological risk factors associated with preterm birth. Br J Obstet Gynaecol 1992; 99(3):190-196.

McDonald HM, O'Loughlin JA, Jolley PT, Vigneswaran R, McDonald PJ. Changes in vaginal flora during pregnancy and association with preterm birth. J Infect Dis 1994; 170(3):724-728.

McDonald HM, O'Loughlin JA, Vigneswaran R, Jolley PT, Harvey JA, Bof A et al. Impact of metronidazole therapy on preterm birth in women with bacterial vaginosis flora (Gardnerella vaginalis): a randomised, placebo controlled trial. Br J Obstet Gynaecol 1997; 104(12):1391-1397.

McDonald HM, Brocklehurst P, Gordon A. Antibiotics for treating bacterial vaginosis in pregnancy. Cochrane Database Syst Rev 2007;(1):CD000262.

McGregor JA, French JI, Richter R, Vuchetich M, Bachus V, Seo K et al. Cervicovaginal microflora and pregnancy outcome: results of a double-blind, placebo-controlled trial of erythromycin treatment. Am J Obstet Gynecol 1990; 163(5 Pt 1):1580-1591.

Morency AM, Bujold E. The effect of second-trimester antibiotic therapy on the rate of preterm birth. J Obstet Gynaecol Can 2007; 29(1):35-44.

Nugent RP, Krohn MA, Hillier SL. Reliability of diagnosing bacterial vaginosis is improved by a standardized method of gram stain interpretation. J Clin Microbiol 1991; 29(2):297-301.

Newbern EC, Foxman B, Leaman D, Sobel JD. Desquamative inflammatory vaginitis: an exploratory case-control study. Ann Epidemiol 2002; 12(5):346-352.

Newton ER. Chorioamnionitis and intraamniotic infection. Clin Obstet Gynecol 1993; 36(4):795-808.

Newton ER, Piper J, Peairs W. Bacterial vaginosis and intraamniotic infection. Am J Obstet Gynecol 1997; 176(3):672-677.

Oakeshott P, Hay P, Hay S, Steinke F, Rink E, Kerry S. Association between bacterial vaginosis or chlamydial infection and miscarriage before 16 weeks' gestation: prospective community based cohort study. BMJ 2002; 325(7376):1334.

Oakeshott P, Kerry S, Hay S, Hay P. Bacterial vaginosis and preterm birth: a prospective community-based cohort study. Br J Gen Pract 2004; 54(499):119-122.

Odendaal HJ, Popov I, Schoeman J, Smith M, Grove D. Preterm labour--is bacterial vaginosis involved? S Afr Med J 2002; 92(3):231-234.

Othman M, Neilson JP, Alfirevic Z. Probiotics for preventing preterm labour. Cochrane Database Syst Rev 2007;(1):CD005941.

Ralph SG, Rutherford AJ, Wilson JD. Influence of bacterial vaginosis on conception and miscarriage in the first trimester: cohort study. BMJ 1999; 319(7204):220-223.

Rezeberga D, Lazdane G, Kroica J, Sokolova L, Donders GG. Placental histological inflammation and reproductive tract infections in a low risk pregnant population in Latvia. Acta Obstet Gynecol Scand 2008; 87(3):360-365.

Rizzo G, Capponi A, Rinaldo D, Tedeschi D, Arduini D, Romanini C. Interleukin-6 concentrations in cervical secretions identify microbial invasion of the amniotic cavity in patients with preterm labor and intact membranes. Am J Obstet Gynecol 1996; 175(4 Pt 1):812-817.

Romero R, Chaiworapongsa T, Kuivaniemi H, Tromp G. Bacterial vaginosis, the inflammatory response and the risk of preterm birth: a role for genetic epidemiology in the prevention of preterm birth. Am J Obstet Gynecol 2004; 190(6):1509-1519.

Romero R, Gotsch F, Pineles B, Kusanovic JP. Inflammation in pregnancy: its roles in reproductive physiology, obstetrical complications, and fetal injury. Nutr Rev 2007; 65(12 Pt 2):S194-S202.

Rosenstein IJ, Morgan DJ, Lamont RF, Sheehan M, Dore CJ, Hay PE et al. Effect of intravaginal clindamycin cream on pregnancy outcome and on abnormal vaginal microbial flora of pregnant women. Infect Dis Obstet Gynecol 2000; 8(3-4):158-165.

Rouse DJ, Hauth JC, Andrews WW, Mills BB, Maher JE. Chlorhexidine vaginal irrigation for the prevention of peripartal infection: a placebo-controlled randomized clinical trial. Am J Obstet Gynecol 1997; 176(3):617-622.

Rouse AG, Gil KM, Davis K. Diagnosis of bacterial vaginosis in the pregnant patient in an acute care setting. Arch Gynecol Obstet 2009; 279(4):545-549.

Shafran I, Burgunder P. Adjunctive antibiotic therapy with rifaximin may help reduce Crohn's disease activity. Dig Dis Sci 2010; 55(4):1079-1084.

Sherman DJ, Tovbin J, Lazarovich T, Avrech O, Reif R, Hoffmann S et al. Chorioamnionitis caused by gram-negative bacteria as an etiologic factor in preterm birth. Eur J Clin Microbiol Infect Dis 1997; 16(6):417-423.

Sobel JD. Desquamative inflammatory vaginitis: a new subgroup of purulent vaginitis responsive to topical 2% clindamycin therapy. Am J Obstet Gynecol 1994; 171(5):1215-1220.

Stevens AO, Chauhan SP, Magann EF, Martin RW, Bofill JA, Cushman J, Morrison JC. Fetal fibronectin and bacterial vaginosis are associated with preterm birth in women symptomatic for preterm labor. Am J Obstet Gynecol 2004;190(6):1582-9.

Tann CJ, Mpairwe H, Morison L, Nassimu K, Hughes P, Omara M et al. Lack of effectiveness of syndromic management in targeting vaginal infections in pregnancy in Entebbe, Uganda. Sex Transm Infect 2006; 82(4):285-289.

Tempera G, Bonfiglio G, Cammarata E, Corsello S, Cianci A. Microbiological/clinical characteristics and validation of topical therapy with kanamycin in aerobic vaginitis: a pilot study. Int J Antimicrob Agents 2004; 24(1):85-88.

Thorp JM, Jr., Dole N, Herring AH, McDonald TL, Eucker B, Savitz DA et al. Alteration in vaginal microflora, douching prior to pregnancy, and preterm birth. Paediatr Perinat Epidemiol 2008; 22(6):530-537.

Ugwumadu A, Manyonda I, Reid F, Hay P. Effect of early oral clindamycin on late miscarriage and preterm delivery in asymptomatic women with abnormal vaginal flora and bacterial vaginosis: a randomised controlled trial. Lancet 2003; 361(9362):983-988.

Vedmedovska N, Rezeberga D, Teibe U, Polukarova S, Donders G. Fetal growth restriction in Latvia. Int J Gynecol obstet 2010; 111 (2): 185-186.

Vedmedovska N, Rezeberga D, Teibe U, Zodzika J, Donders G. Preventable maternal risk factors and association of genital infection with Fetal Growth Restriction. Gynecol Obstet Invest 2010; 70 (4): 291-298.

Verstraelen H, Verhelst R, Roelens K, Claeys G, Weyers S, De BE et al. Modified classification of Gram-stained vaginal smears to predict spontaneous preterm birth: a prospective cohort study. Am J Obstet Gynecol 2007; 196(6):528-6.

Verstraelen H, Verhelst R, Claeys G, De BE, Temmerman M, Vaneechoutte M. Longitudinal analysis of the vaginal microflora in pregnancy suggests that L. crispatus promotes the stability of the normal vaginal microflora and that L. gasseri and/or L. iners are more conducive to the occurrence of abnormal vaginal microflora. BMC Microbiol 2009; 9:116.

Watanabe T, Minakami H, Matsubara S, Honma Y, Uchida A, Sato I. Effect of daily vaginal disinfection on duration of gestation after premature rupture of the membranes and on infant outcome. J Obstet Gynaecol Res 1998; 24(4):285-290.

Waters TP, Denney JM, Mathew L, Goldenberg RL, Culhane JF. Longitudinal trajectory of bacterial vaginosis during pregnancy. Am J Obstet Gynecol 2008; 199(4):431-435.

Weissenbacher ER, Dvorak V, Donders G, Spacek J et al. A Comparison of Dequalinium Chloride Vaginal Tablets (Fluomizin) and Clindaycin Vaginal Cream in Local Treatment of Bacterial Vaginosis. Gynecol Obstet Invest, 2011, in press

Wilson JD, Ralph SG, Rutherford AJ. Rates of bacterial vaginosis in women undergoing in vitro fertilisation for different types of infertility. BJOG 2002; Dec 23, e-pub ahead of press. 109(6):714-717.

Zodzika J, Jermakova I, Rezeberga D, Vasina O, Vedmedovska N, Donders G, Teibe U. Factors related to elevated vaginal pH in the first trimester of pregnancy. Acta Obstet Gynecol Scand 2011; 90: 41-46.

11

Strategies in the Prevention of Preterm Births During and Before Pregnancy

Wolf Kirschner[1] and Klaus Friese[2]
[1]*Forschung, Beratung + Evaluation GmbH c/o Charité, Berlin,*
[2]*Klinik und Poliklinik für Frauenheilkunde und Geburtshilfe, Munich, Germany*

1. Introduction

Preterm birth - defined as a childbirth before 259 days of gestation (<37 weeks) - is the major challenge in obstetrics and gynaecology worldwide. Preterm birth is associated with high perinatal mortality and surviving children often suffer higher morbidity throughout their lives. The incidence of preterm birth is very high in developing countries but also in some developed countries. According to a worldwide WHO report, Africa and North America, with rates of 11.9% and 10.6% in 2005, are the regions with the highest rates of incidence (Beck et al., 2010). Preterm birth not only causes much harm but also is associated with high costs. Despite considerable technical and medical improvements in obstetrics over recent decades, in developed countries preterm birth rates are not decreasing. On the contrary, the incidence continues to increase. In relation to possible preventive and epidemiologically well-founded measures, although onset and aetiology are not completely understood, our epidemiological knowledge concerning risk and protective factors of preterm birth is in no way poor. As regards preventive approaches, a distinction has to be made between primary and secondary preventive interventions, with this chapter focusing on the former.

After presenting some epidemiological and economic data on preterm birth, we will summarise the scope and results of certain programmes aiming to prevent preterm births. Subsequently, we will introduce the framework and methods of our prevention programme BabyCare. Special attention will be given to the evaluative methods and results achieved by our programme in terms of effectiveness and efficiency. While we can register a considerable and stable reduction in the incidence of preterm birth by at least 25% when comparing participants in the programme with a control data set, epidemiological analysis of our data indicates further that certain persistent risk factors of preterm birth observed in relation to programme participants require additional preventive measures which, ideally, should be implemented at the pre-conceptual stage. Consequently, after releasing the BabyCare Program in 2000, the PlanBaby Program was launched in 2007. In conclusion, interventional as well as evaluative problems and limitations of our programmes will be discussed.

2. Epidemiology and costs of preterm births

2.1 Incidence of preterm births

When dealing with the incidence of preterm births, a precise definition of the rates involved is often lacking. Both the numerator and denominator used in compiling rates can be differently defined. We have to distinguish rates referring to birth events from rates referring to infants born (either live births or all births). Logically, the rates referring to infants will be higher than those which refer to events.

		Absolute number		
A	Pregnant women / Birth events	89419		
B	Live births	90704		
C	Live births and still births	90986		
D	Preterm births	7123		
E	Preterm infants born alive	7860		
F	Preterm infants born alive and dead	8046		
		Definition		Incidence
	Birth event rate	D/A	7123/89419	8,0%
	Live birth rate	E/B	7860/90704	8,7%
	Live and still birth rate	F/C	8046/90986	8,8%

Table 1. Definitions of preterm birth rates (Perinatal Data from Medical association of Baden-Wuerttemberg, 2006).

In the United States of America, the incidence of preterm birth increased between 1990 and 2006 by 16%, rising from 10.6% to 12.8%, while since 2007 a slight reduction can be observed (Hamilton, 2010).

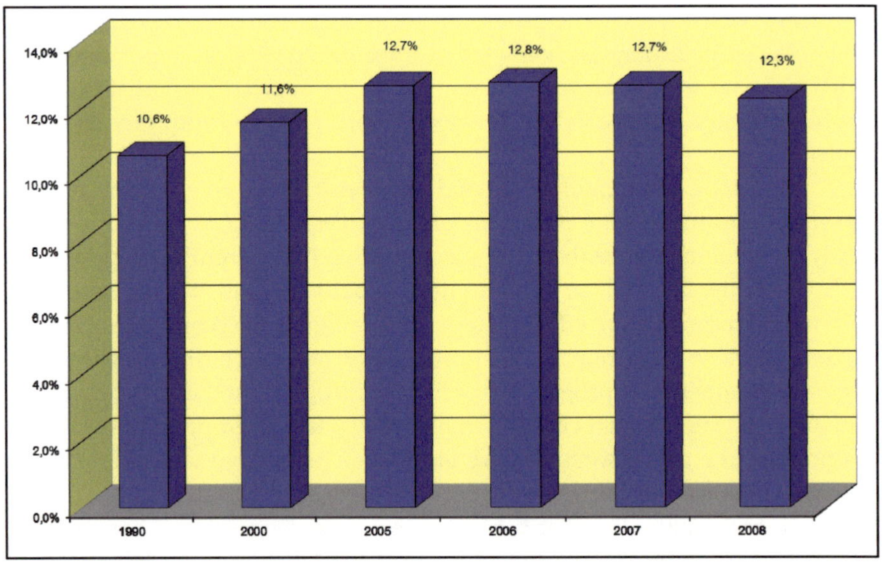

Fig. 1. Incidence of preterm birth in the USA 1990-2008 (Live births).

In the German region of Lower Saxony, we can observe an increase from 7.0% in 1987 to 8.5% in 2009. Again, here, a slight reduction can be seen since 2002. The increased rate can be attributed to the increased age of primiparous women, increased prevalence of risk factors (e.g. smoking, abnormal body weight), iatrogenic effects resulting from saving very preterm infants and fertilisation methods which contribute to preterm birth through a higher incidence of multiple pregnancies. In Germany, at least, the decline in rates may be traced back to the restriction imposed in 2004 on the reimbursement of fertilisation costs which led to a strong reduction of fertility treatments (DIR- Deutsches IVF-Register, Jahresbericht 2009, Annual Report English Version 2009).

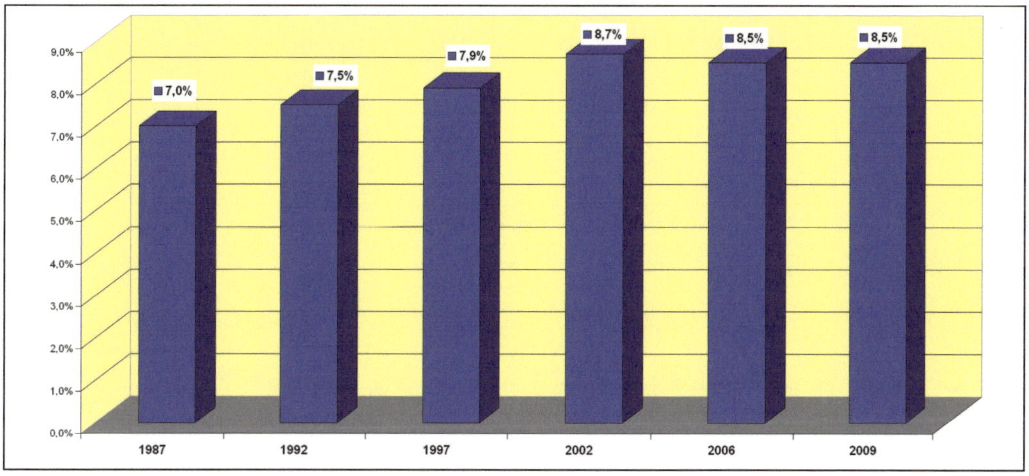

Fig. 2. Incidence of preterm birth in Germany (Lower Saxony) 1987-2009 (Birth events) (Perinatal Data from Medical association of Lower Saxony)

A comparison of preterm birth rates between Europe and North America reveals considerable differences in the incidence of preterm birth. The highest rates are found in the USA, Austria, Germany and Hungary while Ireland and Finland have very low rates (EURO-PERISTAT project, 2008). These differences are probably associated with different risk constellations in the populations (see below), but also differences in the frequency of sonographic determination of gestational age cannot be ruled out completely. "This indicator is defined as the number of live births and fetal deaths at each completed week of gestation (starting from 22 weeks), expressed as a proportion of all live and stillbirths. In most countries, data on gestational age is based on the "best obstetrical estimate", which combines clinical and ultrasound data, but some countries favour use of last menstrual period and others use only ultrasound estimates. There are also differences within countries. The method of determining gestational age can influence the gestational age distribution; use of ultrasound estimates tends to shift the distribution to the left and increase the preterm birth rate, although not all studies have found that this is the case". (European Perinatal Health Report, p. 129)

In addition to the variation in the preterm birth rate between countries, we must also note significant differences within an individual country. For example, in the German region of North Rhine-Westphalia, we can observe variations between municipalities with rates ranging from 9% to 14%, linked to socio-economic differences in the population, and with the highest rates to be found in economically underprivileged regions.

USA	**12,5%**	DNK	7,2%
AUT	**11,6%**	FRA	7,2%
GER	**9,1%**	ITA	7,2%
HUN	**8,9%**	POL	7,1%
CAN	8,2%	PRT	7,0%
BEL / Flanders	8,2%	GBR / NI	7,0%
ESP	8,2%	SWE	6,4%
GBR / Scotland	8,1%	GRC	6,3%
NLD	7,8%	LVA	6,2%
BEL / Brussels	7,4%	LUX	6,2%
MLT	7,4%	EST	6,1%
SVN	7,4%	**IRL**	**5,8%**
CZE	7,3%	**FIN**	**5,8%**
NOR	7,3%	**LTU**	**5,6%**

Table 2. Preterm birth rates in selected countries in Europe and North America, 2004 (Live births).

Looking more closely at the descriptive epidemiology of preterm birth in Germany, using the example of the perinatal database of Lower Saxony,[1] we find that the incidence of preterm birth is greater in primiparous women (9.5%) than in multiparous women (7.5%). In relation to age, we see a typical j-shaped distribution with high rates in very young and older pregnant women. In primiparous women aged 35 years and over the rate of preterm birth is almost 12%.

2.2 Analytical epidemiology of preterm births

Both in relation to the high incidence of preterm birth and the harm and costs involved (see below) the question to be answered is whether preterm birth can be prevented by primary or secondary interventions. In that regard, it must be conceded that the complex process of preterm birth is not completely understood. Nonetheless, epidemiology of preterm birth has identified a stable set of risk and protective factors associated with preterm birth. The epidemiological evidence is comparable, thus, to that which exists in relation to cardiovascular diseases, leading to numerous primary prevention programmes worldwide.

When looking at the medical conditions of an imminent preterm birth, we must first distinguish spontaneous preterm birth (SPB) from elective preterm birth (EPB) by caesarean section. In Lower Saxony, 29% of all deliveries in 2007 were carried out by caesarean section. However, in preterms that proportion rose to 55%. In addition, 16% of all caesarean sections were performed on pregnant women before 37 weeks of gestation.

---

[1]In Germany, perinatal statistics are compiled on a regional basis. A national database has only existed since 2003. For the first evaluation of the BabyCare Program in 2002 (see below), the perinatal database of Lower Saxony was used. Both then and now, in relation to preterm birth rates, the figures for Lower Saxony reflect the average across the whole of Germany.

	Total	Preterm	Term	% Preterm
Vaginal birth	41871	2236	39635	5,3%
Caesarean section	17196	2688	14508	**15,6%**
Total	59067	4924	54143	**8,3%**
% Section	29,1%	**54,6%**	26,8%	

Table 3. Caesarean section and preterm birth (Perinatal Data from Medical association of Lower Saxony, 2008).

The medical conditions at the onset of SPB and EPB are well known and will be illustrated with data from a cohort study of BabyCare participants. Medical conditions associated with preterm birth are placental complications, premature rupture of membranes (PROM), uterine complications, preterm labour and vaginal bleeding. When calculating odds ratios with respect to pregnancy complications in relation to the mode of preterm and term birth, we find PROM to be the strongest risk factor overall and especially for spontaneous preterm birth, whereas preeclampsia and placental complications are strongly associated with elective preterm birth.

	Preterm	**Not Preterm**	**OR**	**CONF 95%***	
n=	67	814			
Placental complications	20.9%	3.6%	7.2	3.9	13.1
Preeclampsia	28.4%	3.1%	12.5	7.3	21.5
Premature rupture of membranes	41.8%	0.5%	145.4	82.9	255.0
Preterm labour	41.8%	13.3%	4.7	2.9	7.6
Vaginal bleeding	25.4%	11.9%	2.5	1.4	4.5
Uterine complications	25.4%	4.5%	7.1	4.1	12.5
**** calculated by Miettinen***					

Table 4. Odds ratios for pregnancy complications (BabyCare Cohort Study).

Prevention of preterm birth is limited, thus, to the prevention of spontaneous preterm birth, as elective preterm birth is actively induced to avoid even greater health risks to the mother or the foetus. This does not imply, however, that preventive interventions are likely to be efficient only in the prevention of SPB because they may also reduce risks of emerging complications leading to EPB. We have to emphasise that at the onset of these medical conditions there is need, at most, for secondary prevention but, normally, urgent therapeutic interventions are required. However, primary prevention of SPB needs to address all medical and in particular non-medical risk factors established by international epidemiological research, ideally, in the earliest stage of pregnancy and, better still, prior to conception. In the context of this chapter, a differentiated analysis or even meta-analysis of analytical epidemiological studies is unnecessary. Quite simply, we wish to emphasise that of the known risk factors over half can either be addressed by preventive interventions or timely diagnosis, supervision of risk patients at close intervals and specific treatment (*italicised* below).

- Age of primiparous >=35 years / < 18 years
- Male sex of infant
- Low educational level
- Prior history of preterm birth

- Prior history of abortion
- *Smoking*
- *Illicit drug use*
- *Overweight / underweight*
- *Vaginal infections, e.g. bacterial vaginosis*
- *Folic acid deficiency*
- *Iron deficiency*
- *Stress in pregnancy*
- *Periodontitis*
- *Diabetes*
- *Hypertension*
- *Thrombosis / clotting disorder*
- *Eating disorders*
- Multifetal pregnancy
- Fertilisation

Spontaneous preterm birth

Age of mother e.g. PP > 35: 2,2	**Sex of fetus** Male: 1,2	**Multiples** 13,4
Low education level 1,1	**Infectious Diseases** e.g. Bacterial Vaginosis:2,2 e.g. Urinary tract infection:4,4	**Chronic Diseases** e.g. Diabetes:4,0 Hypertension:1,9 Thrombosis:1,4
Body Weight /BMI BMI <20:4,0 BMI >25:1,3	**Nutrition** eg. Eating Disorders:3,7 Folic acid deficiency:1,8	**Fertilisation** e.g. IVF : 1,4
Smoking / ill. Drugs e.g. >10 Cigarettes: 1,7	**Stress** **2,6**	**Working Conditions** e.g. hours of work>42:1,3
Reproductive history e.g. induced abortion:1,3 Former preterm birth:3,7	**Gyneacological history** e.g. Abortion / stillbirth:1,7 Gyneacol. Operations: 1,5	**Coffee an tea intake** **> 5 cups** **1,4**

Table 5. Risk factors for SPB with odds ratios and relative risk estimates from different publications (Danielian & Hall, 2005; Holzgreve et al., 2006; BabyCare data).

Thus, having regard to the relationship between risk factors and preterm birth measured by odds ratios or relative risks (an overview is given in Table 5), the interventive potential is anything other than small especially when, in addition, the prevalence of risk factors in the population is taken into account (not shown).

2.3 Costs of preterm births

Preterm birth not only causes harm and in many cases increases morbidity across an individual's life, preterm birth is also expensive. A conservative cost estimate for Germany based on DRG data and calculated by the authors reveals a cost premium in excess of EUR 10 000. In fact, the real costs are much higher as our estimate only includes the first two days in perinatal care. According to our calculations, the costs of preterm birth are EUR 12 800 compared to EUR 2 300 for vaginal deliveries (Kirschner et al., 2009). In the United States of America, the annual cost estimate for preterm birth based on 2005 figures is USD 26.2 billion (Beck et al., 2010). According to a press release of March of Dimes, a non-profit organisation working to reduce the incidence of preterm birth, the average medical cost for healthy full-term babies from birth through to their first birthday was USD 4 551, whereas for infants born preterm the average cost was nearly USD 50 000 (March of Dimes, 2009).

To summarise, preterm birth causes much harm to families and children and is extremely costly to society but there are reasonable possibilities for preventive interventions.

3. Principal strategies in preterm birth prevention and findings of prevention programmes

3.1 Principal strategies

Strategies for preterm birth prevention may differ according to time of intervention, instruments and methods, the target population and the setting chosen. With respect to the time of intervention, we can distinguish:

- preconceptional interventions
- prenatal interventions beginning at best in earliest pregnancy
- antenatal interventions at the onset of labor

Clearly antenatal interventions will not comprise real primary preventive measures and are limited to secondary prevention and the often difficult task of managing imminent preterm birth.

With respect to the instruments, we have to distinguish unifactorial and multifactorial interventions. Multifactorial interventions address a set of risk factors, using specific combinations of health counselling and health promotion measures as well as the application of diagnostic tools (e.g. pH test, oral glucose tolerance test (oGTT)). However, in addition to screening and diagnostics, the main aim of primary interventions is to change risk behaviour.

With respect to the target population, the main differences consist in the choice of risk groups versus interventions which address the whole female population of childbearing age or pregnant women.

The setting of the programmes needs to be organised such that the target population can be easily reached in a timely manner and as comprehensively as possible. Generally, prenatal interventions are likely to be integrated in the existing system of obstetric care provided in a particular country.

3.2 Findings of prevention programmes

In the context of this chapter, it is impossible to paint a concise picture of all the prevention programmes to reduce preterm births or of the evaluative outcomes in that regard. However, preterm birth prevention has a long history reaching back to the 1930s (Papiernik, n.d.). Without a doubt, the national prevention programme operated in France between 1972 and 1988 appears to be the most important intervention in an European country, with a reported reduction in preterm births from 8.2% in 1972 to 4.9% in 1988 (Papiernik, n.d.). Nevertheless, some shortcomings in the evaluation need to be addressed, although the standards of evaluation at the time were slightly different from those in force today.

On the basis of existing assessments of the programmes concerned, we have to conclude that results conflict with respect to effectiveness and efficiency (Alexander et al., 1991; Canadian Task Force on the Periodic Health Examination, 1994; Collaborative group on preterm births prevention, 1993; Dyson et al., 1998; Hueston, 1992; Papiernik, n.d.). However, this result is not surprising as strategies, settings, organisation of obstetric care and the target populations are often very different. In addition, there are shortcomings in evaluation methods, that is, if programmes are indeed documented and rigorously evaluated.

In addition to social policy interventions aiming to reduce preterm birth, there are studies aiming to find biological markers (e.g. cytokines) with high specificity and sensitivity in the prediction of preterm birth risks. However, the predictive values of those markers identified hitherto with respect to the onset of preterm birth are regarded as inadequate (David et al., 2002). As a tool of secondary prevention, they will be excluded from the following discussion.

To reduce complexity in the analysis, we will concentrate firstly on current strategies in Germany and Austria which are unifactorial and address vaginal infections. In this context, in Germany, vaginal pH measurement plays an important role and was recommended for inclusion in obstetric care in the 1990s by Saling, the founder of the Journal of Perinatal Medicine. In several studies, Saling and other researchers reported on the effectiveness and efficiency of pH self-measurement (Hoyme & Saling, 2004). However, the evaluation of these interventions had some shortcomings, the most important of which was the lack of a rigorous case control study. In the wake of the BabyCare Program, as a result of which an increased interest in the prevention of preterm birth especially among health insurance providers could be registered (see below), Saling et al. were successful in establishing programmes based on pH measurement. A pilot project was carried out between 2004 and 2006 by four health insurance providers, which was subject to external evaluation. In addition to this project, the programme "Hallo Baby" was established in 2004 and has since been offered by a number of health insurance providers to their members who are pregnant. This programme also primarily uses the pH measurement supplemented by additional counselling by gynaecologists. However, the latter programme has not been evaluated. In 2010, the evaluation of the pilot project was published. The evaluation did not demonstrate the efficacy of self-testing of vaginal pH for the prevention of preterm delivery. On the contrary, the rate of preterm birth was slightly higher among participants compared to those in control groups (Bitzer et al., 2011).

At this point, it is impossible to identify whether the evaluative conclusion in terms of the 2 x 2 table constitutes a true negative or false negative.[2] As far as we can see, the evaluative methods

[2]For this discussion we refer to Saling (2011).

chosen were not appropriate to reach a final judgement on the efficiency of the instrument. The main shortcomings of the evaluation are an extremely self-selected population of participants and the abandonment of a comprehensive survey concerning the cases and controls, controlling for differences in both samples. Thus, positive interventive effects could not be detected, the reasons for this remain unclear however (Friese et al., 2011).

Another approach to the prevention of preterm birth through screening of vaginal infections was a study of vaginal screening in early pregnancy in Vienna (Kiss et al, 2004). They conclude:

"In the intervention group, the number of preterm births was significantly lower than in the control group (3.0% v 5.3%, 95% confidence interval 1.2 to 3.6; $P = 0.0001$). Preterm births were also significantly reduced in lower weight categories at less than 37 weeks and ≤ 2500 g. Eight late miscarriages occurred in the intervention group and 15 in the control group. Conclusion: Integrating a simple infection screening programme into routine antenatal care leads to a significant reduction in preterm births and reduces the rate of late miscarriage in a general population of pregnant women."(p. 371).

Though the reduction is remarkable, it must be observed that the intervention was a clinical study and the effects have to be confirmed in a non-clinical setting. Additionally, the overall rate of preterm births in the study appears very low which may result from selection. In addition the outcomes of international intervention studies screening vaginal infections with respect to the reduction of preterm birth by antibiotic treatment in asymptomatic pregnant women are conflicting and effects could only be seen in women with prior histories of preterm birth (Riggs, M.A, Klebanoff, M.A., 2004).

4.The BabyCare Program

The BabyCare Program was developed from 1998 to 2000. Following an evaluation of existing national and international prevention projects, we decided to create a multifactorial programme comprising health information and education and health promotion including an important role for nutrition especially in relation to folic acid, iodine and iron.

4.1 Frame and methods

The programme comprises:

- a book covering all the issues arising in pregnancy.
- a self-administered questionnaire addressing all possible risk and protective factors. Part of the questionnaire incorporates the dietary history protocol established by the German Society of Nutrition.
- individual health and nutritional recommendations based on the questionnaire responses given by letter or e-mail.
- optimised recipes especially for women not willing to accept the supplementation of micronutrients.
- individual advice on medication during pregnancy.
- relaxation CD with specially composed music for stress reduction.
- pH test kit - supplied when the number of vaginal infections disclosed in the questionnaire is above average or prior histories of preterm birth or miscarriage are documented.

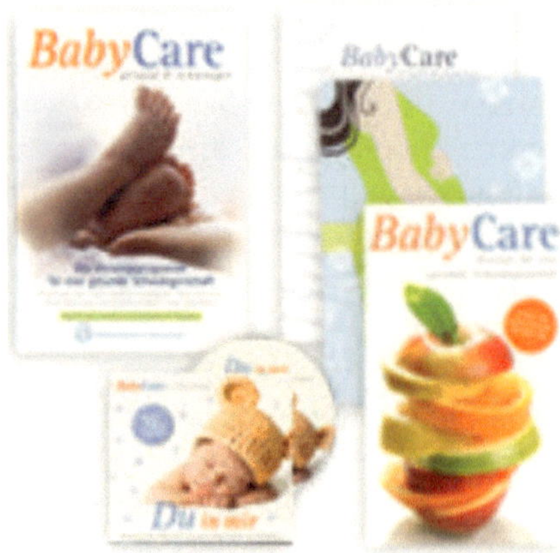

Fig. 3. The BabyCare Program.

For a better understanding of how the programme works, we will first provide some background information on the German health care system. In Germany, medical care outside of hospitals is organised through private practices of general practitioners and medical specialists. In contrast to countries such as the Netherlands, where obstetric care is organised by general practitioners, in Germany, gynaecologists are responsible for obstetric care. There are approximately 7 000 gynaecological practices caring for nearly 750 000 pregnant women annually,[3] and, as a result, on average, each practice sees about 100 pregnant women. Additional care through midwives remains reserved to a few weeks before and after childbirth. Consequently, midwives cannot play an important part in programme implementation, as pregnant women need to be included in the programme as early as possible. In Germany, 90% of the population is a member of a statutory health insurance scheme and, in 2010, there were approximately 150 different insurance providers. In 2010, some 100 or so insurance providers and 1 000 gynaecologists cooperated with BabyCare. The health insurance providers reimburse the programme costs which vary from EUR 30 to EUR 45 depending on the options chosen.

4.2 Evaluative strategies

The programme is evaluated annually with respect to preterm birth rates. For these purposes, the co-operating gynaecologist documents the birth outcomes of a random sample of their participants. This data is compared with the perinatal data of Lower Saxony which reflects the average preterm birth rate for Germany as a whole. An alternative evaluation design involving a prospective case control study with BabyCare participants as cases included in the evaluation and non-participants as controls was rejected both on grounds of excessive costs and anticipated selection effects and biases in the control group. In order to compare cases with controls, the members of the control group would also have to fill in the questionnaire. However, this would lead to uncorrectable intervention effects in the control group. In addition, the comprehensive questionnaire including some 60 questions would probably lead to a sample strongly selected by education, social class and health awareness.

[3]In 2008, there were 658 000 births in Germany. As there are 15% to 20% miscarriages, the number of women diagnosed as pregnant can be estimated as 750 000.

4.3 Evaluative results

4.3.1 Reduction of preterm births

Compared with many other countries, the quantity and quality of epidemiological data in Germany is, in general, not particularly satisfying. This applies also to representative current data on relevant behavioural issues concerning women before and during pregnancy. As already mentioned, perinatal data exists and is collected at a regional level through obstetrics clinics. Therefore, the quality of medical data is good but the quantity and quality of behavioural data only poor. Thus, for example, the prevalence of smoking is likely to be highly underestimated. However, the biggest problem is the fact that the perinatal data does not include socio-demographic variables such as educational level or social class.

Logically, from a statistical point of view, BabyCare participants certainly do not constitute a representative sample of the overall population of pregnant women. They are:

- older
- more often primiparous than multiparous, which is attributable to the fact that amongst women who have already given birth to children without complications acceptance of the programme is likely to be low. In turn, however, this means that multiparous participants will have generally experienced more complications in preceding pregnancies leading them to seek greater advice.
- better educated, something which is a quite normal finding in prevention programmes.
- more often women with multiple pregnancies, a factor which results from a high participation of fertility centres in the programme.

With a view to comparing preterm birth rates of participants with preterm birth rates of Lower Saxony, the structure of our participant group has to be weighted to reflect the structure of the perinatal database which is possible for all variables except the missing educational variable. To correct for education, we have chosen a different approach. As we have representative data on the educational levels of women of childbearing age in Lower Saxony, that distribution is used on the assumption that the distribution of educational levels among pregnant women will not differ significantly - or more importantly, relevantly - from the former group. Although this assumption may be questionable, the weighting procedure gives reasonable estimates and, ultimately, there is no alternative to adopting this approach.

The analysis is based on 12 555 birth documentations produced by cooperating gynaecologists since the year 2000 compiled on the basis of random sampling. The perinatal data used for comparison is the cumulative data for 2005 to 2009 which indicates an overall preterm birth rate of 8.4%, in primiparous women: 9.5% and in multiparous women: 7.5%.

The results of the weighting procedure are shown in Table 6. When weighting for age, a slight variation in the rates can be seen. In primiparous women, there is a reduction due to the fact that older participants with high preterm birth rates are down weighted. Weighting for education increases the rates as preterm birth rates are higher in participants with a basic level of education. After weighting for multiple pregnancy, we have the total weighted rates of 6.9% in primiparous women and 5.1% in multiparous women with an overall reduction of 29%, with a 95% confidence interval between 34% and 24%. Thus, on a conservative estimate, the programme achieves a reduction of about 25%. An analysis by weeks of gestation demonstrates, in addition, that the reduction also takes place in very preterms (<31 weeks). The fact that the preventive effect in multiparous women is even greater than in primiparous women appears particularly striking given their higher risks of prior pregnancy complications. It is possible that this is attributable to the inclusion of the pH testing component for participants with above average rates of vaginal infections and histories of preterm birth and miscarriage. However, this is very difficult to evaluate not least because of the relatively small sample size of multiparous women. There is also no possibility to compare our interventive results with respect to parity with other respective studies as published data does not give informations separated for primi- and multiparous.

	BabyCare data				Perinatal data			
	Unweighted	Weighted for age	Weighted for education	Weighted for multiple pregnancy	cumulative data for 2005-2009	Difference	%	Reduction
n	12555	12555	12555	12438	298158			
PP	**7,4%**	**7,2%**	**7,4%**	**6,9%**	**9,5%**	2,6%	73%	**27,1%**
MP	**5,1%**	**5,3%**	**5,4%**	**5,1%**	**7,5%**	2,4%	68%	**31,6%**
Total	**6,2%**	**6,2%**	**6,3%**	**6,0%**	**8,4%**	2,5%	71%	**29,2%**

95% Confidence interval		
Lower limit		Upper limit
5,6%	**6,0%**	**6,4%**
66,4%	70,8%	75,9%
33,6%	**29,2%**	**24,1%**

Table 6. Reduction in preterm birth rates (Perinatal data from Lower Saxony)

In addition to the factors for which weighting has already been carried out, BabyCare participants may also differ from the overall population of pregnant women in relation to health awareness and health behaviour and in the prevalence of other risks of preterm birth which may possibly be lower in BabyCare participants. However, a recent study suggests that low educational level is only a very low independent risk factor when other risks are controlled. "The lowest-educated pregnant women had a statistically significant higher risk of preterm birth (odds ratio (OR)=1.89 (95% CI 1.28 to 2.80)) than the highest educated women. This increased OR was reduced by up to 22% after separate adjustment for age, height, preeclampsia, intrauterine growth restriction, financial concerns, long-lasting difficulties, psychopathology, smoking habits, alcohol consumption, and body mass index (BMI) of the pregnant women. Joint adjustment for these variables resulted in a reduction of 89% of the increased risk of preterm birth among low-educated pregnant women (fully adjusted OR=1.10)."(Jansen et al., 2009)

Nevertheless, to rule out or to control for this possible selection representative data of a pregnant population would be needed, something which in Germany is currently unavailable. Moreover, even if such data existed, it would have to be treated with caution.

It is well known in social research that many behavioural questions in surveys result in a bias towards "socially desired" answers. This means, for example, both the underreporting of risk behaviour and the overreporting of protective factors. Consequently, alcohol consumption and cigarette smoking are generally underreported in surveys while physical activity and "positive health behaviour" in general (for example, participation in cancer screening programmes for women) is overreported. We assume that in surveys with pregnant women these biases are even stronger, although the effects are difficultly to assess methodologically. It appears logical to assume that by the time of diagnosis of pregnancy women, in general, are more aware of health issues than women of childbearing age. While many will reduce health risks, some will only report doing so. Consequently, the results of behavioural surveys relating to women in the general population of childbearing age cannot be regarded as valid in relation to pregnant women.

Second, the results of surveys, where these exist, carried out with pregnant women pose difficulties for interpretation. To control for a possible bias for positive health awareness among BabyCare participants compared with surveys carried out among the overall population of childbearing age, the following variables had to be excluded:

- alcohol consumption
- cigarette use
- use of illegal drugs

Of the spectrum of indicative variables found in existing female population surveys finally only two remained:

- the body mass index (BMI) and
- the nutritional types

While the first variable does not risk producing a bias as simply weight and height are measured and a ratio obtained, the second item appears even more important in the context of a programme which places particular emphasis on nutrition. Although BabyCare participants more often are underweight to a degree which is statistically significant, because of the high sample size involved in BabyCare the distributions are, however, quite comparable. Moreover, the slightly higher rate of underweight participants in the programme would not constitute a positive selection but a negative selection towards the higher risks of preterm birth.

	BabyCare	German Health Survey 1998
	Women aged 20-29 years	
n=	14765	2015
BMI		
<18.5	6,2%	2,5%
18.5<25	69,2%	71,1%
25<30	16,4%	17,5%
>=30	8,2%	8,9%
	100,0%	100,0%

Table 7. Body mass index of BabyCare participants aged 20-29 years compared to the general female population in Germany 1998 (RKI, 2010).

	BabyCare	Gruner + Jahr Study
n=	8593	10035
completely agree	**13%**	**13%**
agree somewhat	**25%**	**23%**
disagree somewhat	36%	36%
disagree completely	26%	28%
Total	100%	100%

Table 8. Acceptance of nutritional supplements ("For health reasons I take vitamins and/or minerals")

Data analysis shows that in respect of both variables there is no relevant difference in the distribution. As a result, we can conclude that a serious and fundamental bias towards health awareness among BabyCare participants does not exist. The distribution of nutritional types in BabyCare participants is consistent with the distribution in the general population.

In conclusion, significant evidence exists to suggest that the BabyCare questionnaire data reflects the behavioural patterns of pregnant women in Germany, although a final judgement cannot be given in the absence of comparable data.

Reasons for the data displaying this "representativeness" - or, more accurately, only marginal selection effects - may be found in the following facts:

- first, the programme is reimbursed by health insurance providers, hence, women's participation is not influenced by financial factors
- second, health insurance providers with members drawn from weak socio-economic backgrounds are involved in the programme

In summary, the annual evaluation of the programme shows a stable reduction in the rate of PTB of about 25% where, on the basis of the data currently available in Germany, effects of underlying selection and bias can be ruled out.

4.3.2 Remaining risk factors

Although the incidence of preterm birth can be relevantly reduced as a result of the BabyCare programme, even in our population further risk factors of preterm birth are prevalent. An existing epidemiological study suggests that through prevention a target of 5% incidence appears, at best, to be realisable. "Our multi-dimensional analyses revealed rates of prematurity (≤36 weeks) between 5.1% and 27.5% depending on the combination of parameters. We found the highest rate of prematurity of 27.5% in women with the following combination of parameters: ≥1 stillbirth, ≥2 terminations of pregnancy and ≥2 miscarriages. A rather high risk of premature delivery (>11%) was also found for elderly (≥40 years) grand multiparous women as well as small (≤155 cm) and slim women (≤45 kg)" (Voigt et al., 2009, p. 138).

Generally speaking, with a few exceptions, the data on associations presented below do not contain new results but stress the need for and possibilities of additional preventive measures and, in particular, raise issues concerning timing. Some results of the analysis with respect to nutrition require further research, for example, concerning the use of iodine and magnesium. While the latter is plausible in the treatment of preterm labour, the first is not. Also interesting is the betacarotene finding, according to which a high intake constitutes a protective factor. When looking at the other associations we observe, first of all, that certain chronic diseases such as hypertension and thrombosis rarely require closer supervision of risk patients and specific treatment, which, in any event, should start, ideally, even prior to conception. This applies also where women are overweight and smokers. While weight reduction is contraindicated in pregnancy, both risk factors can be reduced more easily and more efficiently before pregnancy. Also improvements to nutritional behaviour and the intake of micronutrients often required, such as, folic acid, iodine and iron, should ideally be implemented before conception in order to be more effective. The same applies to vaccination and the timely diagnosis and treatment of sexually transmitted diseases and the early identification of possible fertility problems.

	Total	PT	NPT	OR	CONF 95%	
	6228	491	5737			
Multiple pregnancy	2,4%	15,3%	1,3%	13,43	17,49	10,31
Diabetes	0,6%	2,0%	0,5%	3,95	7,72	2,03
Eating disorders	1,1%	3,3%	0,9%	3,68	6,26	2,17
Score of pregnancy risks above average	10,6%	21,8%	9,6%	2,62	3,28	2,10
Hypertension	3,7%	6,5%	3,5%	1,92	2,80	1,31
Hospital admission in the last 12 months	15,4%	23,2%	14,7%	1,75	2,18	1,41
History of miscarriage	10,8%	16,1%	10,4%	1,65	2,13	1,28
History of gynaecological operations	20,9%	27,5%	20,3%	1,49	1,83	1,21
Varices and thrombosis	4,0%	5,5%	3,9%	1,44	2,16	0,96
Fertilisation treatment	15,4%	20,2%	15,0%	1,43	1,81	1,14
Daily intake of magnesium in pregnancy	28,1%	34,2%	27,6%	1,36	1,66	1,12
Overweight (BMI >25)	20,8%	25,3%	20,4%	1,32	1,63	1,07
Daily intake of iodine in pregnancy	62,8%	68,4%	62,3%	1,31	1,59	1,07
Folic acid preventive potential known	55,7%	61,3%	55,2%	1,28	1,55	1,06
Smoker on diagnosis of pregnancy	19,9%	23,2%	19,6%	1,24	1,54	1,00
Physically demanding work	18,2%	21,1%	17,9%	1,23	1,56	0,96
Age >=32 years	38,0%	41,5%	37,7%	1,20	1,42	0,98
Betacarotene intake >110% (Sample size reduced n=3025**)	29,3%	23,4%	29,8%	0,72	0,53	0,98
*calculated by Miettinen						
**Diet history questionnaire filled in						

Table 9. Risk factors of preterm birth in primiparous BabyCare participants.

4.3.3 Improvements through an additional preconceptional programme

In the light of our analysis, we decided to develop a preconceptional prevention programme and the PlanBaby programme was launched in 2007. The target groups of the programme are couples planning a baby, couples suspecting fertility problems, and couples undergoing fertilisation treatment. The interventional instruments are the same as in BabyCare but are aimed at both women and men. Although there is growing interest in this programme, it takes time to introduce. As yet, the available data does not permit any firm evaluation.

5. Discussion and conclusion

As we have shown, the number of preterm deliveries can be reduced successfully by at least 25%. After weighting for age, parity, education and multiple pregnancy, the BabyCare participants represent the average population of pregnant women in Germany. With regard to an additional selection bias of participants e.g. towards health awareness or health behaviour, available data on pregnant women and/or representative data of women of childbearing age in Germany are sparse. However, using two lead variables, nutritional types and BMI, does not indicate relevant differences between the data compared. In addition, a specific study dealing with the higher risks of poorly educated women for preterm birth suggests that only a very modest effect comes from education level directly, while the majority of variance is explained by risk behaviour related to educational level, e.g. smoking or physical inactivity. This implies, in turn, that weighting for education, as we have done, does not leave much room for an additional and relevant selection in relation to health awareness or behaviour.

When discussing possible biases in the reduction of the rate of preterm birth, we also have to consider the participating gynaecologists. It is reasonable to assume that they may be more open to prevention issues and, possibly, that the quality of prenatal care may, in any event, be better. On the other hand, there are many reasons to participate in the programme, for example, image of the practice, fees or reduced time needed for consultations. However, we have to concede that there is no possibility whatsoever to evaluate this.

The final indicator that the effect measured is real comes from an independent evaluation produced by a participating health insurance provider. In 2005, the health insurer compared the numbers of preterm birth with those of previous years before the programme was introduced. They registered a reduction from 6.1% to 4.9%, that is, a reduction of 20%. In general, we are interested in external customer evaluations but analyses are often complicated and time-consuming.

Further reductions in the rate of preterm birth are likely to be achieved with a health promotion strategy for the pre-conceptual stage. To meet that need we created the programme PlanBaby, which has been available since 2007. However, as yet, no evaluative results exist and it is much more difficult to develop the appropriate evaluative scheme.

Currently, we are developing a further module for the programme on the choice of maternity clinic. This is intended to address the common situation where women with an increased risk of preterm delivery find themselves giving birth in the delivery unit of a local maternity hospital and not in a clinic offering specialised prenatal, natal and neonatal care.

Finally, we have to mention the most significant obstacle to intervention: programme coverage. In Germany, about 12 000 babies are born every week. Regrettably, however, a pregnancy does not have to be reported to the relevant health insurer at diagnosis, but only six weeks before delivery.

Unlike a disease management programme for a group such as diabetics where the incidence is relatively low and, accordingly, the target population is quite stable, pregnancy is a completely different case. To increase programme coverage would require regular weekly advertising for the target population. However, not even the health insurance providers which currently cooperate with the programme have the necessary financial or, in some cases, technical resources to make this possible.

In recent years we had 30 000 to 50 000 participants annually which means that we reach about 12% to 15% of primiparous pregnant women. To improve programme coverage significantly the legal basis of the programme needs to be modified. At present, the programme is offered by health insurers on a voluntary basis. However, initial discussions are underway to integrate the programme in existing contracts of integrated cooperation between gynaecologists, hospitals and the institutional purchasers/regulators (*kassenärztliche Vereinigungen*). This would increase the participation of gynaecologists and subsequently the number of pregnant women significantly. To summarise for an international audience: the programme can be seen as a positive example in efforts to reduce preterm births.

6. References

Alexander, G.R. et al. (1991). Preterm Birth Prevention - an evaluation of programs in the United States. *Birth*, Vol. 18, No. 3, pp. 160-169, ISSN 0730-7659

Beck, S. et al. (2010). The worldwide incidence of preterm birth: a systematic review of maternal morbidity and mortality. *Bulletin of the World Health Organization*, Vol. 88, No. 1, pp. 31-38, ISSN 0042-9686

Bitzer, E.M. et al. (2011). Self-testing of Vaginal pH to Prevent Preterm Delivery: A Controlled Trial. *Deutsches Ärzteblatt International*, Vol. 108, No. 6, pp. 81-6, ISSN 1866-0452

Canadian Task Force on the Periodic Health Examination. (1994). *The Canadian Guide to Clinical Preventive Health Care: Prenatal and Perinatal Preventive Care: Chapter 4 Prevention of Low Birth Weight/Preterm Birth*. Retrieved from: http://www.phac-aspc.gc.ca/publicat/clinic-clinique/pdf/s1c4e.pdf

Collaborative group on preterm births prevention (1993). Multicenter randomized controlled trial of a preterm prevention program. *American Journal of Obstetrics & Gynecology*, Vol. 169, pp. 352-366, ISSN 0002-9378

Danielian, P. & Hall, M. (2005). The epidemiology of preterm labour and delivery, In: *Preterm Labour: Managing Risk in Clinical Practice*, Norman, J. & Greer, I. (Eds), pp. 1-25, Cambridge University Press, ISBN 0-521-82186-X, Cambridge, UK

David, M.; Pachaly, J. & Vetter, K. (2002). Die Wahrscheinlichkeit einer Spontangeburt - Möglichkeiten und Grenzen von Risikoscores. *Zeitschrift für Geburtshilfe und Neonatologie*, Vol. 206, pp. 219-227, ISSN 0948-2393

DIR- Deutsches IVF-Register, Jahresbericht 2009, Annual Report English Version 2009,*www.deutsches-ivf-register.de/*

Dyson, D.C. et al. (1998). Monitoring Women At Risk For Preterm Labor. *New England Journal of Medicine*, Vol. 338, No. 1, pp. 15-19, ISSN 1533-4406

EURO-PERISTAT project (2008). *European Perinatal Health Report*, Retrieved from http://www.europeristat.com/bm.doc/european-perinatal-health-report.pdf

Friese, K.; Kirschner, W. & Scheffler, A. (2011). Vaginale pH-Selbstmessung zur Verhinderung von Frühgeburten weiterhin gerechtfertigt. *FRAUENARZT*, Vol. 52, No. 4, pp. 336-338, ISSN 0016-0237

Gruner+Jahr, Markenprofile 9, Oktober 2001. Retrieved from http://www.gujmedia.de/_components/markenprofile/index_mapro9.html

Hamilton, B.E. et al. (2010). Births: Preliminary Data for 2008. *National Vital Statistics Reports*, Vol. 58, No. 16, pp. 1-17, ISSN 1551-8922

Holzgreve, W. et al. (2006). Prävention von Frühgeburten. *Der Gynäkologe*, Vol. 29, pp. 293-296, ISSN 0017-5994

Hoyme U.B. & Saling, E. (2004). Efficient prematurity prevention is possible by pH-self measurement and immediate therapy of threatening ascending infection. *European Journal of Obstetrics, Gynecology and Reproductive Biology*, Vol. 115, No. 2, pp. 148–53, ISSN 0301-2115

Hoyme U.B.; Schwalbe N. & Saling, E. (2005). Efficient prematurity prevention is possible by pH-self measurement and immediate therapy of threatening ascending infection. *Journal of Perinatal Medicine*, Vol. 33, (Supplement 1), p. 110, ISSN 0300-5577 http://www.eurekalert.org/pub_releases/2009-03/modf-mcf031309.php

Hueston, W.J. (1992). A critical assessment of preterm labor prevention strategies. *Journal of Family Practice*, Vol. 35, No. 1, pp. 81-9, ISSN 0094-3509

Jansen, P.W. et al. (2009). Explaining educational inequalities in preterm birth: the generation r study. *Archives of Disease in Childhood Fetal & Neonatal Edition* Vol. 94, No. 1, pp. F28-F34, ISSN 1359-2998

Kirschner, W.; Halle, H. & Pogonke, M.A. (2009). Kosten der Früh- und Nichtfrühgeburten und die Effektivität und Effizienz von Präventionsprogrammen am Beispiel von BabyCare: Eine Schätzung auf der Grundlage der Diagnose Related Groups (DRG) unter Berücksichtigung der Primäraufnahmen in der Neonatologie. *Prävention und Gesundheitsförderung*, No. 1, pp. 41-50, ISSN 1861-6755

Kiss, H. et al. (2004). Prospective randomised controlled trial of an infection screening programme to reduce the rate of preterm delivery. *British Medical Journal*, Vol. 329, pp. 371-5, ISSN 0959-8138

March of Dimes (2009). Medical costs for one premature baby could cover a dozen healthy births. Press release 17 March 2009. Retrieved from

Papiernik, E. (n.d.). Prediction and Prevention of Preterm Birth. Inserm-France, Retrieved from http://www.ethique.inserm.fr/ethique/cours.nsf/63ab8071ff4920d5c125685c002b78bf/dd89dd3566ed136980256ae8002ba77b?OpenDocument

Riggs, M.A., Klebanoff, M.A. (2004). Treatment of Vaginal Infections to Prevent Preterm Birth, - A Meta Analysis, *Clinical Obstetrics and Gynecology*, Volume 47, Number 4, 796-807

RKI (2010). Übergewicht und Adipositas. Retrieved from http://www.rki.de/DE/Content/GBE/Auswertungsergebnisse/nichtuebertragbareKrankheiten/Adipositas/adipositas__inhalt.html__nnn=true

Saling, E. (2011). A special comment from the Founder of the Journal of Perinatal Medicine, Editorial, Problems in the prevention of preterm birth - regrettable contradictions. *Journal of Perinatal Medicine*, Vol. 39, pp. 222-225, ISSN 0300-5577

Voigt, M. et al. (2009). Evaluation of Maternal Parameters as Risk Factors for Premature Birth (Individual and Combined Effects). *Zeitschrift für Geburtshilfe und Neonatologie*, Vol. 213, No. 4,pp. 138-146, ISSN 0948-2393

12

Preterm Birth of Extremely Low Birth Weight Infants

Jonathan Muraskas, Lisa DeGregoris,
Colleen Rusciolelli and Christine Sajous
Loyola University Medical Center
USA

1. Introduction

Approximately 13% of births in the United States are preterm, defined as occurring before 37 weeks of gestation. This results in more than 540,000 infants a year born prematurely. In other words, one out of every 8 infants is born premature. Even more disturbing is that despite advances in neonatal and perinatal medicine, the incidence of prematurity has increased by 36% since the 1980's. Over 1 million infants die worldwide every year because of consequences that are related to being born too soon. Every 30 seconds one infant dies of preterm birth. Approximately 1.5% of infants in the United States are born less than 27 weeks gestation which accounts for approximately 100,000 infants annually. Even infants born just a few weeks too soon (34-36 weeks gestations), also known as late preterm birth, have higher rates of death and disability than full term infants. Table 1 describes the evolution of technology in the obstetrical and pediatric management of premature birth in the United States in the last 60 years.

1940-50	Infants < 1 kg were classified as stillborn
1950's	Introduction of Apgar scores made these infants live-born but previable and allowed to die without technologic intervention
1960's	1 kg limit persisted until the widespread use of mechanical ventilation in the late 1960's
1970's	Limit of viability started rolling back
1980's	Survivors with Gestational Age (GA) of 24 weeks and Birth Weight (BW) of 500-600g were rare
1990's	Introduction of Surfactant/antenatal steroids Survivors with GA's of 24 weeks and BW's of 500-600g were common
2000's	Conflict

Table 1. Evolution of Neonatal-Perinatal Medicine

Very low birth weight (VLBW) infants are defined as weighing less than 1500 grams. Extremely low birth weight (ELBW) infants are defined as being less than 1000 grams.
Table 2 correlates GA with BW in appropriate for gestational age (AGA) ELBW infants.

ONE POUND = 454 GRAMS	
AGA	
23 weeks	450 – 550 grams
24 weeks	500 – 650 grams
25 weeks	600 – 750 grams
26 weeks	700 – 850 grams
27 weeks	850 – 950 grams

Table 2. Correlation of Birth Weight with Gestational Age

Introduction of surfactant and antenatal steroids in the early 1990's have dramatically changed the field of neonatal-perinatal medicine. Dramatic increases in the survival of ELBW infants with a concomitant decrease of severe intraventricular hemorrhage (IVH) became the norm. The duration of mechanical ventilation dramatically decreased. In the last two decades, advances in perinatal and neonatal care have reached the point where an infant at 27 weeks gestation weighing 2 pounds (900 grams) has over a 90% chance of surviving and less than a 10% chance of a devastating handicap. Unfortunately, long-term outcomes in infants less than 27 weeks have not shown significant improvement over the years. The application of neonatal intensive care to extremely premature infants less than 27 weeks' gestation is a fundamental controversy in neonatology. Rates of death and numerous morbidities such as chronic lung disease, intracranial hemorrhage, and retinopathy of prematurity are distressingly high. Frequently long-term neurodevelopmental outcomes for these infants born before 27 weeks are very poor. It has been our experience that antenatal exposure to steroids, female gender and delivery by cesarean section have been positive prognostic variables in many extremely low birth weight infants with intact survival.

2. Economics

Although VLBW and ELBW infants account for 1.5% and 0.7% of all live births respectively, these infants contribute disproportionately to neonatal morbidity and to health care costs. Approximately 85% of infants with very low birth weights survive to be discharged from the hospital. Within 2 years after discharge, 2-5% die from medical complications related to preterm birth.

In the United States, approximately 40% of the estimated 6,600 cases of cerebral palsy that are diagnosed each year are a direct result of very low birth weight. Helping these fragile infants survive and thrive comes with a price tag. Preterm birth is a serious health problem that costs the United States more than $26 billion annually. With the incidence of prematurity increasing and smaller and smaller infants being resuscitated, the incidence of cerebral palsy is increasing. There appears to be no reprieve from the extraordinary cost of care that will be needed to manage the medical, educational and special services for this large proportion of extremely low birth weight infants who develop chronic conditions. With increasing discussion of healthcare reform and intensive care for infants exceeding $4000.00 per day, we believe the health care resources currently debated for senior citizens will also lead to rigorous debates at the other end of the spectrum of life in the near future. Many argue that money spent on numerous resources to save the tiniest of infants who develop profound handicaps could be better spent on the education and prenatal care of the pregnant woman, thereby positively impacting the incidence of prematurity and the infant mortality rate.

3. Multiple gestation and preterm birth

Multiple gestations have significantly contributed to the increasing prematurity rate. Since the 1980s, there has been a 65% increase in twin and over 500% increase in triplet births. In the United States, approximately 130,000 infants are born annually of multi-fetal gestation. Roughly 1% of all U.S. infants born annually are conceived by assisted reproductive techniques. Career advancements often delay the starting of a family in early childbearing years. Another reason has also been the significant advancements in the field of infertility and reproductive medicine.

Any multiple gestation is a high-risk pregnancy. Each fetus in multiple gestations shortens the duration of pregnancy by 2 to 3 weeks. A term twin pregnancy is considered 37 weeks gestation. In our experience, the majority of triplets deliver at approximately 33 weeks gestation. Quadruplets and higher order pregnancies sequentially decrease gestational age at delivery by another 2 weeks. Quadruplets would deliver on average at 31 weeks gestation and physiologically, octuplets would be expected to deliver at 23 weeks gestation. The incidence of cerebral palsy and long-term neurologic deficits for twins, triplets and quadruplets are 3.7%, 8.7%, and 11.1%, respectively. With twins the chances of one handicapped child is 7% while triplets and quadruplets are 20 and 50% respectively. The relative risks for severe handicap for twins and triplets is 1.7 and 2.9 compared to singletons The infant mortality rate for singletons, twins and triplets are approximately 9, 57, and 166 per thousand live births, respectively.

4. Initial management

The management of ELBW infants in a neonatal intensive care unit can be stressful. The most common cause of clinical decompensation in these infants is the inability to achieve an adequate airway. In the United States, there are over 4 million births annually. Approximately 10% of all infants born, including low risk deliveries, will require resuscitation. The percentage is significantly higher with extremely low birth weight infants. At least one person skilled in resuscitation should be present at all deliveries. The resuscitation of an ELBW infant requires the teamwork of a physician/neonatal nurse practitioner, neonatal nurse and often a respiratory therapist. The procedural skill of intubation can be difficult even in the most experienced hands. For this reason practitioners in this field should be skilled in bag and mask ventilation. This can be done effectively until someone more skilled with intubation can establish an airway. In a situation of bradycardia and desaturations, practitioners need to assume the endotracheal tube is not in place and be willing to reevaluate, calmly bag and mask and attempt to reintubate. In our experience, chest compressions are rarely indicated in a clinically deteriorating infant. The establishment of adequate airway will usually rectify this clinical decompensation with restoration of normal heart rate and oxygen saturations.

With the advent of surfactant, steroids and gentle ventilation, the incidence of airleak has been significantly reduced in the last two decades. When an adequate airway is achieved and the infant does not respond to resuscitation, one needs to expediently consider a pneumothorax in the differential diagnoses. An unrecognized airleak is one of the most frequent etiologies for sudden death in an unsuccessful infant resuscitation. A tension pneumothorax is an acute life-threatening event that may not allow time for x-ray confirmation. For this reason practitioners should be skilled in needle aspiration of the pleural cavity. Like intubation, placement of chest tubes can be a difficult procedural skill.

The ability to transilluminate and promptly insert a 23-gauge butterfly needle lateral to the nipple can be life-saving. These basic skills are especially in a community or rural hospital when 24/7 neonatal coverage is not feasible.

5. Common complications

5.1 Respiratory distress syndrome

The most common complication of prematurity is respiratory distress syndrome. This is a deficiency of pulmonary surfactant that results in the alveolar collapse, uneven aeration, ventilation/perfusion mismatch and increased alveolar-capillary membrane permeability. These infants can present with tachypnea, grunting, nasal flaring, and substernal retractions. Pathological findings include necrosis of the cell lining of the airways, proteinaceous exudate forming hyaline membranes and infiltration of inflammatory cells within the airway. The incidence and severity of respiratory distress syndrome has been greatly reduced with antenatal steroids and surfactant therapy. Despite this, the incidence of chronic lung disease, as well as neurodevelopmental disability, in an extremely low birth weight infant has not decreased.

5.2 Intraventricular hemorrhage

Intraventricular hemorrhage (IVH) in preterm infants has decreased in recent years in most neonatal centers. The incidence ranges from 29-49% of all infants less than 1500 g. IVH is mainly a complication of infants with a birth weight less than 1000 g and especially those whose weight is less than 750 g. The majority of IVH occurs in the first 72 hours of life. The exact etiology remains unknown although poor cerebral autoregulation is implicated, especially in ELBW infants. IVH is graded from 1 through 4. A grade 1 represents a subependymal hemorrhage while a grade 2 involves IVH without ventricular dilatation. A grade 3 IVH has blood in the ventricle but with concomitant ventricular dilatation. The most severe is a grade 4 IVH in which there is extension of the bleed into the brain parenchyma. Grades 1 and 2 IVH have excellent prognosis for normal development. Grade 3 IVH, especially with hydrocephalus significant enough to require a shunt, has at least a 50% risk of mental retardation or cerebral palsy. A grade 4 IVH carries an 85% risk for a significant devastating handicap. The use of antenatal steroids has positively impacted the incidence of severe grade 3 or grade 4 IVH. However delivery of ELBW infants can be precipitous and usually antenatal steroids take approximately 24 hours to exert accelerated maturation of the germinal matrix and lungs. Cerebral palsy is often not diagnosed well after the first year of life and sometimes not until 2 years of age.

5.3 Retinopathy of prematurity

Retinopathy of prematurity (ROP) is a developmental disease which occurs mainly in the incompletely vascularized retina of premature infants and can progress to retinal detachment. Prematurity is the most important risk factor for ROP. The incidence of retinopathy of prematurity is over 80% in infants less than 1000 g. The incidence of blindness approaches 10%. The international classification of ROP defines the location by zones, the extent by clock hours, and the severity by stages. Special pathologic features are defined by the terms plus disease and threshold disease. The only effective prophylaxis for ROP is the prevention of prematurity. Meticulous oxygen monitoring has not provided a complete solution and various supplements such as vitamin E and selenium therapy have not proven effective. All infants born less than 33 weeks gestation should have an eye exam regardless of oxygen requirement. The first eye exam occurs at 4-6 weeks chronologic age. Frequency of eye exams depends on the severity and rate of progression of retinopathy.

5.4 Patent ductus arteriosus

Patent ductus arteriosus (PDA) is another common complication of extremely low birth weight infants. The Ductus Arteriosus represents an embryological connection between the aorta and pulmonary artery. This duct remains open and clinically presents past the first 3 or 5 days of life in 50% of all ELBW infants, often with increasing oxygen requirements and metabolic acidosis. Infants can present with bounding pulses, wide pulse pressure and a classic machinery-type murmur. Physiologically this duct can augment a left-to-right shunt increasing pulmonary blood flow. Given the potential for decreased blood flow to the intestines, many clinicians are reluctant to feed infants with clinically significant PDAs. Approximately 70-80% of ductuses will respond to medical therapy that has included prostaglandin inhibitors such as indomethacin and ibuprofen. These prostaglandin inhibitors constrict the smooth muscle of the ductus arteriosus. The efficacy of this treatment is greater when initiated within 10 days of life. As with many medications, complications with prostaglandin inhibitors include thrombocytopenia, hyperbilirubinemia and impaired renal function. Prostaglandin inhibitors may further decrease blood flow to the bowel and some studies have reported a higher incidence of spontaneous intestinal perforations and other GI symptoms with this treatment. Ibuprofen is as efficacious as Indomethacin with less renal side effects. Surgical ligation is reserved for those infants who did not respond to medical management concomitant with deteriorating clinical status often with increasing ventilatory requirements because of increased pulmonary blood flow. In most ELBW infants we choose to have ligation performed at the bedside in the NICU. There is recent data now questioning the concept of mandatory closure for all ductuses.

5.5 Sepsis

Maternal chorioamnionitis can have significant effects on the ELBW infant. One of the more common etiologies for preterm birth is maternal infection. Intra-amniotic infection is perhaps the most common cause for an infant born depressed requiring resuscitation. Evidence-based data has demonstrated a strong relationship between chorioamnionitis and subsequent brain damage in both preterm and term infants. Through a cytokine mediated pathway, white matter is especially vulnerable in the infant exposed to maternal infection. Periventricular leukomalacia can result in spastic diplegia and other significant neurodevelopmental disabilities.

A common complication in ELBW infants in the intensive care unit is infection. Approximately 40-50% of ELBW infants will develop an infection. With an already compromised immune system, extremely low birth weight infants undergo multiple instrumentations with endotracheal tubes and central lines. We discuss with parents that it is not unusual for an ELBW infant to have feedings stopped and antibiotics started at least 2-3 times during their neonatal hospital course to rule out an infectious process.

Sepsis neonatorum is defined as any bacterial infection with systemic manifestations which is documented by a positive blood culture during the first month of life. Neonatal sepsis can be classified into 2 categories based on postnatal age at onset: Early onset less than 7 days and late onset greater than 7 days. The incidence of sepsis varies between 1-8 cases per

thousand live births. Prevalence increases inversely with gestational age affecting 25-40% of extremely low birth weight infants. Mortality rates are 10-30% for early onset and 10% for late onset sepsis. Currently group B streptococcus, gram-negative bacilli and Listeria monocytogenes are most commonly associated with early onset sepsis whereas enterococcus, coagulase-negative staphylcoccus and gram-negative bacilli are more frequently responsible for late onset sepsis. Most episodes of early onset sepsis are caused by an ascending infection with the exception of Listeria which is transmitted transplacentally. Infection could also be acquired during vaginal delivery from bacteria colonizing the mother's genital tract. The bacteria causing late onset disease may be transmitted either vertically during the peripartum period or horizontally from all one might see in the environment or from colonized caregivers. Inadequate handwashing can be a major source for the spread of microorganisms from one patient to another. The use of endotracheal tubes, central venous and arterial lines and Foley catheters also significantly increase the risk for neonatal infection.
In our experience, a low WBC count and band/seg ratio > 0.2 is more ominous than a high WBC count. The absolute neutrophil count calculated by WBC x % (Segs and Bands) less than 2000 could suggest an infectious process. Thrombocytopenia is defined as a platelet count less than 150,000/ul. Although thrombocytopenia is present in 80% of cases of sepsis, it has a low sensitivity and specificity. A blood culture is the gold standard to diagnose neonatal sepsis and should be drawn from both central and peripheral lines. If the clinical signs and symptoms are suggesting meningitis or if the blood cultures are positive, a lumbar puncture should always be performed. It seems reasonable not to perform a lumbar puncture on the infant being evaluated only because of maternal risk factors or the infants with respiratory distress syndrome. When the clinical suspicion of sepsis is high, empiric antimicrobial therapy should be started immediately after obtaining the appropriate culture specimens. The choice of empiric therapy is based on several factors including time and setting of the disease, microorganism frequency and susceptibility in your NICU, the site of the suspected infection and penetration of the specific antibiotic to that site, and hepatic and/or renal dysfunction.

5.6 Necrotizing enterocolitis

Another feared complication of preterm birth is necrotizing enterocolitis (NEC). NEC is an inflammatory process resulting from a complex interaction between the mucosal injury caused by a variety of factors such as infection and ischemia and the host response to that injury. NEC is the most common gastrointestinal emergency in the NICU. The incidence of NEC is approximately 10% of all NICU admissions. The majority of NEC manifest between 2-4 weeks of life, usually in the preterm infants who have been fed. Approximately 80% of cases of NEC respond to antibiotics and cessation of feeding while 20% will go on to perforate requiring an operation. Mortality can be as high as 40% despite vigorous therapy. Infection, inflammatory mediators, ischemia and enteral feeds have all been associated with NEC, although the etiology remains elusive despite significant research. Breastmilk macrophages and immunoglobulins were thought to prevent NEC; however exclusively breast-fed infants have occasionally developed NEC. Premature infants can have various presentations with the onset of NEC. These can include vomiting, abdominal distention, apnea, bile stain residuals and bloody stools. Peritoneal signs such as abdominal distention, tenderness and guarding are frequently observed. Radiographically

pneumatosis intestinalis appearing as soap bubbles or linear intramural streaks especially in the right lower quadrant of preterm infants is pathognomonic. Ileal perforation can manifest by abdominal free air. Portal air which represents tracking of air through the bowel wall along the mesenteric vessels and into the portal system can be associated with NEC. In our experience, the presence of thrombocytopenia and metabolic acidosis is highly suggestive of necrotic bowel.
The initial treatment especially with signs of peritonitis includes triple antibiotic therapy and meticulous fluid and electrolyte management. Infants with NEC may develop disseminated intravascular coagulation (DIC) and/or thrombocytopenia requiring blood products. Surgical management has changed over the last decade. More often than not peritoneal drain placement is preferred to stabilize these critically ill infants before considering surgery. Late complications of NEC include intestinal strictures, bowel obstruction and malabsorption. A certain amount of small intestine is necessary for survival. Short gut syndrome is not uncommon and full recovery can take months to years.

5.7 Bronchopulmonary dysplasia

Bronchopulmonary dysplasia (BPD) is a multifactorial disease defined as any infant requiring oxygen beyond 28 days of life or 36 weeks post-conceptional age. Risk factors include barotrauma, prolonged oxygen requirements resulting in free radical induced oxygen toxicity and recurrent infections thought to release cytokine inflammatory mediators. BPD is usually accompanied by an abnormal chest x-ray and clinical signs of respiratory distress. Up to 75% of infants of extremely low birth weight develop BPD. The incidence of BPD has remained unchanged although the severity has declined somewhat. BPD is a spectrum in which there could be minimal oxygen requirement or a ventilator dependency often requiring a tracheostomy in severe cases. Major complications of BPD can include developmental delay, poor growth, heart failure, pulmonary edema and gastrointestinal reflux. Toddlers with the history of BPD have a significantly higher incidence of reactive airway disease and require frequent hospital readmissions. Respiratory syncytial virus (RSV) can be deadly in a neo graduate with BPD. Premature infants that meet criteria for palivizumab (Synagis) administration should receive this throughout the RSV season to help prevent serious infection and respiratory compromise. There are many treatment regimens for BPD. Parents need to be told that many infants who are extremely low birth weight will often require oxygen at home.

5.8 Seizures

Neonatal seizures can complicate the hospital course of an ELBW infant. Newborn seizures can be difficult to clinically diagnose due to subtle abnormal ocular and focal movements. Subtle motor abnormalities with concomitant desaturations and/or apnea often represent seizure activity. One needs to be vigilant and anticipate risk factors such as a difficult resuscitation or the evolution of an intraventricular hemorrhage as a precipitating event leading to seizures. The first line of medication in the treatment of seizures is phenobarbital at a loading dose of 20 mg/kilogram to achieve therapeutic levels of 20-40 mcg/milliliter. Persistent seizures may require the addition of phenytoin or lorazepam (Ativan). Inadequately treated seizures can result in permanent neuronal cell damage due to enhanced metabolic activity.

5.9 Medication errors

Medication errors are preventable events that frequently occur in the NICU. It has been reported that out of every five adverse drug events in pediatric patients, three of those events occurred in the neonatal intensive care. Errors are particularly dangerous in the NICU due to the fragile state of infants. A rapidly changing body weight, different rates of organ development affecting drug pharmacokinetics and the need for dilution of medications contributed to the common occurrence of medication errors in the management of extremely low birth weight infants. Medication errors most commonly result from incorrect dosing, documentation, or processing. With the advent of computerized order entry, reduction of ordering errors is expected due to standardized templates for physicians and nurses. The computerized system also provides an additional way to intercept errors before they affect an infant.

6. Regionalization

Obstetrical and neonatal management of preterm birth often requires advanced services that are not available at all hospitals. Levels I, II, II+ and community hospital Level III intensive care units have set policies and regulations overseen by the regional perinatal center. The lack of experience in a low volume nursery can lead to catastrophic outcomes. Regionalization continues to have a role and is in the best interest of mother and her infant. The best ambulance for ELBW infants is the uterus. An effective maternal transport system in the United States has had a positive impact in the morbidity and mortality of ELBW infants. Studies support delivery of ELBW newborns in tertiary centers with better outcome than Level 2 or 2+ centers.

7. Outcomes

Table 3 describes the neonatal survival and outcomes for infants 22-30 weeks gestation. Clinicians today routinely provide intensive care for infants greater than or equal to 25 weeks gestation and over 750 grams birth weight. The survival rate exceeds 75% and the risk of a devastating handicap as blindness, deafness, cerebral palsy and mental retardation is 15% while the risk of a mild to moderate handicap such as learning disabilities, chronic lung disease, and milder forms of cerebral palsy is approximately 40%. Infants born less than 25 weeks gestation are considered at the threshold of viability. There are many uncertainties regarding resuscitation and management decisions. Currently there is no consensus on early treatment strategies that can currently predict which infants will thrive and which will have severe morbidity based on observations in the delivery room and throughout the first 48 hours of life. With steroid and surfactant technology, many infants after initial stabilization tend to have a honeymoon period where they remain hemodynamically stable often for the first 3 days of life followed by clinical deterioration secondary to a hemodynamically significant patent ductus arteriosus, intraventricular hemorrhage, reduced pulmonary function secondary to surfactant depletion, abnormal electrolytes or sepsis. It can be difficult for parents to get off this treatment train as these ELBW infants survive beyond the first 48 hours of life, regardless of how poor the prognosis is. ELBW infants born prior to 1990 often would die in the first 2 days of life. The median length of stay of ELBW infants who die has increased from 2 to10 days in the last two decades.

Weeks	NICU Survival	Survivors with Severe NDI*	Overall Survival **WITHOUT** Severe NDI*
22	10%	50%	5%
23	30%	33%	20%
24	60%	25%	45%
25	75%	15%	60%
26	80%	15%	70%
27	90%	10%	80%
28	90%	10%	85%
29	95%	5%	90%
30	95%	< 5%	> 90%

*NDI = Neurodevelopmental Impairment

Table 3. Estimated neonatal outcomes
Data derived for Loyola Medical Center, Vermont Oxford Network, and the National Institute of Child Health and Human Development (2010)
Last column reflects both survival and outcome of 100 infants born at given GA, how many will survive and not be severely impaired.
Severe NDI = Any of: significant developmental disability, mental retardation, non-ambulatory CP, blindness, deafness.
Other prenatal factors to consider:

SGA (Small for Gestational Age)/IUGR (Intrauterine Growth Restriction)
Gender
Infection

Approximately 23% of all infants less than 26 weeks gestation will have a severe disability defined as the expectation that a child will never be able to independently perform the activities of daily living. Infants born prematurely at less than 25 weeks gestation continue to present complex and unique medical, social, ethical and economical issues. As noted, despite a dramatic increase in survival, satisfactory long-term outcomes have not kept pace. Numerous studies of long-term follow-up have shown that ELBW infants have over a 50% chance at school age to have a childhood disability, school related disability, and the increased utilization of special educational needs. Low birth weight infants followed into adulthood had lower rates of graduation, a lower mean IQ, and subnormal growth. Extremely low birth weight infants who had the benefit of advanced technologies in the 1990's also continued to have a greater than 50% incidence of continuing to display more cognitive, educational, and behavioral impairments compared to controls. Other studies have shown that infants born in the 1990's had a significantly higher incidence of asthma, cerebral palsy, visual disability, poor cognitive ability, lower academic achievement, decreased motor skills, and poor social adaptive functioning compared to controls.

8. Neonatal viability

TABLE 4 demonstrates some variables that have been used in defining the limits of viability. From an ethical standpoint, most obstetricians and neonatologists consider infants greater than or equal to 25 weeks gestation viable and will intervene and resuscitate independent of parents' wishes on the grounds this is in the best interest of their infant. Where futility and autonomy meet is often described as a gray zone. In neonatal-perinatal medicine, this area is most often encountered at 23-24 weeks gestation with infants 450-600 grams. Different strategies have evolved worldwide to address these issues. The United States has often been criticized for the "wait until certainty" strategy, treating everyone aggressively until it is virtually certain that either death or an irreversible coma will be the result. The United Kingdom tends more towards the individualized prognostic strategy where treatment is initiated and regularly re-evaluated as to its efficacy. In Norway and Sweden, a statistical prognostic strategy is often employed and treatment is withheld from infants who appear to have a grim prognosis. There is no simple solution and this topic will continue to be debated. It has been stated that parents really fear a burdensome outcome more than the death of their infant. Advances in neonatology have far outpaced decision-making practices in the NICU. Past personal experiences, religious perspectives, Baby Doe legislation, and fear of litigation can all influence decision-making.

1) Gestational Age
2) Birth Weight
3) Parents' Desires
4) History of Infertility
5) Method of Payment
6) Infant's Sex
7) Response to Resuscitation
8) Findings on Cranial Ultrasound

Table 4. Defining limits of viability.

Neonatal viability has no consistent definition. Fetal viability is the earliest gestational age at which the potential for long-term survival can be expected. The legal definition of viability is provided by each state rather than the federal government and varies considerably. The ethical definition of viability is described as a gray zone in which long-term survival is desirable but often not possible. In 1992 a survey of maternal fetal medicine specialists in North America found that 100% did not think viability began at less than 24 weeks. A similar survey 10 years later revealed that almost 50% of maternal fetal medicine specialist now believed viability began before 24 weeks.

Many studies can be deceiving in how parents are counseled. The denominator can vary widely to include all births (stillbirths and liveborns), only liveborns or only liveborns that lived long enough to be admitted to NICU. Survival can be overstated by as much as 100% at 23 weeks gestation and 56% at 24 weeks gestation if the denominator included only newborns admitted to NICU versus all fetal deaths and liveborns. The Ballard estimate of gestational age (GA) can yield a GA 10 days older than age determined by best obstetrical estimate. Sex is rarely considered in the numerous studies. The intact survival at 23 weeks GA is 5-10% (approximately 1 pound infant)and increases to near 90% at 27 weeks GA (2 pound infant). One can see how a few days can have significant effect on survival. This 23-24 weeks gestation is filled with ambiguity. We also emphasize that GA and not BW is perhaps the most critical factor in assessing viability. Almost all 100 intact surviving infants in the University of Iowa Hospitals The Tiniest Babies Registry weighing from 260 grams to 400 grams had significant intrauterine growth restriction and were females.

Retrospective nonrandomized studies have consistently failed to document a benefit of cesarean section versus normal spontaneous vaginal delivery for ELBW newborns. A scenario we see is the 23-24 week GA fetus in the breech position where cesarean section (a major surgery) is often not recommended because of poor neonatal outcome.

The National Institute of Health consensus is offering antenatal steroids between 24 and 34 weeks of gestation for a single course. There is controversy and limited data if maternal steroids should be administered prior to 24 weeks GA. If aggressive resuscitation is requested by families at less than 24 weeks GA, we would prefer managing these micropremies with steroids on board.
We believe each case of viability needs to be considered individually. The majority of infants whether born at 18 or 24 weeks will often have a heart rate at birth. The World Health Organization has determined that these infants should be classified as live births. Parents need to be told that infants can have a heart rate for minutes to hours after birth despite being nonviable. This can become problematic in that ELBW infants initially pronounced dead have been later resuscitated after having gasping respirations or being stimulated by a cold steel utility sink, resulting in survival with devastating handicaps. Some institutions continue to use 500 g as the cutoff to initiate or withhold resuscitation.

9. Ethics

Preterm birth has resulted in some interesting landmark ethical cases. In 1995, a 25 week gestational age male was born in Michigan weighing 780 g and was resuscitated against the parents' wishes. The infant was born by C-section after an attempted vaginal birth (VBAC) and came out requiring significant resuscitation. Shortly after birth the parents disconnected the ventilator for fear of having a handicapped child. This infant expired soon afterwards. The physician father was found not guilty of manslaughter. A 1999 case in Texas involved a 23 week gestation 595 g infant male in which resuscitation was attempted but an adequate airway was not achieved. This infant was deemed nonviable. The dilemma arose when this infant was given a large dose of fentanyl to expedite death. Another case involved a 23 week gestation 629 g infant female born in Texas in 1990. The parents refused to sign a consent to allow resuscitation of their 23 week infant daughter. They did not want heroic measures and did not want a neonatologist to attend the delivery. The parents were told the hospital had a policy that all newborns who weighed greater than or equal to 500 g were resuscitated and the parents did not sign the consent to allow resuscitation. The fellow on call resuscitated this infant female with Apgars of 3 and 6. At 7 years of age, this child could not walk, talk, was blind with severe mental retardation and cerebral palsy. This child had seizures, spastic quadriplegia, ventriculoperitoneal shunt and could not be toilet trained. The parents did not sue the physicians but the hospital for battery and negligence saying the doctors did what they were told. The initial jury verdict award was $60 million to the parents. The Texas court of appeals reversed this decision saying the parents could withhold treatment from a child only after their child's medical condition has been certified as terminal under the Texas natural death law. If treatment is urgent, a court order is not necessary to treat.
Medical care, therapy and interventions in the periviable period are based largely on extrapolation of information from infants born at greater gestational ages. Most interventions in the NICU, including resuscitation, can be classified as experimental. All infant cases of viability need to be individualized. We teach our housestaff to resuscitate if any doubt exists. The delivery room is often not the arena to be making decisions on withholding or withdrawing life support.
Good communication between the obstetrician/neonatologist and family is critical. Whenever possible, discussion regarding resuscitation should be initiated before delivery. Survival rates can vary institutionally and one needs to be aware of the local and national data in these discussions. We believe parents should have a significant input in the decisions

concerning the management of their extremely low birth weight infants. Medical, legal and ethical arguments would strongly support clinicians for not practicing defensive medicine. Because of fear of liability, neonatologists, more often than not, respect the parents' wishes regarding their infant's care. The risk of professional liability is minimal for non-aggressive management of infants born less than 25 weeks gestation and less than or equal to 650 grams AGA. Good communication, documentation, and a compassionate caring attitude make professional liability essentially nonexistent.

10. Conclusion

In the last 2 decades survival rates of ELBW infants has plateaued with neurodevelopmental outcomes essentially unchanged. The use of nitric oxide, noninvasive ventilation, more judicious use of steroids, and providing a quieter more family friendly intensive care unit are exciting new developments in our field. The future care of ELBW infants will be exciting for the next generation of practitioners in our field. Will technology keep advancing? How much more can we push the envelope of viability? Caring for the high risk mother and infant is an honor and privilege. If we remain competent, compassionate and caring, we can continue to positively impact future generations.

11. References

Ballard DW, Li Y, Evans J, Ballard RA, Ubel PA. Fear of litigation may increase resuscitation of infants born near the limits of viability. J Pediatr 2002; 140:713-718.

Berghella V. Every 30 seconds a baby dies of preterm birth. What are you doing about it? AJOG 2010; 416-417.

Eichenwald EC, Stark AR. Management and Outcomes of Very Low Birth Weight. N Engl J Med 2008; 358:1700-1711.

Frogel M, et al. Prevention of hospitalization due to respiratory syncytial virus: Results from the Palivizumab Outcomes Registry. J Perinatol 2008; 28:511-517.

Meadow W. 500-Gram Infants - and 800-Pound Gorillas - in the Delivery Room. Pediatrics 2006; 117: 2274-2275.

Meadow W, Lee G, Lin K, Lantos J. Changes in Mortality for Extremely Low Birth Weight Infants in the 1990s: Implications for Treatment Decisions and Resource Use. Pediatrics 2004; 113:1223-1229.

Muraskas J, Carlson N, Halsey C, Frederiksen M, Sabbagha R. Survival of a 280 gram infant. (Correspondence) N Eng J Med 1991; 324:1598-1599.

Muraskas J, Hasson A, Besinger RE. Long Term Follow-Up of a 280 Gram Infant. Correspondence. N Engl J Med 2004; 351(8):836-37.

Rhoden NK. Treating Baby Doe: The Ethic of Uncertainty. Hastings Center Report, August 1986, pp. 34-42.

Singh J, Fanroff J, Andrews B, Caldarelli L, Lagatta J, Plesha-Troyke S, Lantos J, Meadow W. Resuscitation in the "Gray Zone" of Viability: Determining Physician Preferences and Predicting Infant Outcomes. Pediatrics 2007; 120:519-526.

Stephens BE, Tucker R, Vohr BR. Special Health Care Needs of Infants Born at the Limits of Viability. Pediatrics 2010; 125:1152-1158.

University of Iowa, The Tiniest Babies Registry. http://www.medicine.uiowa.edu/tiniestbabies/index.htm

Weiss MG, Muraskas JK, eds. Loyola University of Chicago Stritch School of Medicine Neonatal Intensive Care Unit Resident Physician Manual. 2009.

13

The Protective Role of Erythropoietin in the Developing Brain

Marco Sifringer[1], Angela M. Kaindl[2,4], Stefanie Endesfelder[3], Clarissa von Haefen[1], Ivo Bendix[5] and Ursula Felderhoff-Mueser[5]
[1]*Department of Anaesthesiology and Intensive Care Medicine,*
[2]*Department of Pediatric Neurology,*
[3]*Department of Neonatology,*
[4]*Institute of Cell Biology and Neurobiology,*
Charité - Universitätsmedizin Berlin, Campus Virchow-Klinikum, Berlin,
[5]*Department of Paediatrics I - Neonatology, University Hospital Essen, Essen,*
Germany

1. Introduction

Advances in neonatal intensive care have markedly improved survival of premature and critically ill term infants. Unfortunately, neurologic morbidity did not decrease at the same pace (Johnson et al., 2011; Keller et al., 2010). A substantial proportion of very low birth weight infant survivors have neurologic deficits which affect motor and cognitive function (Hack et al., 2002; Ment et al., 2000; Vohr et al., 2000; Wood et al., 2000). Very common are speech and language difficulties, attention deficit hyperactivity disorder, and dyslexia. Brain imaging studies of survivors of premature birth have demonstrated that motor deficits correlate with white matter damage whereas cognitive deficits correlate with decreased volume of grey matter structures (Abernethy et al., 2002; Ajayi-Obe et al., 2000; Nosarti et al., 2002). These findings suggest that neuronal loss, occurring in the brains of premature infants postnatally, is responsible for their neurologic morbidity. Obvious catastrophic events, such as intracerebral bleeding or parenchymal infarction, only partly explain neurologic disability. An increasing body of evidence casts serious doubts on the primary role of hypoxia and ischemia in injury to the developing brain, particularly in preterm infants, while recent work has emphasized the role of intrauterine and neonatal infections (Murphy et al., 1995; Taylor et al., 1999). Still, in many cases an obvious cause of brain damage is missing. In recent years, we learned about silent triggers of cell death in the developing brain. It has been reported that compounds that are used as sedatives (Ikonomidou et al., 1999, 2000), anesthetics (Jevtovic-Todorovic et al., 2003), or anticonvulsants (Bittigau et al., 2002) in neonatal intensive care units and which alter physiologic synaptic activity, such as antagonists at N-methyl-d-aspartate (NMDA) receptors (ketamine, nitric oxide), agonists at gamma-aminobutyric acid $(GABA)_A$ receptors (barbiturates, benzodiazepines, anesthetics), and sodium channel blockers (phenytoin, valproate), can cause massive apoptotic neurodegeneration in infant rats and mice. This neurotoxic effect in rodents is strictly confined to a developmental period characterized by rapid brain growth, which starts prenatally in humans and expands to several years after birth (Dobbing & Sands, 1979; Ikonomidou et al., 1999, 2000; Olney et al., 2002). This comparison points towards the likely possibility that human infants may be susceptible to and may sustain iatrogenic brain damage from treatments that are considered safe in older patients. Such mechanisms could potentially silently lead to diffuse brain injury in infancy and result in cognitive and motor impairment that will become evident later in life.

Although many findings caution the use of oxygen, its administration cannot always be avoided in neonatal intensive care (e.g. resuscitation and treatment of respiratory distress syndrome, pulmonary hypertension and cardiac surgery) regardless of the dangers this may bear for the developing brain. Hyperoxia has documented toxic effects on premature infants including its implication in the pathogenesis of neonatal lung disease (e.g. bronchopulmonary dysplasia), retinopathy of the prematurity and adverse neurological outcome (Collins et al., 2001; Deulofeut et al., 2006; Hamrick et al., 2004; Maltepe & Saugstad, 2009; Saugstad, 2001; Short et al., 2003). Thus, the search for adjunctive neuroprotective measures that can prevent or ameliorate the toxicity of oxygen for the developing brain is highly warranted.

Erythropoietin (Epo) has a long track record of use in preterm infants to prevent anemia of prematurity (Ghezzi et al., 2010; Ohlsson & Aher, 2006) and has been approved by the US Food and Drug Administration for this clinical use in its recombinant form (rEpo). Erythropoiesis was considered originally to be the sole physiological action of Epo. This premise was changed through the knowledge that Epo and its receptor are expressed in several organs including the central nervous system (CNS) and the subsequent discovery of its neuroprotective properties in ischemic stroke, traumatic brain injury, spinal cord injury and perinatal asphyxia (Juul & Felderhoff-Mueser, 2007; Mammis et al., 2009; McPherson, 2009; Spandou et al., 2005; van der Kooij et al., 2008). However, functions of Epo in different neural injuries have not been clarified in detail, especially for neonatal brain injury. Since there are different responses to the treatment of Epo in neonatal and adult brains, the possible mechanisms of Epo for neonatal brain injury are shown in this context. This chapter overviews the neuroprotective role of Epo on neonatal brain injury in animal and clinical trials. Finally the safety concerns with the use of Epo are highlighted.

2. Epo signaling in the brain

2.1 Epo

Epo is a 30.4 kDa glycoprotein with approximately half of its molecular weight derived from carbohydrates that can vary among species and which was originally identified for its role in erythropoiesis (Koury & Bondurant, 1992; Maiese et al., 2005). The human Epo gene is located on chromosome 7q11-q22, exists as a single copy in a 5.4 kb region of the genomic DNA, and encodes a polypeptide chain containing 193 amino acids (Jacobs et al., 1985; Lee-Huang, 1984). The glycosylated chains are important for the biological activity of Epo and can protect Epo from oxygen radical degradation. Epo is stabilized by the carbohydrate chains (Toyoda et al., 2000) and the oligosaccharides in Epo may protect the protein from oxygen radical activity (Uchida et al., 1997). In addition, the biological activity of Epo also relies on two disulfide bondings formed between cysteines at positions 7 and 160 and at positions 29 and 33 (Li et al., 2004). Reduction of these both bonds results in the loss of its biological activity (Maiese et al., 2008b).

The primary production sites of Epo are the adult kidney and the fetal liver (Zanjani et al., 1977), but also other tissues such as brain (Buemi et al., 2009). The Epo gene expression occurs mainly under the control of an oxygen-sensing, hypoxia-inducible factor 1 (HIF-1) dependent mechanism (Digicaylioglu & Lipton, 2001; Rankin et al., 2007).

2.2 Epo receptor (EpoR)

The principal function of Epo is mediated by its specific receptor, EpoR, which is a membrane receptor that belongs to the cytokine class I receptor superfamily. There are two types of EpoR; EpoR homodimers (EpoR/EpoR) on the cell surface of erythroid precursors and heterodimers of EpoR with other cytokine receptors such as EpoR/CD131, on neurons and glia cells. Epo can bind to both the homodimeric and heterodimeric receptors (Brines et al., 2004). In most cells, high-affinity EpoR homodimers mediate the haematopoietic response, whereas low-affinity heterodimeric receptors mediate the tissue-protective activities (Casals-Pascual et al., 2009). Epo effects in the brain are proposed to involve a heteromeric receptor. Most neurons are likely to express high levels of EpoR (Sanchez et al., 2009). The EpoR is expressed in human fetal and neonatal brains, of which expression levels vary between different ages (Dame et al., 2000; Juul et al., 1999; Sirén et al., 2001). In murine embryonic brains, EpoR expression is 10-fold higher than that in the adult (Knabe et al., 2004; Mazur et al., 2010). EpoR expression gradually decreases after birth but can be upregulated under hypoxic conditions (Bührer et al., 2007; Spandou et al., 2004a; Wen et al., 2004).

2.3 Epo – EpoR signaling pathway

In humans, the capacity of Epo to cross the blood-brain barrier (BBB) depends on the permeability of the BBB. The BBB in premature brains may be dysfunctional or damaged, which increases BBB permeability. In addition, the rate of non-specific transport of blood-borne proteins to the brain remains high in newborn infants (Barnard et al., 1998). Therefore, exogenous Epo can be systematically administered and cross the BBB to reach the CNS of premature infants. Systemic rEpo crosses the BBB in a dose-dependent manner, and is increased after brain injury (Statler et al., 2007). Epo accumulation in spinal fluid depends on its peak serum concentration and injection time (Juul et al., 2004).

Precise signaling transduction through Epo in the neonatal nervous system is not completely understood. Upon binding of exogenous or endogenous Epo, EpoR dimerizes allowing for autophosphorylation of the receptor associated Janus family tyrosine proteinkinase 2 (Jak-2) (Hasselblatt et al., 2006). Then, the receptor functions as a docking complex for intracellular proteins containing Src homology 2 domains to further transducer signals (Foley, 2008). Epo is known to play roles in modulating downstream factors include phosphatidylinositol-3-kinase (PI3K), Akt/protein kinase B, Ras-mitogen-activated protein kinases, signal transducer and activator of transcription (STAT)-5, and nuclear factor-κB (NF-κB) (Hasselblatt et al., 2006; McPherson & Juul, 2008). Initiation of these cascades leads to expression of anti-apoptotic genes and suppression of caspases (Fig. 1). It has been demonstrated that Epo promotes the expression of the anti-apoptotic factors Bcl-2 and Bcl-xL and it has been shown that the anti-apoptotic genes XIAP, c-IAP2, and Bcl-xL are upregulated in animal studies of Epo infusion (Digicaylioglu & Lipton, 2001; Wen et al., 2002).

Epo signaling is terminated by activation of phosphatases which dephosphorylate Jak-2. The ligand-receptor complex is then internalized and degraded by the proteasome (Jelkmann

2007; Youssoufian et al., 1993). In hematopoietic cell lines 60% of the internalized Epo is re-secreted (Gross & Lodish, 2006).

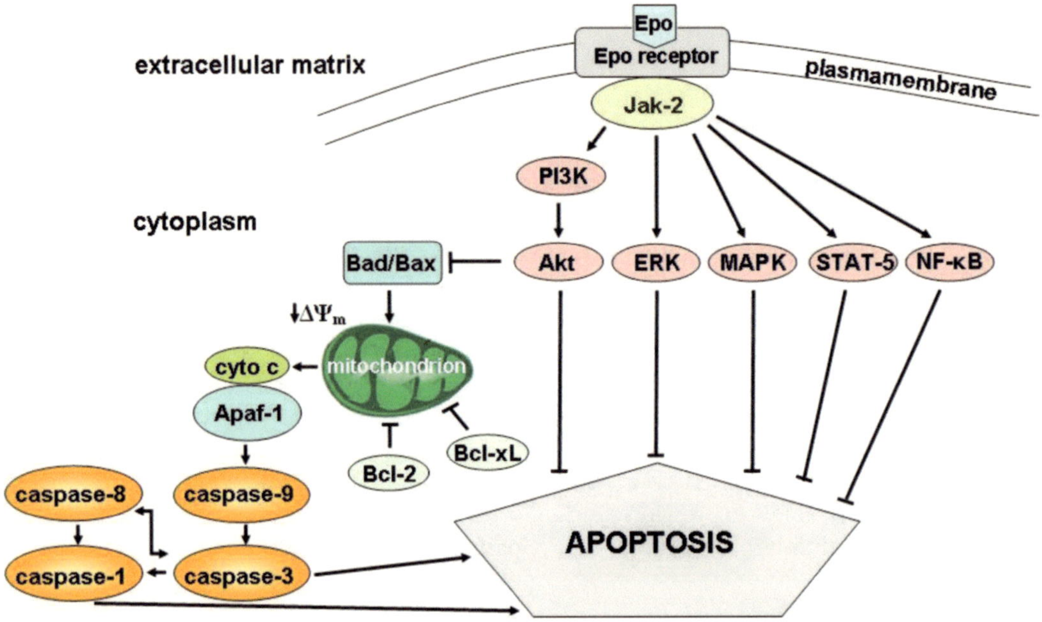

Fig. 1. Epo signaling in the neonatal brain.

Erythropoietin (Epo) prevents apoptotic injury through a series of interconnected cellular pathways. Epo binds to Epo receptor (EpoR) dimer and activates Janus family tyrosine proteinkinase 2 (Jak-2) which results in phosphorylation of Jak-2 and EpoR. Activated Jak-2 initiates signal transduction through several downstream molecules and pathways such as signal transducer and activator of transcription (STAT)-5, mitogen-activated protein kinase (MAPK), extracellular signal-regulated kinases (ERK), phosphatidylinositol-3-kinase (PI3K), protein kinase B (Akt), nuclear factor-κB (NF-κB), mitochondrial membrane potential ($\Delta\Psi_m$), cytochrome *c* (cyto *c*), and caspases. NF-κB and STAT-5 enter into the nucleus, bind to DNA, and transcribe neuroprotective genes such as Bcl-2 and Bcl-xL.

3. Neuroprotective mechanisms of Epo

Epo has been reported to induce a wide range of cellular responses in the brain directed to protect and repair tissue damage. A major mechanism of Epo-induced neuroprotection is its ability to prevent apoptosis (Byts & Sirén, 2009; Chen et al., 2007; Chong et al., 2005; Digicaylioglu & Lipton, 2001; Kaindl et al., 2008; Kumral et al., 2006; Ruscher et al., 2002; Sirén et al., 2001; Villa et al., 2003; Weber et al., 2002; Wen et al., 2002; Wu et al., 2007). Other mechanisms of Epo-induced neuroprotection include anti-inflammatory, anti-oxidative, anti-neurotoxic, angiogenic, neurotrophic effects, neural regeneration, prevention from edema and protecting the white matter (Agnello et al., 2002; Kertesz et al., 2004; Kumral et al., 2005a,b; Maiese et al., 2008a; Pankratova et al., 2010; Rabie & Marti, 2008; Shingo et al., 2001; Sifringer et al., 2009, 2010; Solaroglu et al., 2003; van der Kooij et al., 2008; Wang et al., 2004; Zacharias et al., 2010).

3.1 Anti-apoptotic properties

Epo provides marked neuroprotection against apoptosis in neonatal brain (Yis et al., 2008). Modulation of Bcl-2 family genes is one of the most investigated mechanisms in the anti-apoptotic properties of Epo. Epo consistently increases the expression of the anti-apoptotic gene Bcl-xL, decreases the expression of pro-apoptotic gene Bak and also shifts the Bcl-2/Bax ratio towards an anti-apoptotic effect in microglia cells (Vairano et al., 2002). Bax, a pro-apoptotic molecule, has been shown to be required for apoptotic neuronal cell death during normal development. Bax also plays a role in the regulation of cell death in the CNS following neonatal hypoxic-ischemia (HI) (Gibson et al., 2001; Polster et al., 2003). It has been demonstrated that Epo downregulates Bax gene expression induced by HI and prevents injury-induced Bcl-2 gene downregulation.

Epo significantly prevents hypoxia–ischemia induced Bax mRNA upregulation in brain tissue (Kumral et al., 2006). Exogenous Epo also preserves mitochondrial membrane potential and inhibits the activation of caspase-2, -3, -8 and -9 activities (Chong et al., 2003; Kaindl et al., 2008; Spandou et al., 2004b; Wen et al., 2002).

NF-κB has been shown to induce the expression of the inhibitor of apoptosis (IAP) protein family. These proteins inhibit the active forms of caspase-3 and -9. Induction of IAP activity by NF-κB also suppresses tumor necrosis factor (TNF)-α initiated apoptosis through the inhibition of caspase-8 activity. NF-κB may also prevent apoptosis through the direct activation of Bcl-xL and loss of NF-κB activity negates the neuroprotective effects of Epo suggesting that the activation of NF-κB is necessary for Epo protection in the nervous system (Chong et al., 2002a, 2005).

3.2 Anti-inflammatory effects

Inflammation is an important pathogenic component of brain injury in the newborn, induced either by the production of cytokines and chemokines followed by leukocyte infiltration or glial activation and proliferation. Interleukin (IL)-1β is one of the early-response cytokines that is synthesized and secreted by microglia, astrocytes, and neurons. The biological effects of this pro-inflammatory cytokine include the synthesis of other cytokines and the induction of leukocyte infiltration. Administration of exogenous rEpo before a hyperoxic or after an HI insult prevents rise in IL-1β (Sifringer et al., 2009; Sun et al., 2005). In a mouse model of autoimmune encephalomyelitis, Epo treatment upon onset of paresis was reported to significantly improve neurological functional recovery associated with a significant reduction in inflammatory infiltrates and demyelination (Agnello et al., 2002; Zhang et al., 2006).

3.3 Anti-oxidant effects

Oxidative stress is involved as a crucial mediator in the pathogenesis of several neurodegenerative diseases (Halliwell, 2006; Mariani et al., 2005). The neonatal brain seems particularly vulnerable to oxidative injury because of immature scavenging mechanisms and a relative abundance of iron that acts as a catalyst for the formation of free radicals (Blomgren & Hagberg, 2006). Epo controls a variety of signal transduction pathways during oxidative stress that can involve Jak-2, Akt, STAT cascades, caspases, and NF-κB (Maiese et al., 2008a).

Oxygen-induced cell death in the developing brain is associated with decreased GSH (reduced glutathione) and increased GSSG (oxidized glutathione) levels in which glutathione plays critical roles as an antioxidant (Bains and Shaw, 1997; Dringen, 2000), enzyme cofactor (Chance et al., 1979), cysteine storage form (Cooper and Kristal, 1997; Tateishi et al., 1977) and as a neuromodulator (Janáky et al., 1999) in the CNS. rEpo treatment increased GSH levels and attenuated GSSG to basal levels (Sifringer et al., 2010). Moreover, rEpo reduces NO-mediated formation of free radicals or antagonizes their toxicity through an increase in the activity of antioxidant enzymes in neurons (Sakanaka et al., 1998) and inhibits lipid peroxidation by increasing the activities of cytosolic anti-oxidant enzymes such as glutathione peroxidase (GPX) (Chattopadhyay et al., 2000; Kumral et al., 2005a,b; Solaroglu et al., 2003). Furthermore, rEpo stimulates GPX production in astrocyte cultures (Genc et al. 2002), protects microglia from oxidative stress-induced cell death (Li et al., 2006), and restores brain mitochondrial function after traumatic brain injury (Xiong et al., 2009).

3.4 Neurotrophic properties and neural regeneration

The reported neurotrophic effects of Epo include the ability to stimulate neurite formation, axonal regrowth, dendritic sprouting, electrical activity and modulate intracellular calcium and neurotransmitter synthesis and release (Byts et al., 2008; Byts & Sirén, 2009; Campana et al., 1998; Kawakami et al., 2000, 2001; Konishi et al., 1993; Koshimura et al., 1999; Lipton, 2004; Tabira et al., 1995; Tsai et al., 2006; Viviani et al., 2005; Weber et al., 2002; Yamamoto et al., 2000). Epo activates the cAMP response element binding protein (CREB) transcription pathway and increases brain-derived neurotrophic factor (BDNF) expression and production in primary hippocampal neurons, which contributes to neuroprotection (Viviani et al., 2005). Furthermore, Epo was shown to improve functional outcomes by modulating plasticity, synaptic connectivity and activity of memory-related neuronal networks (Adamcio et al., 2008; Weber et al., 2002).

The developing brain possesses a greater capacity to recover from injury than the adult brain. HI injury in the neonatal brain initiates an enduring regenerative response from the subventricular zone (SVZ) (Yang et al., 2007). Epo may contribute to the brain repair process after insult as it has a promoting capacity on neurogenesis both *in vitro* and *in vivo* (Shingo et al., 2001). Repeated doses of Epo treatment immediately after HI contribute to neurovascular remodeling by promoting tissue protection, revascularization, and neurogenesis in the neonatal injured brain and improve neurobehavioral outcomes (Iwai et al., 2007). If hippocampal progenitor cultures were stimulated into differentiation, Epo directed cells to a neuronal cell fate (Osredkar et al., 2010). In a neonatal stroke model, Epo has been shown to decrease SVZ morphologic changes following brain injury, which is thought to be associated with directing cell fate toward neurogenesis and away from gliogenesis (Gonzalez et al., 2007). Epo can promote differentiation of neuronal stem cells into astrocytes, which may be associated with the activation of NF-κB (Lee et al., 2004). Delayed administration of Epo also promotes oligodendrogenesis and attenuates white matter injury concurrently with increased neurogenesis. These effects are likely to contribute to the observed improvement in neurological functional outcomes (Iwai et al., 2010). Moreover, Epo was found to induce elongation of neurite outgrowth, thereby enhancing and modulating the regenerative effect in spiral ganglion cells (Berkingali et al., 2008).

3.5 Angiogenic potential

In the vascular system, Epo not only offers direct preservation of endothelial cell integrity, but also promotes new capillary formation from existing vessels into an avascular area, a process known as angiogenesis (Chong et al., 2002b; Maiese et al., 2008b). Angiogenesis by Epo offers an additional level of cytoprotection in various cell systems. In models of cerebral ischemia, Epo promotes factors for angiogenesis such as Tie-2 and Angiopoietin-2 that may assist with the restoration of cerebral blood flow to pre-ischemic levels (Li et al., 2007). Epo

has been shown to upregulate expression of several genes involved in vascular function, signal transduction, and energy transfer, in cultured endothelial cells (Banerjee et al., 2000; Carlini et al., 1995; Födinger et al., 2000; Wang & Vaziri, 1999). In angiogenesis, Epo stimulates proliferation of endothelial precursor cells, production of matrix metalloproteinase-2, migration of endothelial cells into vascular sites and formation of capillary tubes (Jaquet et al., 2002; Ribatti et al., 2003; Wang et al., 2006). Epo controlled angiogenesis also may play a role during renal inflammation and prevention of allograft rejection (Reinders et al., 2006). Moreover, Epo may promote the viability of transplanted bone marrow stromal cells and enhance capillary density during experimental cardiac ischemia (Zhang et al., 2007). In clinical studies, Epo serum levels are significantly associated with the number and function of circulating endothelial progenitor cells and Epo can stimulate postnatal neovascularization by increasing endothelial progenitor cell mobilization from the bone marrow (Heeschen et al., 2003).
One concern specific to preterm infants is that the angiogenic effects of Epo might affect the development of retinopathy of prematurity (ROP) (McPherson & Juul, 2008).

3.6 Anti-neurotoxic properties

Glutamate, a principal excitatory neurotransmitter in the brain, participates in the pathogenesis of the neuronal cell loss associated with several neurological diseases. The neurotoxicity of glutamate is mediated by the NMDA receptor. Epo protects the brain from glutamate toxicity through the crosstalk between Jak-2/STAT and PI3K/Akt signaling (Byts et al., 2008). The GABAergic system undergoes profound changes during development and is particularly susceptible to modulation by endogenous factors. In cultured cells, Epo exerts a modulatory action on GABAergic transmission of the development of hippocampal neurons (Wójtowicz & Mozrzymas, 2008). In newborn rats, Epo can completely abolished neuronal degeneration associated with the GABA-mimetic agent propofol administration (Zacharias et al., 2010). In addition, simultaneous administration of rEpo along with ethanol attenuated the lipid peroxidation process and restored the levels of antioxidants, indicating rEpo may be potentially beneficial in treating ethanol-induced brain injury (Kumral et al., 2005b). In a newborn mouse model of periventricular leukomalacia, Epo upregulates EpoR and reduce NMDA receptor mediated excitotoxic damage (Keller et al., 2006).

3.7 Prevention from edema

Epo has demonstrated neuroprotective effects against HI, subarachnoid haemorrhage (SAH) and traumatic brain injury by decreasing brain edema and cellular swelling (Brissaud et al., 2010; Jin et al., 2011; Zhang et al., 2010). The treatment with rEpo markedly upregulated the mRNA expression of the anti-oxidant transcription factor, nuclear factor erythroid 2-related factor 2 (Nrf2) and its downstream cytoprotective enzymes heme oxygenase-1 (HO-1), NAD(P)H:quinone oxidoreductase-1 (NQO1), and glutathione S-transferase α-1 (GST-α1) (Jin et al., 2011; Zhang et al., 2010).
Another possible mechanism by which rEpo decreases brain edema could be through better clearance of excess water in brain tissue by upregulation of the water channel protein aquaporin-4 (AQP4) (Brissaud et al., 2010).

3.8 Protecting the white matter

Periventricular leukomalacia (PVL) is the most common cause of brain injury in preterm infants associated with motor and cognitive deficits observed later (Deng et al., 2008; Volpe,

2009). Activated microglia trigger white matter damage and play a major role in the development of PVL. Epo treatment decrease microglia activation, oligodendrocyte damage and myelin depletion in mouse models of PVL, and is associated with decreased poly-(ADP-ribose) polymerase-1 (PARP-1) activity (Liu et al., 2011). In rat PVL models rEpo attenuates lipopolysaccharide (LPS)-induced white matter injury in the neonatal brain (Kumral et al., 2007) and protects late oligodendrocyte progenitors from HI injury (Mizuno et al., 2008). Given to newborn mice, Epo upregulates EpoR and reduce NMDA receptor mediated excitotoxic damage in PVL (Keller et al., 2006). After transient intrauterine ischemia, Epo reduces white matter injury as evidenced by myelin preservation in neonatal rats (Mazur et al., 2010). In addition, Epo-containing nanoparticles can ameliorate drug-induced liquefaction in a model of PVL (He et al., 2010).

3.9 Enhancement of neurodevelopmental outcome

The improved neurodevelopmental outcomes in rEpo treated animals have been observed in multiple settings. Activation of Epo signaling pathways can inhibit apoptosis, neurotoxicity, inflammation, brain edema, white matter injury and can increase neural regeneration. Epo increases latency and reduces duration of seizures in rat pups after a hypoxic event (Mazur et al., 2010; Mikati et al., 2007) and improves hippocampal dependent memory by modulating plasticity, synaptic connectivity and activity of memory-related neuronal networks. In a neonatal rat model of middle cerebral artery occlusion, rats treated with 3 doses of Epo performed better on tests of cognitive function than either rats treated with a single dose or vehicle-treated injured rats (Gonzalez et al., 2009). Moreover, treatment of newborn rats with rEpo also prevented HI induced learning impairment and substantia nigra neuron loss (McPherson et al., 2007) and improves long-term spatial memory deficits (Kumral et al., 2004). Neonatal HI can cause rapid auditory processing deficits which have been suggested to play a role in later language impairments. Fortunately, a low dose of Epo had novel effects in neuroprotection of auditory deficits, which may have an encouragement in clinical trial (McClure et al., 2006).

4. Effects of Epo in clinical trials

In clinical studies the safety and efficacy of Epo for improving the neurological outcome in preterm infants have been tested (Table 1).

Reference	n_{total}	n_{Epo}	Epo dose (U/kg)	Epo dosing frequency
Newton et al., 1999	40	20	100 or 200	2-7 per week for 6 weeks
Ohls et al., 2004	172	87	ambiguous	23 ± 10 for 8 to 10 weeks
Bierer et al., 2006	16	7	400	3 per week for 6 weeks
He et al., 2008	44	22	250	3 per week for 4 weeks
Juul et al., 2008	60	30	500, 1.000 or 2.500	3 at 24 h intervalls
Fauchère et al., 2008	45	30	3.000	3 within 42 h after birth
Brown et al., 2009	324	82	250-400	3 per week
Neubauer et al., 2010	146	89	8.574 (average cumulative dose)	15 to 121 days

Table 1. Summary of clinical trials of erythropoietin in preterm infants.

4.1 Epo benefits the neural outcome of preterm infants

The neurodevelopmental outcomes of preterm infants treated with rEpo has been evaluated (Newton et al., 1999). There was no adverse effect of Epo on neurologic outcome, growth patterns and the rate of cognitive deficits. Posterior, developmental outcomes at 18-22 months' corrected age in extremely low birth weight (ELBW) infants treated with Epo were compared (Ohls et al., 2004). There was no difference between groups with respect to the percentage of infants with blindness, deafness or hearing loss, moderate to severe cerebral palsy found.

The neuroprotective potential of Epo may be cumulative dose-dependent. In a randomized blinded trial, the concentration of serum Epo was measured in 15 ELBW infants and it was found that infants with elevated Epo concentrations (≥500 mU/mL) had higher mental development index (MDI) scores than those with lower Epo concentrations (<500 mU/mL) (Bierer et al., 2006).

In a study with 366 infants (<1500 g and ≤30 weeks), multivariate analysis revealed that cumulative doses of rEpo were associated with adjusted MDI scores. However, this study has several limitations since the loss of follow-up population was high (>70%) and there was no true placebo-treated or control group. Even though, an advantage of this study is that the statistical analysis included a wide range of cumulative rEpo doses, which indicated the possibility of a threshold effect for Epo (Brown et al., 2009).

The safety of Epo in preterm infants has been established by its high dose administration in two trials. In a randomized, double-blinded trial, the safety of administration of high-dose Epo (3.000 U/kg) to preterm infants has been investigated and no side effect of Epo such as intraventricular hemorrhage, retinopathy, and necrotizing enterocolitis has been found (Fauchère et al., 2008). In another trial of high-dose rEpo in ELBW infants 30 infants who were treated with high-dose rEpo (500, 1.000, or 2.500 U/kg at 24-h intervals) were compared with 30 concurrent control subjects (Juul et al., 2008). Early high-dose rEpo is well tolerated by ELBW infants, causing no excess mortality. Both studies provide an important insight into the safety of preterm infants who received early high-dose rEpo and suggest that an early high-dose administration of rEpo to preterm infants to improve neurodevelopmental outcome is feasible.

The effects of rEpo on neurobehavioral development in preterm infants have been evaluated (He et al., 2008). 44 preterm infants were randomly divided into rEpo treatment and control group. From postnatal day 7, the rEpo treatment group received intravenous rEpo (250 IU/kg 3 times weekly) for 4 weeks. The neonatal behavioral neurological assessment (NBNA) score in the rEpo treatment group was significantly higher than that in the control group at 40 weeks of corrected gestational age. 12 months after birth, the developmental quotient of motor and language in the rEpo group was significantly higher than that in the control group. Hence, early use of rEpo may mediate better neurobehavioral development in preterm infants. A long-term retrospective study has confirmed the neuroprotective benefits of rEpo for ELBW infants at school age (Neubauer et al., 2010). ELBW infants receiving rEpo scored significantly better than untreated children in the overall developmental assessment as well as in the psychological examination (Hamburg-Wechsler Intelligence Test for Children-III (HAWIK-III) intelligence quotient (IQ) score, 90.8 versus 81.3). Moreover, rEpo treatment works well even when given days after the onset of brain injury, which suggests a broader window of therapy.

5. Possible adverse reactions of Epo

Speculations on the benefit of Epo treatment has to be weighed against potential harm. Although Epo treatment for premature infants with anemia has a long history and seems to be safe, there are several issues remaining about its possible adverse reactions in neonate clinical application.

5.1 Haemangioma

Haemangioma is the most common benign neoplasm of infancy (Chiller et al., 2002). The ability of rEpo to induce haemangiomas in very low birth weight preterm infants may partly be attributed to the high proliferation potential of endothelial cells in neonates. In a case report of a preterm infant, the proliferative effects of rEpo in the development of haemangiomas have been reported (Leung, 2000). The haemangiomas in this infant were multiple, shortly after starting rEpo treatment. Similarly, rEpo was assumed to cause the development of haemangiomas in three preterm neonates after 3-4 weeks administration with rEpo (Zaffanello et al., 2003). However, the prevalence of haemangiomas in premature infants is reported as high as 13% (Atherton, 1998). Therefore, it is hard to prove that haemangioma is induced by Epo in the above reports.

5.2 Hypertension

While there have been reports of Epo-associated hypertension in adults (Aher & Ohlsson, 2006b; Klipp et al., 2007; Ohls et al., 2001), those on Epo-related neonatal hypertension are scarce. In a case report, an extremely premature infant developed hypertension after Epo treatment for a period of time, but then hypertension seemed to have improved after Epo was discontinued (Chen et al., 2008).

5.3 Coagulation

Studies in animals and healthy adults show that Epo interacts with platelet function and thrombopoiesis, and as a procoagulant Epo can induce coagulation disorders. In a randomized-controlled trial, ELBW infants received Epo during the first weeks of life. Epo therapy was found to have a short effect on improving platelet activity and functions without changing the total platelet count (Haiden et al., 2005).

5.4 Retinopathy of prematurity (ROP)

One doubt about Epo is its possible effect of enhancing ROP due to its role in promoting vessels growth. Epo has been shown to be a target gene responsible for experimental ROP in mice (Morita et al., 2003). So far, clinical trials have not rendered uniform results. The systematic review of Cochrane Collaboration suggests that neither early Epo (<8 days of age) nor late Epo (>8 days of age) application significantly increase any important adverse outcomes except a significant increase in the rate of ROP for early Epo treatment (Aher & Ohlsson, 2006a,b; Ohlsson & Aher, 2006). The cumulative effects of rEpo at a high dose may increase the incidence of ROP (Shah et al., 2010).

5.5 Neurological recovery and development

Epo can improve neurological outcome in the neonate after HI. But, Epo administration may also have adverse effects for normal neuronal development. First, the expression of Epo and

EpoR is significant during brain development. It is conceivable that exogenous Epo administration may inhibit endogenous Epo expression (Poveshchenko et al., 2001; Strunk et al., 2004). In addition, Epo inhibits apoptosis, which may be a necessary physiological component for normal brain development. Furthermore, Epo induces the proliferation of neuronal stem cells, which may have a negative impact on multipotent progenitor cells (Shingo et al., 2001).

6. Conclusion

The protective potential of Epo has been demonstrated in *in vitro* studies and in animal models of neonatal brain injury. Clinical studies have suggested favorable results about the neuroprotective effects of Epo in neonates. Anyway, many questions still remain unanswered. More information is needed regarding the optimal dose, dosing frequency and length of Epo treatment.

A concern unique to the preterm population remains whether Epo might increase the risk or severity of ROP. To avoid possible adverse effects of Epo, other non-haematopoietic variants, such as asialo-Epo and carbamoylated Epo (Sirén et al., 2009) may hold great promise for future treatments of focal and global cerebral injury. These novel neuroprotective non-haematopoietic Epo mimetics may offer new opportunities for the treatment of neurological disorders in clinic and as candidates for adjunctive neuroprotective therapy of preterm infants.

7. References

Abernethy, L.J.; Palaniappan, M. & Cooke, R.W. (2002). Quantitative magnetic resonance imaging of the brain in survivors of very low birth weight. *Archives of Disease in Childhood,* Vol. 87, No. 4, (October 2002), pp. 279-283, ISSN 1359-2998

Adamcio, B.; Sargin, D.; Stradomska, A.; Medrihan, L.; Gertler, C.; Theis, F.; Zhang, M.; Müller, M.; Hassouna, I.; Hannke, K.; Sperling, S.; Radyushkin, K.; El-Kordi, A.; Schulze L.; Ronnenberg, A.; Wolf, F.; Brose, N.; Rhee, J.S.; Zhang, W. & Ehrenreich H. (2008). Erythropoietin enhances hippocampal long-term potentiation and memory. *BMC Biology,* Vol. 6, No. 37, (September 2008), ISSN 1741-7007

Agnello, D.; Bigini, P.; Villa, P.; Pennini, T.; Cerami, A.; Brines, M.L. & Ghezzi P. (2002). Erythropoietin exerts an anti-inflammatory effect on the CNS in a model of experimental autoimmune encephalomyelitis. *Brain Research,* Vol. 952, No. 1, (October 2002), pp. 128-134, ISSN 0006-8993

Aher, S. & Ohlsson, A. (2006a). Late erythropoietin for preventing red blood cell transfusion in preterm and/or low birth weight infants. *The Cochrane Database of Systematic Reviews,* Vol. 19, No. 3, (July 2006), CD004868, ISSN 1469-493X

Aher, S.M. & Ohlsson, A. (2006b). Early versus late erythropoietin for preventing red blood cell transfusion in preterm and/or low birth weight infants. *The Cochrane Database of Systematic Reviews,* Vol. 19, No. 3, (July 2006), CD004865, ISSN 1469-493X

Ajayi-Obe, M.; Saeed, N.; Cowan, F.M.; Rutherford, M.A. & Edwards, A.D. (2000). Reduced development of cerebral cortex in extremely preterm infants. *Lancet,* Vol. 356, No. 9236, (September 2000), pp. 1162-1163, ISSN 0140-6736

Atherton, D. (1998). Infantile haemangiomas: a review. *Hong Kong Journal of Paediatrics (New Series),* Vol. 3, No. 2, (1998), pp. 89-102, ISSN 1013-9923

Bains, J.S. & Shaw, C.A. (1997). Neurodegenerative disorders in humans: the role of glutathione in oxidative stress-mediated neuronal death. *Brain Research. Brain Research Reviews,* Vol. 25, No. 3, (December 1997), pp. 335-358, ISSN 0165-0173

Banerjee, D.; Rodriguez, M.; Nag, M. & Adamson, J.W. (2000). Exposure of endothelial cells to recombinant human erythropoietin induces nitric oxide synthase activity. *Kidney International,* Vol. 57, No.5, (May 2000), pp. 1895-1904, ISSN 0085-2538

Barnard, K.; Herold, R.; Siemes, H. & Siegert, M. (1998). Quantification of cerebrospinal fluid proteins in children by high-resolution agarose gel electrophoresis. Journal *of Child Neurology,* Vol. 13, No. 2, (February 1998), pp. 51-58, ISSN 0883-0738

Berkingali, N.; Warnecke, A.; Gomes, P.; Paasche, G.; Tack, J.; Lenarz, T. & Stöver, T. (2008). Neurite outgrowth on cultured spiral ganglion neurons induced by erythropoietin. *Hearing Research,* Vol. 243, No. 1-2, (September 2008), pp. 121-126, ISSN 0378-5955

Bierer, R.; Peceny, M.C.; Hartenberger, C.H. & Ohls, R.K. (2006). Erythropoietin concentrations and neurodevelopmental outcome in preterm infants. *Pediatrics,* Vol. 118, No. 3, (September 2006), pp. e635-640, ISSN 0031-4005

Bittigau, P.; Sifringer, M.; Genz, K.; Reith, E.; Pospischil, D.; Govindarajalu, S.; Dzietko, M.; Pesditschek, S.; Mai, I.; Dikranian, K.; Olney, J.W. & Ikonomidou, C. (2002). Antiepileptic drugs and apoptotic neurodegeneration in the developing brain. *Proceedings of the National Academy of Sciences of the United States of America,* Vol. 99, No. 23, (November 2002), pp. 15089-15094, ISSN 0027-8424

Blomgren, K. & Hagberg H. (2006). Free radicals, mitochondria, and hypoxia-ischemia in the developing brain. *Free Radical Biology & Medicine,* Vol. 40, No. 3, (February 2006), pp. 388-397, ISSN 0891-5849

Brines, M.; Grasso, G.; Fiordaliso, F.; Sfacteria, A.; Ghezzi, P.; Fratelli, M.; Latini, R.; Xie, Q.W.; Smart, J.; Su-Rick, C.J.; Pobre, E.; Diaz, D.; Gomez, D.; Hand, C.; Coleman, T. & Cerami, A. (2004). Erythropoietin mediates tissue protection through an erythropoietin and common beta-subunit heteroreceptor. *Proceedings of the National Academy of Sciences of the United States of America,* Vol. 101, No. 41, (October 2004), pp. 14907-14912, ISSN 0027-8424

Brissaud, O.; Villega, F.; Pieter Konsman, J.; Sanchez, S.; Raffard, G.; Franconi, J.M.; Chateil, J.F. & Bouzier-Sore, A.K. (2010). Short-term effect of erythropoietin on brain lesions and aquaporin-4 expression in a hypoxic-ischemic neonatal rat model assessed by magnetic resonance diffusion weighted imaging and immunohistochemistry. *Pediatric Research,* Vol. 68, No. 2, (August 2010), pp. 123-127, ISSN 0031-3998

Brown, M.S.; Eichorst, D.; Lala-Black, B. & Gonzalez, R. (2009). Higher cumulative doses of erythropoietin and developmental outcomes in preterm infants. *Pediatrics,* Vol. 124, No. 4, (October 2009), pp. e681-687, ISSN 0031-4005

Bührer, C.; Felderhoff-Mueser, U. & Wellmann, S. (2007). Erythropoietin and ischemic conditioning—why two good things may be bad. *Acta Paediatrica,* Vol. 96, No. 6, (June 2007), pp. 787-789, ISSN 0803-5253

Buemi, M.; Lacquaniti, A.; Maricchiolo, G.; Bolignano, D.; Campo, S.; Cernaro, V.; Sturiale, A.; Grasso, G.; Buemi, A.; Allegra, A.; Donato, V. & Genovese, L. (2009). Regenerative medicine: does Erythropoietin have a role? *Current Pharmaceutical Design,* Vol. 15, No. 17, (2009), pp. 2026-2036, ISSN 1381-6128

Byts, N.; Samoylenko, A.; Fasshauer, T.; Ivanisevic, M.; Hennighausen, L.; Ehrenreich, H. & Sirén A.L. (2008). Essential role for Stat5 in the neurotrophic but not in the neuroprotective effect of erythropoietin. *Cell Death and Differentiation*, Vol. 15, No. 4, (April 2008), pp. 783-792, ISSN 1350-9047

Byts, N. & Sirén, A.L. (2009). Erythropoietin: a multimodal neuroprotective agent. *Experimental & Translational Stroke Medicine*, Vol. 1, No. 4, (October 2009), ISSN 2040-7378

Campana, W.M.; Misasi, R. & O'Brien, J.S. (1998). Identification of a neurotrophic sequence in erythropoietin. *International Journal of Molecular Medicine*, Vol. 1, No. 1, (January 1998), pp. 235-241, ISSN 1107-3756

Carlini, R.G.; Reyes, A.A. & Rothstein M. (1995). Recombinant human erythropoietin stimulates angiogenesis in vitro. *Kidney International*, Vol. 47, No. 3, (March 1995), pp. 740-745, ISSN 0085-2538

Casals-Pascual, C.; Idro, R.; Picot, S.; Roberts, D.J. & Newton, C.R. (2009). Can erythropoietin be used to prevent brain damage in cerebral malaria? *Trends in Parasitology*, Vol. 25, No. 1, (January 2009), pp. 30-36, ISSN 1471-4922

Chance, B.; Sies, H. & Boveris, A. (1979). Hydroperoxide metabolism in mammalian organs. *Physiological Reviews*, Vol. 59, No. 3, (July 1979), pp. 527-605, ISSN 0031-9333

Chattopadhyay, A.; Choudhury, T.D.; Bandyopadhyay, D. & Datta, A.G. (2000). Protective effect of erythropoietin on the oxidative damage of erythrocyte membrane by hydroxyl radical. *Biochemical Pharmacology*, Vol. 59, No. 4, (February 2000), pp. 419-425, ISSN 0006-2952

Chen, Z.Y.; Asavaritikrai, P.; Prchal, J.T. & Noguchi C.T. (2007). Endogenous erythropoietin signaling is required for normal neural progenitor cell proliferation. *The Journal of Biological Chemistry*, Vol. 282, No. 35, (August 2007), pp. 25875-25883, ISSN 0021-9258

Chen, J.M.; Jeng, M.J.; Chiu, S.Y.; Lee, Y.S.; Soong, W.J.; Hwang, B. & Tang, R.B. (2008). Conditions associated with hypertension in a high-risk premature infant. *Journal of the Chinese Medical Association*, Vol. 71, No. 9, (September 2008), pp. 485-490, ISSN 1726-4901

Chiller, K.G.; Passaro, D. & Frieden, I.J. (2002). Hemangiomas of infancy: clinical characteristics, morphologic subtypes, and their relationship to race, ethnicity, and sex. *Archives of Dermatology*, Vol. 138, No. 12, (December 2002), pp. 1567-1576, ISSN 0003-987X

Chong, Z.Z.; Kang, J.Q. & Maiese, K. (2002a). Angiogenesis and plasticity: role of erythropoietin in vascular systems. *Journal of Hematotherapy & Stem Cell Research*, Vol. 11, No. 6, (December 2002), pp. 863-871, ISSN 1525-8165

Chong, Z.Z.; Kang, J.Q. & Maiese, K. (2002b). Hematopoietic factor erythropoietin fosters neuroprotection through novel signal transduction cascades. *Journal of Cerebral Blood Flow & Metabolism*, Vol. 22, No. 5, (May 2002), pp. 503-514, ISSN 0271-678X

Chong, Z.Z.; Kang, J.Q. & Maiese, K. (2003). Apaf-1, Bcl-xL, cytochrome c, and caspase-9 form the critical elements for cerebral vascular protection by erythropoietin. *Journal of Cerebral Blood Flow & Metabolism*, Vol. 23, No. 3, (March 2003), pp. 320-330, ISSN 0271-678X

Chong, Z.Z.; Li, F. & Maiese, K.. (2005). Erythropoietin requires NF-kappaB and its nuclear translocation to prevent early and late apoptotic neuronal injury during beta-amyloid toxicity. *Current Neurovascular Research,* Vol. 2, No. 5, (December 2005), pp. 387-399, ISSN 1567-2026

Collins, M.P.; Lorenz, J.M.; Jetton, J.R. & Paneth, N. (2001). Hypocapnia and other ventilation-related risk factors for cerebral palsy in low birth weight infants. *Pediatric Research,* Vol. 50, No. 6, (December 2001), pp. 712-719, ISSN 0031-3998

Cooper, A.J. & Kristal, B.S. (1997). Multiple roles of glutathione in the central nervous system. *Biological Chemistry,* Vol. 378, No. 8, (August 1997), pp. 793-802, ISSN 1431-6730

Dame, C.; Bartmann, P.; Wolber, E.; Fahnenstich, H.; Hofmann, D. & Fandrey, J. (2000). Erythropoietin gene expression in different areas of the developing human central nervous system. *Brain Research. Developmental Brain Research,* Vol. 125, No. 1-2, (December 2000), pp. 69-74., ISSN 0165-3806

Deng, W.; Pleasure, J. & Pleasure, D. (2008). Progress in periventricular leukomalacia. *Archives of Neurology,* Vol. 65, No. 10, (October 2008), pp. 1291-1295, ISSN 0003-9942

Deulofeut, R.; Critz, A.; Adams-Chapman, I. & Sola, A. (2006). Avoiding hyperoxia in infants < or = 1250 g is associated with improved short- and long-term outcomes. *Journal of Perinatology,* Vol. 26, No. 11, (November 2006), pp. 700-705, ISSN 0743-8346

Digicaylioglu, M. & Lipton, S.A. (2001). Erythropoietin-mediated neuroprotection involves cross-talk between Jak2 and NF-kappaB signalling cascades. *Nature,* Vol. 412, No. 6847, (August 2001), pp. 641-647, ISSN 0028-0836

Dobbing, J. & Sands, J. (1979). Comparative aspects of the brain growth spurt. *Early Human Development,* Vol. 3, No. 1, (March 1979), pp. 79-83, ISSN 0378-3782

Dringen, R. (2000). Metabolism and functions of glutathione in brain. *Progress in Neurobiology,* Vol. 62, No. 6, (December 2000), pp. 649-671, ISSN 0301-0082

Fauchère, J.C.; Dame, C.; Vonthein, R.; Koller, B.; Arri, S.; Wolf, M. & Bucher, H.U. (2008). An approach to using recombinant erythropoietin for neuroprotection in very preterm infants. *Pediatrics,* Vol. 122, No. 2, (August 2008), pp. 375-382, ISSN 0031-4005

Födinger, M.; Fritsche-Polanz, R.; Buchmayer, H.; Skoupy, S.; Sengoelge, G.; Hörl, W.H. & Sunder-Plassmann, G. (2000). Erythropoietin-inducible immediate-early genes in human vascular endothelial cells. *Journal of Investigative Medicine,* Vol. 48, No. 2, (March 2000), pp. 137-149, ISSN 1081-5589

Foley, R.N. (2008). Erythropoietin: physiology and molecular mechanisms. *Heart Failure Reviews,* Vol. 13, No. 4, (December 2008), pp. 405-414, ISSN 1382-4147

Genc, S.; Akhisaroglu, M.; Kuralay, F. & Genc, K. (2002). Erythropoietin restores glutathione peroxidase activity in 1-methyl-4-phenyl-1,2,5,6-tetrahydropyridine-induced neurotoxicity in C57BL mice and stimulates murine astroglial glutathione peroxidase production in vitro. *Neuroscience Letters,* Vol. 321, No. 1-2, (March 2002), pp. 73-76, ISSN 0304-3940

Ghezzi, P.; Bernaudin, M.; Bianchi, R.; Blomgren, K.; Brines, M.; Campana, W.; Cavaletti, G.; Cerami, A.; Chopp, M.; Coleman, T.; Digicaylioglu, M.; Ehrenreich, H.; Erbayraktar, S.; Erbayraktar, Z.; Gassmann, M.; Genc, S.; Gokmen, N.; Grasso, G.; Juul, S.; Lipton, S.A.; Hand, C.C.; Latini, R.; Lauria, G.; Leist, M.; Newton, S.S.; Petit, E.; Probert, L.; Sfacteria, A.; Siren, A.L.; Talan, M.; Thiemermann, C.; Westenbrink, D.; Yaqoob, M. & Zhu, C. (2010). Erythropoietin: not just about erythropoiesis. *Lancet,* Vol. 375, No. 9732, (June 2010), pp. 2142, ISSN 0140-6736

Gibson, M.E.; Han, B.H.; Choi, J.; Knudson, C.M.; Korsmeyer, S.J.; Parsadanian, M. & Holtzman D.M. (2001). BAX contributes to apoptotic-like death following neonatal hypoxia–ischemia: evidence for distinct apoptosis pathways. *Molecular Medicine,* Vol. 7, No. 9, (September 2001), pp. 644-655, ISSN 1076-1551

Gonzalez, F.F.; McQuillen, P.; Mu, D.; Chang, Y.; Wendland, M.; Vexler, Z. & Ferriero, D.M. (2007). Erythropoietin enhances long-term neuroprotection and neuroge- nesis in neonatal stroke. *Developmental Neuroscience,* Vol. 29, No. 4-5, (2007), pp. 321-330, ISSN 0378-5866

Gonzalez, F.F.; Abel, R.; Almli, C.R.; Mu, D.; Wendland, M. & Ferriero, D.M. (2009). Erythropoietin sustains cognitive function and brain volume after neonatal stroke. *Developmental Neuroscience,* Vol. 31, No. 5, (2009), pp. 403-411, ISSN 0378-5866

Gross, A.W. & Lodish, H.F. (2006). Cellular trafficking and degradation of erythropoietin and novel erythropoiesis stimulating protein (NESP). *The Journal of Biological Chemistry,* Vol. 281, No. 4, (January 2006), pp. 2024-2032, ISSN 0021-9258

Hack, M.; Flannery, D.J.; Schluchter, M.; Cartar, L.; Borawski, E. & Klein, N. (2002). Outcomes in young adulthood for very-low-birth-weight infants. *The New England Journal of Medicine,* Vol. 346, No. 3, (January 2002), pp. 149-157, ISSN 0028-4793

Haiden, N.; Cardona, F.; Schwindt, J.; Berger, A.; Kuhle, S.; Homoncik, M.; Jilma-Stohlawetz, P.; Pollak, A. & Jilma, B. (2005). Changes in thrombopoiesis and platelet reactivity in extremely low birth weight infants undergoing erythropoietin therapy for treatment of anaemia of prematurity. *Thrombosis and haemostasis,* Vol. 93, No. 1, (January 2005), pp. 118-123, ISSN 0340-6245

Halliwell, B. (2006). Oxidative stress and neurodegeneration: where are we now? *Journal of Neurochemistry,* Vol. 97, No. 6, (June 2006), pp. 1634-1658, ISSN 0022-3042

Hamrick, S.E.; Miller, S.P.; Leonard, C.; Glidden, D.V.; Goldstein, R.; Ramaswamy, V.; Piecuch, R. & Ferriero, D.M. (2004). Trends in severe brain injury and neurodevelopmental outcome in premature newborn infants: the role of cystic periventricular leukomalacia. *The Journal of Pediatrics,* Vol. 145, No. 5, (November 2004), pp. 593-599, ISSN 0022-3476

Hasselblatt, M.; Ehrenreich, H. & Sirén, A.L. (2006). The brain erythropoietin system and its potential for therapeutic exploitation in brain disease. *Journal of Neurosurgical Anesthesiology,* Vol. 18, No. 2, (April 2006), pp. 132-138, ISSN 0898-4921

He, J.S.; Huang, Z.L.; Yang, H.; Weng, K.Z. & Zhu, S.B. (2008). Early use of recombi- nant human erythropoietin promotes neurobehavioral development in preterm infants. *Chinese Journal of Contemporary Pediatrics,* Vol. 10, No. 5, (October 2008), pp. 586-588, ISSN 1008-8830

He, N.; Wang, T.; Jiang, L.; Wang, D.; Hu, Y. & Zhang, L. (2010). Therapy for cerebral ischemic injury with erythropoietin-containing nanoparticles. *Journal of Nanoscience and Nanotechnology,* Vol. 10, No. 8, (August 2010), pp. 5320-5323, ISSN 1533-4880

Heeschen, C.; Aicher, A.; Lehmann, R.; Fichtlscherer, S.; Vasa, M.; Urbich, C.; Mildner-Rihm, C.; Martin, H.; Zeiher, A.M. & Dimmeler, S. (2003). Erythropoietin is a potent physiologic stimulus for endothelial progenitor cell mobilization. *Blood,* Vol. 102, No. 4, (August 2003), pp. 1340-1346, ISSN 0006-4971

Ikonomidou, C.; Bosch, F.; Miksa, M.; Vöckler, J.; Bittigau, P.; Dikranian, K.; Tenkova, T.; Turski, L. & Olney, J.W. (1999). Blockade of NMDA receptors and apoptotic neurodegeneration in the developing brain. *Science,* Vol. 283, No. 5398, (January 1999), pp. 70-74, ISSN 0036-8075

Ikonomidou, C.; Bittigau, P.; Ishimaru, M.J.; Wozniak, D.F.; Koch, C.; Genz, K.; Price, M.T.; Stefovska, V.; Hörster, F.; Tenkova, T.; Dikranian, K. & Olney, J.W. (2000). Ethanol-induced apoptotic neurodegeneration and fetal alcohol syndrome. *Science*, Vol. 287, No. 5455, (February 2000), pp. 1056-1060, ISSN 0036-8075

Iwai, M.; Cao, G.; Yin, W.; Stetler, R.A.; Liu, J. & Chen J. (2007). Erythropoietin promotes neuronal replacement through revascularization and neurogenesis after neonatal hypoxia/ischemia in rats. *Stroke,* Vol. 38, No. 10, (October 2007), pp. 2795-2803, ISSN 0039-2499

Iwai, M.; Stetler, R.A.; Xing, J.; Hu, X.; Gao, Y.; Zhang, W.; Chen, J. & Cao, G. (2010). Enhanced oligodendrogenesis and recovery of neurological function by erythropoietin after neonatal hypoxic/ischemic brain injury. *Stroke,* Vol. 41, No. 5, (May 2010), pp. 1032-1037, ISSN 0039-2499

Jacobs, K.; Shoemaker, C.; Rudersdorf, R.; Neill, S.D.; Kaufman, R.J.; Mufson, A.; Seehra, J.; Jones, S.S.; Hewick, R.; Fritsch, E.F.; Kawakita, M.; Shimizu, T. & Miyake, T. (1985). Isolation and characterization of genomic and cDNA clones of human erythropoietin. *Nature,* Vol. 313, No. 6005, (February-March 1985), pp. 806-810, ISSN 0028-0836

Janáky, R.; Ogita, K.; Pasqualotto, B.A.; Bains, J.S.; Oja, S.S.; Yoneda, Y. & Shaw, C.A. (1999). Glutathione and signal transduction in the mammalian CNS. *Journal of Neurochemistry,* Vol. 73, No. 3, (September 1999), pp. 889-902, ISSN 0022-3042

Jaquet, K.; Krause, K.; Tawakol-Khodai, M.; Geidel, S. & Kuck, K.H. (2002). Erythropoietin and VEGF exhibit equal angiogenic potential. *Microvascular Research,* Vol. 64, No. 2, (September 2002), pp. 326-333, ISSN 0026-2862

Jelkmann, W. (2007). Erythropoietin after a century of research: younger than ever. *European Journal of Haematology,* Vol. 78, No. 3, (March 2007), pp. 183-205, ISSN 0902-4441

Jevtovic-Todorovic, V.; Hartman, R.E.; Izumi, Y.; Benshoff, N.D.; Dikranian, K.; Zorumski, C.F.; Olney, J.W. & Wozniak, D.F. (2003). Early exposure to common anesthetic agents causes widespread neurodegeneration in the developing rat brain and persistent learning deficits. *The Journal of Neuroscience,* Vol. 23, No. 3, (February 2003), pp. 876-882, ISSN 0270-6474

Jin, W.; Kong, J.; Lu, T.; Wang, H.; Ni, H.; Wu, J.; Dai, Y.; Jiang, J. & Liang, W. (2011). Erythropoietin prevents secondary brain injury induced by cortical lesion in mice: possible involvement of Nrf2 signaling pathway. *Annals of Clinical and Laboratory Science,* Vol. 41, No. 1, (Fall 2011), pp. 25-32, ISSN 0091-7370

Johnson, S.; Wolke, D.; Hennessy, E. & Marlow, N. (2011). Educational outcomes in extremely preterm children: neuropsychological correlates and predictors of attainment. *Developmental Neuropsychology,* Vol. 36, No. 1, (January 2011), pp. 74-95, ISSN 8756-5641

Juul, S.E.; Yachnis, A.T.; Rojiani, A.M. & Christensen, R.D. (1999). Immunohistochemical localization of erythropoietin and its receptor in the developing human brain. *Pediatric and Developmental Pathology,* Vol. 2, No. 2, (March-April 1999), pp. 148-158, ISSN 1093-5266

Juul, S.E.; McPherson, R.J.; Farrell, F.X.; Jolliffe, L.; Ness, D.J. & Gleason, C.A. (2004). Erytropoietin concentrations in cerebrospinal fluid of nonhuman primates and fetal sheep following high-dose recombinant erythropoietin. *Biology of the Neonate,* Vol. 85, No. 2, (2004), pp. 138-144, ISSN 0006-3126

Juul, S. & Felderhoff-Mueser, U. (2007). Epo and other hematopoietic factors. *Seminars in Fetal & Neonatal Medicine,* Vol. 12, No. 4, (August 2007), pp. 250-258, ISSN 1744-165X

Juul, S.E.; McPherson, R.J.; Bauer, L.A.; Ledbetter, K.J.; Gleason, C.A. & Mayock, D.E. (2008). A phase I/II trial of high-dose erythropoietin in extremely low birth weight infants: pharmacokinetics and safety. *Pediatrics,* Vol. 122, No. 2, (August 2008), pp. 383-391, ISSN 0031-4005

Kaindl, A.M.; Sifringer, M.; Koppelstaetter, A.; Genz, K.; Loeber, R.; Boerner, C.; Stuwe, J.; Klose, J. & Felderhoff-Mueser, U. (2008). Erythropoietin protects the developing brain from hyperoxia-induced cell death and proteome changes. *Annals of Neurology,* Vol. 64, No. 5, (November 2008), pp. 523-534, ISSN 0364-5134

Kawakami, M.; Iwasaki, S.; Sato, K. & Takahashi, M. (2000). Erythropoietin inhibits calcium-induced neurotransmitter release from clonal neuronal cells. *Biochemical and Biophysical Research Communications,* Vol. 279, No. 1, (December 2000), pp. 293-297, ISSN 0006-291X

Kawakami, M.; Sekiguchi, M.; Sato, K.; Kozaki, S. & Takahashi, M. (2001). Erythropoietin receptor-mediated inhibition of exocytotic glutamate release confers neuroprotection during chemical ischemia. *The Journal of Biological Chemistry,* Vol. 276, No. 42, (October 2001), pp. 39469-39475, ISSN 0021-9258

Keller, M.; Yang, J.; Griesmaier, E.; Gorna, A.; Sarkozy, G.; Urbanek, M.; Gressens, P. & Simbruner, G. (2006). Erythropoietin is neuroprotective against NMDA-receptor-mediated excitotoxic brain injury in newborn mice. *Neurobiology of Disease,* Vol. 24, No. 2, (November 2006), pp. 357-366, ISSN 0969-9961

Keller, M.; Felderhoff-Mueser, U.; Lagercrantz, H.; Dammann, O.; Marlow, N.; Hüppi, P.; Buonocore, G.; Poets, C.; Simbruner, G.; Guimaraes, H.; Mader, S.; Merialdi, M. & Saugstad, O.D. (2010). Policy benchmarking report on neonatal health and social policies in 13 European countries. *Acta Paediatrica,* Vol. 99, No. 11, (November 2010), pp. 1624-1629, ISSN 0803-5253

Kertesz, N.; Wu, J.; Chen, T.H.; Sucov, H.M. & Wu, H. (2004). The role of erythropoietin in regulating angiogenesis. *Developmental Biology,* Vol. 276, No. 1, (December 2004), pp. 101-110, ISSN 0012-1606

Klipp, M.; Holzwarth, A.U.; Poeschl, J.M.; Nelle, M. & Linderkamp, O. (2007). Effects of erythropoietin on erythrocyte deformability in non-transfused preterm infants. *Acta Paediatrica,* Vol. 96, No. 2, (February 2007), pp. 253-256, ISSN 0803-5253

Knabe, W.; Knerlich, F.; Washausen, S.; Kietzmann, T.; Sirén, A.L.; Brunnett, G.; Kuhn, H.J. & Ehrenreich, H. (2004). Expression patterns of erythropoietin and its receptor in the developing midbrain. *Anatomy and Embryology,* Vol. 207, No. 6, (March 2004), pp. 503-512, ISSN 0340-2061

Konishi, Y.; Chui, D.H.; Hirose, H.; Kunishita, T. & Tabira, T. (1993). Trophic effect of erythropoietin and other hematopoietic factors on central cholinergic neurons in vitro and in vivo. *Brain Research,* Vol. 609, No. 1-2, (April 1993), pp. 29-35, ISSN 0006-8993

Koshimura, K.; Murakami, Y.; Sohmiya, M.; Tanaka, J. & Kato, Y. (1999). Effects of erythropoietin on neuronal activity. *Journal of Neurochemistry,* Vol. 72, No. 6, (June 1999), pp. 2565-2572, ISSN 0022-3042

Koury, M.J. & Bondurant, M.C. (1992). The molecular mechanism of erythropoietin action. *European Journal of Biochemistry,* Vol. 210, No. 3, (December 1992), pp. 649-663, ISSN 0014-2956

Kumral, A.; Uysal, N.; Tugyan, K.; Sonmez, A.; Yilmaz, O.; Gokmen, N.; Kiray, M.; Genc, S.; Duman, N.; Koroglu, T.F.; Ozkan, H. & Genc, K. (2004). Erythropoietin improves long-term spatial memory deficits and brain injury following neonatal hypoxia-ischemia in rats. *Behavioural Brain Research,* Vol. 153, No. 1, (August 2004), pp. 77-86, ISSN 0166-4328

Kumral, A.; Gonenc, S.; Acikgoz, O.; Sonmez, A.; Genc, K.; Yilmaz, O.; Gokmen, N.; Duman, N. & Ozkan, H. (2005a). Erythropoietin increases glutathione peroxidase enzyme activity and decreases lipid peroxidation levels in hypoxic–ischemic brain injury in neonatal rats. *Biology of the Neonate,* Vol. 87, No. 1, (2005), pp. 15-18, ISSN 0006-3126

Kumral, A.; Tugyan, K.; Gonenc, S.; Genc, K.; Genc, S.; Sonmez, U.; Yilmaz, O.; Duman, N.; Uysal, N. & Ozkan, H. (2005b). Protective effects of erythropoietin against ethanol-induced apoptotic neurodegenaration and oxidative stress in the developing C57BL/6 mouse brain. *Brain Research. Developmental Brain Research,* Vol. 160, No. 2, (December 2005), pp. 146-156, ISSN 0165-3806

Kumral, A.; Genc, S.; Ozer, E.; Yilmaz, O.; Gokmen, N.; Koroglu, T.F.; Duman, N.; Genc, K. & Ozkan, H. (2006). Erythropoietin downregulates bax and DP5 proapoptotic gene expression in neonatal hypoxic–ischemic brain injury. *Biology of the Neonate,* Vol. 89, No. 3, (2006), pp. 205-210, ISSN 0006-3126

Kumral, A.; Baskin, H.; Yesilirmak, D.C.; Ergur, B.U.; Aykan, S.; Genc, S.; Genc, K.; Yilmaz, O.; Tugyan, K.; Giray, O.; Duman, N. & Ozkan H. (2007). Erythropoietin attenuates lipopolysaccharide-induced white matter injury in the neonatal rat brain. *Neonatology,* Vol. 92, No. 4, (2007), pp. 269-278, ISSN 1661-7800

Lee, S.M.; Nguyen, T.H.; Park, M.H.; Kim, K.S.; Cho, K.J.; Moon, D.C.; Kim, H.Y.; Yoon, D.Y. & Hong, J.T. (2004). EPO receptor-mediated ERK kinase and NF-kappaB activation in erythropoietin-promoted differentiation of astrocytes. *Biochemical and Biophysical Research Communications,* Vol. 320, No. 4, (August 2004), pp. 1087-1095, ISSN 0006-291X

Lee-Huang, S. (1984). Cloning and expression of human erythropoietin cDNA in Escherichia coli. *Proceedings of the National Academy of Sciences of the United States of America,* Vol. 81, No. 9, (May 1984), pp. 2708-2712, ISSN 0027-8424

Leung, S.P. (2000). Multiple strawberry haemangiomas-side effect of rhuEpo? *Acta Paediatrica,* Vol. 89, No. 7, (July 2000), pp. 890, ISSN 0803-5253

Li, F.; Chong, Z.Z. & Maiese, K. (2004). Erythropoietin on a tightrope: balancing neuronal and vascular protection between intrinsic and extrinsic pathways. *Neurosignals,* Vol. 13, No. 6, (November-December 2004), pp. 265-289, ISSN 1424-862X

Li, F.; Chong, Z.Z. & Maiese, K. (2006). Microglial integrity is maintained by erythropoietin through integration of Akt and its substrates of glycogen synthase kinase-3beta, beta-catenin, and nuclear factor-kappaB. *Current Neurovascular Research,* Vol. 3, No. 3, (August 2006), pp. 187-201, ISSN 1567-2026

Li, Y.; Lu, Z.; Keogh, C.L.; Yu, S.P. & Wei, L. (2007). Erythropoietin-induced neurovascular protection, angiogenesis, and cerebral blood flow restoration after focal ischemia in mice. *Journal of Cerebral Blood Flow & Metabolism,* Vol. 27, No. 5, (May 2007), pp. 1043-1054, ISSN 0271-678X

Lipton, S.A. (2004). Erythropoietin for neurologic protection and diabetic neuropathy. *The New England Journal of Medicine,* Vol. 350, No. 24, (June 2004), pp. 2516-2517, ISSN 0028-4793

Liu, W.; Shen, Y.; Plane, J.M.; Pleasure, D.E. & Deng, W. (2011). Neuroprotective potential of erythropoietin and its derivative carbamylated erythropoietin in periventricular leukomalacia. *Experimental Neurology,* Vol. 230, No. 2, (August 2011), pp. 227-239, ISSN 0014-4886

Maiese, K.; Li, F. & Chong, Z.Z. (2005). New avenues of exploration for erythropoietin. *The Journal of the American Medical Association,* Vol. 293, No. 1, (January 2005), pp. 90-95, ISSN 0098-7484

Maiese, K.; Chong, Z.Z.; Hou, J. & Shang, Y.C. (2008a). Erythropoietin and oxidative stress. *Current Neurovascular Research,* Vol. 5, No. 2, (May 2008), pp. 125-142, ISSN 1567-2026

Maiese, K.; Chong, Z.Z.; Li, F. & Shang, Y.C. (2008b). Erythropoietin: elucidating new cellular targets that broaden therapeutic strategies. *Progress in Neurobiology,* Vol. 85, No. 2, (June 2008), pp. 194-213, ISSN 0301-0082

Maltepe, E. & Saugstad, O.D. (2009). Oxygen in health and disease: regulation of oxygen homeostasis-clinical implications. *Pediatric Research,* Vol. 65, No. 3, (March 2009), pp. 261-268, ISSN 0031-3998

Mammis, A.; McIntosh, T.K. & Maniker, A.H. (2009). Erythropoietin as a neuroprotective agent in traumatic brain injury. *Surgical Neurology,* Vol. 71, No. 5, (May 2009), pp. 527-531, ISSN 0090-3019

Mariani, E.; Polidori, M.C.; Cherubini, A. & Mecocci, P. (2005). Oxidative stress in brain aging, neurodegenerative and vascular diseases: an overview. *Journal of Chromatography. B, Analytical Technologies in the Biomedical and Life Sciences,* Vol. 827, No. 1, (November 2005), pp. 65-75, ISSN 1570-0232

Mazur, M.; Miller, R.H. & Robinson, S. (2010). Postnatal erythropoietin treatment mitigates neural cell loss after systemic prenatal hypoxic-ischemic injury. *Journal of Neurosurgery. Pediatrics,* Vol. 6, No. 3, (September 2010), pp. 206-221, ISSN 1933-0707

McClure, M.M.; Threlkeld, S.W. & Fitch, R.H. (2006). The effects of erythropoietin on auditory processing following neonatal hypoxic-ischemic injury. *Brain Research,* Vol. 1087, No. 1, (May 2006), pp. 190-195, ISSN 0006-8993

McPherson, R.J. (2009). Can erythropoietin improve developmental outcomes for preterm infants? *Pediatrics,* Vol. 124, No. 4, (October 2009), pp. e805-806, ISSN 0031-4005

McPherson, R.J.; Demers, E.J. & Juul, S.E. (2007). Safety of high-dose recombinant erythropoietin in a neonatal rat model. *Neonatology,* Vol. 91, No. 1, (2007), pp. 36-43, ISSN 1661-7800

McPherson, R.J. & Juul S.E. (2008). Recent trends in erythropoietin mediated neuroprotection. *International Journal of Developmental Neuroscience,* Vol. 26, No. 1, (February 2008), pp. 103-111, ISSN 0736-5748

Ment, L.R.; Schneider, K.C.; Ainley, M.A. & Allan, W.C. (2000). Adaptive mechanisms of developing brain. The neuroradiologic assessment of the preterm infant. *Clinics in Perinatology,* Vol. 27, No. 2, (June 2000), pp. 303-323, ISSN 0095-5108

Mikati, M.A.; El Hokayem, J.A. & El Sabban, M.E. (2007). Effects of a single dose of erythropoietin on subsequent seizure susceptibility in rats exposed to acute hypoxia at P10. *Epilepsia,* Vol. 48, No. 1, (January 2007), pp. 175-181, ISSN 0013-9580

Mizuno, K.; Hida, H.; Masuda, T.; Nishino, H. & Togari, H. (2008). Pretreatment with low doses of erythropoietin ameliorates brain damage in periventricular leukomalacia by targeting late oligodendrocyte progenitors: a rat model. *Neonatology,* Vol. 94, No. 4, (2008), pp. 255-266, ISSN 1661-7800

Morita, M.; Ohneda, O.; Yamashita, T.; Takahashi, S.; Suzuki, N.; Nakajima, O.; Kawauchi, S.; Ema, M.; Shibahara, S.; Udono, T.; Tomita, K.; Tamai, M.; Sogawa, K.; Yamamoto, M. & Fujii-Kuriyama, Y. (2003). HLF/HIF-2alpha is a key factor in retinopathy of prematurity in association with erythropoietin. *The EMBO Journal,* Vol. 22, No. 5, (March 2003), pp. 1134-1146, ISSN 0261-4189

Murphy, D.J.; Sellers, S.; MacKenzie, I.Z.; Yudkin, P.L. & Johnson, A.M. (1995). Case-control study of antenatal and intrapartum risk factors for cerebral palsy in very preterm singleton babies. *Lancet,* Vol. 346, No. 8988, (December 1995), pp. 1449-1454, ISSN 0140-6736

Neubauer, A.P.; Voss, W.; Wachtendorf, M. & Jungmann, T. (2010). Erythropoietin improves neurodevelopmental outcome of extremely preterm infants. *Annals of Neurology,* Vol. 67, No. 5, (May 2010), pp. 657-666, ISSN 0364-5134

Newton, N.R.; Leonard, C.H.; Piecuch, R.E. & Phibbs, R.H. (1999). Neurodevelopmental outcome of prematurely born children treated with recombinant human erythropoietin in infancy. *Journal of Perinatology,* Vol. 19, No. 6 Pt 1, (September 1999), pp. 403-406, ISSN 0743-8346

Nosarti, C.; Al-Asady, M.H.S.; Frangou, S.; Stewart, A.L.; Rifkin, L. & Murray, R.-M. (2002). Adolescents who were born very preterm have decreased brain volumes. *Brain,* Vol. 125, No. 7, (July 2002), pp. 1616-1623, ISSN 0006-8950

Ohls, R.; Ehrenkranz, R.; Wright, L.; Lemons, J.; Korones, S.; Stoll, B.; Stark, A.; Shankaran, S.; Donovan, E. & Close, N. (2001). Effects of early erythropoietin therapy on the transfusion requirements of preterm infants below 1250 grams birth weight: a multicenter, randomized, controlled trial. *Pediatrics,* Vol. 108, No. 4, (October 2001), pp. 934-942, ISSN 0031-4005

Ohls, R.K.; Ehrenkranz, R.A.; Das, A.; Dusick, A.M.; Yolton, K.; Romano, E.; Delaney-Black, V.; Papile, L.A.; Simon, N.P.; Steichen, J.J. & Lee, K.G. (2004). Neurodevelopmental outcome and growth at 18 to 22 months' corrected age in extremely low birth weight infants treated with early erythropoietin and iron. *Pediatrics,* Vol. 114, No. 5, (November 2004), pp. 1287-1291, ISSN 0031-4005

Ohlsson, A. & Aher, S.M. (2006). Early erythropoietin for preventing red blood cell transfusion in preterm and/or low birth weight infants. *The Cochrane Database of Systematic Reviews,* Vol. 19, No. 3, (July 2006), CD004863, ISSN 1469-493X

Olney, J.W.; Wozniak, D.F.; Jevtovic-Todorovic, V.; Farber, N.B.; Bittigau, P. & Ikonomidou, C. (2002). Drug induced apoptotic neurodegeneration in the developing brain. *Brain Pathology,* Vol. 12, No. 4, (October 2002), pp. 488-498, ISSN 1015-6305

Osredkar, D.; Sall, J.W.; Bickler, P.E. & Ferriero, D.M. (2010). Erythropoietin promotes hippocampal neurogenesis in in vitro models of neonatal stroke. *Neurobiology of Disease,* Vol. 38, No. 2, (May 2010), pp. 259-265, ISSN 0969-9961

Pankratova, S.; Kiryushko, D.; Sonn, K.; Soroka, V.; Kohler, L.B.; Rathje, M.; Gu, B.; Gotfryd, K.; Clausen, O.; Zharkovsky, A.; Bock, E. & Berezin, V. (2010). Neuroprotective properties of a novel, nonhaematopoietic agonist of the erythropoietin receptor. *Brain,* Vol. 133, No. 8, (August 2010), pp. 2281-2294, ISSN 0006-8950

Polster, B.M.; Robertson, C.L.; Bucci, C.J.; Suzuki, M. & Fiskum, G. (2003). Postnatal brain development and neural cell differentiation modulate mitochondrial Bax and BH3 peptide-induced cytochrome c release. *Cell Death and Differentiation,* Vol. 10, No. 3, (March 2003), pp. 365-370, ISSN 1350-9047

Poveshchenko, A.F.; Filimonov, P.N.; Abramov, V.V.; Korotkova, N.A.; Iakushenko, E.V. & Kozlov, V.A. (2001). Expression of erythropoietin receptor mRNA in mouse brain hemispheres. *Tsitologiia,* Vol. 43, No. 3, (2001), pp. 279-283, ISSN 0041-3771

Rabie, T. & Marti, H.H. (2008). Brain protection by erythropoietin: a manifold task. *Physiology,* Vol. 23, No. 5, (October 2008), pp. 263-274, ISSN 1548-9213

Rankin, E.B.; Biju, M.P.; Liu, Q.; Unger, T.L.; Rha, J.; Johnson, R.S.; Simon, M.C.; Keith, B. & Haase, V.H. (2007). Hypoxia-inducible factor-2 (HIF-2) regulates hepatic erythropoietin in vivo. *The Journal of Clinical Investigation,* Vol. 117, No. 4, (April 2007), pp. 1068-1077, ISSN 0021-9738

Reinders, M.E.; Rabelink, T.J. & Briscoe, D.M. (2006). Angiogenesis and endothelial cell repair in renal disease and allograft rejection. *Journal of the American Society of Nephrology,* Vol. 17, No. 4, (April 2006), pp. 932-942, ISSN 1046-6673

Ribatti, D.; Vacca, A.; Roccaro, A.M.; Crivellato, E. & Presta, M. (2003). Erythropoietin as an angiogenic factor. *European Journal of Clinical Investigation,* Vol. 33, No. 10, (October 2003), pp. 891-896, ISSN 0014-2972

Ruscher, K.; Freyer, D.; Karsch, M.; Isaev, N.; Megow, D.; Sawitzki, B.; Priller, J.; Dirnagl, U. & Meisel, A. (2002). Erythropoietin is a paracrine mediator of ischemic tolerance in the brain: evidence from an in vitro model. *The Journal of Neuroscience,* Vol. 22, No. 23, (December 2002), pp. 10291-10301, ISSN 0270-6474

Sakanaka, M.; Wen, T.C.; Matsuda, S.; Masuda, S.; Morishita, E.; Nagao, M. & Sasaki, R. (1998). In vivo evidence that erythropoietin protects neurons from ischemic damage. *Proceedings of the National Academy of Sciences of the United States of America,* Vol. 95, No. 8, (April 1998), pp. 4635-4640, ISSN 0270-6474

Sanchez, P.E.; Navarro, F.P.; Fares, R.P.; Nadam, J.; Georges, B.; Moulin, C.; Le Cavorsin, M.; Bonnet, C.; Ryvlin, P.; Belmeguenai, A.; Bodennec, J.; Morales, A. & Bezin, L. (2009). Erythropoietin receptor expression is concordant with erythropoietin but not with common beta chain expression in the rat brain throughout the life span. *The Journal of Comparative Neurology,* Vol. 514, No. 4, (June 2009), pp. 403-414, ISSN 0021-9967

Saugstad, O.D. (2001). Is oxygen more toxic than currently believed? *Pediatrics,* Vol. 108, No. 5, (November 2001), pp. 1203-1205, ISSN 0031-4005

Shah, N.; Jadav, P.; Jean-Baptiste, D.; Weedon, J.; Cohen, L.M. & Kim, M.R. (2010). The effect of recombinant human erythropoietin on the development of retinopathy of prematurity. *American Journal of Perinatology,* Vol. 27, No. 1, (January 2010), pp. 67-71, ISSN 0735-1631

Shingo, T.; Sorokan, S.T.; Shimazaki, T. & Weiss, S. (2001). Erythropoietin regulates the in vitro and in vivo production of neuronal progenitors by mammalian forebrain neural stem cells. *The Journal of Neuroscience,* Vol. 21, No. 24, (December 2001), pp. 9733-9743, ISSN 0270-6474

Short, E.J.; Klein, N.K.; Lewis, B.A.; Fulton, S.; Eisengart, S.; Kercsmar, C.; Baley, J. & Singer, L.T. (2003). Cognitive and academic consequences of bronchopulmonary dysplasia and very low birth weight: 8-year-old outcomes. *Pediatrics,* Vol. 112, No. 5, (November 2003), pp. e359-366, ISSN 0031-4005

Sifringer, M.; Genz, K.; Brait, D.; Brehmer, F.; Löber, R.; Weichelt, U.; Kaindl, A.M.; Gerstner, B. & Felderhoff-Mueser, U. (2009). Erythropoietin attenuates hyperoxiainduced cell death by modulation of inflammatory mediators and matrix metalloproteinases. *Developmental Neuroscience,* Vol. 31, No. 5, (2009), pp. 394-402, ISSN 0378-5866

Sifringer, M.; Brait, D.; Weichelt, U.; Zimmerman, G.; Endesfelder, S.; Brehmer, F.; von Haefen, C.; Friedman, A.; Soreq, H.; Bendix, I.; Gerstner, B. & Felderhoff-Mueser U. (2010). Erythropoietin attenuates hyperoxia-induced oxidative stress in the developing rat brain. *Brain, Behavior, and Immunity,* Vol. 24, No. 5, (July 2010), pp. 792-799, ISSN 0889-1591

Sirén, A.L.; Fratelli, M.; Brines, M.; Goemans, C.; Casagrande, S.; Lewczuk, P.; Keenan, S.; Gleiter, C.; Pasquali, C.; Capobianco, A.; Mennini, T.; Heumann, R.; Cerami, A.; Ehrenreich, H. & Ghezzi, P. (2001). Erythropoietin prevents neuronal apoptosis after cerebral ischemia and metabolic stress. *Proceedings of the National Academy of Sciences of the United States of America,* Vol. 98, No. 7, (March 2001), pp. 4044-4049, ISSN 0027-8424

Sirén, A.L.; Fasshauer, T.; Bartels, C. & Ehrenreich, H. (2009). Therapeutic potential of erythropoietin and its structural or functional variants in the nervous system. *Neurotherapeutics,* Vol. 6, No. 1, (January 2009), pp. 108-127, ISSN 1933-7213

Solaroglu, I.; Solaroglu, A.; Kaptanoglu, E.; Dede, S.; Haberal, A.; Beskonakli, E. & Kilinc, K. (2003). Erythropoietin prevents ischemia-reperfusion from inducing oxidative damage in fetal rat brain. *Child's Nervous System*, Vol. 19, No. 1, (January 2003), pp. 19-22, ISSN 0256-7040

Spandou, E.; Papoutsopoulou, S.; Soubasi, V.; Karkavelas, G.; Simeonidou, C.; Kremenopoulos, G. & Guiba-Tziampiri, O. (2004a). Hypoxia-ischemia affects erythropoietin and erythropoietin receptor expression pattern in the neonatal rat brain. *Brain Research*, Vol. 1021, No. 2, (September 2004), pp. 167-172, ISSN 0006-8993

Spandou, E.; Soubasi, V.; Papoutsopoulou, S.; Karkavelas, G.; Simeonidou, C.; Kaiki-Astara, A. & Guiba-Tziampiri, O. (2004b). Erythropoietin prevents hypoxia/ischemia-induced DNA fragmentation in an experimental model of perinatal asphyxia. *Neuroscience Letters*, Vol. 366, No. 1, (August 2004), pp. 24-28, ISSN 0304-3940

Spandou, E.; Papadopoulou, Z.; Soubasi, V.; Karkavelas, G.; Simeonidou, C.; Pazaiti, A. & Guiba-Tziampiri, O. (2005). Erythropoietin prevents longterm sensorimotor deficits and brain injury following neonatal hypoxia–ischemia in rats. *Brain Research*, Vol. 1045, No. 1-2, (May 2005), pp. 22-30, ISSN 0006-8993

Statler, P.A.; McPherson, R.J.; Bauer, L.A.; Kellert, B.A. & Juul, S.E. (2007). Pharmacokinetics of high-dose recombinant erythropoietin in plasma and brain of neonatal rats. *Pediatric Research*, Vol. 61, No. 6, (June 2007), pp. 671-675, ISSN 0031-3998

Strunk, T.; Hartel, C. & Schultz, C. (2004). Does erythropoietin protect the preterm brain? *Archives of Disease in Childhood. Fetal and Neonatal Edition*, Vol. 89, No. 4, (July 2004), pp. F364-366, ISSN 1359-2998

Sun, Y.; Calvert, J.W. & Zhang, J.H. (2005). Neonatal hypoxia/ischemia is associated with decreased inflammatory mediators after erythropoietin administration. *Stroke*, Vol. 36, No. 8, (August 2005), pp. 1672-1678, ISSN 0039-2499

Tabira, T.; Konishi, Y. & Gallyas, F.Jr. (1995). Neurotrophic effect of hematopoietic cytokines on cholinergic and other neurons in vitro. *International Journal of Developmental Neuroscience*, Vol. 13, No. 3-4, (June-July 1995), pp. 241-252, ISSN 0736-5748

Tateishi, N.; Higashi, T.; Naruse, A.; Nakashima, K. & Shiozaki, H. (1977). Rat liver glutathione: possible role as a reservoir of cysteine. *The Journal of Nutrition*, Vol. 107, No. 1, (January 1977), pp. 51-60, ISSN 0022-3166

Taylor, D.L.; Edwards, D. & Mehmet, H. (1999). Oxidative metabolism, apoptosis and perinatal brain injury. *Brain Pathology*, Vol. 9, No. 1, (January 1999), pp. 93-117, ISSN 1015-6305

Toyoda, T.; Itai, T.; Arakawa, T.; Aoki, K.H. & Yamaguchi, H. (2000). Stabilization of human recombinant erythropoietin through interactions with the highly branched N-glycans. *Journal of Biochemistry*, Vol. 128, No. 5, (November 2000), pp. 731-737, ISSN 0021-924X

Tsai, P.T.; Ohab, J.J.; Kertesz, N.; Groszer, M.; Matter, C.; Gao, J.; Liu, X.; Wu, H. & Carmichael, S.T. (2006). A critical role of erythropoietin receptor in neurogenesis and post-stroke recovery. *The Journal of Neuroscience*, Vol. 26, No. 4, (January 2006), pp. 1269-1274, ISSN 0270-6474

Uchida, E.; Morimoto, K.; Kawasaki, N.; Izaki, Y.; Abdu Said, A. & Hayakawa, T. (1997). Effect of active oxygen radicals on protein and carbohydrate moieties of recombinant human erythropoietin. *Free Radical Research,* Vol. 27, No. 3, (September 1997), pp. 311-323, ISSN 1071-5762

Vairano, M.; Dello Russo, C.; Bozzoli, G.; Battaglia, A.; Scambia, G.; Tringali, G.; Aloe-Spiriti, M.A.; Preziosi, P. & Navarra, P. (2002). Erythropoietin exerts anti-apoptotic effects on rat microglial cells in vitro. *The European Journal of Neuroscience,* Vol. 16, No. 4, (August 2002), 584-592, ISSN 0953-816X

van der Kooij, M.A.; Groenendaal, F.; Kavelaars, A.; Heijnen, C.J. & van Bel, F. (2008). Neuroprotective properties and mechanisms of erythropoietin in in vitro and in vivo experimental models for hypoxia/ischemia. *Brain Research Reviews,* Vol. 59, No. 1, (November 2008), pp. 22-33, ISSN 0165-0173

Villa, P.; Bigini, P.; Mennini, T.; Agnello, D.; Laragione, T.; Cagnotto, A.; Viviani, B.; Marinovich, M.; Cerami, A.; Coleman, T.R.; Brines, M. & Ghezzi, P. (2003). Erythropoietin selectively attenuates cytokine production and inflammation in cerebral ischemia by targeting neuronal apoptosis. *The Journal of Experimental Medicine,* Vol. 198, No. 6, (September 2003), pp. 971-975, ISSN 0022-1007

Viviani, B.; Bartesaghi, S.; Corsini, E.; Villa, P.; Ghezzi, P.; Garau, A.; Galli, C.L. & Marinovich, M. (2005). Erythropoietin protects primary hippocampal neurons increasing the expression of brain-derived neurotrophic factor. *Journal of Neurochemistry,* Vol. 93, No. 2, (April 2005), pp. 412-421, ISSN 0022-3042

Vohr, B.R.; Wright, L.L.; Dusick, A.M.; Mele, L.; Verter, J.; Steichen, J.J.; Simon, N.P.; Wilson, D.C.; Broyles, S.; Bauer, C.R.; Delaney-Black, V.; Yolton, K.A.; Fleisher, B.E.; Papile, L.A. & Kaplan, M.D. (2000). Neurodevelopmental and functional outcomes of extremely low birth weight infants in the National Institute of Child Health and Human Development Neonatal Research Network 1993–1994. *Pediatrics,* Vol. 105, No. 6, (June 2000), pp. 1216-1226, ISSN 0031-4005

Volpe, J.J. (2009). Brain injury in premature infants: a complex amalgam of destructive and developmental disturbances. *Lancet Neurology,* Vol. 8, No. 1, (January 2009), pp. 110-124, ISSN 1474-4422

Wang, X.Q. & Vaziri, N.D. (1999). Erythropoietin depresses nitric oxide synthase expression by human endothelial cells. *Hypertension,* Vol. 33, No. 3, (March 1999), pp. 894-899, ISSN 0194-911X

Wang, L.; Zhang, Z.G.; Wang, Y.; Zhang, R.L. & Chopp, M. (2004). Treatment of stroke with erythropoietin enhances neurogenesis and angiogenesis and improves neurological function in rats. *Stroke,* Vol. 35, No. 7, (July 2004), pp. 1732-1737, ISSN 0039-2499

Wang, L.; Zhang, Z.G.; Zhang, R.L.; Gregg, S.R.; Hozeska-Solgot, A.; LeTourneau, Y.; Wang, Y. & Chopp, M. (2006). Matrix metalloproteinase 2 (MMP2) and MMP9 secreted by erythropoietin-activated endothelial cells promote neural progenitor cell migration. *The Journal of Neuroscience,* Vol. 26, No. 22, (May 2006), pp. 5996-6003, ISSN 0270-6474

Weber, A.; Maier, R.F.; Hoffmann, U.; Grips, M.; Hoppenz, M.; Aktas, A.G.; Heinemann, U.; Obladen, M. & Schuchmann, S. (2002). Erythropoietin improves synaptic transmission during and following ischemia in rat hippocampal slice cultures. *Brain Research,* Vol. 958, No. 2, (December 2002), pp. 305-311, ISSN 0006-8993

Wen, T.C.; Sadamoto, Y.; Tanaka, J.; Zhu, P.X.; Nakata, K.; Ma, Y.J.; Hata, R. & Sakanaka, M. (2002). Erythropoietin protects neurons against chemical hypoxia and cerebral ischemic injury by up-regulating Bcl-x(L) expression. *Journal of Neuroscience Research,* Vol. 67, No. 6, (March 2002), pp. 795-803, ISSN 0360-4012

Wen, T.C.; Rogido, M.; Genetta, T. & Sola, A. (2004). Permanent focal cerebral ischemia activates erythropoietin receptor in the neonatal rat brain. *Neuroscience Letters,* Vol. 355, No. 3, (January 2004), pp. 165-168, ISSN 0304-3940

Wójtowicz, T. & Mozrzymas, J.W. (2008). Erythropoietin affects GABAergic transmission in hippocampal neurons in vitro. *Cellular & Molecular Biology Letters,* Vol. 13, No. 4, (2008), pp. 649-655, ISSN 1425-8153

Wood, N.S.; Marlow, N.; Costeloe, K.; Gibson, A.T. & Wilkinson, A.R. (2000). Developmental disability after extremely preterm birth. *The New England Journal of Medicine,* Vol. 343, No. 6, (August 2000), pp. 378-384, ISSN 0028-4793

Wu, Y.; Shang, Y.; Sun, S.; Liang, H. & Liu, R. (2007). Erythropoietin prevents PC12 cells from 1-methyl-4-phenylpyridinium ion-induced apoptosis via the Akt/GSK-3beta/caspase-3 mediated signaling pathway. *Apoptosis,* Vol. 12, No. 8, (August 2007), pp. 1365-1375, ISSN 1360-8185

Xiong, Y.; Chopp, M. & Lee, C.P. (2009). Erythropoietin improves brain mitochondrial function in rats after traumatic brain injury. *Neurological Research,* Vol. 31, No. 5, (June 2009), pp. 496-502, ISSN 0161-6412

Yamamoto, M.; Koshimura, K.; Kawaguchi, M.; Sohmiya, M.; Murakami, Y. & Kato, Y. (2000). Stimulating effect of erythropoietin on the release of dopamine and acetylcholine from the rat brain slice. *Neuroscience Letters,* Vol. 292, No. 2, (October 2000), pp. 131-133, ISSN 0304-3940

Yang, Z.; Covey, M.V.; Bitel, C.L.; Ni, L.; Jonakait, G.M. & Levison S.W. (2007). Sustained neocortical neurogenesis after neonatal hypoxic/ischemic injury. *Annals of Neurology,* Vol. 61, No. 3, (March 2007), pp. 199-208, ISSN 0364-5134

Yiş, U.; Kurul, S.H.; Kumral, A.; Tuğyan, K.; Cilaker, S.; Yilmaz, O.; Genç, S. & Genç, K. (2008). Effect of erythropoietin on oxygen-induced brain injury in the newborn rat. *Neuroscience Letters,* Vol. 448, No. 3, (December 2008), pp. 245-249, ISSN 0304-3940

Youssoufian, H.; Longmore, G.; Neumann, D.; Yoshimura, A. & Lodish, H.F. (1993) Structure, function, and activation of the erythropoietin receptor. *Blood,* Vol. 81, No. 9, (May 1993), pp. 2223-2236, ISSN 0006-4971

Zacharias, R.; Schmidt, M.; Kny, J.; Sifringer, M.; Bercker, S.; Bittigau, P.; Bührer, C.; Felderhoff-Müser, U. & Kerner, T. (2010). Dose-dependent effects of erythropoietin in propofol anesthetized neonatal rats. *Brain Research,* Vol. 1343, No., (July 2010), pp. 14-19, ISSN 0006-8993

Zaffanello, M.; Franchini, M. & Rugolotto, S. (2003). Recombinant human erythropoietin might induce strawberry haemangiomas in very-low-birthweight preterm infants. *Acta Paediatrica,* Vol. 92, No. 11, (November 2003), pp. 1353-1354, ISSN 0803-5253

Zanjani, E.D.; Poster, J.; Burlington, H.; Mann, L.I. & Wasserman, L.R. (1977). Liver as the primary site of erythropoietin formation in the fetus. *The Journal of Labaratory and Clinical Medicine,* Vol. 89, No. 3, (March 1977), pp. 640-644, ISSN 0022-2143

Zhang, J.; Randall, M.S.; Loyd, M.R.; Li, W.; Schweers, R.L.; Persons, D.A.; Rehg, J.E.; Noguchi, C.T.; Ihle, J.N. & Ney, P.A. (2006). Role of erythropoietin receptor signaling in Friend virus-induced erythroblastosis and polycythemia. *Blood,* Vol. 107, No. 1, (January 2006), pp. 73-78, ISSN 0006-4971

Zhang, D.; Zhang, F.; Zhang, Y.; Gao, X.; Li, C.; Ma, W. & Cao, K. (2007). Erythropoietin enhances the angiogenic potency of autologous bone marrow stromal cells in a rat model of myocardial infarction. *Cardiology,* Vol. 108, No. 4, (2007), pp. 228-236, ISSN 0008-6312

Zhang, J.; Zhu, Y.; Zhou, D.; Wang, Z. & Chen, G. (2010). Recombinant human erythropoietin (rhEPO) alleviates early brain injury following subarachnoid hemorrhage in rats: possible involvement of Nrf2-ARE pathway. *Cytokine,* Vol. 52, No. 3, (December 2010), pp. 252-257, ISSN 1043-4666

14

Preterm Birth and Long-Term Pulmonary Function

Indra Narang and Amal Al-Naimi
The Division of Respiratory Medicine,
The Hospital for Sick Children, Toronto,
Canada

1. Introduction

1.1 Lung development

To understand the pathophysiology and the outcome of chronic lung disease of infancy, it is essential to understand normal lung development and the host of cofactors that will interfere with both antenatal and postnatal lung development. Lung growth starts in utero and continues to early adolescence going through different phases (Burri, 2006). The embryonic phase, between the 4th and 7th week, begins with the formation of a groove in the ventral lower pharynx and a bud at the lower part of the groove. After further elongation and subdivision of the bud, the two main bronchi are formed. Between the 7th and 16th week of gestation, known as the pseudoglandular phase, the air conducting trees continue to subdivide to form the terminal bronchioles. During the canalicular phase from the 17th to the 26th week of gestation, airway branching is complete with the formation of the primitive saccules. It is also during this phase that the cuboidal epithelium lining the saccules differentiates into type I and type II pneumocytes with concomitant increases in peripheral mesenchyme vascularization. From 27 weeks onwards, during the saccular phase, the lung will begin to prepare for birth with thinning of the connective tissue, secondary septation subdividing the sacculi into smaller subunits or alveoli and the presence of a single capillary layer characteristic of mature alveoli (Hislop et al., 1986; Langston et al., 1984; Post & Copland, 2002). Alveoli continue to increase in number until and beyond birth. At 29 weeks gestation, there are approximately 30 million alveoli and this will increase to some 150 million alveoli by term, one third to half the adult number(Hislop et al., 1986; Langston et al., 1984).

1.2 Chronic lung disease of infancy

Chronic lung disease of infancy (CLDI) is a heterogeneous group of diseases that usually evolves from an acute newborn respiratory disorder. These disorders, such as respiratory distress syndrome secondary to preterm birth, meconium aspiration, sepsis, persistent pulmonary hypertension, congenital heart disease and their subsequent treatments, may predispose the infant to the development of CLDI. Bronchopulmonary dysplasia (BPD), the most significant long-term pulmonary complication of preterm birth (Eber & Zach, 2001) was initially defined as the continued dependence on supplementary oxygen for greater than 28 days postpartum (Northway, 1979). However, BPD has been redefined as we approach a new era of survivors of extreme preterm birth due to important advances in all aspects of neonatal care including surfactant treatment, new ventilator strategies, improved nutrition and other treatments leading an increase in incidence of live preterm birth (Tracy et al., 2007). However, despite these treatments, the overall incidence of BPD has not changed over the past decade (Smith et al., 2005). The 'new BPD' is defined as the need for supplemental oxygen for at least 28 days after birth, and its severity is graded according to the respiratory support required at 36 weeks post-natal age for infants born at gestational ages of less than 32 weeks (Jobe & Bancalari, 2001).

1.3 Pathogenesis of BPD

Old BPD was characterized by diffuse airway damage, alternating areas of overinflation with atelectasis, fibrosis and smooth muscle hypertrophy and prominent vascular hypertensive lesions. Pathologically, the new BPD is different. Unlike the original form of the disease, this 'new' BPD develops in extreme preterm newborns who may have only required minimal ventilator support and low inspired oxygen concentrations during the early postnatal days (Rojas et al., 1995). However, the birth of the extremely immature infant leads to an interruption of alveolarization at a very early stage, with fewer, larger alveoli with subsequent alveolar capillary hypoplasia as a prominent feature. It is important to briefly consider the factors implicated in the pathogenesis of BPD. It is well recognized that those treatments that are necessary for the survival of the preterm infant, such as antenatal steroids, mechanical intermittent positive pressure ventilation (IPPV) and oxygen therapy, may further affect normal pulmonary vascular and alveolar development (Hislop, 1997; Hislop et al., 1987; Rojas et al., 1995). Choriomnoititis, post natal infection and patent ductus arteriosus are also implicated in BPD (Speer, 2006; Watterberg et al., 1996). Abnormalities of gene expression for surfactant synthesis, vascular development and inflammatory regulation are thought to play a role in the development of the new BPD (Bhandari et al., 2006). Although the diagnosis of BPD identifies most patients at increased risk for long-term respiratory sequelae, there is no linear relationship between respiratory support early in life and subsequent respiratory outcome (Greenough, 2006). Indeed, infants with BPD may have a full clinical and functional recovery, and late respiratory symptoms and pulmonary function abnormalities may appear even in young adults who did not require prolonged oxygen supplementation in the neonatal period (Narang et al., 2008).

The aim of this chapter is to review the long-term follow-up of respiratory outcomes in adolescents and adults who were born premature with and without chronic lung disease and will focus on the current available data on respiratory symptoms, pulmonary function, exercise capacity and on structural lung disease. Unless otherwise stated in the manuscript and the tables, all the studies reviewed with BPD subjects refer to the 'old BPD.'

1.4 Long-term respiratory outcome following preterm birth

1.4.1 Respiratory symptoms

1.4.1.1 Childhood

In infancy, there is a wealth of evidence indicating that subjects who are born premature are symptomatic with cough, wheeze and recurrent chest infections in mid-childhood (Chan et al., 1989b; McLeod et al., 1996; Mitchell & Teague, 1998; Palta et al., 2001; Rona et al., 1993) with evidence of an increased rate of hospitalization in the first 2 years of life for a respiratory illness (Mahon et al., 2007).

Multiple studies have been undertaken to look for predictors of wheezing and asthma diagnosis in preterm children (Greenough et al., 2005; Grischkan et al., 2004; Holditch-Davis et al., 2008). Most of these studies were based on questionnaires not validated in preterms with a lack of a universal definition for wheeze and asthma. However, low birth weight per se may predispose to an increased risk of wheeze and lower lung function which may increase the likelihood of a wheezing response to viral infections in early childhood (Greenough et al., 2005; Lewis et al., 1995). Other risk factors for wheeze and asthma in later life in preterm children include male sex (Palta et al., 2001) and African-American ethnicity (Kumar et al., 2008). Despite the increased risk of wheezing in preterms, there is a balance of evidence showing improvement of respiratory symptoms with age.

1.4.1.2 Adolescence and adulthood

See Table 1. Adolescents (defined here as >12 years of age) and young adults, who were preterm either with or without subsequent BPD have excess respiratory symptoms, including cough, wheeze and asthma (Halvorsen et al., 2004; Narang et al., 2008). In one of the oldest studies to date, Northway et al (Northway et al., 1990) studied a group of young adults, mean age 18.3 years (mean birth weight of 1.9kg), with a previous history of BPD. They had a history of more wheezing, episodes of pneumonia and long-term medication use when compared with non-ventilated BPD babies. In one of the most recent studies with longitudinal follow up from childhood to adulthood, preterm infants (mean birth weight of 1.4 kg), the majority of whom had no history of BPD, there was an excess of respiratory symptoms (either cough, wheeze or asthma) compared with controls, 27% vs. 8%, respectively (Narang et al., 2008). Of significance the overall prevalence of respiratory symptoms in this cohort had decreased with time (Narang et al., 2008). Interestingly, the presence of respiratory symptoms did not necessarily translate to abnormal pulmonary function, an increase in the prevalence of airway hyper-responsiveness or an abnormal exercise tolerance (Narang et al., 2008). However, in a recent population-based case-control study, low birth weight (LBW, less than 1500 g, gestational age not given) did translate to increased hospitalization rates in adulthood (Walter et al., 2009). Specifically, LBW adults aged 18–27 years had 83% higher odds of hospitalization for asthma, respiratory infections and respiratory failure as young adults when compared with those who were of normal birth weight (Walter et al., 2009). Similarly, using inhaled corticosteroids (ICS) as a surrogate marker of respiratory symptoms and asthma, a national cohort study in Sweden, found that ICS use increased with the degree of immaturity at birth (Vogt et al., 2011). By contrast, Vrijlandt et al. (Vrijlandt et al., 2006) did not observe an excess of respiratory symptoms, however, the questionnaire focused only on previous and current history of asthma and no recurrent hospitalization data were given. Therefore, the true prevalence of respiratory symptoms may be under-represented in this cohort. It must also be considered that the variability of respiratory symptoms between the studies may be attributed to the use of different definitions. The term 'asthma' is used very imprecisely and furthermost studies do not employ objective cough monitoring (Archer & Simpson, 1985; Falconer et al., 1993; Munyard et al., 1994). Only the international study of asthma and allergies in children (ISAAC) questionnaire (Asher & Weiland, 1998) has been rigorously validated, and the sensitivity, reproducibility and validity of other questionnaires are not known. However, even the use of the ISAAC questionnaire in a preterm population may be debatable since it was not exclusively designed or validated for this unique population.

Author	Age (years)	Number of Subjects	BW (g)	Gestation (weeks)	Number of Controls	Methods	Results
Anand et al.(Anand et al., 2003)	15.0	128 [BPD=8]	1249	30.7	128	Questionnaire	28% had cough# 31% had wheeze# 19% had asthma#
Doyle et al.(Doyle et al., 2006)	18.9	147 [BPD=33]	<1500	<32	37	Use of bronchodilator for wheeze= asthma	22% had asthma#
Halvorsen et al.(Halvorsen et al., 2004)	17.7	46 [BPD=36]	1014	27.3	46	ISAAC Questionnaire	35% had history of asthma#
Narang et al.(Narang et al., 2008)	21.7	60 [BPD=7]	1435	31.5	50	Questionnaire	27% had either cough, wheeze or asthma #
Northway et al.(Northway et al., 1990)	18.3	26 [all BPD]	1894	33.2	26 no-BPD 53 term	Questionnaire	Respiratory symptoms persisted in 23%#
Vrijlandt et al.(Vrijlandt et al., 2006)	19.0	42 [BPD=9]	1246	30.0	48	Questionnaire	No excess history of current asthma
Wong et al.(Wong et al., 2008)	19.0	21 [all BPD]	895	27 (24-30)	None	Questionnaire	71% had either wheeze/cough/ SOB

BW=birth weight; g =grams; BPD = bronchopulmonary dysplasia; SOB = shortness of breath.
All values are mean unless otherwise indicated. # Increased when compared with controls.

Table 1. Studies in adolescence seeking associations between prematurity and subsequent reported respiratory symptoms.

1.4.2 Pulmonary function

1.4.2.1 Childhood

In infants, Friedrich and colleagues using the raised volume rapid thoracic compression (RVRTC) technique showed that even healthy asymptomatic preterm infants have low expiratory flows with normal expired volume measured from a point near total lung capacity to residual volume, thus suggesting that lung growth is proportional to somatic growth in preterm infants (Fawke et al., 2010). The low expiratory flow measurements observed in these preterm infants is thought to be secondary to improper airway development and a reduction in airway caliber secondary to inflammation and/or airway thickening (Friedrich et al., 2006). In childhood, several studies have now documented abnormal pulmonary function in those born preterm, with evidence of significant airflow obstruction, with the mean forced expired volume in 1 second (FEV_1) values between 70% and 80% of the predicted levels (Baraldi et al., 1991; Chan et al., 1990; McLeod et al., 1996; Mitchell & Teague, 1998). Recently, the extremely premature infant cure (EPICure) study assessed pulmonary function in children at an average age of 11 years following preterm birth. They found that preterms compared to controls had higher residual volume (RV) and RV/total lung capacity (TLC), lower FEV_1 and lower forced vital capacity (FVC) z scores compared with controls, the effect being more pronounced in preterms with a history of BPD compared with those preterms without a history of BPD (Fawke et al., 2010).

Author	Age (years)	Number of Subjects	BW (g)	Gestation (weeks)	Number of Controls	Methods	Results	Significance
Anand et al. (Anand et al., 2003)	15	128 [BPD=8]	1249	30.7	128	Spirometry	FVC % = 109.5 FEV_1 % = 94.9 $FEF_{25-75\%}$ % = 88.1# FEV_1/FVC % = 87.0#	#p<0.001 compared to controls
Doyle et al. (Doyle et al., 2006)	18.9	147 [BPD=33]	<1500	<32	37	Spirometry Lung volumes	BPD group data only FVC % = 98.4 FEV_1 % = 81.6#$ $FEF_{25-75\%}$ % = 57.5$ FEV_1/FVC % = 73.9#$ RV % = 108.7 TLC % = 99.6	#p< 0.05 compared to controls $ p<0.05 compared to no-BPD group
Halvorsen et al. (Halvorsen et al., 2004)	17.7	46 [BPD=36]	1014	27.3	46	Spirometry Plethysmography	Data for the moderate to severe BPD group FVC % = 101.0 FEV_1 % = 87.8 $FEF_{75\%}$ % = 78.4# RV % = 123.5 TLC % = 108.3	#p< 0.001 compared to controls
Narang et al. (Narang et al., 2008)	21.7	60 [BPD=7]	1435	31.5	50	Spirometry	FVC % = 96.4 FEV_1 % = 92.6 $FEF_{25-75\%}$ % = 78.6	p=NS compared to controls
Northway et al. (Northway et al., 1990)	18.3	26 [all BPD]	1894	33.2	26 no-BPD 53 term	Spirometry Plethysmography	FVC % =96.8# FEV_1 % = 74.8#$ $FEF_{25-75\%}$ % = 46.5#$ TLC % = 108.6	#p< 0.01 compared to controls $ p<0.01 compared to no-BPD group
Vrijlandt et al.(Vrijlandt et al., 2006)	19.0	42 [BPD=9]	1246	30.0	48	Spirometry Whole body plethysmography	FVC % = 97.7# FEV_1 % = 95.4# $FEF_{75\%}$ % = 75.3# FEV_1/FVC % = 82.2# RV % = 99.4 TLC % = 100.1	#p<0.01 compared to controls
Wong et al.(Wong et al., 2008)	20.3	21 [all BPD]	895	27	None	Spirometry Lung volumes	FVC % = N/A FEV_1 % = 89.0 $FEF_{25-75\%}$ % = 63.7 RV % = 95.8 TLC % = 106	

All values are mean data unless otherwise indicated. Unless otherwise stated, the spirometry data given are for the entire pre-term cohort. All spirometry values shown are % predicted unless otherwise indicated. BW, birth weight; g, grams; BPD, bronchopulmonary dysplasia; FVC, forced vital capacity; FEV_1, forced expired volume in one second; $FEF_{25-75\%}$, forced expiratory flow at 25-75% of forced vital capacity; $FEF_{75\%}$, forced expiratory flow at 75% of forced vital capacity; NS, non-significant; RV, residual volume; TLC, total lung capacity.

Table 2. Lung function in adolescence and adulthood following preterm birth.

Many studies have now observed that the main risk factors cited for impaired lung function in ex-preterm children are intermittent positive pressure ventilation (IPPV), prolonged oxygen therapy, male sex and maternal smoking (Chan et al., 1990; McLeod et al., 1996; Mitchell & Teague, 1998).

1.4.2.2 Adolescence and adulthood

There are fewer studies that have now documented pulmonary function in adolescence and adulthood (see Table 2). Furthermore, there is a paucity of relevant longitudinal data. Whether 'catch-up' growth of pulmonary function occurs from mid-childhood to adulthood is highly debated. In the longest follow-up to date, Northway and colleagues (Northway et al., 1990) found that the mean percentage predicted FEV_1, FVC and forced mid-expiratory flow at 25% to 75% of FVC (FEF_{25-75}) were significantly lower in the BPD group compared with the preterm and term controls. BPD was considered the major risk factor for reduced airflow as there was no apparent association with neonatal variables. However, the small numbers of subjects, relatively high birth weights (mean > 1800 g) and maturity (mean gestational age >33 weeks) in the BPD preterm groups may have resulted in the lack of any association. It must also be borne in mind that in the present day, those considered to be at high risk of respiratory morbidity probably did not survive in the late 1960s. In more recent studies in adolescents, Anand and colleagues after adjusting for self-reported smoking both in the subjects and their mothers, found a reduction in FEF_{25-75} in their very low birth weight group (defined as less than 1500 g) compared with the controls, suggesting distal airflow obstruction (Friedrich et al., 2006). However, distal airflow obstruction was not associated with either low birth weight, respiratory support or BPD; the key risk factor cited was preterm birth per se (Friedrich et al., 2006). Interestingly, Halvorsen and colleagues (Halvorsen et al., 2004) also observed a lower FEV_1 when compared with controls, with the discrepancies in pulmonary function increasing significantly with the increasing severity of BPD. Doyle and colleagues (Doyle et al., 2006) found that pulmonary function was mostly normal in the three groups they studied, term, preterms with BPD and preterms without BPD. However, a significantly greater proportion of children with BPD compared with those preterm children without BPD had a clinically important reduction in their mean percentage predicted FEV_1 (81.6 and 92.9, respectively) and FEV_1/FVC ratios (73.9 and 83.2, respectively). It should be noted that the mean percentage predicted FEF_{25-75} in the Doyle study was lower than that of the preterm group studied by Anand et al (Anand et al., 2003). The different conclusions may be due to the different reference values used, again underscoring the need for appropriate controls. Similarly, Vrijlandt and colleagues (Vrijlandt et al., 2006) demonstrated pulmonary function values that were within normal range in their expreterm population, most of whom did not have BPD. However, the percentage predicted values of FVC, FEV_1 and FEV_1/FVC were lower than that in the controls, the majority of who were medical students, which might select for a healthier and higher socioeconomic class population and reflect the results observed. In a more recent study and one of the largest longitudinal follow-up studies from birth to adulthood, there was evidence of airway obstruction in children aged 7–9 years (Chan et al., 1989b). This same cohort in adulthood did not show any significant differences between FEV_1, FVC and FEF_{25-75} when compared with controls, implying catch-up growth (Narang et al., 2008). The authors were also able to show some evidence of tracking, in that mid childhood spirometry was predictive of adult values (relationship between z scores for FEV_1 in childhood and adulthood was $p < 0.001$ and $r^2 = 0.34$) (Narang et al., 2008). However, the low incidence of

BPD and maternal smokers, both risk factors for poorer airway function, may have created a bias towards improved airway function in adulthood (Northway et al., 1990).

1.4.3 Airway Hyperresponsiveness (AHR)

1.4.3.1 Childhood

Atopy and AHR are thought to be associated, even in asymptomatic subjects (Boulet et al., 1983; Sears et al., 1991). It is debated whether AHR, which was repeatedly reported to occur in long-term survivors of BPD, is a consequence of BPD or contributes to the pathophysiology of BPD in genetically predisposed patients following preterm birth (Northway et al., 1990; Wohl, 1995). In one study reported baseline spirometry was significantly reduced in BPD and non-BPD groups compared with term controls, and the provocative dose of histamine to cause a 15% fall in FEV_1 (PD15) was lower in the BPD compared with the non-BPD preterm group (Pelkonen et al., 1997). There was a strong association between respiratory symptoms and AHR (Chan et al., 1989a). In young adults with a history of BPD, AHR was more prevalent in the BPD than the ex-preterm no-BPD population and further, AHR was not related to respiratory symptoms, atopy, or a family history of asthma (Northway et al., 1990). In the Hammersmith cohort, increased AHR was seen in 71% of the index study group, compared with 43% of controls ($p<0.01$) (Chan et al., 1989a). There was a significant association between a personal or family history of asthma and increased AHR in both the index study group and controls and further, for the index study group, there was also an association between AHR and duration of oxygen treatment (Chan et al., 1989a). Increased AHR in the index study group was also observed more in those subjects with a positive skin-prick test to house dust mite, grass pollens, or cat fur ($p<0.01$), although skin-prick tests were not performed in the control group (Chan et al., 1989a). However, to elucidate the pathophysiological basis for the increased prevalence of AHR in the index study group, 35 of the mothers of the index study group also underwent a histamine challenge. Using the same protocol, 8.6% of mothers of the index study group had a PD15 (using histamine) of 3.9 mmol, which was similar to the 10.5% reported in an adult population using the same methods to determine AHR. In a second study, 15 subjects participated in a double-blind, placebo controlled, crossover design with 4-week-long treatment periods with inhaled steroids or placebo. There was no significant difference in respiratory symptom score, baseline airway function, or airway response to histamine between the two treatment periods. From these studies, the authors concluded that abnormal AHR was related to abnormal pulmonary development and not to an effect of chronic inflammation or maternal factors. However, the authors assumed that any preexisting inflammation would be steroid-sensitive, which may not necessarily be true.

1.4.3.2 Adolescence and adulthood

There are very few studies assessing AHR in ex-preterm adolescents and young adults. In a longitudinal follow up study involving 52 subjects from the Hammersmith cohort (Chan et al., 1989a), there was no significant difference in the prevalence of AHR in the index study group compared with controls (23% vs 19% respectively, p=NS). The finding of a decrease in AHR prevalence in this study is similar to that of a larger longitudinal study with more than 800 subjects, in which AHR declined from childhood to adolescence, paralleling the increase in lung function during this period (Forastiere et al., 1996).

1.4.4 Exercise capacity

Because cardiopulmonary limitations may not be clinically evident while the child is at rest, exercise testing may be useful in children born preterm and who developed BPD to determine the presence and extent of any dysfunction of gas exchange secondary to alveolar growth impairment. During exercise, cardiac output may increase fivefold as a result of increases in both heart rate and stroke volume; minute ventilation may increase 25-fold in healthy individuals, depending on the intensity of the exercise. Carbon monoxide transfer (DL_{CO}) increases by up to 50% during exercise, because of recruitment and distension of the pulmonary capillaries, particularly in the upper parts of the lung. Maximum oxygen consumption (VO_2 max) is the best index for aerobic capacity and is the gold standard for cardiorespiratory fitness (ATS/ACCP, 2003). It is related to oxygen availability and provides information regarding aerobic metabolism in response to exercise stress.

1.4.4.1 Childhood

During mid-childhood, there are conflicting data regarding exercise performance in ex-preterm children. Some have demonstrated normal exercise ability (Baraldi et al., 1991; Jacob et al., 1997; Northway et al., 1990) while others have shown abnormal cardiopulmonary responses to exercise (Bader et al., 1987; Mitchell & Teague, 1998). Some explanations for the variability seen between these studies include different methods of exercise testing, differing exercise protocols and variation in the motivation of study subjects. The EPIcure study demonstrated that ex-preterm subjects had baseline lower tidal volumes, lower oxygen consumption, lower anaerobic threshold, lower minute ventilation and 20% lower workload; however, these changes were not associated with a significant reduction in oxygen saturation but were associated with an increased likelihood of self-reported difficulties in breathing during exercise (Welsh et al., 2010).

1.4.4.2 Adolescence and adulthood

See Table 3. In the only adult study to date that has assessed both exercise performance as well as gas transfer at both rest and exercise (using an incremental protocol and a cycle ergometer), there were no significant differences in exercise capacity between the ex-preterm subjects and controls (Narang et al., 2009). Interestingly, the main abnormal findings were that ex-preterm subjects in adulthood had reduced DL_{CO} and effective pulmonary blood flow (Qpeff) at rest, which normalized during exercise and was again reduced after a recovery period. These results do not suggest true alveolar capillary hypoplasia as DL_{CO} was appropriate for Qpeff (Narang et al., 2009). Vrijlandt et al. in their study of 42 adults reported resting and exercise data also using an incremental protocol with a cycle ergometer (Vrijlandt et al., 2006). They too found a significantly low DL_{CO} at rest compared with controls, 88% and 96% predicted, respectively ($p = 0.003$). However, the DL_{CO} values were not corrected for Qpeff or body surface area, both important determinants of DL_{CO}, and significantly, there were no DL_{CO} measurements undertaken during exercise or during recovery, thus posing difficulties with the interpretation of these results. Furthermore, this ex-preterm group reached a 15% lower workload than healthy peers; however, closer analyses of the results suggest that the ex-preterm subjects may have muscular deconditioning accounting for these results (Vogt et al., 2011). Indeed, these ex-preterms also reported fewer hours of exercise per week than the control subjects, which might explain their lower level of fitness (Vogt et al., 2011). In a group of adolescents assessed at 17 years of age using a step test and muscle strength tests, there were significant differences in motor performance in the

Author	Age (years)	Number of subjects	BW (g)	Gestation (weeks)	Number of controls	Methods	Results
Narang et al.(Narang et al., 2009)	21.7	60 [BPD=7]	1435	31.5	50	1) VO_2 max using cycle ergometer 2) Acetylene rebreathing to determine Qpeff.	No difference in exercise capacity between ex-preterm subjects and controls. Decreased DL_{co} compared to controls but normal DL_{co} during exercise.
Vrijlandt et al.(Vrijlandt et al., 2006)	19.0	42 [BPD=9]	1246	30.0	48	1) Incremental exercise test using cycle ergometer	Wmax 15% lower in ex-preterms. Decreased DLco compared to controls.
Rogers et al.(Rogers et al., 2005)	17.3	53	720	26	31	1) Step test 2) Muscle strength tests 3) Activity-lead questionnaire	Decreased aerobic capacity, muscle strength and activity level.

BW, birthweight; g, grams; BPD, bronchopulmonary dysplasia; VO2 max, maximum oxygen consumption; Qpeff, effective pulmonary blood flow; DLco, transfer factor for carbon monoxide; Wmax, maximum workload. All values are mean data unless otherwise indicated.

Table 3. Exercise capacity in adolescents and adulthood following preterm birth.

ex-preterm group compared with healthy term subjects reflected in aerobic capacity, strength, endurance, flexibility, and activity level (Rogers et al., 2005). However, similar to the study by Vrijlandt et al., the differences in fitness and physical activity were possibly related to the interaction of effects of preterm birth on the motor system, together with a more inactive lifestyle (Vrijlandt et al., 2006). Burns and colleagues (Burns et al., 2009) compared 54 non-disabled ex-preterms aged 11-13 years (mean birth weight of 769 grams and mean gestational age of 26.6 weeks) with 55 children born at term. Ex-preterm adolescents had significantly lower motor coordination, 72.2% compared with 21.8% of the control group (Vogt et al., 2011). VO_2 max calculated from a 20m Shuttle Run test, was lower in the ex-preterm group compared with the controls ($p = 0.001$).

1.5 Structural lung disease

In 1967, Northway based his BPD description on chest x-rays giving chest imaging a central role in diagnosing BPD. However, despite that, there is still a lack information in regards to structural abnormalities in ex-preterm children and adults with and without BPD (See Table 4). High resolution computed tomography (HRCT) images of the chest have been reported to be abnormal and thus useful in the diagnosis of BPD (Howling et al., 2000; Oppenheim et al., 1994). In one cohort of children with a median age of 10 years, 20/26 (77%) of the subjects had reduced lung attenuation (Aquino et al., 1999). The children had abnormalities of pulmonary function, which we now understand to be associated with BPD (median FEV_1 was 64% predicted) which correlates with abnormal HRCT findings. Aukland et al. studied HRCT images in 72 ex-preterm subjects which included two birth cohorts, children (mean age 10 years) and adults (mean age 18 years) (Aukland et al., 2006). Their main abnormal findings were linear and triangular opacities, gas trapping and mosaic perfusion, especially in the 56/72 (78%) survivors with severe BPD, which represented subjects with old and new BPD (Aukland et al., 2006). No subject had evidence of emphysema. The same authors also demonstrated a reduction in FEV_1 in subjects with a high HRCT chest score (Wong et al., 2008). Subjects with hypoattenuation had a lower FEV_1 than those without hypoattenuation (mean FEV_1 80.9% vs. 89.8%, respectively) (Aukland et al., 2006). Increased number of days with oxygen treatment also predicted an increase in the total HRCT score (Wong et al., 2008). In a more recent study of adults only, all with a previous history of BPD, simultaneous pulmonary function and HRCT chest evaluation was undertaken (Wong et al., 2008). The main abnormal finding, observed in 84% of the subjects, was the presence of emphysema, the severity of which also correlated with abnormal z scores for FEV_1 in this population ($p < 0.001$and $r^2 = 0.50$) (Baraldi et al., 1991). Other HRCT abnormalities included architectural distortion, bronchial wall thickening and gas trapping. The presence of emphysema could not be predicted by perinatal or postnatal factors or a personal history of smoking. The differences in the findings with the study by Aukland et al. (Aukland et al., 2006) may be attributed to the fact that the study by Wong et al. (Wong et al., 2008) represents a group of adults who were highly selected, constituting 19 subjects (14%) with severe perinatal disease from the original cohort of 133 subjects. These subjects all had moderate/severe BPD compared to the other studies that had included ex-preterm subjects with no or mild BPD. The lack of correlation with perinatal factors may be due to the fact that perinatal factors become less important with age or simply that the study was under-powered to seek such associations. However, what is clear is that structural abnormalities, as determined by HRCT scans, do exist in an ex-preterm population, even in the absence of overt clinical disease. More intriguing is the association of radiological findings with perinatal data. Further studies are required to delineate factors, perinatal or otherwise, that impact on the structure of the immature lungs.

Author	Age (years)	Number of subjects	BW (g)	Gestation (weeks)	Methods	Results
Wong et al.(Wong et al., 2008)	19.0	19 [all BPD]	895	27	Expiratory and inspiratory HRCT chest	84% had emphysema 36% had gas trapping 42% had bronchial wall thickening
Aquino et al.(Aquino et al., 1999)	5-18	26	900	28	Expiratory and inspiratory HRCT chest	77% reduced lung attenuation 92% had gas trapping
Auckland et al. (Aukland et al., 2006; Aukland et al., 2009)	40 adults (Age 18.0) 32 children (Age 10.0)	72 [BPD=56]	991	27.2	Expiratory and inspiratory HRCT chest	72% linear capacity 58% triangular capacity 26% gas trapping 13% mosaic perfusion 10% bronchiectasis * Higher (abnormal) HRCT significantly associated with increased number of days with oxygen treatment.

BW, birthweight; g, grams; BPD, bronchopulmonary dysplasia; HRCT, high resolution computed tomography. All values are mean data unless otherwise indicated.

Table 4. Studies assessing structural lung disease in adolescence and adulthood following preterm birth.

2. Summary and implications

Following preterm birth, there is evidence for respiratory symptoms in infancy and childhood. While these symptoms do improve with time, the evidence does suggest that respiratory symptoms in ex-preterm subjects remain prevalent in adulthood. With regards to pulmonary function, the studies suggest evidence for catch-up growth and normalization of pulmonary function from childhood to adulthood in ex-preterm subjects without BPD. However, pulmonary function abnormalities appear to persist in those who had a more severe neonatal course and who had a diagnosis of BPD. Exercise capacity, although not overtly abnormal, may be affected by the reduced physical activity levels of ex-preterm subjects. It is postulated that the reduced DL_{CO} at rest observed in the studies may suggest the prolonged influence of antenatal programming (Narang et al., 2009). Certainly, pulmonary circulatory abnormalities have been observed in adult subjects with a transient history of lung injury secondary to persistent fetal circulation in the neonatal period (Sartori et al., 1999). These subjects, with normal pulmonary artery pressure at rest, demonstrated an exaggerated pulmonary artery pressure increase at high altitude compared with controls (Sartori et al., 1999). Structural lung disease, as determined by HRCT scans are prevalent in these subjects and further, are associated with pulmonary function abnormalities. What are the likely explanations for the respiratory morbidity of ex-preterm subjects in adulthood? It is certainly likely to be multifactorial. It is plausible that there is sustained vulnerability of the airways secondary to a host of factors related to preterm birth. Additionally, there is disruption of normal lung development as a result of preterm birth and the subsequent adaptation to extra-uterine life. This adverse disruption may be exacerbated by perinatal factors, particularly prolonged oxygen requirement and subsequent development of BPD, both of which have been identified as causal in functional and structural respiratory sequelae. It is unclear how oxygen mediates these effects. The prolonged use of oxygen in this vulnerable population may represent the final common pathway of a cascade of events related to preterm birth and lung injury. Alternatively, neonatal factors such as oxygen therapy become less important and it is possible that a host of environmental influences such as smoking dominate on more vulnerable airways. However, while it is virtually impossible to unpick the relationship between the environment, perinatal factors and prematurity on adulthood respiratory function, other investigators have demonstrated that BPD infants are particularly susceptible to lower respiratory illnesses in childhood and that these may be related to chronic airflow obstruction in adulthood (Samet et al., 1983). The improvement in pulmonary function observed may be a result of increased lung volumes as seen with somatic growth or indeed physiologic remodeling of the airway. Or could it simply be that the studies describing apparent normalization of lung function do not truly reflect 'catch-up' of lung growth? Perhaps, the results merely reflect decreased sensitivity of spirometry in this age group. Spirometry has long been known to be insensitive to distal airway obstruction until the very late phases. Sophisticated methods to assess lung ventilation and lung growth, such as the lung clearance index (LCI), a marker of ventilation inhomogeneity, may be necessary to provide more accurate information (Aurora et al., 2005). However, in one recent study assessing lung function using both spirometry and LCI in ex-preterm children aged 11 years, spirometry was more discriminative than LCI in detecting pulmonary function abnormalities (Lum et al., 2011). Recently, hyperpolarised gas MRI has demonstrated regional ventilation abnormalities in young cystic fibrosis patients with normal lung function (Bannier et al., 2010) and is known to be particularly sensitive to early changes in emphysema (Yablonskiy et al., 2009). Perhaps, the non-invasive longitudinal assessment of lung growth with the use of labeled carbon monoxide (Rosenthal & Bush, 1998; Rosenthal & Bush, 1999) and hyperpolarized gases in magnetic resonance may provide further answers with regard to lung growth and ventilation abnormalities (Eberle et al., 2001).

3. Chronic lung disease of prematurity and chronic obstructive pulmonary disease in adulthood

It is important to consider the long-term implications of abnormal functional and structural lung disease for survivors of preterm birth in adulthood. Specifically, is BPD a significant risk factor for chronic obstructive pulmonary disease (COPD)? It has long been hypothesized that COPD has its origin in fetal life (Stein et al., 1997). Additional childhood risk factors for COPD in adulthood include maternal smoking, maternal genetics, history of asthma, respiratory infections, environmental pollution and childhood nutrition (Bush, 2008; Franssen et al., 2008; Stein et al., 1997). Similarly, poorer lung function in ex-BPD subjects is associated with childhood respiratory infections and asthma. Indeed, BPD and COPD share some similar pathophysiological features; both disorders are subject to oxidant stress, inflammation and accelerated cell death resulting in complex distal lung injury. Although there are no studies evaluating lung function in BPD subjects in old age, BPD and subsequent impaired pulmonary function in adulthood, whether latent or overt, could result in an accelerated decline in ventilatory reserve that could further increase the risk of COPD like phenotype in later life. Loss of pulmonary function may be further accelerated in smokers as smoking is a well-known risk factor for a steeper age-related decline in pulmonary function and subsequent emphysema (Fletcher & Peto, 1977). The high prevalence of emphysema observed in HRCT scans in one study (Wong et al., 2008) is of greater concern given that up to 50% of preterm survivors smoke in adulthood (Doyle et al., 2006; Narang et al., 2008).

Thus it would not be unreasonable to assume that survivors of preterm birth are likely to be a cohort of subjects prone to COPD. Hence until preterm birth and its complications cease to be a problem, the prevalence of COPD or COPD like phenotype is likely to increase in the next few decades.

4. Conclusions and future directions

The respiratory sequelae associated with preterm birth can no longer be a cause for concern just for pediatricians. Adult physicians will need to become increasingly aware of the long-term consequences of preterm birth, with recognition of both functional and structural lung disease associated with prematurity, as a reduced respiratory reserve could increase the risk of a COPD-like phenotype in later life. Further, because impaired airway function in adult life is an important and independent indicator of mortality risk (Barker et al., 1991), continued surveillance of these subjects into late adulthood, particularly of the active smokers, will be vital. Finally, as the etiology of chronic lung disease of prematurity remains elusive, the burden of chronic lung disease in infancy, childhood and adulthood both to the individual and in health care resources is significantly high. Thus, large long-term longitudinal studies are urgently required with subjects recruited antenatally not only to evaluate structural and functional lung disease but also to delineate the pathogenesis, diagnosis and subsequent clinical management of lung disease of prematurity, specifically the 'new BPD.' However, future research must not be unifocal. We now understand that there is no linear relationship between neonatal factors and subsequent respiratory sequelae and that prematurity in the absence of both neonatal disease and treatments may result in long-term respiratory morbidity. Therefore, the ultimate priority for future research must be to determine preventative factors to diminish preterm birth.

5. References

ATS/ACCP. (2003). ATS/ACCP Statement on cardiopulmonary exercise testing. *American Journal of Respiratory and Critical Care Medicine,* 167, 2, (Jan 15), pp. 211-77, 1073-449X (Print) 1073-449X (Linking)

Anand, D., Stevenson, C.J., West, C.R. & Pharoah, P.O. (2003). Lung function and respiratory health in adolescents of very low birth weight. *Archives of Disease in Childhood,* 88, 2, (Feb), pp. 135-8, 1468-2044 (Electronic) 0003-9888 (Linking)

Aquino, S.L., Schechter, M.S., Chiles, C., Ablin, D.S., Chipps, B. & Webb, W.R. (1999). High-resolution inspiratory and expiratory CT in older children and adults with bronchopulmonary dysplasia. *AJR. American Journal of Roentgenology,* 173, 4, (Oct), pp. 963-7, 0361-803X (Print) 0361-803X (Linking)

Archer, L.N. & Simpson, H. (1985). Night cough counts and diary card scores in asthma. *Archives of Disease in Childhood,* 60, 5, (May), pp. 473-4, 1468-2044 (Electronic) 0003-9888 (Linking)

Asher, M.I. & Weiland, S.K. (1998). The International Study of Asthma and Allergies in Childhood (ISAAC). ISAAC Steering Committee. *Clinical and Experimental Allergy,* 28 Suppl 5, (Nov), pp. 52-66; discussion 90-1, 0954-7894 (Print) 0954-7894 (Linking)

Aukland, S.M., Halvorsen, T., Fosse, K.R., Daltveit, A.K. & Rosendahl, K. (2006). High-resolution CT of the chest in children and young adults who were born prematurely: findings in a population-based study. *AJR. American Journal of Roentgenology,* 187, 4, (Oct), pp. 1012-8, 1546-3141 (Electronic) 0361-803X (Linking)

Aukland, S.M., Rosendahl, K., Owens, C.M., Fosse, K.R., Eide, G.E. & Halvorsen, T. (2009). Neonatal bronchopulmonary dysplasia predicts abnormal pulmonary HRCT scans in long-term survivors of extreme preterm birth. *Thorax,* 64, 5, (May), pp. 405-10, 1468-3296 (Electronic) 0040-6376 (Linking)

Aurora, P., Bush, A., Gustafsson, P., Oliver, C., Wallis, C., Price, J., Stroobant, J., Carr, S. & Stocks, J. (2005). Multiple-breath washout as a marker of lung disease in preschool children with cystic fibrosis. *American Journal of Respiratory and Critical Care Medicine,* 171, 3, (Feb 1), pp. 249-56, 1073-449X (Print) 1073-449X (Linking)

Bader, D., Ramos, A.D., Lew, C.D., Platzker, A.C., Stabile, M.W. & Keens, T.G. (1987). Childhood sequelae of infant lung disease: exercise and pulmonary function abnormalities after bronchopulmonary dysplasia. *Journal of Pediatrics,* 110, 5, (May), pp. 693-9, 0022-3476 (Print) 0022-3476 (Linking)

Bannier, E., Cieslar, K., Mosbah, K., Aubert, F., Duboeuf, F., Salhi, Z., Gaillard, S., Berthezene, Y., Cremillieux, Y. & Reix, P. (2010). Hyperpolarized 3He MR for sensitive imaging of ventilation function and treatment efficiency in young cystic fibrosis patients with normal lung function. *Radiology,* 255, 1, (Apr), pp. 225-32, 1527-1315 (Electronic) 0033-8419 (Linking)

Baraldi, E., Zanconato, S., Zorzi, C., Santuz, P., Benini, F. & Zacchello, F. (1991). Exercise performance in very low birth weight children at the age of 7-12 years. *European Journal of Pediatrics,* 150, 10, (Aug), pp. 713-6, 0340-6199 (Print) 0340-6199 (Linking)

Barker, D.J., Godfrey, K.M., Fall, C., Osmond, C., Winter, P.D. & Shaheen, S.O. (1991). Relation of birth weight and childhood respiratory infection to adult lung function and death from chronic obstructive airways disease. *BMJ,* 303, 6804, (Sep 21), pp. 671-5, 0959-8138 (Print) 0959-535X (Linking)

Bhandari, V., Bizzarro, M.J., Shetty, A., Zhong, X., Page, G.P., Zhang, H., Ment, L.R. & Gruen, J.R. (2006). Familial and genetic susceptibility to major neonatal morbidities in preterm twins. *Pediatrics,* 117, 6, (Jun), pp. 1901-6, 1098-4275 (Electronic) 0031-4005 (Linking)

Boulet, L.P., Cartier, A., Thomson, N.C., Roberts, R.S., Dolovich, J. & Hargreave, F.E. (1983). Asthma and increases in nonallergic bronchial responsiveness from seasonal pollen exposure. *Journal of Allergy and Clinical Immunology,* 71, 4, (Apr), pp. 399-406, 0091-6749 (Print) 0091-6749 (Linking)

Burns, Y.R., Danks, M., O'Callaghan, M.J., Gray, P.H., Cooper, D., Poulsen, L. & Watter, P. (2009). Motor coordination difficulties and physical fitness of extremely-low-birthweight children. *Developmental Medicine and Child Neurology,* 51, 2, (Feb), pp. 136-42, 1469-8749 (Electronic) 0012-1622 (Linking)

Burri, P.H. (2006). Structural aspects of postnatal lung development - alveolar formation and growth. *Biology of the Neonate,* 89, 4, pp. 313-22, 0006-3126 (Print) 0006-3126 (Linking)

Bush, A. (2008). COPD: a pediatric disease. *COPD,* 5, 1, (Feb), pp. 53-67, 1541-2555 (Print) 1541-2563 (Linking)

Chan, K.N., Wong, Y.C. & Silverman, M. (1990). Relationship between infant lung mechanics and childhood lung function in children of very low birthweight. *Pediatric Pulmonology,* 8, 2, pp. 74-81, 8755-6863 (Print) 1099-0496 (Linking)

Chan, K.N., Elliman, A., Bryan, E. & Silverman, M. (1989a). Clinical significance of airway responsiveness in children of low birthweight. *Pediatric Pulmonology,* 7, 4, pp. 251-8, 8755-6863 (Print) 1099-0496 (Linking)

Chan, K.N., Elliman, A., Bryan, E. & Silverman, M. (1989b). Respiratory symptoms in children of low birth weight. *Archives of Disease in Childhood,* 64, 9, (Sep), pp. 1294-304, 1468-2044 (Electronic) 0003-9888 (Linking)

Doyle, L.W., Faber, B., Callanan, C., Freezer, N., Ford, G.W. & Davis, N.M. (2006). Bronchopulmonary dysplasia in very low birth weight subjects and lung function in late adolescence. *Pediatrics,* 118, 1, (Jul), pp. 108-13, 1098-4275 (Electronic) 0031-4005 (Linking)

Eber, E. & Zach, M.S. (2001). Long term sequelae of bronchopulmonary dysplasia (chronic lung disease of infancy). *Thorax,* 56, 4, (Apr), pp. 317-23, 0040-6376 (Print) 0040-6376 (Linking)

Eberle, B., Markstaller, K., Schreiber, W.G. & Kauczor, H.U. (2001). Hyperpolarised gases in magnetic resonance: a new tool for functional imaging of the lung. *Swiss Med Wkly,* 131, 35-36, (Sep 8), pp. 503-9, 1424-7860 (Print) 0036-7672 (Linking)

Falconer, A., Oldman, C. & Helms, P. (1993). Poor agreement between reported and recorded nocturnal cough in asthma. *Pediatric Pulmonology,* 15, 4, (Apr), pp. 209-11, 8755-6863 (Print) 1099-0496 (Linking)

Fawke, J., Lum, S., Kirkby, J., Hennessy, E., Marlow, N., Rowell, V., Thomas, S. & Stocks, J. (2010). Lung function and respiratory symptoms at 11 years in children born extremely preterm: the EPICure study. *American Journal of Respiratory and Critical Care Medicine,* 182, 2, (Jul 15), pp. 237-45, 1535-4970 (Electronic) 1073-449X (Linking)

Fletcher, C. & Peto, R. (1977). The natural history of chronic airflow obstruction. *British Medical Journal,* 1, 6077, (Jun 25), pp. 1645-8, 0007-1447 (Print) 0007-1447 (Linking)

Forastiere, F., Corbo, G.M., Dell'Orco, V., Pistelli, R., Agabiti, N. & Kriebel, D. (1996). A longitudinal evaluation of bronchial responsiveness to methacholine in children: role of baseline lung function, gender, and change in atopic status. *American Journal of Respiratory and Critical Care Medicine,* 153, 3, (Mar), pp. 1098-104, 1073-449X (Print) 1073-449X (Linking)

Franssen, F.M., O'Donnell, D.E., Goossens, G.H., Blaak, E.E. & Schols, A.M. (2008). Obesity and the lung: 5. Obesity and COPD. *Thorax,* 63, 12, (Dec), pp. 1110-7, 1468-3296 (Electronic) 0040-6376 (Linking)

Friedrich, L., Stein, R.T., Pitrez, P.M., Corso, A.L. & Jones, M.H. (2006). Reduced lung function in healthy preterm infants in the first months of life. *American Journal of Respiratory and Critical Care Medicine,* 173, 4, (Feb 15), pp. 442-7, 1073-449X (Print) 1073-449X (Linking)

Greenough, A. (2006). Bronchopulmonary dysplasia--long term follow up. *Paediatr Respir Rev,* 7 Suppl 1, pp. S189-91, 1526-0542 (Print) 1526-0542 (Linking)

Greenough, A., Limb, E., Marston, L., Marlow, N., Calvert, S. & Peacock, J. (2005). Risk factors for respiratory morbidity in infancy after very premature birth. *Archives of Disease in Childhood. Fetal and Neonatal Edition,* 90, 4, (Jul), pp. F320-3, 1359-2998 (Print) 1359-2998 (Linking)

Grischkan, J., Storfer-Isser, A., Rosen, C.L., Larkin, E.K., Kirchner, H.L., South, A., Wilson-Costello, D.C., Martin, R.J. & Redline, S. (2004). Variation in childhood asthma among former preterm infants. *Journal of Pediatrics,* 144, 3, (Mar), pp. 321-6, 0022-3476 (Print) 0022-3476 (Linking)

Halvorsen, T., Skadberg, B.T., Eide, G.E., Roksund, O.D., Carlsen, K.H. & Bakke, P. (2004). Pulmonary outcome in adolescents of extreme preterm birth: a regional cohort study. *Acta Paediatrica,* 93, 10, (Oct), pp. 1294-300, 0803-5253 (Print) 0803-5253 (Linking)

Hislop, A.A. (1997). Bronchopulmonary dysplasia: pre- and postnatal influences and outcome. *Pediatric Pulmonology,* 23, 2, (Feb), pp. 71-5, 8755-6863 (Print) 1099-0496 (Linking)

Hislop, A.A., Wigglesworth, J.S. & Desai, R. (1986). Alveolar development in the human fetus and infant. *Early Human Development,* 13, 1, (Feb), pp. 1-11, 0378-3782 (Print) 0378-3782 (Linking)

Hislop, A.A., Wigglesworth, J.S., Desai, R. & Aber, V. (1987). The effects of preterm delivery and mechanical ventilation on human lung growth. *Early Human Development,* 15, 3, (May), pp. 147-64, 0378-3782 (Print) 0378-3782 (Linking)

Holditch-Davis, D., Merrill, P., Schwartz, T. & Scher, M. (2008). Predictors of wheezing in prematurely born children. *Journal of Obstetric, Gynecologic, and Neonatal Nursing,* 37, 3, (May-Jun), pp. 262-73, 0884-2175 (Print) 0090-0311 (Linking)

Howling, S.J., Northway, W.H., Jr., Hansell, D.M., Moss, R.B., Ward, S. & Muller, N.L. (2000). Pulmonary sequelae of bronchopulmonary dysplasia survivors: high-resolution CT findings. *AJR. American Journal of Roentgenology,* 174, 5, (May), pp. 1323-6, 0361-803X (Print) 0361-803X (Linking)

Jacob, S.V., Lands, L.C., Coates, A.L., Davis, G.M., MacNeish, C.F., Hornby, L., Riley, S.P. & Outerbridge, E.W. (1997). Exercise ability in survivors of severe bronchopulmonary dysplasia. *American Journal of Respiratory and Critical Care Medicine,* 155, 6, (Jun), pp. 1925-9, 1073-449X (Print) 1073-449X (Linking)

Jobe, A.H. & Bancalari, E. (2001). Bronchopulmonary dysplasia. *American Journal of Respiratory and Critical Care Medicine,* 163, 7, (Jun), pp. 1723-9, 1073-449X (Print) 1073-449X (Linking)

Kumar, R., Yu, Y., Story, R.E., Pongracic, J.A., Gupta, R., Pearson, C., Ortiz, K., Bauchner, H.C. & Wang, X. (2008). Prematurity, chorioamnionitis, and the development of recurrent wheezing: a prospective birth cohort study. *Journal of Allergy and Clinical Immunology,* 121, 4, (Apr), pp. 878-84 e6, 1097-6825 (Electronic) 0091-6749 (Linking)

Langston, C., Kida, K., Reed, M. & Thurlbeck, W.M. (1984). Human lung growth in late gestation and in the neonate. *The American Review of Respiratory Disease,* 129, 4, (Apr), pp. 607-13, 0003-0805 (Print) 0003-0805 (Linking)

Lewis, S., Richards, D., Bynner, J., Butler, N. & Britton, J. (1995). Prospective study of risk factors for early and persistent wheezing in childhood. *European Respiratory Journal,* 8, 3, (Mar), pp. 349-56, 0903-1936 (Print) 0903-1936 (Linking)

Lum, S., Kirkby, J., Welsh, L., Marlow, N., Hennessy, E. & Stocks, J. (2011). Nature and severity of lung function abnormalities in extremely pre-term children at 11 years of age. *European Respiratory Journal,* 37, 5, (May), pp. 1199-207, 1399-3003 (Electronic) 0903-1936 (Linking)

Mahon, B.E., Ehrenstein, V., Norgaard, M., Pedersen, L., Rothman, K.J. & Sorensen, H.T. (2007). Perinatal risk factors for hospitalization for pneumococcal disease in childhood: a population-based cohort study. *Pediatrics,* 119, 4, (Apr), pp. e804-12, 1098-4275 (Electronic) 0031-4005 (Linking)

McLeod, A., Ross, P., Mitchell, S., Tay, D., Hunter, L., Hall, A., Paton, J. & Mutch, L. (1996). Respiratory health in a total very low birthweight cohort and their classroom controls. *Archives of Disease in Childhood,* 74, 3, (Mar), pp. 188-94, 1468-2044 (Electronic) 0003-9888 (Linking)

Mitchell, S.H. & Teague, W.G. (1998). Reduced gas transfer at rest and during exercise in school-age survivors of bronchopulmonary dysplasia. *American Journal of Respiratory and Critical Care Medicine,* 157, 5 Pt 1, (May), pp. 1406-12, 1073-449X (Print) 1073-449X (Linking)

Munyard, P., Busst, C., Logan-Sinclair, R. & Bush, A. (1994). A new device for ambulatory cough recording. *Pediatric Pulmonology,* 18, 3, (Sep), pp. 178-86, 8755-6863 (Print) 1099-0496 (Linking)

Narang, I., Bush, A. & Rosenthal, M. (2009). Gas transfer and pulmonary blood flow at rest and during exercise in adults 21 years after preterm birth. *American Journal of Respiratory and Critical Care Medicine,* 180, 4, pp. 339-345,

Narang, I., Rosenthal, M., Cremonesini, D., Silverman, M. & Bush, A. (2008). Longitudinal evaluation of airway function 21 years after preterm birth. *American Journal of Respiratory and Critical Care Medicine,* 178, 1, (Jul 1), pp. 74-80, 1535-4970 (Electronic) 1073-449X (Linking)

Northway, W.H., Jr. (1979). Observations on bronchopulmonary dysplasia. *Journal of Pediatrics,* 95, 5 Pt 2, (Nov), pp. 815-8, 0022-3476 (Print) 0022-3476 (Linking)

Northway, W.H., Jr., Moss, R.B., Carlisle, K.B., Parker, B.R., Popp, R.L., Pitlick, P.T., Eichler, I., Lamm, R.L. & Brown, B.W., Jr. (1990). Late pulmonary sequelae of bronchopulmonary dysplasia. *New England Journal of Medicine,* 323, 26, (Dec 27), pp. 1793-9, 0028-4793 (Print) 0028-4793 (Linking)

Oppenheim, C., Mamou-Mani, T., Sayegh, N., de Blic, J., Scheinmann, P. & Lallemand, D. (1994). Bronchopulmonary dysplasia: value of CT in identifying pulmonary sequelae. *AJR. American Journal of Roentgenology,* 163, 1, (Jul), pp. 169-72, 0361-803X (Print) 0361-803X (Linking)

Palta, M., Sadek-Badawi, M., Sheehy, M., Albanese, A., Weinstein, M., McGuinness, G. & Peters, M.E. (2001). Respiratory symptoms at age 8 years in a cohort of very low birth weight children. *American Journal of Epidemiology,* 154, 6, (Sep 15), pp. 521-9, 0002-9262 (Print) 0002-9262 (Linking)

Pelkonen, A.S., Hakulinen, A.L. & Turpeinen, M. (1997). Bronchial lability and responsiveness in school children born very preterm. *American Journal of Respiratory and Critical Care Medicine,* 156, 4 Pt 1, (Oct), pp. 1178-84, 1073-449X (Print) 1073-449X (Linking)

Post, M. & Copland, I. (2002). Overview of lung development. *Acta Pharmacologica Sinica,* S23, pp. 4-7,

Rogers, M., Fay, T.B., Whitfield, M.F., Tomlinson, J. & Grunau, R.E. (2005). Aerobic capacity, strength, flexibility, and activity level in unimpaired extremely low birth weight (<or=800 g) survivors at 17 years of age compared with term-born control subjects. *Pediatrics,* 116, 1, (Jul), pp. e58-65, 1098-4275 (Electronic) 0031-4005 (Linking)

Rojas, M.A., Gonzalez, A., Bancalari, E., Claure, N., Poole, C. & Silva-Neto, G. (1995). Changing trends in the epidemiology and pathogenesis of neonatal chronic lung disease. *Journal of Pediatrics,* 126, 4, (Apr), pp. 605-10, 0022-3476 (Print) 0022-3476 (Linking)

Rona, R.J., Gulliford, M.C. & Chinn, S. (1993). Effects of prematurity and intrauterine growth on respiratory health and lung function in childhood. *BMJ,* 306, 6881, (Mar 27), pp. 817-20, 0959-8138 (Print) 0959-535X (Linking)

Rosenthal, M. & Bush, A. (1998). Haemodynamics in children during rest and exercise: methods and normal values. *European Respiratory Journal,* 11, 4, (Apr), pp. 854-65, 0903-1936 (Print) 0903-1936 (Linking)

Rosenthal, M. & Bush, A. (1999). The effects of surgically treated pulmonary stenosis on lung growth and cardiopulmonary function in children during rest and exercise. *European Respiratory Journal,* 13, 3, (Mar), pp. 590-6, 0903-1936 (Print) 0903-1936 (Linking)

Samet, J.M., Tager, I.B. & Speizer, F.E. (1983). The relationship between respiratory illness in childhood and chronic air-flow obstruction in adulthood. *The American Review of Respiratory Disease,* 127, 4, (Apr), pp. 508-23, 0003-0805 (Print) 0003-0805 (Linking)

Sartori, C., Allemann, Y., Trueb, L., Delabays, A., Nicod, P. & Scherrer, U. (1999). Augmented vasoreactivity in adult life associated with perinatal vascular insult. *Lancet,* 353, 9171, (Jun 26), pp. 2205-7, 0140-6736 (Print) 0140-6736 (Linking)

Sears, M.R., Burrows, B., Flannery, E.M., Herbison, G.P., Hewitt, C.J. & Holdaway, M.D. (1991). Relation between airway responsiveness and serum IgE in children with asthma and in apparently normal children. *New England Journal of Medicine,* 325, 15, (Oct 10), pp. 1067-71, 0028-4793 (Print) 0028-4793 (Linking)

Sell, M., Cotton, R., Hirata, T., Guthrie, R., LeBlanc, M., Mammel, M. & Long, W. (1995). One-year follow-up of 273 infants with birth weights of 700 to 1100 grams after prophylactic treatment of respiratory distress syndrome with synthetic surfactant or air placebo. American Exosurf Neonatal Study Group I. *Journal of Pediatrics,* 126, 5 Pt 2, (May), pp. S20-5, 0022-3476 (Print) 0022-3476 (Linking)

Smith, V.C., Zupancic, J.A., McCormick, M.C., Croen, L.A., Greene, J., Escobar, G.J. & Richardson, D.K. (2005). Trends in severe bronchopulmonary dysplasia rates between 1994 and 2002. *Journal of Pediatrics,* 146, 4, (Apr), pp. 469-73, 0022-3476 (Print) 0022-3476 (Linking)

Speer, C.P. (2006). Pulmonary inflammation and bronchopulmonary dysplasia. *Journal of Perinatology,* 26 Suppl 1, (May), pp. S57-62; discussion S63-4, 0743-8346 (Print) 0743-8346 (Linking)

Stein, C.E., Kumaran, K., Fall, C.H., Shaheen, S.O., Osmond, C. & Barker, D.J. (1997). Relation of fetal growth to adult lung function in south India. *Thorax,* 52, 10, (Oct), pp. 895-9, 0040-6376 (Print) 0040-6376 (Linking)

Tracy, S.K., Tracy, M.B., Dean, J., Laws, P. & Sullivan, E. (2007). Spontaneous preterm birth of liveborn infants in women at low risk in Australia over 10 years: a population-based study. *BJOG,* 114, 6, (Jun), pp. 731-5, 1471-0528 (Electronic) 1470-0328 (Linking)

Vogt, H., Lindstrom, K., Braback, L. & Hjern, A. (2011). Preterm birth and inhaled corticosteroid use in 6- to 19-year-olds: a Swedish national cohort study. *Pediatrics,* 127, 6, (Jun), pp. 1052-9, 1098-4275 (Electronic) 0031-4005 (Linking)

Vrijlandt, E.J., Gerritsen, J., Boezen, H.M., Grevink, R.G. & Duiverman, E.J. (2006). Lung function and exercise capacity in young adults born prematurely. *American Journal of Respiratory and Critical Care Medicine,* 173, 8, (Apr 15), pp. 890-6, 1073-449X (Print) 1073-449X (Linking)

Walter, E.C., Ehlenbach, W.J., Hotchkin, D.L., Chien, J.W. & Koepsell, T.D. (2009). Low birth weight and respiratory disease in adulthood: a population-based case-control study. *American Journal of Respiratory and Critical Care Medicine,* 180, 2, (Jul 15), pp. 176-80, 1535-4970 (Electronic) 1073-449X (Linking)

Watterberg, K.L., Demers, L.M., Scott, S.M. & Murphy, S. (1996). Chorioamnionitis and early lung inflammation in infants in whom bronchopulmonary dysplasia develops. *Pediatrics,* 97, 2, (Feb), pp. 210-5, 0031-4005 (Print) 0031-4005 (Linking)

Welsh, L., Kirkby, J., Lum, S., Odendaal, D., Marlow, N., Derrick, G. & Stocks, J. (2010). The EPICure study: maximal exercise and physical activity in school children born extremely preterm. *Thorax,* 65, 2, (Feb), pp. 165-72, 1468-3296 (Electronic) 0040-6376 (Linking)

Wohl, M.E. (1995). Pulmonary sequelae of insults to the lung in early life. *Pediatric Pulmonology,* 19, 2, (Feb), pp. 90-5, 8755-6863 (Print) 1099-0496 (Linking)

Wong, P.M., Lees, A.N., Louw, J., Lee, F.Y., French, N., Gain, K., Murray, C.P., Wilson, A. & Chambers, D.C. (2008). Emphysema in young adult survivors of moderate-to-severe bronchopulmonary dysplasia. *European Respiratory Journal,* 32, 2, (Aug), pp. 321-8, 1399-3003 (Electronic) 0903-1936 (Linking)

Yablonskiy, D.A., Sukstanskii, A.L., Woods, J.C., Gierada, D.S., Quirk, J.D., Hogg, J.C., Cooper, J.D. & Conradi, M.S. (2009). Quantification of lung microstructure with hyperpolarized 3He diffusion MRI. *Journal of Applied Physiology,* 107, 4, (Oct), pp. 1258-65, 1522-1601 (Electronic) 0161-7567 (Linking)

15

Cardiovascular Consequences of Preterm Birth in the First Year of Life

Karinna Fyfe, Stephanie R. Yiallourou and Rosemary S.C. Horne
The Ritchie Centre, Monash Institute for Medical Research, Monash University, Melbourne, Australia

1. Introduction

The definition of a premature infant includes any infant born less than 37 completed weeks of gestation (Beck et al., 2009). This can be further divided into extremely, early and late preterm birth with those infants being born before 26 weeks of gestation being regarded as extremely preterm, between 26 and 34 weeks of gestation regarded as early preterm and those born between 34 and 37 weeks regarded as late preterm (Thilo and Rosenberg, 2010). Due to their reduced gestation, preterm infants are often born with a low birth weight (LBW) defined as a birth weight of less than 2500g, preterm infants are frequently also categorised as very low birth weight (VLBW), defined as less than 1500g and extremely low birth weight (ELBW), defined as less than 1000g (WHO, 2007). The worldwide rate of preterm birth is estimated to be 9.6% of all births, a total of almost 13 million births annually (Beck et al., 2009). Rates of premature birth vary between countries, but are around 10.6% in the USA, 6.2% in Europe and 6.4% in Australia (Beck et al., 2009). Despite a slight decrease in the last 4 years, the number of preterm births has been steadily increasing with a rise of greater than 30% over the past 30 years (Thilo and Rosenberg, 2010). This is due to a combination of factors including changing obstetric practices with a shift towards earlier delivery via either induction of labour or caesarean section and an increase in the number of multiple births (Thilo and Rosenberg, 2010). With improvements in neonatal intensive care techniques, the percentage of infants surviving premature birth has increased dramatically over the last two decades however, premature birth still has a significant impact on infant health and is associated with numerous neonatal problems both in the short and long term (Saigal et al., 2008). This review will focus on the problems associated with the cardiovascular system and its control during the first year of life.

1.1 Preterm birth and sleep

During infancy, the risks of cardiovascular instabilities are most marked during sleep, which has a marked influence on cardio-respiratory control (Gaultier, 1995). Sleep-related instability is of particular importance in infancy, as term infants spend up to 70% of each 24 hours asleep, while preterm infants devote almost 90% of their day to sleeping (Curzi-Dascalova and Challamel, 2000). In infants, two sleep states are defined, active sleep, the precursor to adult rapid eye movement sleep, and quiet sleep, the precursor to adult non rapid eye movement sleep. Postnatal maturation of sleep is one of the most important physiological changes occurring during the first six months after birth, and infants spend the majority of the time in active sleep, a state where cardio-respiratory control is most unstable (Gaultier, 1995). Significant differences in sleep patterns and the structure of sleep exist between term and preterm infants with preterm infants spending a much larger amount of time in active sleep. Thus studies of cardio-respiratory development and control in preterm infants have predominantly been carried out during sleep. As sleep state has a marked effect on the cardio-respiratory system it is also critical that the sleep state of the infant be taken into account when the results are interpreted.

2. Development of cardiovascular control

The formation of the cardiovascular system begins in early embryological development when the heart and blood vessels first appear (Guyton, 1991, Larson, 2001), and continues to develop and mature throughout fetal life. The cardiovascular system remains immature and continues to develop for several weeks after term birth (Larson, 2001). DNA synthesis and mitotic divisions of the myocardium have been found to continue for several weeks after birth and the mechanical performance of the myocardium improves with postnatal age (Davis et al., 1975, Friedman, 1972). Furthermore, the sympathetic nerve supply to the myocardium is thought to be immature at term (Tynan et al., 1977). In addition to the rapid maturation of the cardiovascular system after birth, the newborn circulation undergoes critical structural changes whereby circulatory shunts, including the ductus arteriosus, ductus venosus and foramen ovale close and transform the system from having a placental oxygen source to a pulmonary source (Guyton, 1991). In infants born preterm, circulatory shunts do not always close immediately after birth (Rhoades and Pflanzer, 1996), adding to the immaturity of the cardiovascular system and placing these infants at a significant risk of circulatory complications.

The autonomic nervous system (ANS) is responsible for control of the involuntary organs of the body and has a huge variety of functions. It is particularly important in the control of cardiovascular parameters such as heart rate, heart rate variability (HRV) and blood pressure. It consists of two opposing arms, the sympathetic which is responsible for 'fight or flight' responses and parasympathetic which plays the 'rest and digest' role. Autonomic function has been demonstrated to increase with gestational age in the fetus during pregnancy (Gagnon et al., 1987, Karin et al., 1993). The sympathetic arm is believed to develop at a consistent rate throughout gestation, while the parasympathetic arm undergoes a period of accelerated development at around 37 to 38 weeks conceptional age (Clairambault et al., 1992). Autonomic function has been demonstrated to be immature in preterm infants compared with term infants at term corrected age, and this is inversely related to gestational age at birth (Gournay et al., 2002, Lagercrantz et al., 1990). To perform effective cardio-respiratory and thermoregulatory functions the autonomic nervous system (ANS) needs to be mature and it has been suggested that this is why preterm infants are at a greater risk of cardiovascular instability.

2.1 Heart rate and blood pressure after preterm birth

It has recently been shown that immediately after birth, heart rate is lower amongst preterm infants than those infants born at term (Dawson et al., 2010). Heart rate also rises more slowly, taking a median time of 1.9 minutes to reach a heart rate of 100 beats per minute, which is considered normal (Dawson et al., 2010). This is important as heart rate is a commonly used indicator of the health of a newborn infant and reflects the infant's ability to transition from intra to extra-uterine life. Although heart rate may be lower initially amongst preterm infants, once haemodynamic stability is achieved preterm infants display a higher heart rate as a result of ANS immaturity.

Early studies which examined heart rate over gestation found heart rate differences between healthy preterm (born at 29-36 wks gestational age (GA)) and term infants at matched corrected ages (CA) HR was elevated in preterm infants compared with term infants in both active sleep and quiet sleep and these differences in quiet sleep persisted until a chronological age of 7 months (Katona et al., 1980). More recent studies, which followed infants born at 28 weeks PMA and studied longitudinally at weekly intervals until term equivalent age, have also shown that heart rate is elevated in preterm infants compared to term born infants (Patural et al., 2008). In support of these findings, studies comparing preterm and term infants at term have also shown that preterm infants had elevated heart rate in both sleep states compared with term infants (Eiselt et al., 1993). In contrast, other studies have demonstrated no heart rate differences between term and preterm infants (born at 26-32 wks GA) when compared at 2-3 weeks and 2-3 months CA (Tuladhar et al., 2005b) or when followed up to 6 months CA in infants born 28-32 wks GA (Witcombe et al., 2008). The differences between studies may have been due to the neonatal history of the infants. However, the marked sleep state difference in heart rate observed in term infants where heart rate is significantly elevated in active sleep compared with quiet sleep was not present in the preterm infants (Tuladhar et al., 2005b) and did not appear until 5-6 months of age (Witcombe et al., 2008) indicating that there may be a delay in the maturation of sleep state related autonomic control of heart rate.

Blood pressure measured longitudinally with an oscillometric device has also been shown to increase with gestational age and postnatal age in preterm infants over the first month of life (Pejovic et al., 2007). Blood pressure increased more rapidly in the preterm infants than in term infants and was higher in the groups with higher birth weight (Pejovic et al., 2007). There have been limited studies on blood pressure in preterm infants past term equivalent age. This has been primarily because of the difficulty of measuring blood pressure continuously and non-invasively in infants. Recent studies have validated the use of a photoplethysmographic cuff designed for an adult finger for use around the infant wrist (Andriessen et al., 2004b, Drouin et al., 1997, Yiallourou et al., 2006). This technique has been shown to provide an accurate beat-to-beat measure of blood pressure when compared to an arterial catheter (Yiallourou et al., 2006). Studies have shown that blood pressure is lower in preterm infants born at 28-32 weeks GA and studied longitudinally across the first six months after term CA compared to age matched term infants in both active sleep and quiet sleep (Witcombe et al., 2008). In contrast when awake a recent study has reported that systolic blood pressure in VLBW infants was elevated at one year of age compared to published reference values when adjusted for age, gender and height (Duncan et al., 2011). These findings suggest that the elevated blood pressure reported in adolescence and adulthood born preterm appears as early as the first year of life. Furthermore, there was no age related rise in blood pressure between one and three years of age (Duncan et al., 2011).

In summary, it appears that heart rate and blood pressure are altered after preterm birth and these differences persist across the first year after term CA. These differences may underpin the increased risk for cardiovascular problems later in life.

2.2 Heart rate and blood pressure control after preterm birth

Autonomic function can be assessed by examining fluctuations in heart rate termed heart rate variability (HRV). Traditionally, HRV has been analysed using two methods: time domain analyses and frequency domain analyses. Time domain analysis usually calculates the standard deviation of the variability between successive heart beats. The standard deviation of the change in R-R interval from one beat to the next (SDR-R) which relates to the variance of the R-R histogram data projected on the x-axis and the standard deviation of the difference between R-R intervals (SDΔR-R) which relates the variance of the R-R interval histogram data points parallel to the line of identity can be calculated (Galland et al., 1998). HRV reflect changes in efferent excitatory and inhibitory autonomic activity. Computerised spectral analysis of HRV shows that these rhythmical oscillations are concentrated in two main frequency ranges (Task Force of the European Society of Cardiology and the North American Society of Pacing and Electrophysiology, 1996). The long term or low frequency (LF) component (in adults 0.04-0.15 Hz) depends on both sympathetic and parasympathetic branches of the ANS and reflects baroreflex mediated changes in heart rate (Malliani et al., 1991, Pagani et al., 1986, Task Force of the European Society of Cardiology and the North American Society of Pacing and Electrophysiology, 1996). The short term or high frequency (HF) peak occurring above 0.15-0.4 Hz (in adults) is related to parasympathetic vagal activity and corresponds to the respiratory frequency (Malliani et al., 1991, Pagani et al., 1986, Task Force of the European Society of Cardiology and the North American Society of Pacing and Electrophysiology, 1996). These adult values are not appropriate for infants because of their higher respiratory rates which may range between 30 and 90 breaths per minute, similar to 0.5 and 1.5 Hz respectively and heart rates which may range between 100 and 200 beats per minute (similar to 1.7 and 3.3 Hz respectively) (De Beer et al., 2004). In the past, neonatal studies have used different spectral divisions for defining LF and HF components to account for these heart and respiratory rate differences from adults and this different band width used may explain some of the differences in findings of these studies. Recently it has been proposed that based on previous studies and taking into account the ranges of neonatal heart and respiratory rates that the spectral divisions for neonates be 0.04-0.15Hz for LF and 0.4-1.5 Hz for HF (De Beer et al., 2004). In adults, the ratio of low to high spectral power (LF/HF) has been used to reflect sympathovagal balance(Task Force of the European Society of Cardiology and the North American Society of Pacing and Electrophysiology, 1996) and this has also been used in neonates (Franco et al., 2003, Kluge et al., 1988).

2.2.1 Heart rate variability in healthy preterm infants

There have been a number of studies examining the development of cardiovascular control by assessing HRV in low risk healthy preterm infants, however the majority of studies have studied infants cross-sectionally, usually placing infants in gestational age groups. The effects of preterm birth on autonomic control prior to term has been studied in healthy preterm infants (born at 26 – 37 wks GA with birth weights of 795 – 1600g) and studied at 31 – 38 wks CA. The study demonstrated a decrease in heart rate in quiet sleep with increasing chronological age. In addition, in both quiet sleep and active sleep there was an increase in both time and frequency domain measures of HRV, indicating that there was a maturation of autonomic cardiovascular control during this period before term (Patural et al., 2004).

In a comparative study of healthy low risk preterm infants at term CA and term infants, Eiselt et al (Eiselt et al., 1993) demonstrated that in both active sleep and quiet sleep heart rate was elevated and HRV as measured by spectral analysis, was lower in the preterm group. In addition, in contrast to the term group where heart rate was lower in quiet sleep with higher HF power and lower LF power compared with active sleep, there were no sleep state differences in heart rate or HRV in the preterm group. In a later study by the same group in which 3 groups of infants were compared, a preterm group 31-36 wks conceptional age (ConA), an intermediate group 37-38 wks ConA and a term group 39-41 wks ConA the HF power, mid frequency (MF) power, LF power and mean RR interval all increased with age and the differences were more marked in active sleep compared with quiet sleep. In addition, HF power showed the greatest increase from the preterm to term group, while LF power showed equal differences from preterm to intermediate and intermediate to term indicating that there is a steep increase in vagal tone at 37-38 wks ConA which plateaux to term and a steady increase in sympathetic tone from 31-41 wks (Clairambault et al., 1992). In a similar study of preterm infants divided into groups of 25-27, 28-31, and 32-37 weeks GA and studied at term CA compared with full term infants, it was found that all three groups of preterm infants had significantly lower HF power values in quiet sleep compared to the term infants (Patural et al., 2004). Furthermore, preterm infants had lower parasympathetic activity at term CA. The authors suggested that preterm birth may prevent the maturation of parasympathetic activity, or alternatively low ANS activity may be involved in premature delivery (Patural et al., 2004). In a study of healthy preterm infants born at 29-35 weeks GA there was no affect of behavioural state (quiet sleep or active sleep) or gender in the group. The authors also did not identify any correlation between HRV parameters and birth-weight or length (Longin et al., 2006). When the group was divided into those infants born <32 weeks and those >32 weeks GA there was an increase in all HRV parameters in the older group. When compared to a group of healthy term infants studied at 1-7 days of age (Longin et al., 2005) the preterm infants had higher heart rates and lower HRV in all parameters measured (Longin et al., 2006). In a study of preterm infants born at 26-32 weeks GA and studied within 36h of birth spectral analysis was performed before and after administration of atropine sulphate a parasympathetic blocker. Atropine increased heart rate without altering systolic blood pressure, decreased HRV, and the decrease in LF power was larger than the decrease in HF power. These findings suggest that although the higher heart rate of preterm infants indicate relatively low vagal tone, the response to provides evidence that that a significant amount of vagal tone is present shortly after birth (Andriessen et al., 2004a). A recent study which followed 31 low risk preterm infants born at 28 weeks PMA to 34 weeks PMA at weekly intervals found no significant changes in the total, HF or ratio of LF/HF HRV components in the group overall. However, female infants had increased HF power compared to male infants from 31 weeks PMA onwards suggesting a more mature ANS (Krueger et al., 2010).

In a novel study where HRV was compared between fetuses who were 26-35 weeks PMA and prematurely born infants of 24-36 weeks PMA Padhye et al., reported that HF HRV was elevated and multiscale entropy (a measure of heart rate irregularity) were higher in the fetuses, suggesting that autonomic balance was poorer in the premature neonates than in the fetuses of identical PMA (Padhye et al., 2008). In a longitudinal study of preterm infants born 25-37 weeks GA and studied at term equivalent age both HF and LF power were significantly lower in the preterm groups compared to age matched term born infants, however the LF/HF ratio was not different (De Rogalski Landrot et al., 2007). When the subjects were re-studied at 2-3 years of age there was no difference between the groups for any of the variables measured suggesting that maturation of the ANS was faster in the preterm group and that by this age was fully mature (De Rogalski Landrot et al., 2007).

In summary these studies provide evidence of a reduced ability to control heart rate in healthy low risk preterm infants and suggest that there is a delayed maturation of the ANS and control of the cardiovascular system in this group of infants which may place them at risk for increased cardiovascular instability particularly during sleep in the early period after term equivalent age. Recent studies however suggest that control is equivalent to that of infants born at term by 2-3 years of age.

2.2.2 Heart rate variability in high risk preterm infants

There are somewhat fewer studies examining the development of cardiovascular control in high risk preterm infants. A study of 38 high risk VLBW infants from 23-38 weeks PMA where HRV was assessed weekly or biweekly found that there was an increase in LF power with PMA and that ventilated infants had lower HRV (Khattak et al., 2007). In the same group of infants, heart rate responses to blood sampling were also assessed (Padhye et al., 2009). A reduction in HRV was observed in both HF and LF bands during the heel lance procedure together with an increase in heart rate. As found in the previous study those infants who were mechanically ventilated showed substantially reduced heart rate responses to pain. Similar findings were reported by Patural et al., (Patural et al., 2008) in a similarly designed study which also compared preterm infants to those born at term. Compared to term born infants preterm infants had lower values of all HRV indices at term equivalent age (Patural et al., 2008).

In summary, these limited studies also suggest that cardiovascular control is impaired in high risk preterm infants, however further studies are required to elucidate if these deficits persist past term equivalent age and into infancy and childhood and if high risk preterm infants have increased impairment compared to age matched "healthy" preterm infants.

2.2.3 Effects of apnoea of prematurity on heart rate variability

Apnoea of prematurity is the most common disorder affecting infants born prematurely and the incidence and severity of apnoea are also inversely related to gestational age (Henderson-Smart, 1981). Apnoea is associated with bradycardia and hence these infants exhibit increased cardiovascular instability. In a comparative study of preterm infants born at 24 - 35 wks ConA with a neonatal history of persistent apnoea of prematurity and term infants it was found that heart rate was higher and HRV reduced at term age in the preterm group (Henslee et al., 1997). Furthermore, in infants born prior to 30 wks ConA these differences persisted over the next 6 months as did the differences in HRV in infants born at 30 - 35 wks ConA who had experienced respiratory distress syndrome (RDS). In a later study by the same group, infants with apnoea of prematurity (born at 31 - 35 wks ConA) were compared with both healthy term infants and term infants with persistent apnoea (Schechtman et al., 1998). It was found that the preterm infants showed similar alterations in cardiovascular control to the term group with apnoea in that heart rate was lower and HRV increased. These studies suggest that the mechanisms associated with apnoea have long lasting alterations on autonomic control.

2.2.4 Reflex heart rate responses

Stimulation of the trigeminal area of the face can induce arousal in sleeping infants and the tachycardia following arousal has been used as an index of autonomic function in term (Tuladhar et al., 2003) and preterm infants (Tuladhar et al., 2005b). When trigeminal stimulation does not evoke arousal, a reflex bradycardia is elicited (Ramet et al., 1990) which, together with apnoea and peripheral vasoconstriction, is a feature of the diving reflex. Non-arousing trigeminal cutaneous stimulation has been used to assess autonomic function in both preterm (Lagercrantz et al., 1990, Ramet et al., 1990, Tuladhar et al., 2005b) and term infants (Goksor et al., 2002, Harrington et al., 2001, Tuladhar et al., 2005b).

In studies comparing heart rate responses at arousal following trigeminal stimulation in term and preterm infants (born at 26 - 32 wks GA) with a neonatal history of apnoea of prematurity it was found that although there was no difference in the maximum value of heart rate, the normalized heart rate response (ΔHR%) was significantly greater in the term infants compared to the preterm infants at 2-3 weeks of CA in quiet sleep (Tuladhar et al., 2005b). This finding suggests a reduction of autonomic function in preterm infants at 2-3 weeks of age and supports the hypothesis that the postnatal maturation of autonomic function is delayed in preterm infants. The study also demonstrated that in the preterm infants the relative tachycardia following arousing stimuli (ΔHR%) was significantly greater at 2-3 months of CA compared to 36 weeks GA in active sleep, suggesting a maturation of autonomic control with increasing chronological age. In contrast, there was no evidence of maturation in the term infants (Tuladhar et al., 2005b). In addition, there was no difference between sleep states in maximum heart rate at either 36 weeks GA or 2-3 weeks CA in the preterm infants, however term infants had significantly greater maximum heart rate responses in active sleep at 2-3 weeks, indicated the effects of sleep state on heart rate control appear to be delayed in preterm infants.

In studies examining heart rate responses following trigeminal stimulation in which there was no arousal there is a fall in heart rate or bradycardia. Studies by Ramet et al., (Ramet et al., 1990) in preterm and term infants aged 26.5 - 40.5 wks GA in active sleep showed a significant maturation of the bradycardic response with post conceptual age, suggesting a dominance of vagal influences on autonomic regulation of the heart in preterm infants. Studies comparing this bradycardic response between term and preterm infants found no differences at either 2-3 weeks or 2-3 months CA (Tuladhar et al., 2005a). In active sleep no maturation in heart rate responses was observed in either preterm or term infants, however in quiet sleep the magnitude of the heart rate response increased with chronological age in both preterm and term infants (Tuladhar et al., 2005b). These findings are in contrast to other studies which have reported that the bradycardic reflex decreases with age after birth in both preterm and term infants in responses to trigeminal air-stream stimulation to the face, ocular compression and esophageal dilation and during active sleep and that by term responses were minimal (Ramet et al., 1995, Ramet et al., 1988, Ramet et al., 1990). The authors suggested that this bradycardic reflex may be inappropriate and increase the risk of the Sudden Infant Death Syndrome (SIDS) in preterm infants. The studies were however, not carried out longitudinally in the same infant and the tests performed only in active sleep up to term CA. The findings of Tuladhar et al.,(Tuladhar et al., 2005a) that a bradycardic reflex occurred until 2-3 months post term age are supported by a recent study of awake term infants between 4 and 12 months of age which found that the reflex bradycardia in response to submersion, although decreasing with chronological age, was still present at 12 months of age (Goksor et al., 2002). Despite these conflicting findings as to the age at which the bradycardic reflex response to trigeminal stimulation disappears, it appears that the response is increased in preterm infants which may contribute to their vulnerability to cardiovascular instability.

Heart rate responses after spontaneous cortical and sub-cortical arousal from sleep have also been compared between term and preterm infants (Hanzer et al., 2007). In term infants heart rate increased after arousal and this was greater after cortical arousal compared with sub-cortical. In contrast heart rate significantly decreased in the preterm infants and there was no difference in responses between cortical and sub-cortical arousal. However, the infants were not studied at matched ages with the preterm infants being studied at around 35 weeks PCA and the term infants at 45±12 days after birth, thus the findings could simply be that the preterm group was less mature when studied (Hanzer et al., 2007).

In summary, it appears that preterm infants have immature or impaired heart rate responses to both trigeminal stimulation and after arousal from sleep further suggesting that they are at increased risk of cardiovascular instability.

2.2.5 Baroreflex control of heart rate and blood pressure

The arterial baroreflex is the most important autonomic regulatory mechanism for short term control of arterial pressure, heart rate and cardiac contractility. This reflex corrects fluctuations in arterial pressure principally by altering both heart rate and arterial vascular tone. Thus, when there is an increase in arterial pressure this is countered by a decrease in both heart rate and arterial vascular tone. The responses of heart rate and vascular tone are mediated by the efferent parasympathetic and sympathetic limb of the baroreflex respectively. As both systems are involved, studies of the baroreflex provide information on the sympathovagal balance of control of the autonomic nervous system. Head-up and head-down tilting has also been used as a simple non-invasive method of assessing baroreflex control. In adults, it has been shown that head-up tilting results in a small transient decrease in arterial blood pressure, which in turn evokes a peripheral vasoconstriction and heart rate acceleration (Borst et al., 1984, Borst et al., 1982). Tilting also results in an increase in the LF component of HRV and a decrease in the HF component, the size of the changes being correlated to the degree of the tilt (Montano et al., 1994).

Early studies in preterm infants demonstrated that head up tilting (45°) did not produce significant tachycardia in infants between 28 - 40 wks GA (Holden et al., 1985, Waldman et al., 1979) or in infants 25 - 36 wks GA studied between 1-11 wks chronological age (Lagercrantz et al., 1990), however these studies combined a number of ages of preterm infants with differing clinical histories which may have effected results. In the latter study, blood pressure was also unchanged on tilting however peripheral vascular resistance increased significantly, and there was no correlation between cardiovascular parameters and gestational or chronological age (Lagercrantz et al., 1990). In contrast, Finley et al., (Finley et al., 1984) showed that both term infants studied in the first week after birth and preterm infants (born at 33 -37 week GA) studied at 2 -29 d had significant increases in heart rate on head-up tilting (30°) and significant decreases on head-down tilting, results were however very variable between infants. In addition, there was no difference in responses between sleep states, and they concluded that control of heart rate was well developed at term. In healthy preterm infants (born at 28-32 wks GA) heart rate responses to tilting (45°) in quiet sleep were studied serially at 1-5 weeks chronological age. The study found that at the first age there was no significant change in heart rate following the tilts and that the change in heart rate increased with increasing chronological age (Mazursky et al., 1998). In addition the LF/HF ratio progressively decreased with increasing chronological age indicating maturation of sympathovagal balance (Mazursky et al., 1998). In a study where heart rate responses to head up tilting (45°) and baseline heart rate values in active sleep were compared between healthy preterm infants (30-34 wks ConA) and term infants at term corrected age no differences were found, however responses in both groups were immature with half of the infants not exhibiting the tachycardia observed in older infants (Massin et al., 2002). Overall, these studies suggest that that there is maturation of baroreflex control of heart rate prior to term however control is still immature in preterm infants at term CA when compared with term infants.

There have been a limited number of studies of baroreflex control of blood pressure in the newborn infant, mainly due to the limited means of inducing and recording blood pressure changes in neonates. With advances in non-invasive and continuous recording of blood pressure in preterm infants (Andriessen et al., 2004b, Gournay et al., 2002, Yiallourou et al., 2006) using beat-beat analyses of spontaneously occurring changes in heart rate and systolic blood pressure (Gournay et al., 2002) have demonstrated that baroreflex sensitivity in preterm infants (born at 24-36 wks GA) increased with both gestational and chronological age. However, it was still lower in preterm infants at term corrected age compared to infants born at term, suggesting an immaturity of baroreflex control in the preterm infants (Gournay et al., 2002). In a cross-sectional study of preterm and term infants born at 28-32 wks postmenstrual age (PMA), 32-37 wks PMA and 37-42 wks PMA Andriesson et al., (Andriessen et al., 2005) also found that baroreflex sensitivity increased with PMA and suggested that this was an effect of a progressive increase in parasympathetic activity. They suggested that the very low BRS in the very preterm infants may be of importance in the clinical management of blood pressure in these infants.

There have been limited studies assessing baroreflex control of blood pressure after term equivalent age. Studies using a 15° head up tilt demonstrated that preterm infants born at 28-32 weeks GA and studied longitudinally at 2-4 weeks, 2-3 months and 5-6 months CA had similar heart rate and blood pressure responses to age matched term infants, i.e. initial increase in both heart rate and blood pressure followed by a bradycardia and subsequent return of blood pressure and heart rate to baseline values. However, return of blood pressure to baseline following the tilt was considerably delayed in the preterm group ~37 beats post-tilt compared to the term infants ~23 beats post-tilt at both 2-3 weeks and 2-3 months CA (Witcombe et al., 2010). These findings suggest that control of blood pressure is immature or maturationally delayed until 5-6 months post term corrected age in preterm infants. These studies support earlier reports of abnormal responses to circulatory stress induced by hypercapnia (4% CO_2 administered during quiet sleep) of healthy preterm infants born at 27-34 weeks GA and preterm infants diagnosed with bronchopulmonary dysplasia born at 23-33 weeks GA and studied at 36 weeks and 40 weeks PMA (Cohen et al., 2007). In a later study, the same group also performed 60° head up tilts in addition to hypercapnia exposure and also found that responses of preterm infants studied at term equivalent age to be markedly different to term infants, with a 3-4 fold greater rise in blood pressure following the tilt and a reduced heart rate response to hypercapnia (Cohen et al., 2008). Preterm infants with bronchopulmonary dysplasia have also been demonstrated to display abnormal cardiovascular responses to side motion and head up tilt (45°) tests when studied at 2-4 months CA (Viskari et al., 2007).

3. Preterm infants and the Sudden Infant Death Syndrome (SIDS)

In recent years, the incidence of SIDS has been more than halved by world-wide public health campaigns introduced in the early 1990's which published the known major risk factors of prone sleeping, maternal smoking and overheating (Moon et al., 2007). However, despite this dramatic decline in incidence, SIDS still remains the major cause of unexpected death in infants in western countries contributing to 47% of all post-neonatal deaths (Byard and Krous, 2003, Carpenter et al., 2004). SIDS was the third leading cause of infant death in the United States in 2007 (Xu et al., 2010) and was the fourth leading cause of infant death in Australia in 2005 (Australian Bureau of Statistics, 2009, Linacre, 2007).

Preterm infants have been shown to be at increased risk for SIDS, with approximately 20% of all SIDS cases occurring in the preterm population (Blair et al., 2006, Thompson and Mitchell, 2006). The most recent study showed that this risk was 4 times greater than for an infant born at term (Blair et al., 2006). The risk for SIDS in preterm infants has also been shown to be inversely related to gestational age (Grether and Schulman, 1989, Hoffman et al., 1988, Hoffman and Hillman, 1992, Malloy and Freeman, 2000, Malloy and Hoffman, 1995, Peterson, 1966, Standfast et al., 1979), with one study demonstrating that the incidence of SIDS in infants born at 24-28 weeks, 29-32 weeks, 33-36 weeks and more than 37 weeks was 3.52, 3.01, 2.27 and 1.06 deaths / 1000 live births respectively (Malloy and Hoffman, 1995). Recent studies of data collected following the introduction of public awareness campaigns of the risks for SIDS have shown that risk factors for preterm infants are similar to those of term infants (Blair et al., 2006, Thompson and Mitchell, 2006).

Although the exact causal mechanisms remain an enigma, it is commonly believed that the final event of SIDS involves a failed or impaired arousal response from sleep to a life-threatening cardio-respiratory challenge (Harper, 1996, Kahn et al., 2002, Phillipson and Sullivan, 1978). In further support of this hypothesis, studies have identified disturbances in the cholinergic and serotonergic systems of SIDS victims (Kinney et al., 1995, Paterson et al., 2006), as well as structural abnormalities in medullary nuclei intimately involved in the central control of cardio-respiratory defensive responses and sleep/wake states (Lavezzi et al., 2004, Machaalani and Waters, 2008). Over 20 years ago it has been suggested that autonomic dysfunction may be a possible cause of SIDS (Kahn et al., 1983). More recently, studies have demonstrated that infants at increased risk for SIDS such as those sleeping prone (Franco et al., 1996, Galland et al., 1998), exposed to maternal smoking (Franco et al., 2000a) or to high ambient temperatures (Franco et al., 2000b) had reduced parasympathetic activity as measured from HRV. Additionally, infants who had been studied previously and who subsequently died from SIDS had higher baseline heart rates (Kelly et al., 1986), lower HRV (Schechtman, 1998), prolonged QT indexes (Schwartz et al., 1998) low parasympathetic tone and/or high sympathovagal balance (Franco et al., 2003, Kluge et al., 1988).

3.1 SIDS risk factors and preterm birth

Prone sleeping is the major risk factor for SIDS with some studies suggesting a causal relation between prone sleep and SIDS (Moon et al., 2007). LBW preterm infants (born at 26-34 wks GA) and studied at 30-38 wks had higher heart rate and respiratory rate together with lower HRV and respiratory variability when they slept prone compared to supine in both active sleep and quiet sleep (Sahni et al., 1999a). Healthy preterm infants born at 27 - 36 wks CA were studied at around 36 wks CA prior to discharge from hospital whilst sleeping both prone and supine (Goto et al., 1999). Heart rate was found to be higher in the supine position compared with the prone position in active sleep. In addition maximum heart rate was higher in both sleep states and HRV was increased in quiet sleep in the supine position. In a later study by the same group healthy preterm infants born at 28 - 36 wks CA were studied at 1 and 3 months CA age at home whist sleeping prone and supine (Ariagno et al., 2003). In active sleep, heart rate and HRV were not different between sleeping positions at either 1 or 3 months of age. In contrast, in quiet sleep heart rate was higher at 3 months and time domain estimates of HRV were increased at both 1 and 3 months in the supine position. Frequency domain analysis showed that HF power was elevated at 1 month in quiet sleep in the supine position. In addition, both JTc and QTc were shorter at 1 month in quiet sleep in the supine position. A study of low birth weight preterm infants (born at 26 - 37 wks GA and weighing 795-1600g) found that when placed to sleep prone these infants had higher heart rate with lower time and frequency domain measures of HRV than when sleeping supine in both active sleep and quiet sleep (Sahni et al., 1999b). There were also fewer sustained accelerations or decelerations of heart rate in the prone position. In addition, the positional differences in heart rate increased in quiet sleep with increasing postnatal age and the differences in HRV increased in both sleep states (Sahni et al., 2000).

Maternal smoking during pregnancy is associated with preterm birth and is also an independent risk factor for SIDS. When HRV in preterm infants whose mothers had smoked during pregnancy was compared with that in age matched preterm infants whose mother had not smoked, at 33-34 weeks PCA the infants in the smoking group had lower LF power. In addition, in contrast to the non-smoking group, there was no correlation between heart rate and total power with gestational age at birth in the smoking group (Thiriez et al., 2009).

Current theories for the final mechanism of SIDS propose that an infant fails to arouse from sleep after a prolonged cardio-respiratory event (Moon et al., 2007). Arousal from sleep is a vital protective response to a life-threatening challenge as simply by arousing from sleep heart rate, blood pressure and respiration are increased and most importantly a behavioural response can be initiated (Phillipson and Sullivan, 1978). Studies from our laboratory have shown that preterm infants have abnormal or impaired arousal responses compared to term born infants. Compared to healthy term infants (37-42 weeks gestation), preterm infants born at 31-35 weeks gestation have a delay in the maturation of sleep-state-related difference in arousability between active sleep and quiet sleep; this difference only appeared at 2-3 months of age as compared to 2-3 weeks for term infants (Horne et al., 2002). Moreover, preterm infants (26-32 weeks of gestation) with a history of apnoea and bradycardia of prematurity showed decreased responses in both active sleep and quiet sleep at term, and in quiet sleep at 2-3 months post-term (Horne et al., 2001). After a mild hypoxia challenge (15% oxygen), preterm infants had a longer arousal latency in active sleep at 2-3 weeks of age and reached significantly lower SpO_2 levels at 2-5 weeks in both active sleep and quiet sleep and at 2-3 months in quiet sleep (Verbeek et al., 2008). The greater desaturation during the hypoxic challenge combined with the longer arousal latency suggested that in preterm infants there was an impairment or inadequate response to hypoxia during sleep, which may explain the enhanced risk for SIDS in this group. Recently in studies by our group we have investigated the link between impaired cardiovascular control in the prone sleeping position and the decreased arousability which is also associated with this position. Using Near Infrared Spectroscopy techniques in conjunction with continuous blood pressure measurements we showed that in health term infants the prone position was associated with lower cerebral oxygenation in both quiet sleep and active sleep at 2-3 months of age and in quiet sleep at 2-3 months of age (Wong et al., 2011). We suggest that this reduction may underpin the reduced arousability from sleep exhibited by normal infants when sleeping prone, and provides new insight into potential risks of prone sleeping and mechanisms of SIDS. Further studies are currently underway to determine if preterm infants show similar or greater reductions in cerebral oxygenation when they sleep prone and if this is related to gestational age at birth.

It has been suggested that monitoring of infants at increased risk for SIDS may be useful in identifying infants with abnormal cardiorespiratory control so that these infants could be targeted for interventions to prevent their deaths. In the 1980's Andre Kahn initiated a unique study which brought over 45,000 infants into 10 sleep laboratories across Belgian for an overnight sleep study. Of these, 40 infants subsequently died from SIDS some days or weeks after their study. Results from various sub-groups of this study have been published. In the first report which examined the sleep studies of 30 of the infants who died and compared their sleep and respiratory characteristics to 60 controls matched for age, postnatal age, gestational age and weight at birth the only two polysomnographic characteristics which identified the infants who subsequently died were that they moved less during sleep and had more obstructive breathing events (Kahn et al., 1992). Subsequently it was shown in a subset of 16 of these infants that they had fewer cortical arousals during both active sleep and quiet sleep and that the duration and frequency of sub cortical activation was significantly greater, findings suggestive of an incomplete arousal response (Kato et al., 2003). The differences in the sleep and arousal characteristics of the infants who subsequently died were subtle and as such a large number of studies resulted in such a few infant deaths the cost of studying infants with overnight polysomnography is probably not warranted to try to identify infants who might subsequently die. To test the effectiveness of monitoring infants who were perceived at increased risk for SIDS the Collaborative Home Infant Monitoring Evaluation (CHIME) study was funded by the National Institutes of Health in the USA. Between May 1994 to February 1998 over 1000 infants were monitored with a device which recorded both heart rate and breathing in the home. Preterm infants, siblings of infants who had died from SIDS and infants who had suffered an apparent life threatening event (ALTE) were studied and results compared to healthy term controls. It was hypothesised that those infants in the "at risk groups" would have more frequent cardiorespiratory events and that these would be related to PCA. 1079 infants were studied with over 700,000 hours of recordings. Events were divided into "conventional" which were defined as apnoeas lasting <20s duration, bradycardias <60 bpm for 5s in infants < 44 weeks PMA or <80 bpm for 15s in infants <44 weeks PMA or bradycardias <50bpm for 5s or <60 bpm for at least 15s in infants ≤ 44 weeks PMA. "Extreme events" were defined as apnoeas persisting <30s duration or bradycardia <60 bpm for at least 10s in infants ≤ 44 weeks PMA. Either of these events could be accompanied by oxygen desaturation. The initial report found that conventional events were quite common even in term control infants. Extreme events were only common in the preterm group but their timing which peaked before 43 weeks PCA did not coincide with the peak risk period for SIDS and it was concluded that these events were not likely to be precursors of SIDS (Ramanathan et al., 2001). Subsequent analyses of the data set have concluded that the extreme events are associated with immaturity of autonomic control of the cardiorespiratory system rather than risk factors for SIDS and do not seem to be causally related to SIDS (Hoppenbrouwers et al., 2008, Hunt et al., 2008). Thus it would appear that home cardiorespiratory monitoring is unlikely to identify abnormal events before the SIDS event and is also unlikely to prevent a SIDS death. At risk infants are frequently monitored at home but apart from providing reassurance to the parents there seems to be little evidence to support this practice as preventative for SIDS. However to date no home monitoring studies have examined autonomic control using such methods as heart rate variability analysis which could perhaps be a marker of infants at increased risk.

In summary, preterm infants are at significantly increased risk for SIDS and the factors which increase the risk in healthy term infants also increase the risk in preterm infants. Immature cardiovascular control may underpin this increased risk which may be further exacerbated by prone sleep or maternal smoking. The importance of alerting parents and health professionals to this increased risk must be stressed as preterm infants are often nursed prone in the intensive care setting to enhance respiratory mechanics. It has been demonstrated that very prematurely born infants studied before neonatal unit discharge slept longer, had fewer arousals from sleep, and more central apnoeas when sleeping prone (Bhat et al., 2006). However, other studies have shown no differences in the incidence of clinically significant apnoea, bradycardia or desaturations in preterm infants (Keene et al., 2000). A recent study has also shown no effect of sleep position on oxygen saturation levels in preterm infants and after 36 weeks GA there was no additional requirement for oxygen (Elder et al., 2011). Thus it is critical that premature infants be placed supine as soon as is medically safe, and well before hospital discharge, to ensure that the infant and parents are accustomed to supine placement. However, further studies are required to define the exact age at which this can be done and whether or not high risk infants are able to be placed supine safely at the same age as healthy preterm infants.

4. Conclusions

Preterm birth is associated with immaturity of autonomic nervous system control of the cardiovascular system. This is manifest with higher heart rates, reduced heart rate variability, decreased baroreflex sensitivity, lower parasympathetic activity, decreased reflex heart rate responses to trigeminal stimulation and at arousal from sleep and lower blood pressure. There also appears to be a significant relationship between gestational age at birth and reduced autonomic control, with infants born at younger gestation ages having more immature responses at equivalent PCA. The most rapid maturation of autonomic control appears to be in the last 8-10 weeks of gestation. This reduced autonomic control compared to age matched term infants appears to last for several months post term, however there are few longitudinal studies to confirm the exact age at which preterm infants "catch-up" with term infants. When preterm birth is associated with apnoea of prematurity this immaturity appears to be more severe and prolonged, however there are also limited longitudinal studies in these infants. It is well known that infants born preterm go on to have cardiovascular complications later in life including elevated blood pressure and increased arterial stiffness (Bonamy et al., 2005, Irving et al., 2000). It appears that abnormalities in cardiovascular control can be identified very early in postnatal life in preterm infants but further studies are needed to identify the role these play in the development of cardiovascular complications later in life.

The major risk factors for SIDS namely prone sleeping and maternal smoking have been shown to exert a major influence on autonomic function during sleep in term infants and this is also the case in preterm infants, although there are fewer studies. The immaturity of the autonomic nervous system in preterm infants may explain the increased risk of SIDS in this group and assessment of autonomic control could also provide insights into the underlying mechanisms of preterm problems such as the propensity for apnoea-bradycardia and provide new methods of assessment of risk for sudden and unexplained death.

5. References

Andriessen, P., Janssen, B. J., Berendsen, R. C., Oetomo, S. B., Wijn, P. F. and Blanco, C. E. (2004a). Cardiovascular autonomic regulation in preterm infants: the effect of atropine. *Pediatric Research*, Vol.56, No. 6, pp. 939-946.

Andriessen, P., Oetomo, S. B., Peters, C., Vermeulen, B., Wijn, P. F. and Blanco, C. E. (2005). Baroreceptor reflex sensitivity in human neonates: the effect of postmenstrual age. *The Journal of Physiology*, Vol.568, No. Pt 1, pp. 333-341.

Andriessen, P., Schoffelen, R. L., Berendsen, R. C., De Beer, N. A., Oei, S. G., Wijn, P. F. and Blanco, C. E. (2004b). Noninvasive assessment of blood pressure variability in preterm infants. *Pediatric Research*, Vol.55, No. 2, pp. 220-223.

Ariagno, R. L., Mirmiran, M., Adams, M. M., Saporito, A. G., Dubin, A. M. and Baldwin, R. B. (2003). Effect of position on sleep, heart rate variability, and QT interval in preterm infants at 1 and 3 months' corrected age. *Pediatrics*, Vol.111, No. 3, pp. 622-625.

Australian Bureau of Statistics Causes of Death, Australia, 2007. In. Australian Bureau of Statistics, Canberra, 2009.

Beck, S., Wojdyla, D., Say, L., Betran, A. P., Merialdi, M., Requejo, J. H., Rubens, C., Menon, R. and Van Look, P. F. (2009). The worldwide incidence of preterm birth: a systematic review of maternal mortality and morbidity. *Bull World Health Organ*, Vol.88, No. 1, pp. 31-38.

Bhat, R. Y., Hannam, S., Pressler, R., Rafferty, G. F., Peacock, J. L. and Greenough, A. (2006). Effect of prone and supine position on sleep, apneas, and arousal in preterm infants. *Pediatrics*, Vol.118, No. 1, pp. 101-107.

Blair, P. S., Platt, M. W., Smith, I. J. and Fleming, P. J. (2006). Sudden infant death syndrome and sleeping position in pre-term and low birth weight infants: an opportunity for targeted intervention. *Archives of Diseases in Childhood*, Vol.91, No. 2, pp. 101-106.

Bonamy, A. K., Bendito, A., Martin, H., Andolf, E., Sedin, G. and Norman, M. (2005). Preterm birth contributes to increased vascular resistance and higher blood pressure in adolescent girls. *Pediatr Res*, Vol.58, No. 5, pp. 845-849.

Borst, C., Van Brederode, J. F., Wieling, W., Van Montfrans, G. A. and Dunning, A. J. (1984). Mechanisms of initial blood pressure response to postural change. *Clinical Science (London)*, Vol.67, No. 3, pp. 321-327.

Borst, C., Wieling, W., Van Brederode, J. F., Hond, A., De Rijk, L. G. and Dunning, A. J. (1982). Mechanisms of initial heart rate response to postural change. *American Journal of Physiology*, Vol.243, No. 5, pp. H676-681.

Byard, R. W. and Krous, H. F. (2003). Sudden infant death syndrome: overview and update. *Pediatric and Development Pathology*, Vol.6, No. 2, pp. 112-127.

Carpenter, R. G., Irgens, L. M., Blair, P. S., England, P. D., Fleming, P., Huber, J., Jorch, G. and Schreuder, P. (2004). Sudden unexplained infant death in 20 regions in Europe: case control study. *The Lancet*, Vol.363, No. 9404, pp. 185-191.

Clairambault, J., Curzi-Dascalova, L., Kauffmann, F., Medigue, C. and Leffler, C. (1992). Heart rate variability in normal sleeping full-term and preterm neonates. *Early Human Development*, Vol.28, No., pp. 169-183.

Cohen, G., Lagercrantz, H. and Katz-Salamon, M. (2007). Abnormal circulatory stress responses of preterm graduates. *Pediatric Research*, Vol.61, No. 3, pp. 329-334.

Cohen, G., Vella, S., Jeffery, H., Lagercrantz, H. and Katz-Salamon, M. (2008). Cardiovascular stress hyperreactivity in babies of smokers and in babies born preterm. *Circulation*, Vol.118, No. 18, pp. 1848-1853.

Curzi-Dascalova, L. and Challamel, M. (2000). *Sleep and Breathing in Children* Marcel Dekker, New York

Davis, P., Dewar, J., Tynan, M. and Ward, R. (1975). Post-natal developmental changes in the length-tension relationship of cat papillary muscles. *J Physiol*, Vol.253, No., pp. 95-102.

Dawson, J. A., Kamlin, C. O., Wong, C., Te Pas, A. B., Vento, M., Cole, T. J., Donath, S. M., Hooper, S. B., Davis, P. G., Morley, C. J. and Kamlin, C. O. F. (2010). Changes in heart rate in the first minutes after birth. *Archives of Disease in Childhood Fetal & Neonatal Edition*, Vol.95, No. 3, pp. F177-181.

De Beer, N. A., Andriessen, P., Berendsen, R. C., Oei, S. G., Wijn, P. F. and Oetomo, S. B. (2004). Customized spectral band analysis compared with conventional Fourier analysis of heart rate variability in neonates. *Physiological Measurement*, Vol.25, No. 6, pp. 1385-1395.

De Rogalski Landrot, I., Roche, F., Pichot, V., Teyssier, G., Gaspoz, J. M., Barthelemy, J. C. and Patural, H. (2007). Autonomic nervous system activity in premature and full-term infants from theoretical term to 7 years. *Autonomic Neuroscience*, Vol.136, No. 1-2, pp. 105-109.

Drouin, E., Gournay, V., Calamel, J., Mouzard, A. and Roze, J. C. (1997). Feasibility of using finger arterial pressure in neonates. *Archives of Disease in Childhood: Fetal and Neonatal Edition*, Vol.77, No. 2, pp. F139-140.

Duncan, A. F., Heyne, R. J., Morgan, J. S., Ahmad, N. and Rosenfeld, C. R. (2011). Elevated systolic blood pressure in preterm very-low-birth-weight infants </=3 years of life. *Pediatric Nephrology*, Vol.26, No. 7, pp. 1115-1121.

Eiselt, M., Curzi-Dascalova, L., Clairambault, J., Kauffmann, F., Medigue, C. and Peirano, P. (1993). Heart-rate variability in low-risk prematurely born infants reaching normal term: a comparison with full-term newborns. *Early Human Development*, Vol.32, No. 2-3, pp. 183-195.

Elder, D. E., Campbell, A. J. and Galletly, D. (2011). Effect of position on oxygen saturation and requirement in convalescent preterm infants. *Acta Paediatrica*, Vol.100, No. 5, pp. 661-665.

Finley, J. P., Hamilton, R. and Mackenzie, M. G. (1984). Heart rate response to tilting in newborns in quiet and active sleep. *Biology of the Neonate*, Vol.45, No. 1, pp. 1-10.

Franco, P., Chabanski, S., Szliwowski, H., Dramaix, M. and Kahn, A. (2000a). Influence of maternal smoking on autonomic nervous system in healthy infants. *Pediatric Research*, Vol.47, No. 2, pp. 215-220.

Franco, P., Grosswasser, J., Sottiaux, M., Broadfield, E. and Kahn, A. (1996). Decreased cardiac responses to auditory stimulation during prone sleep. *Pediatrics*, Vol.97, No., pp. 174-178.

Franco, P., Szliwowski, H., Dramaix, M. and Kahn, A. (2000b). Influence of ambient temperature on sleep characteristics and autonomic nervous control in healthy infants. *Sleep*, Vol.23, No. 3, pp. 401-407.

Franco, P., Verheulpen, D., Valente, F., Kelmanson, I., De Broca, A., Scaillet, S., Groswasser, J. and Kahn, A. (2003). Autonomic responses to sighs in healthy infants and in victims of sudden infant death. *Sleep Medicine*, Vol.4, No. 6, pp. 569-577.

Friedman, W. F. (1972). The intrinsic physiologic properties of the developing heart. *Progress in Cardiovascular Diseases*, Vol.XV, No. 1, pp. 87-111.

Gagnon, R., Campbell, K., Hunse, C. and Patrick, J. (1987). Patterns of human fetal heart rate accelerations from 26 weeks to term. *American Journal of Obstetrics and Gynecololgy*, Vol.157, No., pp. 743-748.

Galland, B., Reeves, G., Taylor, B. J. and Bolton, D. P. G. (1998). Sleep position, autonomic function and arousal. *Archives of Disease in Childhood Fetal & Neonatal Edition*, Vol.78, No. 3, pp. F189-F194.

Gaultier, C. (1995). Cardiorespiratory Adaptation During Sleep in Infants and Children. *Pediatric Pulmonology*, Vol.19, No., pp. 105-117.

Goksor, E., Rosengren, L. and Wennergren, G. (2002). Bradycardic response during submersion in infant swimming. *Acta Paediatrica*, Vol.91, No. 3, pp. 307-312.

Goto, K., Mirmiran, M., Adams, M. M., Longford, R. V., Baldwin, R. B., Boeddiker, M. A. and Ariagno, R. L. (1999). More awakenings and heart rate variability during supine sleep in preterm infants. *Pediatrics*, Vol.103, No., pp. 603-609.

Gournay, V., Drouin, E. and Roze, J. C. (2002). Development of baroreflex control of heart rate in preterm and full term infants. *Archives of Disease in Childhood Fetal & Neonatal Edition*, Vol.86, No. 3, pp. F151-154.

Grether, J. K. and Schulman, J. (1989). Sudden infant death syndrome and birth weight. *Journal of Paediatrics*, Vol.114, No., pp. 561-567.

Guyton, A. C. (1991). *Textbook of Medical Physiology* (8th), W.B Saunders Company, Philadelphia

Hanzer, M., Reinhold, K., Urlesberger, B., Mueller, W., Pichler, G. and Zotter, H. (2007). Comparison of heart rate responses during cortical and subcortical arousals in term and preterm infants. *Early Human Development*, Vol.83, No., pp. 511-515.

Harper, R. M. (1996). The Cerebral regulation of Cardiovascular and respiratory function. *Seminars in Pediatric Neurology*, Vol.3, No. 1, pp. 13-22.

Harrington, C., Kirjavainen, T., Teng, A. and Sullivan, C. E. (2001). Cardiovascular responses to three simple, provocative tests of autonomic activity in sleeping infants. *Journal of Applied Physiology*, Vol.91, No. 2, pp. 561-568.

Henderson-Smart, D. J. (1981). The effect of gestational age on the incidence and duration of recurrent apnoea in newborn babies. *Australian Paediatric Journal*, Vol.17, No. 4, pp. 273-276.

Henslee, J. A., Schechtman, V. L., Lee, M. Y. and Harper, R. M. (1997). Developmental patterns of heart rate and variability in prematurely-born infants with apnea of prematurity. *Early Human Development*, Vol.47, No., pp. 35-50.

Hoffman, H. J., Damus, K., Hillman, L. and Krongrad, E. (1988). Risk factors for SIDS: Results of the National Institute of Child Health and Human Development SIDS cooperative epidemiology study. *Annals of the New York Academy of Sciences*, Vol.533, No., pp. 13-30.

Hoffman, H. J. and Hillman, L. S. (1992). Epidemiology of the sudden infant death syndrome: maternal , neonatal, and postneonatal risk factors. *Clinics in Perinatology*, Vol.19, No. 4, pp. 717-737.

Holden, K., Morgan, J. S., Krauss, A. N. and Auld, P. A. (1985). Incomplete baroreceptor responses in newborn infants. *American Journal of Perinatology*, Vol.2, No. 1, pp. 31-34.

Hoppenbrouwers, T., Hodgman, J. E., Ramanathan, A. and Dorey, F. (2008). Extreme and conventional cardiorespiratory events and epidemiologic risk factors for SIDS. *J Pediatr*, Vol.152, No. 5, pp. 636-641.

Horne, R. S., Andrew, S., Mitchell, K., Sly, D. J., Cranage, S. M., Chau, B. and Adamson, T. M. (2001). Apnoea of prematurity and arousal from sleep. *Early Human Development*, Vol.61, No. 2, pp. 119-133.

Horne, R. S., Bandopadhayay, P., Vitkovic, J., Cranage, S. M. and Adamson, T. M. (2002). Effects of age and sleeping position on arousal from sleep in preterm infants. *Sleep*, Vol.25, No. 7, pp. 746-750.

Hunt, C. E., Corwin, M. J., Lister, G., Weese-Mayer, D. E., Ward, S. L., Tinsley, L. R., Neuman, M. R., Willinger, M., Ramanathan, R. and Rybin, D. (2008). Precursors of cardiorespiratory events in infants detected by home memory monitor. *Pediatr Pulmonol*, Vol.43, No. 1, pp. 87-98.

Irving, R. J., Belton, N. R., Elton, R. A. and Walker, B. R. (2000). Adult cardiovascular risk factors in premature babies. *Lancet*, Vol.355, No. 9221, pp. 2135-2136.

Kahn, A., Groswasser, J., Rebuffat, E., Sottiaux, M., Blum, D., Foerster, M., Franco, P., Bochner, A., Alexander, M., Bachy, A., Richard, P., Verghote, M., Polain, D. L. and Wayenberg, J. L. (1992). Sleep and Cardiorespiratory Characteristics of Infant Victims of Sudden Death: A Prospective Case-Control Study. *Sleep*, Vol.15, No. 4, pp. 287-292.

Kahn, A., Riazi, J. and Blum, D. (1983). Oculocardiac reflex in near miss for sudden infant death syndrome infants. *Pediatrics*, Vol.71, No. 1, pp. 49-52.

Kahn, A., Sawaguchi, T., Sawaguchi, A., Groswasser, J., Franco, P., Scaillet, S., Kelmanson, I. and Dan, B. (2002). Sudden infant deaths: from epidemiology to physiology. *Forensic Science International*, Vol.130 Suppl, No., pp. S8-20.

Karin, J., Hirsch, M. and Akselrod, S. (1993). An estimate of fetal autonomic state by spectral analysis of fetal heart rate fluctuations. *Pediatric Research*, Vol.34, No., pp. 134-138.

Kato, I., Franco, P., Groswasser, J., Scaillet, S., Kelmanson, I., Togari, H. and Kahn, A. (2003). Incomplete arousal processes in infants who were victims of sudden death. *Am J Respir Crit Care Med*, Vol.168, No. 11, pp. 1298-1303.

Katona, P. G., Frasz, A. and Egbert, J. (1980). Maturation of cardiac control in full-term and preterm infants during sleep. *Early Human Development*, Vol.4, No. 2, pp. 145-159.

Keene, D. J., Wimmer, J. E., Jr. and Mathew, O. P. (2000). Does supine positioning increase apnea, bradycardia, and desaturation in preterm infants? *J Perinatol*, Vol.20, No. 1, pp. 17-20.

Kelly, D. H., Golub, H., Carley, D. and Shannon, D. C. (1986). Pneumograms in infants who subsequently died of sudden infant death syndrome. *Journal of Pediatrics*, Vol.109, No. 2, pp. 249-254.

Khattak, A. Z., Padhye, N. S., Williams, A. L., Lasky, R. E., Moya, F. R. and Verklan, M. T. (2007). Longitudinal assessment of heart rate variability in very low birth weight infants during their NICU stay. *Early Human Development*, Vol.83, No. 6, pp. 361-366.

Kinney, H., Filiano, J., Sleeper, L., Mandell, F., Valdes-Dapena, M. and White, W. (1995). Decreased muscarinic receptor binding in the arcuate nucleus in sudden infant death syndrome. *Science*, Vol.269, No. 5229, pp. 1146-1150.

Kluge, K. A., Harper, R. M., Schechtman, V. L., Wilson, A. J., Hoffman, H. J. and Southall, D. P. (1988). Spectral analysis assessment of respiratory sinus arrhythmia in normal infants and infants who subsequently died of sudden infant death syndrome. *Pediatric Research*, Vol.24, No. 6, pp. 677-682.

Krueger, C., Van Oostrom, J. H. and Shuster, J. (2010). A longitudinal description of heart rate variability in 28--34-week-old preterm infants. *Biological Research for Nursing*, Vol.11, No. 3, pp. 261-268.

Lagercrantz, H., Henderson-Smart, D. and Jeffrey, H. (1990). Autonomic Reflexes in Preterm Infants. *Acta Paediatrica Scandinavica*, Vol.79, No., pp. 721-728.

Larson, W. J. (2001). *Human Embryology* (3rd ed), Churchill Livingstone, Philadelphia

Lavezzi, A. M., Ottaviani, G., Mauri, M. and Matturri, L. (2004). Hypoplasia of the arcuate nucleus and maternal smoking during pregnancy in sudden unexplained perinatal and infant death. *Neuropathology*, Vol.24, No. 4, pp. 284-289.

Linacre, S. (2007). Australia's Babies. *ABS: Australian Social Trends*, Vol.4102.0, No., pp.

Longin, E., Gerstner, T., Schaible, T., Lenz, T. and Konig, S. (2006). Maturation of the autonomic nervous system: differences in heart rate variability in premature vs. term infants. *Journal of Perinatal Medicine*, Vol.34, No. 4, pp. 303-308.

Longin, E., Schaible, T., Lenz, T. and Konig, S. (2005). Short term heart rate variability in healthy neonates: normative data and physiological observations. *Early Human Development*, Vol.81, No. 8, pp. 663-671.

Machaalani, R. and Waters, K. A. (2008). Neuronal cell death in the Sudden Infant Death Syndrome brainstem and associations with risk factors. *Brain*, Vol.131, No., pp. 218-228.

Malliani, A., Pagani, M., Lombardi, F. and Cerutti, S. (1991). Cardiovascular neural regulation explored in the frequency domain. *Circulation*, Vol.84, No. 2, pp. 482-492.

Malloy, M. H. and Freeman, D. H., Jr. (2000). Birth weight- and gestational age-specific sudden infant death syndrome mortality: United States, 1991 versus 1995. *Pediatrics*, Vol.105, No. 6, pp. 1227-1231.

Malloy, M. H. and Hoffman, M. A. (1995). Prematurity, sudden infant death syndrome and age of death. *Pediatrics*, Vol.96, No. 3, pp. 464-471.

Massin, M. M., Maeyns, K., Lombet, J., Rigo, J. and Gerard, P. (2002). Heart rate response profiles to tilting in healthy and unhealthy neonates. *Medical Science Monitor*, Vol.8, No. 5, pp. CR321-325.

Mazursky, J. E., Birkett, C. L., Bedell, K. A., Ben-Haim, S. A. and Segar, J. L. (1998). Development of baroreflex influences on heart rate variability in preterm infants. *Early Human Development*, Vol.53, No., pp. 37- 52.

Montano, N., Ruscone, T. G., Porta, A., Lombardi, F., Pagani, M. and Malliani, A. (1994). Power spectrum analysis of heart rate variability to assess the changes in sympathovagal balance during graded orthostatic tilt. *Circulation*, Vol.90, No. 4, pp. 1826-1831.

Moon, R. Y., Horne, R. S. and Hauck, F. R. (2007). Sudden infant death syndrome. *The Lancet*, Vol.370, No. 9598, pp. 1578-1587.

Padhye, N. S., Verklan, M., Brazdeikis, A., Williams, A. L., Khattak, A. Z. and Lasky, R. E. (2008). A comparison of fetal and neonatal heart rate variability at similar post-menstrual ages. *Conference Proceedings IEEE Engineering in Medicine and Biology Society*, Vol.2008, No., pp. 2801-2804.

Padhye, N. S., Williams, A. L., Khattak, A. Z. and Lasky, R. E. (2009). Heart rate variability in response to pain stimulus in VLBW infants followed longitudinally during NICU stay. *Developmental Psychobiology*, Vol.51, No. 8, pp. 638-649.

Pagani, M., Lombardi, F., Guzzetti, S., Rimoldi, O., Furlan, R., Pizzinelli, P., Sandrone, G., Malfatto, G., Dell'orto, S., Piccaluga, E. and Et Al. (1986). Power spectral analysis of heart rate and arterial pressure variabilities as a marker of sympatho-vagal interaction in man and conscious dog. *Circulation Research*, Vol.59, No. 2, pp. 178-193.

Paterson, D. S., Trachtenberg, F. L., Thompson, E. G., Belliveau, R. A., Beggs, A. H., Darnall, R., Chadwick, A. E., Krous, H. F. and Kinney, H. C. (2006). Multiple serotonergic brainstem abnormalities in sudden infant death syndrome. *Journal of the American Medical Association*, Vol.296, No. 17, pp. 2124-2132.

Patural, H., Barthelemy, J. C., Pichot, V., Mazzocchi, C., Teyssier, G., Damon, G. and Roche, F. (2004). Birth prematurity determines prolonged autonomic nervous system immaturity. *Clinical Autonomic Research*, Vol.14, No. 6, pp. 391-395.

Patural, H., Pichot, V., Jaziri, F., Teyssier, G., Gaspoz, J. M., Roche, F. and Barthelemy, J. C. (2008). Autonomic cardiac control of very preterm newborns: a prolonged dysfunction. *Early Human Development*, Vol.84, No. 10, pp. 681-687.

Pejovic, B., Peco-Antic, A. and Marinkovic-Eric, J. (2007). Blood pressure in non-critically ill preterm and full-term neonates. *Pediatric Nephrology*, Vol.22, No. 2, pp. 249-257.

Peterson, D. R. (1966). Sudden, unexpected death in infants. An epidemiologic study. *American Journal of Epidemiology*, Vol.84, No. 3, pp. 478-482.

Phillipson, E. A. and Sullivan, C. E. (1978). Arousal: The Forgotten Response to Respiratory Stimuli. *American Review of Respiratory Disease*, Vol.118, No., pp. 807-809.

Ramanathan, R., Corwin, M. J., Hunt, C. E., Lister, G., Tinsley, L. R., Baird, T., Silvestri, J. M., Crowell, D. H., Hufford, D., Martin, R. J., Neuman, M. R., Weese-Mayer, D. E., Cupples, L. A., Peucker, M., Willinger, M. and Keens, T. G. (2001). Cardiorespiratory events recorded on home monitors: Comparison of healthy infants with those at increased risk for SIDS. *Jama*, Vol.285, No. 17, pp. 2199-2207.

Ramet, J., Hauser, B., Dehan, M., Curzi-Dascalova, L. and Gaultier, C. (1995). Effect of State of Alertness on the Heart Rate Response to Ocular Compression in Human Infants. *Biology of the Neonate*, Vol.68, No., pp. 270-275.

Ramet, J., Praud, J., D'allest, A., Carofilis, A., Dehan, M. and Guilleminault, C. (1988). Effect of Maturation on Heart Rate Response to Ocular Compression Test during Rapid Eye Movement Sleep in Human Infants. *Pediatric Research*, Vol.24, No. 4, pp. 477-480.

Ramet, J., Praud, J. P., D'allest, A. M., Dehan, M. and Gaultier, C. (1990). Trigeminal airstream stimulation. Maturation-related cardiac and respiratory responses during REM sleep in human infants. *Chest*, Vol.98, No. 1, pp. 92-96.

Rhoades, R. and Pflanzer, R. (1996). *Human Physiology* Saunders College Publishing, USA

Sahni, R., Schulze, K. F., Kashyap, S., Ohira-Kist, K., Fifer, W. P. and Myers, M. M. (1999a). Postural differences in cardiac dynamics during quiet and active sleep in low birthweight infants. *Acta Paediatr*, Vol.88, No. 12, pp. 1396-1401.

Sahni, R., Schulze, K. F., Kashyap, S., Ohira-Kist, K., Fifer, W. P. and Myers, M. M. (2000). Maturational changes in heart rate and heart rate variability in low birth weight infants. *Developmental Psychobiology*, Vol.37, No. 2, pp. 73-81.

Sahni, R., Schulze, K. F., Kashyap, S., Ohira-Kist, K., Myers, M. M. and Fifer, W. P. (1999b). Body position, sleep states, and cardiorespiratory activity in developing low birth weight infants. *Early Human Development*, Vol.54, No. 3, pp. 197-206.

Saigal, S., Doyle, L. W., Saigal, S. and Doyle, L. W. (2008). An overview of mortality and sequelae of preterm birth from infancy to adulthood. *Lancet*, Vol.371, No. 9608, pp. 261-269.

Schechtman, V. L., Henslee, J. A. and Harper, R. M. (1998). Developmental patterns of heart rate and variability in infants with persistant apnea of infancy. *Early Human Development*, Vol.50, No., pp. 251- 262.

Schechtman, V. L., Henslee, J.A., Harper, R.M. (1998). Developmental patterns of heart rate and variability in infants with persistant apnea of infancy. *Early Human Development*, Vol.50, No., pp. 251- 262.

Schwartz, P. J., Stramba-Badiale, M., Segantini, A., Austoni, P., Bosi, G., Giorgetti, R., Grancini, F., Marni, E. D., Perticone, F., Rosti, D. and Salice, P. (1998). Prolongation of the QT interval and the sudden infant death syndrome. *The New England Journal of Medicine*, Vol.338, No. 24, pp. 1709- 1714.

Standfast, S. J., Jereb, S. and Janerich, D. T. (1979). The epidemiology of sudden infant death in upstate New York. *Journal of the American Medical Association*, Vol.241, No. 11, pp. 1121-1124.

Task Force of the European Society of Cardiology and the North American Society of Pacing and Electrophysiology (1996). Heart rate variability: Standards of measurement, physiological interpretation, and clinical use. *Circulation*, Vol.93, No. 5, pp. 1043-1065.

Thilo, E. H. and Rosenberg, A. A. (2010) The Late Preterm Infant In: *Current Diagnosis and Treatment: Pediatrics* W. HAY, M. LEVIN, J. SONDHEIMER and R. DETERDING (Eds), *Current Diagnosis and Treatment: Pediatrics*. McGraw-Hill Aurora, Colorado

Thiriez, G., Bouhaddi, M., Mourot, L., Nobili, F., Fortrat, J. O., Menget, A., Franco, P. and Regnard, J. (2009). Heart rate variability in preterm infants and maternal smoking during pregnancy. *Clinical Autonomic Research*, Vol.19, No. 3, pp. 149-156.

Thompson, J. M. and Mitchell, E. A. (2006). Are the risk factors for SIDS different for preterm and term infants? *Archives of Diseases in Childhood*, Vol.91, No. 2, pp. 107-111.

Tuladhar, R., Harding, R., Adamson, T. M. and Horne, R. S. (2005a). Heart rate responses to non-arousing trigeminal stimulation in infants: effects of sleep position, sleep state and postnatal age. *Early Human Development*, Vol.81, No. 8, pp. 673-681.

Tuladhar, R., Harding, R., Cranage, S. M., Adamson, T. M. and Horne, R. S. (2003). Effects of sleep position, sleep state and age on heart rate responses following provoked arousal in term infants. *Early Human Development*, Vol.71, No. 2, pp. 157-169.

Tuladhar, R., Harding, R., Michael Adamson, T. and Horne, R. S. (2005b). Comparison of postnatal development of heart rate responses to trigeminal stimulation in sleeping preterm and term infants. *Journal of Sleep Research*, Vol.14, No. 1, pp. 29-36.

Tynan, M., Davis, P. and Sheridan, D. (1977). Postnatal maturation of noradrenaline uptake and release in cat papillary muscles. *Cardiovascular Research*, Vol.11, No., pp. 206-209.

Verbeek, M. M., Richardson, H. L., Parslow, P. M., Walker, A. M., Harding, R. and Horne, R. S. (2008). Arousal and ventilatory responses to mild hypoxia in sleeping preterm infants. *Journal of Sleep Research*, Vol.17, No. 3, pp. 344-353.

Viskari, S., Andersson, S., Hytinantti, T. and Kirjavainen, T. (2007). Altered cardiovascular control in preterm infants with bronchopulmonary dysplasia. *Pediatric Research*, Vol.61, No. 5 Pt 1, pp. 594-599.

Waldman, S., Krauss, A. N. and Auld, P. A. (1979). Baroreceptors in preterm infants: their relationship to maturity and disease. *Developmental Medicine and Child Neurology*, Vol.21, No. 6, pp. 714-722.

WHO (2007) Certain conditions originating in the perinatal period, In: *International Statistical Classification of Diseases and Related Health Problems*), *International Statistical Classification of Diseases and Related Health Problems*. World Health Organization Geneva

Witcombe, N. B., Yiallourou, S. R., Walker, A. M. and Horne, R. S. (2008). Blood pressure and heart rate patterns during sleep are altered in preterm-born infants: implications for sudden infant death syndrome. *Pediatrics*, Vol.122, No. 6, pp. e1242-1248.

Witcombe, N. B., Yiallourou, S. R., Walker, A. M. and Horne, R. S. C. (2010). Delayed blood pressure recovery after head-up tilting during sleep in preterm infants. *Journal of Sleep Research*, Vol.19, No., pp. 93-102.

Wong, F. Y., Witcombe, N. B., Yiallourou, S. R., Yorkston, S., Dymowski, A. R., Krishnan, L., Walker, A. M. and Horne, R. S. (2011). Cerebral oxygenation is depressed during sleep in healthy term infants when they sleep prone. *Pediatrics*, Vol.127, No. 3, pp. e558-565.

Xu, J., Kochanek, K. D., Murphy, S. L. and Tejada-Vera, B. (2010). Deaths: Final Data for 2007. *National Vital Statistics Reports*, Vol.58, No. 19, pp.

Yiallourou, S. R., Walker, A. M. and Horne, R. S. (2006). Validation of a new noninvasive method to measure blood pressure and assess baroreflex sensitivity in preterm infants during sleep. *Sleep*, Vol.29, No. 8, pp. 1083-1088.

16

The Effect of Preterm Birth on Kidney Development and Kidney Function over Time

M.G. Keijzer-Veen and A.J. van der Heijden
Erasmus University Medical Center Rotterdam, Sophia Children's Hospital
The Netherlands

1. Introduction

In the last decades the survival of (extremely) preterm born and small for gestational age individuals has improved significantly.(Faranoff 2003; EXPRESS 2009) Many articles have been published showing a relation between unfavourable perinatal factors (*eg* growth restriction, maternal factors, maternal and postnatal medication use such as antenatal steroids and nephrotoxic agents) and increased risk for diseases in later life, like cardiovascular disease, diabetes mellitus, unfavourable lipid profile (together: the metabolic syndrome) and renal impairment. Recently, an increasing amount of studies have been published concerning the effects of preterm birth and these adult diseases as well. This chapter discusses the normal kidney development and the effect of premature and small for gestational age birth on kidney development and kidney function over time.

2. Developmental origins of health and diseases

Since several decades epidemiological research is performed to elucidate the pathophysiological mechanisms in the 'developmental origins of health and diseases' hypothesis, also known as the Barker hypothesis, or the fetal origins of adult disease hypothesis. In 1986 Barker first suggested a correlation between birth weight and ischaemic heart disease in adults in England and Wales. (Barker & Osmond, 1986) In this study the neonatal mortality in the period of 1921 - 1925 was positively related to the ischaemic heart disease in the same regions in the period of 1968-1978. Also other diseases were related to infant mortality, suggesting that poor living conditions, including poor nutrition, in early life is an important factor in development of disease on the short and long run. Furthermore, weight at the age of 1 year was negatively related to cardiovascular mortality at adult age. Therefore, it was suggested that processes linked to growth and acting in prenatal or early postnatal life strongly influence the risk of ischaemic heart disease. Many studies concerning the developmental origins of health and diseases are published in the years thereafter.(Barker & Osmond, 1988; Barker et al. 1993; Irving et al., 2000; Langley et al., 1994) Hypertension, hyperlipidemia, diabetes mellitus type II, stroke, coronary heart disease and renal impairment all seem to be related to low birth weight. (Barker & Bagby, 2005)
Still, the pathophysiological mechanisms are not preciously elucidated yet. Both genetic and environmental factors seem important. Genetic variation and gene expression will influence organogenesis. If unfavourable environmental factors are present at the crucial time of organ development (the critical window of development) it is likely that organ structure is

altered and function may be influenced in a negative way as well. In addition is has been postulated that accelerated postnatal growth in these subjects will aggravate the negative effect on organ function and risk of diseases over time (figure 1).

In a large cohort of middle ages adults (50-58 yr), who were exposed to undernutrition during the dutch famine it was shown that undernutrition in early gestation (first trimester) increases the risk for coronary heart disease and a more atherogenic plasma lipid profile. (Roseboom et al., 2006) Microalbuminuria and obstructive lung disease were more prevalent in those subjects who were exposed to undernutrition in mid gestation. Late gestation undernutrition increased the risk for glucose intolerance. Accererated postnatal growth is thought to further increases risk of disease in adult life, but it has not been demonstrated whether this growth is the cause or consequence of earlier growth restriction-related adult diseases. (Hales & Ozanne, 2002) In addition, catch up growth probably amplifies this effect by accelerated cellular aging (telomere shortening). This was suggested in a rat model: low protein diet offspring pups had significantly fewer large telomeres compared to control (normal diet offspring pups). (Jennings et al., 1999; Tarry-Adkins et al., 2009)

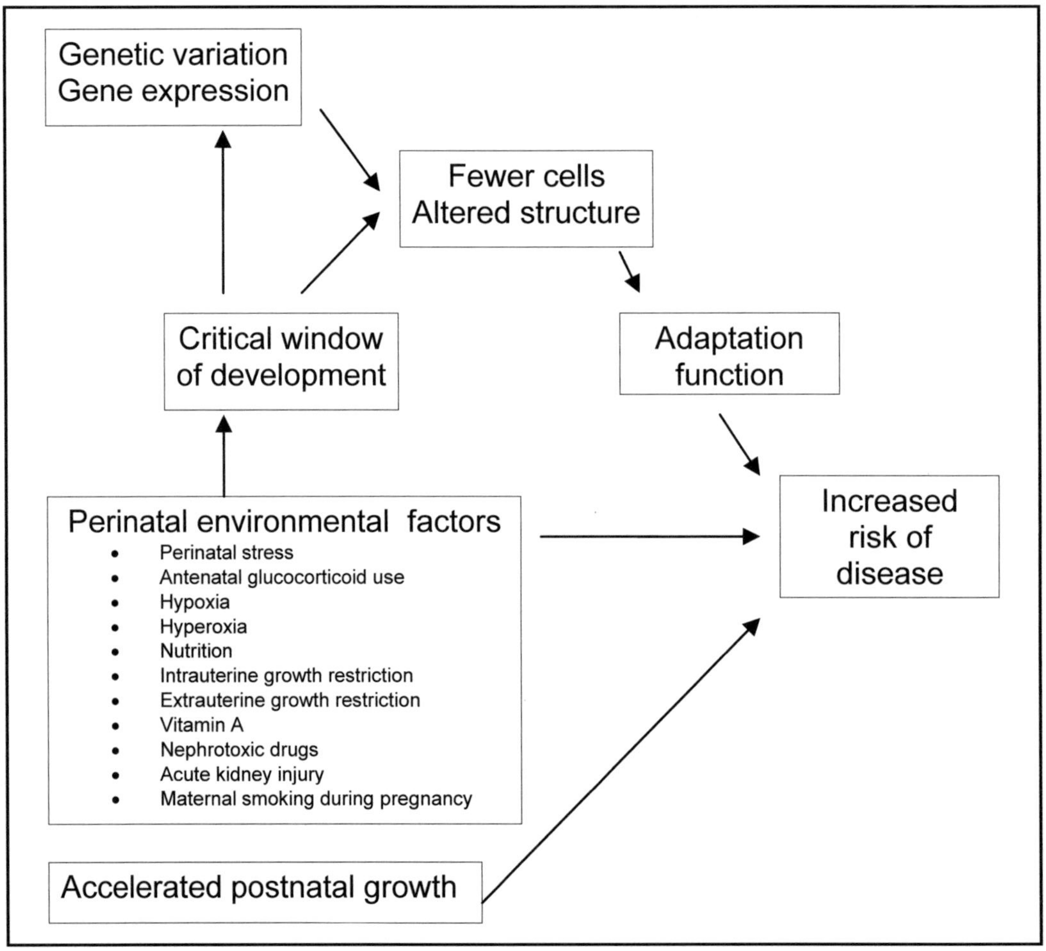

Fig. 1. Factors in Developmental Origins of adult Health and Disease (DOHaD).

The role of decreased renal development has been studied increasingly. Nephron endowment may result in glomerular and systemic hypertension, and in a decreased renal functional reserve capacity leading to a higher risk for decrease in renal function in later life (see below: hyperfiltration theory). Also, endothelial dysfunction and underdevelopment of the kidneys may be related to changes in the renin-angiotensin-system (RAS) and therefore increase blood pressure.

Low birth weight is mainly caused by malnutrition of the fetus, due to placenta insufficiency or maternal malnutrition, leading to redistribution of nutrients in favour of the development of the brain. Changes in cardiac output, hormone production, and sensitivity to hormones are thought to be altered and affect organs like lungs, pancreas and kidneys. This adaptation to the 'low nutrient' situation (programming), may lead to an increased susceptibility for malfunction of these specific organs after birth when the 'low nutrient' situation is discontinued. Other environmental factors, as hypoxia, hyperoxia, nephrotoxic medications, vitamin A deficiency, and variation in genes and genetic expression are also important in the context of the 'developmental origins of health and diseases' hypothesis. The effect of these factors on renal development are described in more detail below.

Lungs, pancreas and kidney are known to develop until the last few weeks of gestation. It is not completely elucidated whether premature birth decreases final development of these organs. Premature birth itself may therefore play an additional role in the increased risk for diseases in later life. In a Swedish study lower gestational age (GA) was associated with an increased blood pressure at the age of 49 years in 44 men. This correlation was stronger in the lower range of gestation (GA 30-38 weeks) (Siewert-Delle et al., 1998). In a study of 24 year old subjects born prematurely an increased blood pressure and insulin concentration was shown compared to subjects born at term. There was no difference in blood pressure between small for gestational age (SGA) preterm subjects and appropriate for gestational age (AGA) preterm subjects. In 2005 and 2008 we described an increased systolic blood pressure at 19 and 20 years of age in both SGA and AGA preterms (GA < 32 weeks) compared to the general population and to term born controls of the same age.(Keijzer-Veen et al, 2005; Keijzer-Veen et al, 2008) Ex-utero growth and development during the third trimester of the preterm infant was suggested to be more important in development of cardiovascular risk factors than growth retardation alone.(Irving et al, 2000) This was also demonstrated in women born preterm (GA < 32 weeks), at term SGA subjects and at term controls between 23 and 30 years of age in Sweden. Systolic blood pressure was only increased in the preterm subjects. Also the number of hypertensive blood pressure readings were higher in the preterm group (Kistner et al., 2000).

3. Hyperfiltration theory

It is suggested that the kidneys also are 'programmed' in intrauterine growth restricted fetuses. A deficit of nephrons is measured in several studies, possibly affecting long term renal function.(Langley-Evans et al., 1999; Lucas et al., 1997; Merlet-Benichou et al., 1994; Zeman, 1968) Also alterations in the renin-angiotensin-system (RAS) are thought to be important to increase blood pressure at adult life in these individuals.

In 1992 Brenner postulated the 'hyperfiltration theory', which enables to understand the possible mechanical pathway in the hypothesis that renal diseases at adult age is associated with intrauterine growth restriction (figure 2). Malnutrition of the fetus can lead to intrauterine growth restriction and impairment of renal development including deficit in nephron numbers (Hinchliffe et al, 1992), which causes a decreased filtration surface area. Renal hemodynamic alterations, like hyperfiltration, are needed to improve the glomerular filtration in order to maintain normal renal function. This phenomenon is accompanied with glomerular and systemic hypertension. Glomerular hypertension may cause damage of nephrons leading to acquired glomerular sclerosis which decreases nephron numbers and filtration surface (vicious circle).(Brenner & Anderson, 1992; Brenner & Chertow, 1994; Martyn et al., 1996) Major criticism exists that no study confirmed the presence of an increased renal and systemic blood pressure as a consequence of hyperfiltration in growth restricted individuals. Brenner implicates that all kinds of nephron deficit are associated with the development of hypertension. He refers to studies in persons with unilateral agenesis and ablative surgery as in kidney donors. (Hakim et al., 1984; Thorner et al., 1984) Other studies show normal blood pressures ranges after 20 years of follow up in healthy kidney donors. (Goldfarb et al., 2001; Iglesias-Marquez et al., 2001) These individuals however, seem more healthy than the general population in first place. It seems more likely that hypertension is an additional factor in the pathway of impaired renal function in low birth weights.

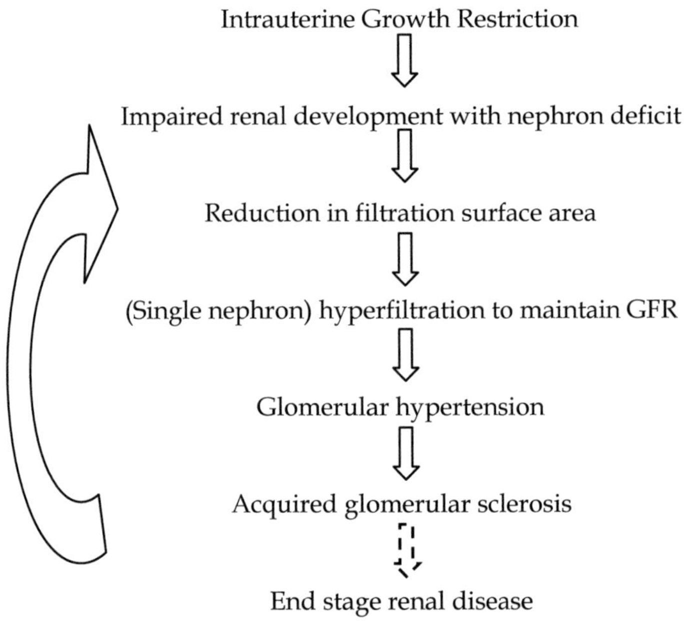

Fig. 2. Hyperfiltration theory. GFR: glomerular filtration rate. (adapted from Brenner & Chertow, 1994)

A strong relation between birth weight and renal size, nephron number, albuminuria and systolic blood pressure is shown in Aboriginal communities.(Singh & Hoy, 2004) In these communities diseases like type II diabetes, cardiovascular diseases and renal diseases take epidemic proportions. In another study in deceased 56 African Americans and Caucasians the kidneys were microscopically investigated.(Hoy et al., 2003) Nephron number was measured by stereologic estimation. Here, also nephron number was related to birth weight. Also, nephron number was inversely related to glomerular volume, suggesting that glomerulomegaly is a marker of an increased risk of groups of patients or populations with progressive renal disease. These findings support the 'hyperfiltration theory' saying that birth weight is a risk factor for the development of progressive renal disease. (Singh & Hoy, 2004; Hughson, 2003)

4. Kidney development

4.1 Normal kidney development

In mammals, three different pair of renal organ system exist through embryologic development. The pronephros and mesonephros develop within the first 5 weeks of pregnancy and regress during development. They have no or limited renal function. The permanent kidney development start at approximately the 7th week of gestation with the outgrowth of the ureteric but from caudal end of the mesonephric duct, meeting the metanephric blastema which together will differentiate into nephrons. (Moritz & Wintour, 1999) In addition, integration of small vessel growth is required in nephron formation. The first urine producing nephrons are developed within the first ten weeks of gestation and the amount is increasing with age. Driving forces to the outgrowth of the ureteric epithelium are direct cell-to-cell interactions, which are dependent of mesenchymal growth factors. These factors induce intracellular signalling and the expression of several gene products. (Jahnukainen et al., 2001) Many regulatory factors are involved, like fibroblast growth factor (FGF)-2, endothelial growth factor (EGF), bone morphogenetic protein-7, retinoic acid receptor expression, and PAX2, WT1, Wnt-11 genes. (Burrow et al., 2000; Burrow et al., 2007) PAX2 and WT1 are important in the proliferation and cell survival of the metanephric development. (Jahnukainen et al., 2001) Most nephrons are formed after the 20th week and at the age of 34-36 weeks the nephrogenesis is finished. At term birth, no new nephrons are formed. On average 750,000 nephrons per kidney are formed with a wide inter-individual range (250,000 to 2,000,000). (Hughson 2003, 2006, Nyengaard et al., 1992; Keller et al., 2003) The intrauterine renal blood flow and glomerular filtration rate is low, due to high vascular resistance. The urine production increases with fall in renal vascular resistance after birth maintained by a delicate balance in vasodilatory and vasoconstricting factors which is easily disturbed by illness of the neonatal infant (sepsis, cardiovascular distress, medications). Plasma creatinin levels fall from maternal levels to neonatal levels within three weeks. (Drukker & Guignard, 2002)

Also renal tubular function is recognised at early gestation (12-14 weeks) and rapidly developing. Tubular function in the neonate is characterized by reduced renal concentration and acidification ability, which improves in the first year of life. This phenomenon is more pronounced in preterm born subjects and in newborns suffering obstructive uropathy. (Chevalier, 1996) Urine calcium excretion is high, which can be aggravated by calciuric drugs, such as furosemide and glucocorticoids. In neonates, urine production and sodium excretion is relatively high compared to older children and adults, but fractional sodium excretions normalises within a few weeks. The concentrating capacity of the distal convolute tubule and collecting ducts increase within the first year of life.

4.2 Kidney development in preterm born individuals

As nephrogenesis is ongoing until the gestational age of 34-36 weeks, preterm born individuals suffer a diminished number of nephrons at birth. Many studies have shown lower renal volume in growth restricted subjects, both in animals and humans. Question is:

Is the premature infant capable of ongoing nephrogenesis after birth? and which factors may disturb this phenomenon?
From a study in 56 deceased extremely premature human infants and 10 deceased full term born controls it appeared that nephron number was highly correlated to gestational age and that glomerulogenesis had stopped after 40 days postnatal. (Rodriguez et al., 2004) A limited postnatal glomerulogenesis in preterm born individuals was shown and postnatal renal failure further inhibited the glomerulogenesis. In a small Italian study an active glomerulogenesis at preterm birth was seen but also ceased after a short period. (Faa et al. 2010) Therefore, nephron deficit (oligonephronia) in preterm born individuals probably exists throughout life placing the patient at risk for renal function deterioration. (Hughson et al., 2003: Singh et al., 2004)
In addition, histological changes are seen as well in the preterm born kidney. Animal studies in premature born baboons have shown abnormal glomeruli in the outer renal cortex, which contain the most newly formed glomeruli. Enlargement of the Bowman's space and shrinkage of the glomerular tuft are described. (Sutherland 2009) Glomerulomegaly and sausage shape kidneys may be a compensatory mechanism through hyperfiltration in oligonephronia. (Konje et al., 1996 Konje et al., 1997) Several studies have shown a reduced renal length and volume after SGA and preterm birth. (Konje et al., 1997; Spencer et al., 2001; Singh et al., 2004; Keijzer-Veen et al., 2010a) Konje showed lower renal volume in SGA born individuals compared to AGA. Differences were already shown at 26-28 weeks of gestation. (Konje et al., 1997) An Australian study showed lower renal volume in LBW aboriginal children (5-18 yr). (Spencer et al., 2001) Singh et al. also described that lower renal volume in aboriginals represents kidneys with reduced nephron number (Singh et al., 2004). We described decreased renal size in very preterm born individuals compared with full term born controls. (Keijzer-Veen et al., 2010a) Also, an increased number of renal anomalies was suggested in this study population.

4.3 Factors affecting kidney development

Both antenatal, perinatal and postnatal factors have been associated with impaired renal development in the neonate. Maternal factors like use of antenatal steroids, antihypertensive medication are studied. In addition, the infant may also suffer other conditions affecting postnatal renal development, like hypoxia, hyperoxia, use of nephrotoxic medications, acute kidney injury, vitamin A deficiency, and variation in genes and genetic expression. Effects of these factors are describes in more detail below.
Variation in genes and genetic expression: Epigenetic mechanisms are capable to induce important changes in the tissue-specific gene expression. Unfavorable environmental factors may influence promoter methylation, genetic imprinting and metastable epialleles and may alter tissue function. The critical window for epigenetic changes is not known. (Gluckman et al., 2008 and Wadhwa et al., 2009) Additional population based studies are conducted and results awaiting.
Antenatal steroid use: Glucocorticoids are important regulators of fetal growth and development. They affect gene transcription and cell differentiation and maturation in at least 15 different tissues. (Ballard et al., 1995) With the use of antenatal glucocorticoids preterm survival has improved significantly by accelerated maturation of lungs and surfactant production, increase in blood pressure and renal blood flow and GFR, with a decrease in urinary sodium excretion. (Kari et al., 1994) Increased nephrogenesis is

suggested when glucocorticoids are used at late pregnancy, while early administration was affecting nephrogenesis in a negative way in several animal studies. (Jahnukainen et al., 2001) (Gughaju et al., 2011).

Hypoxia: Perinatal hypoxia is a common feature in preterm born individuals. Underdevelopment of the lungs, and unfavourable perinatal conditions (sepsis, cardiovascular instability, metabolic changes) all increase the risk for hypoxic periods. Also spontaneous hypoxic events occur often in premature born infants. Hypoxia-induced tissue injury increase the risk for neurological but also renal morbidity. (Petrova & Metha, 2011) Renal ultrasound shows an increased hyperreflectivity of the renal parenchyma after hypoxic episodes. (Streitman et al., 2001) Hypoxia may lead to acute tubulus necrosis and *acute kidney injury* and deterioration of renal function. Mostly, the damage seems reversible, but loss of nephrons is not repaired and therefore is likely to increase the risk for renal disease in later life. (Askenazi et al., 2006)

Hyperoxia: Impaired angiogenesis is a wellknown result from hyperoxic state in preterm neonates leading to an increased risk for retinopathy of prematurity and bronchopulmonary dysplasia. It is suggested that an impaired renal angiogenesis may contribute a decreased renal development. (Gughaju et al. 2011) Further studies are needed to elucidate the effect of hyperoxia on renal development.

Nephrotoxic medications: Use of nephrotoxic medication in preterm neonates quite common. Aminoglycosides (gentamycin) are associated with nephron endowment and acute tubulus necrosis. (Gilbert 1996) Drug therapeutic monitoring strategies should be performed. Indomethacin (prostaglandin synthetase inhibitor) is also known to decrease renal blood flow due to decrease in prostaglandin production and vasoconstriction. Diuresis and natriuresis decreases and serum creatinine levels may rise. Ibuprofen exerts less effect on kidney function. (Giniger et al., 2007) The effect seems temporary, but it is not known if renal function over time is influenced if these medications are prescribed in early life.

Intrauterine growth restriction (IUGR): As describes above, many studies have shown an effect of (very) low birth weight and adult diseases. However, low birth weight subjects are not per definition exposed to growth restriction. Subjects born prematurely have lower birth weights than subjects born at term, but they both may have grown normally until that period of gestation. The extent of intra uterine growth restriction can therefore be expressed best by adjusting birth weight for gestational age. (Arnold et al., 1991) The most common way to describe (birth) weight is to express weight as a standard deviation score (SDS), which in fact is a z-score for birth weight, instead of using the SI units like (kilo)grams. A birth weight SDS of zero means that the subject's birth weight is the equal to the mean birth weight of all subjects born at the same gestational age. Lower birth weight than would be expected given that certain gestational age leads to a birth weight (SDS) below zero (also known as small for gestational age or SGA). Subjects with higher birth weights than would be expected given their gestational age will have a birth weight (SDS) above zero (also known as appropriate for gestational age or AGA). Normally the SDS ranges mainly between -3 and +3. The definition of IUGR is an arbitrary value between 0 and minus infinity, depending on the reference population, which is used to calculate the SDS. IUGR is most commonly defined as a birth weight (SDS) < 0 or < -2.

Extrauterine growth restriction (EUGR): Poor postnatal growth is known as a serious problem in very prematurely born individuals. In a large study including the data of 24,371 premature neonates it was shown that the incidence of EUGR was common (28%, 34% and

16% for weight, length and head circumference) and the incidence increased with gestational age and birth weight. (Clark et al., 2003) More recently it was shown that also postnatal growth restriction affected renal function over time in children born prematurely. At the age of 7 years blood pressure was slightly increased and renal size decreased in both 23 IUGR and 16 EUGR children in a study from France. (Bachetta et al., 2009)

Vitamin A deficiency: Vitamin A (retinoid acid) plays a critical role in fetal organogenesis, and it suggested that deficiency may induce malformations. Vitamin A is involved in normal branching of the ureteric. In a rat model a 50% reduction of vitamin A levels reduced nephron number by 20%. (Lelievre-Pegorier et al., 1998) However, postnatal supplementation of Vitamin A did not improve nephrogenesis in preterm born rats suggesting that vitamin A supplementation is of more importance during pregnancy. (Sutherland et al., 2009) Human studies seem scarce. In 2007 it was suggested that maternal vitamin A deficiency may induce kidney hypoplasia in their children. (Goodyer et al., 2007) Adequate Vitamin A intake should be undertaken.

Salt overload: Cardoso et al has suggested an increased risk for hypertension and reduced GFR after postnatal sodium overload in a study of 27 Wistar rats. (Cardoso et al.,2009) Offspring of the sodium overloaded pregnant rats had higher blood pressure, proteinuria and decreased renal function 90 days postnatally. Lipid profile was also disturbed and changes in the renin-angiotensin system was observed.

Renin-Angiotensin-System: A low renal blood flow leads to an increase in renin production by juxta-glomerular apparatus, which increases blood pressure by renin-angiotensin-system (RAS) in two ways. First renin converts angiotensinogen into angiotensin I (AT I), which is converted to angiotensin II (AT II) by angiotensin-converted enzyme (ACE). AT II stimulates α-receptors causing vasoconstriction in small vessels leading to an increase in blood pressure. Second, AT II stimulates aldosterone hormone production in the adrenal glands that stimulates sodium resorption and water retention in the distal convolute tubulus leading to an increase of circulating volume and blood pressure. In addition to the role to regulate blood pressure, the RAS is also thought to be an important factor in the renal development. Renal abnormalities are shown in animals in which RAS was blocked during renal development.(Guron & Friberg, 2000) Use of ACE inhibiting or AT II receptor blockage are therefore contraindicated during pregnancy.

Konje studied the active renin levels and AT I levels in the umbilical vein in preterms and IUGR fetuses. (Konje et al., 1996) AT I levels were increased in intra uterine growth restricted infants born preterm. Explanation could be hypoxia, increased sympatic nerve activity and catecholamin production (all present in growth restricted fetuses), but also a proliferation of juxta-glomerular cells (and thus renin producing cells). Protein restriction in pregnant rats leads to suppression of RAS in the fetus, associated with a inhibition of nephrogenesis and development of the ascending limb of Henle. (Lasaitiene et al., 2004) Also an increased $ATII_1$ receptor expression is shown in undernutritioned fetal rats. This may be a direct effect of protein restriction or a response to a decreased ATII concentration.(Sahajpal & Ashton, 2003) Martyn showed a decrease in inactive renine levels in adults exposed to malnutrition and intrauterine growth restriction.(Martyn et al., 1996) Fetal alterations in RAS activity may affect blood pressure in adult life. However, data are limited and not convincing. Further investigation is needed to elucidate the role of RAS in nephrogenesis and hypertension in adult life and the consequences for preterms and intrauterine growth restricted subjects.

5. Preterm birth and renal function over time

The plasma creatinin levels inversely correlate with the birth weight and gestational age during the first days of life. Creatinine falls within the first three weeks of life. (Bueva & Guignard, 1994) The normal fall in fractional sodium excretion is delayed in preterm born individuals. (Drukker & Guignard, 2002) Normal maturation of urine concentrating capacity takes about 1 year. Newer laboratory methods for renal function, like Cystatin C and Urinary Neutrophil gelatinase-assiciated lipocalin (*N-GAL*) are under investigation for the prediction of renal damage in this patient group as well. Further studies are upcoming.

With the knowledge that renal development is likely to be unfinished in preterm born individuals, and further development may be impaired, and that the preterm subject may suffer severe co-morbidity, and other risk factors for renal function impairment, the question rises what the implications are for renal health over time?

To elucidate the effect of preterm birth over time the information from long term follow up cohort studies are crucial. However, neonatal intensive care and general pediatric care are improving significantly. Therefore, extrapolation of the data from the older cohort studies to current time is not justified. On the other hand, more recent cohort studies only describe short period of follow up, and large cohorts are needed to demonstrate small differences between these 'younger' groups. In addition, most studies are limited because of small sample size and very low birth weight criteria are used instead of birth weight adjusted for gestational age. (Arnold et al., 1991)

Recently, Zanardo described an increased urinary microalbumin to creatinin ratio in 23 Italian toddlers (age 18 months) born after intra uterine growth restriction compared to 21 AGA born subjects. (Zanardo et al., 2011) Also, arterial intima media thickness and systolic blood pressure were increased in the SGA group. In this study the SGA group was born much more premature (mean gestational age 32 weeks compared to 38 weeks in the AGA group). Gestational age could have influenced the results. No blood samples were taken in this study. (Zanardo et al., 2011) A Polish study in 78 subjects born with a birth weight < 1,000 gr showed higher Cystatin C levels in the ELBW group compared to 38 controls at the mean age of 6.7 years. Renal volume was also significantly lower in the ELBW group. (Kwinta et al., 2011) Iacobelli found that neonatal hypotension was an independent risk factor for the development of microalbuminuria at the age of 7 years in 48 very preterm born individuals. (Iacobelli et al., 2007) No significant difference in renal function, size and blood pressure was seen between preterms and controls. In contrast, in a Swedish study renal function was not different between preterm born AGA (*N*= 29) and at term SGA (*N*= 39) children at the age of 9-12 yrs. Absolute renal volume was lower in the preterms, but after adjustment for body surface area the difference disappeared. (Rakow et al., 2008). Kistner et al. described blood pressure and renal function in 50 women born preterm and AGA, at term born SGA and at term born controls at the age of 29 years. Casual and ambulatory systolic blood pressure was increased in the preterm born group. No significant differences between groups were found in renal function. (Kistner et al. 2000; Kistner et al., 2002)

In the Netherlands two large prospective cohorts are available and ongoing. Additional studies are planned. The first large cohort study in the Netherlands is the **POPS study** (Project Of Preterms and Small for gestational age infants), which includes 94% of all individuals born with a gestational age < 32 weeks and/or a birth weight < 1500 grams in the Netherlands in 1983 (*N*=1338). At the ages of 3, 6, 12 and 24 months and 5, 10, 14, and 19 years of age these subjects were tested for general health, cognitive development and motor skills and disabilities and quality of life. At the age of 19 years blood pressure, blood samples and urine samples were taken to evaluate the risk factors for cardiovascular disease, diabetes type 2, lipid profile deterioration and renal impairment. Pulse wave velocity and intima media thickness were measured. Of 1338 study subjects, 962 survived until the age of 14 years and 28 were lost to follow up. At the age of 19 years 934 were eligible for inclusion in the POPS19 study. Five hundred and ninety six subjects participated in this study (64%). Of these 596 subjects, 422 were born very preterm (GA < 32 weeks) and 174 had a very low birth weight < 1500 gram and a GA > 32 weeks. Blood pressure was significantly higher in all preterm born, independent of the birth weight. (Keijzer-Veen et al., 2005a) Renal function was normal, but not in favour of the small for gestational age born subgroups with higher levels of serum creatinine and increased microalbuminuria. (Keijzer-Veen et al., 2005b) No difference in intima-media thickness nor pulse wave velocity was found. (Finken et al, 2006a) Also the lipid profile was equal in all groups. (Euser et al., 2005) Insulin resistance was predicted by rapid postnatal weight gain until 3 months post term and by adult body composition. (Finken et al, 2006b)

An additional study in a subset of premature infants, comparing small for gestational age (SGA), appropriate for gestational age (AGA) and at term born controls. In this study renal function was measured in more detail. Inulin and para-aminohippuric acid clearances were measured with a continuous infusion, as well as renal reserve capacity. Renal ultrasound and 24 hour blood pressure monitoring were also performed. This study showed that blood pressure is increased in preterm born individuals compared to at term born controls. (Keijzer-Veen et al. 2010b) No differences between SGA and AGA infants was found. Renal function was normal in all individuals but lower in SGA preterm subjects. (Keijzer-Veen et al. 2007) Also the renal reserve capacity and effective renal plasma flow was reduced in SGA preterm subjects. The number of renal anomalies (mainly ectasia of the urinary system) was higher in preterm born individuals, and the renal size was decreased compared to controls. There was a difference in left and right kidney, and renal size differed between gender. (Keijzer-Veen et al. 2010a)

More recently, the **Generation R study**, a population based prospective cohort study from fetal life until young adulthood in Rotterdam, the Netherlands is conducted. (Jaddoe et al. 2010) In total, 9,778 mothers with a delivery date from April 2002 until January 2006 were enrolled in the study. Of all eligible children at birth, 61% participate in the study. General follow up rates exceed 75% at age 4 years. In addition, more detailed assessments are conducted in a subgroup of 1,232 pregnant women and their children. Data collection in the prenatal phase and postnatal phase until the age of 4 years includes questionnaires, detailed physical and ultrasound examinations, behavioral observations and biological samples. (Jaddoe et al. 2007) Renal ultrasound was performed antenatal and postnatal.

Results in regard to renal development and function: Maternal smoking was associated with reduced kidney size in the offspring. A curved shaped association between the number of cigarettes smoked in the third trimester of pregnancy and fetal kidney size was found. Small kidney size in fetal life tends to persist in early childhood. (Geelhoed et al. 2009 and Taal 2011) Preferential fetal blood flow to the brain was also associated with smaller kidneys in late pregnancy. (Verburg et al. 2007)

6. Clinical implications and future perspectives

The survival of extremely preterm birth, even at gestational age of 22-23 weeks has improved tremendously. One-year survival rates of 9.8% in 22 weeks of gestation and 53% in 23 weeks of gestation have been described in Sweden in the period 2004-2007. (EXPRESS group 2009) In this study the overall mortality was 30% in all 22-26 weeks of gestation at the age of 1 year and only 45% of survivors had no major morbidity at the age of 1 year. To improve normal ex-utero growth (like in-utero) and development the ESPGHAN guidelines recommend a high protein intake of at least 3 g/kg/day, a phosphate intake of 60-90 mg/kg/day and a calciumintake of 120-140 mg/kg/day. (Agostoni et al. 2009) However, it is to be investigated if renal development also benefits this protein, calcium- and phosphate load. Follow-up of these children should include the evaluation of nephrocalcinosis incidence and glomerular and tubular function over time. Moreover, the extremely preterm born subjects (gestational age 22-24 weeks) are likely to have an increased exposure to factors depriving kidney development in the neonatal intensive care unit. It is hypothesized that renal function loss will become evident at even younger age compared with individuals born less premature or in the early eighties or nineties.

In addition, with increasing prevalence of obesity and increased salt intake in adults and children, the risk for the metabolic syndrome and renal function loss is increasing in the general population. It has been shown that the risk for renal function loss was twofold in children obese born prematurely compared to obese children born at term. (Abitbol et al 2009) Therefore, childhood obesity and salt intake overload should be avoided in all children, especially when born premature.

It is important to acknowledge the problem of disturbed nephrogenesis in the preterm born infant, and to prevent further disturbed development by good clinical practice. Primary prevention of preterm birth and IUGR and secondary prevention of other factors affecting renal development like hyperoxia, hypoxia, infection with decreased renal blood flow (blood pressure regulation and toxins), nephrotoxic medications and extra-uterine growth restriction should be addressed daily at the neonatal intensive care units. Clinicians should evaluate the effects of their actions. Long term follow-up is advised by simple urinary test (proteinuria/microalbuminuria) and blood pressure screening. Patients with abnormalities should be referred to a paediatrician for more detailed renal function measurement.

7. Conclusion

This chapter has shown the normal kidney development and the effect of premature birth. Nephron endowment is a risk factor for glomerular hyperfiltration and renal function deterioration over time. Prevention of premature birth and intrauterine growth restriction, prevention of childhood obesity and salt and protein overload should be highly advocated in all populations and health care organizations. The importance of prevention of further renal damage in premature born individuals is not to be underestimated.

8. References

Abitbol CL, Chandar J, Rodriguez MM; Berho M; Seeherunvong M; Freundlich M; Zilleruelo G. (2009) Obesity and preterm birth: additive risks in the progression of kidney disease in children. Ped Nephrol Vol.24, No.7, pp. 1363-1370.

Agostoni, C. ESPGHAN Guidelines. (2009) Enteral Nutrient supply for preterm infants. *J Pediatr Gastroenterol Nutr,* Vol.50, pp.1-9

Arnold,C.C.; Kramer,M.S.; Hobbs,C.A.; McLean,F.H.; Usher,R.H.(1991). Very low birth weight: a problematic cohort for epidemiologic studies of very small or immature neonates. *Am J Epidemiol,* Vol. 134, No. 6, pp. 604-613

Askenazi, D.J.; Feig, D.I.; Graham, N.M.; Hui-Stickle, S.; Goldstein, S.L. (2006). 3-5 year longitudinal follow up of pediatric patients after acute renal failure. Kidney Int, Vol. 69, pp. 184-189

Cardoso, H.D., Cabral, E.V.; Vieira-Filho, L.D.; Vieyra, A.; Paixao, A.D.O. (2009). Fetal development and renal function in adult rats prenatally subjected to sodium overload. *Ped Nephrol* Vol. 24, pp. 1959-1965

Chevalier RH. (1996). Developmental renal physiology of the low birth weight preterm newborn. *J Urol,* Vol.156, No.2, pp.714-719

Clark, R.H.; Thomas, P. & Piebody J. (2003). Extrauterine growth restriction remains a serious problem in prematurely born neonates. *Pediatrics,* Vol. 111, No 5, pp.986-990

Bachetta, J.; Harambat, J.; Dubourg, L., (2009) Both extrauterine and intrauterine growth restriction impair renal function in children born very preterm. Kidney Int Vol.76, No.4, pp.445-452

Ballard PL & Ballard RA (1995) Scientific basis and therapeutic regimens for use of antenatal glucocorticoids. Am J Obstet Gynaecol. Vol.173, No.1, pp.254-262

Barker DJ, Osmond C (1986). Infant mortality, childhood nutrition, and ischaemic heart disease in England and Wales. Lancet 1:1077-1081

Barker DJ, Osmond C (1988). Low birth weight and hypertension. British Medical Journal 297:134-135

Barker DJ, Gluckman PD, Godfrey KM, Harding JE, Owens JA, Robinson JS (1993) Fetal nutrition and cardiovascular disease in adult life. Lancet 341:938-941

Barker,D.J.; Bagby,S.P. (2005) Developmental Antecedents of Cardiovascular Disease: A Historical Perspective. *J Am Soc Nephrol,* Vol.16, No. 9, Pp.2537-2544

Brenner BM, Anderson S (1992) The interrelationships among filtration surface area, blood pressure, and chronic renal disease. J Cardiovasc Pharmacol 19 Suppl 6:S1-S7

Brenner BM, Chertow GM (1994) Congenital oligonephropathy and the etiology of adult hypertension and progressive renal injury. Am J Kidney Dis 23:171-175

Bueva A; Guignard JP. (1994). Renal function in preterm neonates. *Ped Research,* Vol.36. No.5, pp.572-577

Burrow, C.R. (2007). Regulatory molecules in kidney development. *Pediatr Nephrol,* Vol. 14, pp. 240-253

Burrow, C.R. (2000). Retinoids and renal development. *Exp Nephrol,* Vol. 8, pp. 219-225

Drukker, A. & Guignard, J.P. (2002). Renal aspects of the term and preterm infants: a selective update. *Curr Opin Pediatr,* Vol.14, pp.175-182

Euser AM, Finken MJJ, Keijzer-Veen MG, Hille ETM, Wit JM, Dekker FW (2005) Associations between prenatal and infancy weight gain and BMI, fat mass, and fat distribution in young adulthood: a prospective cohort study in males and females born very preterm. Am J Clin Nutr 81:480-487

EXPRESS Group, Fellman V, Hellström-Westas L, Norman M, Westgren M, Källén K, Lagercrantz H, Marsál K, Serenius F, Wennergren M. (2009) One-year survival of extremely preterm born infants after active perinatal care in Sweden. JAMA, Vol.301, No.21 pp.2225-2233

Fanaroff,A.A.; Hack,M.; Walsh,M.C. (2003). The NICHD neonatal research network: changes in practice and outcomes during the first 15 years *Semin Perinatol,* Vol. 27, No. 4, pp. 281-287

Finken MJ, Inderson A, Van Montfoort N, Keijzer-Veen MG, van Weert AW, Carfil N, Frolich M, Hille ET, Romijn JA, Dekker FW, Wit JM (2006a) Lipid profile and carotid intima-media thickness in a prospective cohort of very preterm subjects at age 19 years: effects of early growth and current body composition. *Pediatr Res* 59:604-609

Finken MJ, Keijzer-Veen MG, Dekker FW, Frolich M, Hille ET, Romijn JA, Wit JM (2006b) Preterm birth and later insulin resistance: effects of birth weight and postnatal growth in a population based longitudinal study from birth into adult life. *Diabetologia* 49:478-485

Geelhoed JJ; Verburg BO; Nauta J; Lequin M; Hofman A; Moll HA; Witteman JCM; van der Heijden AJ; Steegers EAP; Jaddoe VWV. (2009) Tracking and determinants of kidney size from fetal life until the age of 2 years: The Generation R study. Am J Kidney Dis. Vol. 53, No.2 ;pp248-258

Gilbert,T.; Cibert,C.; Moreau,E.; Geraud,G.; Merlet-Benichou,C. (1996) Early defect in branching morphogenesis of the ureteric bud in induced nephron deficit. *Kidney Int* Vol. 50, No. 3; pp 783-795

Giniger RP; Buffat C; Millet V; Simeoni U. (2007) Renal effects of ibuprofen for the treatment of patent ductus arteriosus in premature infants. *J Matern Fetal Neonatol Med,* Vol.20, No.4, Pp 275-83.

Gluckman PD; Hanson MA; Cooper C; Thornburg KL. (2008) Effect of in utero and early-life conditions on adult health and disease. *N Eng J Med,* Vol 359, No. 1, pp. 61-73

Goldfarb DA, Matin SF, Braun WE, Schreiber MJ, Mastroianni B, Papajcik D, Rolin HA, Flechner S, Goormastic M, Novick AC (2001) Renal outcome 25 years after donor nephrectomy. J Urol 166:2043-2047

Gughaju, L.; Sutherland, M.R. & Black, M.J. (2011). Preterm birth and the kidney: Implications for long-term renal health. *Reproductive Sciences.* Vol.18, No.4, pp. 322-333.

Guron G, Friberg P (2000) An intact renin-angiotensin system is a prerequisite for normal renal development. J Hypertens 18:123-137

Hakim RM, Goldszer RC, Brenner BM (1984) Hypertension and proteinuria: long-term sequelae of uninephrectomy in humans. Kidney Int 25:930-936

Hales CN; Ozanne SE. (2002) The dangerous road of cath-up growth. J Physiol, Vol. 547. No. 1, pp.5-10

Hinchliffe, S.A.; Lynch,M.R.; Sargent,P.H.; Howard,C.V.; van Velzen,D. (1992) The effect of intrauterine growth retardation on the development of renal nephrons. *Br J Obstet Gynaecol,* Vol. 99, No, 4, pp. 296-301

Hoy WE, Douglas-Denton R, Hughson M, Cass MD, Johnson K, Bertram JF (2003) A stereological study of glomerular number and volume: Preliminary findings in a multiracial study of kidneys at autopsy. Kidney Int Suppl 63:S31-S37

Hughson, M.; Farris, A.B.; Douglas-Denton, R. Hoy, W.E. & Bertram, J. (2003). Glomerular number and size in autopsy kidneys : The relationship to birth weight. *Kidney Int*, Vol.63, pp. 2113-2122

Hughson, M.; Douglas-Denton, R.; Bertram, J. & Hoy, W.E. (2006). Hypertension, glomerular number, and birth weight in African American and white subjects in the southeastern United States. *Kidney Int*, Vol.69, pp.671-678

Iacobelli, S.M.D.; Loprieno, S.M.D.; Bonsante, F.M.D.; Latorre G.M.D.; Esposito L.M.D.; Gouyon J.M.D.B.; (2007) Renal function in early childhood in very low birthweight infants. *Am J Perinatol*, Vol. 10, pp. 587-592

Iglesias-Marquez RA, Calderon S, Santiago-Delpin EA, Rive-Mora E, Gonzalez-Caraballo Z, Morales-Otero L 2001 The health of living kidney donors 20 years after donation. Transplant Proc 33:2041-2042

Ingelfinger,J.R.; Schnaper,H.W. (2005) Renal Endowment: Developmental Origins of Adult Disease. *J Am Soc Nephrol*, Vol.16, No. 9, Pp.2533-2536

Irving RJ, Belton NR, Elton RA, Walker BR (2000) Adult cardiovascular risk factors in premature babies. Lancet 355:2135-2136

Jaddoe VWV; van Duijn CM; van der Heijden AJ; Mackenbach JP; Moll HA; Steegers EAP; Tiemeier H; Uitterlinen AG; Verhulst FC; Hofman A. (2007) The generation R study: design and cohort update until the age of 4 years. *Eur J Epidemiol*, Vol. 23, pp. 801-811

Jaddoe VWV; van Duijn CM; van der Heijden AJ; Mackenbach JP; Moll HA; Steegers EAP; Tiemeier H; Uitterlinen AG; Verhulst FC; Hofman A. (2010) The generation R study: design and cohort update 2010. *Eur J Epidemiol*, Vol. 25, No.11, pp. 823-841

Jahnukainen, T.; Chen, M.; Berg, U. & Celsi, G. (2001). Antenatal glucocorticoids and renal function after birth. *Semin Neonatol*, Vol.6, pp. 351-355

Kari, M.; Hallma, M.; Eronen, M. (1994) Prenatal dexamethasone treatment in conjuction with rescue therapy of human surfactant: a randomized placebo-controlled multicenter study. Pediatrics Vol.93, No.5, pp.730-736.

Keijzer-Veen, M.G.; Finken MJ, Nauta J, Dekker FW, Hille ET, Frölich M, Wit JM, van der Heijden AJ; Dutch POPS-19 Collaborative Study Group. (2005) Is blood pressure increased 19 years after intrauterine growth restriction and preterm birth? A prospective follow-up study in The Netherlands.Pediatrics. Vol.116, No.3, pp.725-731.

Keijzer-Veen MG; Schrevel M, Finken MJ, Dekker FW, Nauta J, Hille ET, Frölich M, van der Heijden BJ; Dutch POPS-19 Collaborative Study Group. (2005a) Microalbuminuria and lower glomerular filtration rate at young adult age in subjects born very premature and after intrauterine growth retardation.J Am Soc Nephrol. Vol.16, No.9, pp.2762-2768.

Keijzer-Veen MG, Kleinveld HA, Lequin MH, Dekker FW, Nauta J, de Rijke YB, van der Heijden BJ (2007) Renal function and size at young adult age after intrauterine growth restriction and very premature birth. Am J Kidney Dis 50:542-551

Keijzer-Veen, M.G.; Dülger A, Dekker FW, Nauta J, van der Heijden BJ. (2010a) Very preterm birth is a risk factor for increased systolic blood pressure at a young adult age. Pediatr Nephrol. Vol. 25, No.3, pp.509-16.

Keijzer-Veen, M.G.; Devos, A.; Meradji, M.; Dekker FW, Nauta J, van der Heijden BJ. (2010b) Reduced renal length and volume 20 years after very preterm birth. Pediatr Nephrol. Vol. 25, No.3, pp.499-507.

Keller, G. ; Zimmer, G.; Mall G; Ritz E; Amann K. (2003). Nephron number in patients with primary hypertension. *N Eng J Med*, Vol.348, No.2, pp.101-108

Kistner,A.; Celsi,G.; Vanpee,M.; Jacobson,S.H. (2000). Increased blood pressure but normal renal function in adult women born preterm. *Pediatr Nephrol,* Vol 15, No. 3-4, pp 215-220

Kistner,A.; Celsi,G.; Vanpee,M.; Jacobson,S.H. (2005). Increased systolic daily ambulatory blood pressure in adult women born preterm. *Pediatr Nephrol,* Vol 20, No. 2, pp 232-233

Konje,J.C.; Bell,S.C.; Morton,J.J.; de Chazal,R.; Taylor,D.J. (1996) Human fetal kidney morphometry during gestation and the relationship between weight, kidney morphometry and plasma active renin concentration at birth. *Clin Sci (Lond),* Vol. 91, No. 2, pp. 169-175

Konje,J.C.; Okaro,C.I.; Bell,S.C.; de Chazal,R.; Taylor,D.J. (1997) A cross-sectional study of changes in fetal renal size with gestation in appropriate- and small-for-gestational-age fetuses *Ultrasound Obstet Gynecol,* Vol. 10, No. 1, pp. 22-26

Langley SC, Browne RF, Jackson AA (1994) Altered glucose tolerance in rats exposed to maternal low protein diets in utero. Comp Biochem Physiol Physiol 109:223-9

Langley-Evans SC, Welham SJ, Jackson AA (1999) Fetal exposure to a maternal low protein diet impairs nephrogenesis and promotes hypertension in the rat. Life Sci 64:965-974

Lasaitiene D, Friberg P, Sundelin B, Chen Y (2004) Neonatal RAS inhibition changes the phenotype of the developing thick ascending limb of Henle. Am J Physiol Renal Physiol 286:F1144-F1153

Lucas SR, Costa S, V, Miraglia SM, Zaladek GF (1997) Functional and morphometric evaluation of offspring kidney after intrauterine undernutrition. Pediatr Nephrol 11:719-723

Martyn CN, Lever AF, Morton JJ (1996) Plasma concentrations of inactive renin in adult life are related to indicators of foetal growth. J Hypertens 14:881-886

Merlet-Benichou C, Gilbert T, Muffat-Joly M, Lelievre-Pegorier M, Leroy B (1994) Intrauterine growth retardation leads to a permanent nephron deficit in the rat. Pediatr Nephrol 8:175-180

Moritz, K.M.& Wintour, E.M. (1999). Functional development of the meso- and metanephros. *Pediatr Neprhol,* Vol 13, pp.171-178

Nyengaard, J.R. & Bendtsen, T.F. (1992). Glomerular number and size in relation to age, kidney weight, and body surface area ub birnak nab, *Anat Rec,* Vol.232, pp.194-201

Petrova, A. & Mehta, R. (2010) Regional tissue oxygenation in association with duration of hypoxaemia and haemodynamic variability in preterm neonates. *Arch Dis Child Fetal Neonatal Ed,* Vol.95, pp.F213-219

Rakow A; Johansson S; Legnevall L; Sevastik R; Celsi G; Normal L; Vanpee M. (2008). Renal volume and function in school-ages children born preterm or small for gestational age. *Ped Nephrol,* Vol.23 pp. 1309-1315

Roseboom T; de Rooij S; Painter R. (2006) The Dutch famine and its long-term consequences for adult health.

Singh, G.R.& Hoy, W.H. (2004). Kidney volume, blood pressure, and albuminuria: findings in an Australian aboriginal community. *Am J Kidney Dis,* Vol.43, No.2, pp. 253-259

Sahajpal V, Ashton N (2003) Renal function and angiotensin AT1 receptor expression in young rats following intrauterine exposure to a maternal low-protein diet. Clin Sci (Lond) 104:607-614

Siewert-Delle A, Ljungman S (1998) The impact of birth weight and gestational age on blood pressure in adult life: a population-based study of 49-year-old men. Am J Hypertens 11:946-53

Streitman, K.; Toth, A.; Horvath, I.; Talosi, G. (2001). Renal injury in perinatal hypoxia: ultrasonography and changes in renal function. *Eur J Pediatr,* Vol. 160, pp. 473-477

Sutherland MR; Gubhaju L; Stahlman MT; Black MJ. (2009). The effects of postnatal retinoid acid administration on nephron endowment in the preterm baboon kidney. *Ped Research* Vol. 65. No. 4. pp.397-402

Taal HR; Geelhoed JJM; Steegers EAP; Hofman A; Moll HA; Lequin M; van der Heijden AJ, Jaddoe VWV. (2011) Maternal smoking during pregnancy and kidney volume in the offspring: the Generation R study. *Ped Nephrol,* Vol. 26, pp.1275-1283

Thorner PS, Arbus GS, Celermajer DS, Baumal R 1984 Focal segmental glomerulosclerosis and progressive renal failure associated with a unilateral kidney. Pediatrics 73:806-810

Gubhaju, L.; Sutherland, M.R.; Yoder BA; Zulli A; Bertram JF; Black MJ. (2009) Is nephrogenesis affected by preterm birth? Studies in a non-human primate model. *Am J Physiol Renal Physiol,* Vol. 297, pp. F1668-1677

Verburg BO; Geelhoed JJ; Steegers EAP; Hofman A; Moll HA; Witteman JC; Jaddoe VW. (2007) Fetal kidney volume and its association with growth and blood flow in fetal life: The Generation R study. Kidney Int, Vol. 72. No. 6, pp. 754-761

Wadhwa PD; Buss C; Enrtinger S; Swanson JM (2009). Developmental origins of health and disease: Brief history of the approach and current focus on epigenetic mechanisms. *Semin Reprod,* Med Vol. 27, No.5, pp 358-368

Zanardo V; Fanelli T; Weiner G; Fanos V; Zaninotto M; Visentin S; Cavallin F; Trevisanuto D; Cosmi E; (2011) Intrauterine growth restriction is associated with persistent aortic wall thickening and glomerular proteinuria during infancy. *Kidney Int,* Vol. April 13, EPub ahead of print. doi:10.1038/ki.2011.99

Zeman FJ (1968) Effects of maternal protein restriction on the kidney of the newborn young of rats. J Nutr 94:111-116